PharmPrep:

ASHP's NAPLEX® Review

Fourth Edition

Lea S. Eiland, Pharm.D., BCPS
Associate Clinical Professor and Associate Department Head
Department of Pharmacy Practice
Auburn University, Harrison School of Pharmacy
Clinical Associate Professor of Pediatrics
UAB School of Medicine Huntsville Regional Medical Campus
Huntsville, Alabama

Diane B. Ginsburg, M.S., R.Ph., FASHP
Clinical Professor
Assistant Dean for Student Affairs
Regional Director, Internship Program
The University of Texas at Austin
College of Pharmacy
Austin, Texas

American Society of Health-System Pharmacists®
Bethesda, Maryland

Any correspondence regarding this publication should be sent to the publisher, American Society of Health-System Pharmacists, 7272 Wisconsin Avenue, Bethesda, MD 20814, attention: Special Publishing.

The information presented herein reflects the opinions of the contributors and advisors. It should not be interpreted as an official policy of ASHP or as an endorsement of any product.

Because of ongoing research and improvements in technology, the information and its applications contained in this text are constantly evolving and are subject to the professional judgment and interpretation of the practitioner due to the uniqueness of a clinical situation. The editors, contributors, and ASHP have made reasonable efforts to ensure the accuracy and appropriateness of the information presented in this document. However, any user of this information is advised that the editors, contributors, advisors, and ASHP are not responsible for the continued currency of the information, for any errors or omissions, and/or for any consequences arising from the use of the information in the document in any and all practice settings. Any reader of this document is cautioned that ASHP makes no representation, guarantee, or warranty, express or implied, as to the accuracy and appropriateness of the information contained in this document and specifically disclaims any liability to any party for the accuracy and/or completeness of the material or for any damages arising out of the use or non-use of any of the information contained in this document.

Director, Special Publishing: Jack Bruggeman

Senior Editorial Project Manager: Dana Battaglia

Editorial Resources Manager: Bill Fogle

Design and Layout: David A.Wade

ISBN 978-1-58528-255-5

Dedication

This edition is dedicated to my grandmother, Minnie Lee Conner, due to her faith, strong mind, and eagerness to help others succeed.

Lea S. Eiland

And to all those who have been great teachers and role models in our lives, including my mother, Phyllis B. Ginsburg.

Diane B. Ginsburg

Table of Contents

Disease Management Sections and Cases

Cardiac and Vascular Diseases

Section Editor: James A. Karboski

Respiratory and Pulmonary Diseases

Section Editor: Michelle Condren

Gastrointestinal Disorders

Section Editors: Pramodini Kale-Pradhan,
Sheila M. Wilhelm

Hepatic and Pancreatic Disorders

Section Editor: Robert MacLaren

Table of Contents

Acknowledgments

I have been honored to be able to serve as Managing Editor for the Fourth Edition. This book means so much to me as the first edition was released when I graduated and I used it to study for the board exams. I recall Diane working so hard on this book and telling me about it when I was a student. I was honored when she asked me to become an author for the second edition and then a section editor for the third edition. I truly believe in the educational tool this book provides. Not only did I use it as a student to assess my learning, but I have used it to teach students during my times as an educator. I have seen the light bulb "turn on" when a student was working on a case. The words *Thank you* are not enough to tell Diane how grateful I am to have been able to serve *PharmPrep* this year the way it has served me in the past.

I greatly appreciate all of the section editors who graciously agreed to work on the fourth edition. Your work and contributions make this textbook be the strong caliber it is today. The time and effort each one of the authors spent creating and revising the cases this year shows the dedication our outstanding practitioners have for the profession.

A special thank you to the ASHP staff, especially Dana Battaglia, Jack Bruggeman, Rebecca Olson, Bill Fogle, Moyo Myers, and Oedi Rice for the time and patience you had with me this first year. I appreciate the time you spent answering all of my questions and orienting me to the role as managing editor. You all do an outstanding job and have a wonderful commitment and pride in the ASHP publications.

Lea S. Eiland

In addition to the acknowledgments of our incredible staff at ASHP, special thanks to Lea S. Eiland for her efforts and commitment to this project. It is students (former) like Lea that are a major part of the reason I do what I do on a daily basis. It has truly been my privilege to work with her and I am honored to have her as principle in this text.

Diane B. Ginsburg

Diane Ginsburg is one of the most dynamic pharmacy educators in the United States. It is evident that her effervescence in the classroom is poured into this, her fourth edition of *PharmPrep*. She is joined by co-editor Lea S. Eiland, a top practitioner and educator whose positive influence on new practitioners and exceptional clinical practice in pediatrics is setting the pace in our rapidly advancing profession. Together the editors have made *PharmPrep* an essential self-evaluation and learning tool for the new graduate, as well as the mature practitioner.

For the last decade, *PharmPrep* has been a top choice of new graduates preparing for the NAPLEX® examination. The case presentation and question format is both stimulating and challenging for the reader. Case simulation not only enhances the learning experience, but assists with retention. After all, we all remember the most interesting cases we have encountered. The same is true with *PharmPrep*! The introduction of *PharmPrep Online* in 2008 enabled anytime, anyplace access to the 244 cases that comprise this essential learning resource.

PharmPrep is an equally important reference for the experienced practitioner. As practice advances, it is essential for pharmacists to continue to develop professionally. In my own practice setting, we will use *PharmPrep* as a competency assessment tool. It will be a resource provided for those practitioners preparing a personal development plan for advanced clinical practice in our new practice model.

As drug therapy becomes more complex, *PharmPrep* has continued to update and revise cases so they reflect contemporary clinical practice. All *PharmPrep* cases have been created by an elite group of pharmacy clinicians from across America. This fourth edition of *PharmPrep*: ASHP's NAPLEX® Review includes 77 cases from the revised and refreshed *PharmPrep Online*.

Every day I'm impressed by many of the pharmacists and students with whom I work. Their desire for practice excellence is evident from their work on the patient care unit, in the outpatient clinic, and at each medical staff meeting. With this book, Ginsburg and Eiland have given us the ability to evaluate ourselves and sharpen our skills so we can maintain the rightful role of being the medication expert in our individual practice setting.

Kevin Coigan, M.A., FASHP
Corporate Director of Pharmacy
Rush University Medical Center
Chicago, Illinois

In the profession of pharmacy, as students we are educated on "real" yet paper patient cases. Frustration can arise when there is not a right or wrong answer, but several options of care are correct. On clerkships it is easier to recognize and consider these options as a "real "patient is sitting right before you. However, as you develop a practice of your own after you earn your Doctor of Pharmacy degree, you realize that very few patient cases present with an easy right or wrong decision. Multiple factors such as age, condition of health, and patient and health care resources all influence the clinical decision-making we do in patient care.

PharmPrep: *ASHP's NAPLEX® Review* Fourth Edition, is a case-based board review which provides a comprehensive review of disease states that are covered on the North American Pharmacy Licensure Examination (NAPLEX®). The student is provided a patient case accompanied by 10 questions which addresses NAPLEX® competency statements. This text, like the first three editions, is an unique board review book in that it is case-based. The textbook should help students identify areas requiring additional study as well as provide a comprehensive review of the types of disease states and therapeutic related issues that pharmacists encounter in a wide variety of pharmacy practices. In addition, this review guide serves as an excellent tool for the practitioner who would like to update his or her knowledge in a specific disease state or organ system, practice calculations, or review the federal law.

The authors of *PharmPrep*: *ASHP's NAPLEX® Review* Fourth Edition, have used real patient cases to emphasize that patients seen in practice rarely present in a textbook/black-and-white manner. The goal for the student is to be able to prepare not only for the NAPLEX® but for real practice by exposure to actual patients. The student is able to practice their clinical decision-making skills on the cases in the text, knowing an incorrect answer will not result in harm to the patient. In addition to cases, *PharmPrep* includes a Compounding and Calculations section as well as a Federal Law review. Each of these sections has related questions to assess learning.

The fourth edition comes with new cases and expanded sections as well as all cases have been revised to reflect today's standard of practice. New disease states cases are included such as cystic fibrosis, lung transplantation, conjunctivitis, and rosacea. The online (software) edition encompasses all of the cases and sections. Cases selected for the book include those that are commonly seen in the community and hospital settings. The online edition and textbook are organized by therapeutic areas of focus, and then tailored into more specific disease states. There are 126 different disease management areas with approximately 2 cases per topic for a total of 244 patient cases. The textbook includes 77 of these cases. The Compounding and Calculations section has been expanded with additional questions for this edition. The Federal Law section has been revised. The questions in this section mirror those on the Multistate Pharmacy Jurisprudence Examination (MJPE®). There continues to be a revised section on "Successful Test-Taking Strategies."

The layout of each case is presented similar to a medical chart and includes 10 questions with the NAPLEX® competency statement designated in the answer section. The correct answer is fully explained, including why other answers are incorrect. The online (software) version will allow the student to simulate taking the NAPLEX® or enable the student to review a specific therapeutic area or disease state.

The authors who have contributed to the fourth edition represent all facets of pharmacy practice and are experts in their respective disciplines. A board-certified physician in psychiatry and neurology has also authored cases. The cases, questions, and answers all represent information that the practitioners have taken from their clinical experiences. The authors have been careful to recommend therapies that are reflective of current standards and treatment guidelines; however, there may be more than one manner in which to treat the patients seen in this textbook.

PharmPrep: *ASHP's NAPLEX® Review,* Fourth Edition, is designed not only to assist the student in preparing for licensure, but also to facilitate life-long learning. As professionals, we as pharmacists are dedicated to providing our patients with the best patient care. However, this requires us to stay abreast with current treatment recommendations as well as ensure understanding of the disease state. Reviewing this type of information to maintain competency is imperative. We hope this book will assist you with your learning, and we wish you the best in your practice.

Lea S. Eiland and *Diane B. Ginsburg*

Editors-in-Chief

Lea S. Eiland, Pharm.D., BCPS
Associate Clinical Professor and Associate Department Head
Department of Pharmacy Practice
Auburn University, Harrison School of Pharmacy
Clinical Associate Professor of Pediatrics
UAB School of Medicine Huntsville Regional Medical Campus
Huntsville, Alabama

Diane B. Ginsburg, M.S., R.Ph., FASHP
Clinical Professor
Assistant Dean for Student Affairs
Regional Director, Internship Program
The University of Texas at Austin
College of Pharmacy
Austin, Texas

Section Editors

Over-the-Counter Medication
W. Reneé Acosta, R.Ph., M.S.
Clinical Associate Professor
The University of Texas College of Pharmacy
Austin, Texas

Transplant
Rebecca Brady, Pharm.D., BCPS
Assistant Professor, Pharmacy Practice
Feik School of Pharmacy
University of the Incarnate Word
San Antonio, Texas

Pamela R. Maxwell, Pharm.D., BCPS
Clinical Pharmacy Manager, University Transplant Center
University Health System
San Antonio, Texas

Neoplastic Disorders
Joseph Bubalo Pharm.D., BCPS, BCOP
Assistant Professor of Medicine
Oncology Clinical Specialist and Oncology Lead
OHSU Hospital and Clinics
Portland, Oregon

Neurological Disorders
Jack J. Chen, Pharm.D., FCCP, BCPS, CGP
Associate Professor (Neurology)
Schools of Medicine and Pharmacy, Loma Linda University
Loma Linda, California

Psychiatric Disorders
Lawrence J. Cohen, Pharm.D., BCPP, FASHP, FCCP
Professor, Departments of Pharmacotherapy and Health Policy and
Administration
Washington State University College of Pharmacy
Assistant Director for Psychopharmacology Research and Training
Washington Institute for Mental Health Research and Training
Spokane, Washington

Respiratory and Pulmonary Disorders

Michelle Condren, Pharm.D., AE-C, CDE
Associate Professor
University of Oklahoma College of Pharmacy
And School of Community Medicine
Tulsa, Oklahoma

Urological Disorders

Lourdes M. Cuellar, M.S., R.Ph., FASHP
Administrative Director of Pharmacy & Clinical Support Services
TIRR Memorial Hermann
Houston, Texas

Skin Disorders

Ellen R. DeGrasse, Pharm.D.
Clinical Assistant Professor of Pharmacy Practice
University of Washington
Seattle, Washington

Pediatric Therapy

Lea S. Eiland, Pharm.D., BCPS
Associate Clinical Professor
Associate Department Head
Department of Pharmacy Practice
Auburn University, Harrison School of Pharmacy
Huntsville, Alabama

Perioperative Care

Julie Golembiewski, Pharm.D.
Clinical Assistant Professor, Pharmacy Practice
University of Illinois College of Pharmacy
Clinical Associate Professor, Anesthesiology
University of Illinois College of Medicine
Chicago, Illinois

Blood Disorders

Lori B. Hornsby, Pharm.D.
Assistant Clinical Professor of Pharmacy Practice
Auburn University
Huntsville, Alabama

Anne Marie Liles, Pharm.D., BCPS
Assistant Clinical Professor
Auburn University Harrison School of Pharmacy
Auburn, Alabama

Fluid, Electrolytes, and Nutrition

Charles W. Jastram, Jr., Pharm.D., FASHP
Associate Professor and Department Head
Clinical & Administrative Sciences
College of Pharmacy
University of Louisiana at Monroe
Monroe, Louisiana

Geriatric Disorders

Rebecca A. Rottman-Sagebiel, Pharm.D., BCPS, CGP
Geriatrics Clinical Pharmacy Specialist
PGY1 Pharmacy Residency Program Director
South Texas Veterans Health Care System
San Antonio, Texas

Sharon Jung Tschirhart, Pharm.D., BCPS
Residency Coordinator
Geriatrics Clinical Pharmacy Specialist

PGY2 Geriatric Pharmacy Residency Program Director
South Texas Veterans Health Care System
San Antonio, Texas

Gastrointestinal Disorders

Pramodini Kale-Pradhan, Pharm.D.
Associate Professor
Department of Pharmacy Practice
Eugene Applebaum College of Pharmacy and Health Sciences
Wayne State University
Detroit, Michigan

Sheila M. Wilhelm, Pharm.D., BCPS
Clinical Assistant Professor
Wayne State University Eugene Applebaum College of Pharmacy and
Health Sciences
Harper University Hospital
Detroit, Michigan

Cardiac and Vascular Disease

James A. Karboski, Pharm.D.
Clinical Associate Professor
University of Texas at Austin
College of Pharmacy
Austin, Texas

Hepatic and Pancreatic Disorders

Robert MacLaren, Pharm.D.
Associate Professor
University of Colorado School of Pharmacy
Aurora, Colorado

Endocrine and Metabolic Disorders

Dannielle O'Donnell, B.S., Pharm.D.
Sr. Medical Science Liaison
Genentech
Austin, Texas

Infectious Diseases

Catherine M. Oliphant, Pharm.D.
Associate Professor of Pharmacy Practice
College of Pharmacy
Idaho State University
Meridian, Idaho

John L. Woon, Pharm.D., FASHP
Manager, Pharmacy Informatics
Providence Sacred Heart Medical Center & Children's Hospital
Providence Holy Family Hospital
Spokane, Washington

Diseases of the Eye and Ear

Celtina K. Reinert, Pharm.D.
Integrative Pharmacist
Sastun Center of Integrative Health Care
Overland Park, Kansas

Rheumatic Disorders

Terry L. Schwinghammer, Pharm.D., BCPS
Chair and Professor
Department of Clinical Pharmacy
West Virginia University School of Pharmacy
Morgantown, West Virginia

Renal Disorders

Holli Temple, Pharm.D., BCPS
Clinical Pharmacist
North Austin Medical Center
Adjunct Assistant Professor
The University of Texas at Austin
College of Pharmacy
Austin, Texas

Compounding and Calculations Review

Jason M. Vaughn, Ph.D.
Director of Research
Enavail LLC
Austin, Texas

Robert O. (Bill) Williams III, Ph.D., R.Ph.
Johnson & Johnson Centennial Professor, Pharmaceutics
College of Pharmacy
University of Texas at Austin
Austin, Texas

Federal Law Review

Jesse Vivian, R.Ph., JD
Professor of Pharmacy Practice
Wayne State University
Detroit, Michigan

OB/GYN Disorders and Women's Health

C. Brock Woodis, Pharm.D., BCPS, CPP
Assistant Professor of Pharmacy Practice
Campbell University College of Pharmacy and Health Sciences
Clinical Pharmacy Specialist in Family Medicine
Assistant Professor
Duke Family Medicine
Duke University Medical Center
Durham, North Carolina

Contributors

W. Reneé Acosta, R.Ph., M.S.
Clinical Associate Professor
The University of Texas College of Pharmacy
Austin, Texas

Jennifer A. Buxton, B.S., Pharm.D., CPP
Pharmacist
New Hanover Regional Medical Center
Wilmington, North Carolina

Yeshewaneh Beyene. B.Sc. Pharm. D.
Clinical Science Consultant
Boehringer Ingelheim Pharmaceuticals
Baltimore, Maryland

Edward P. Bornet, M.S., RPh.
Director of Pharmacy Services
San Jacinto Methodist Hospital
Baytown, Texas

Rebecca Brady, Pharm.D., BCPS
Assistant Professor, Pharmacy Practice
Feik School of Pharmacy
University of the Incarnate Word
San Antonio, Texas

Susan P. Bruce, Pharm.D., BCPS
Associate Professor & Chair, Pharmacy Practice
Northeastern Ohio Universities Colleges of Medicine & Pharmacy
Rootstown, Ohio

Bruce R. Canaday, Pharm.D., FASHP, FAPhA
Professor & Chair
Department of Pharmacy Practice & Pharmacy Administration
Philadelphia College of Pharmacy
University of the Sciences
Philadelphia, Pennsylvania

Jack J. Chen, Pharm.D., FCCP, BCPS, CGP
Associate Professor (Neurology)
Schools of Medicine and Pharmacy, Loma Linda University
Loma Linda, California

Vincent Chia, Pharm.D.
Clinical Manager
Novartis Pharmaceuticals Corporation
East Hanover, New Jersey

Michelle Condren, Pharm.D., AE-C, CDE
Associate Professor
University of Oklahoma College of Pharmacy & School of Community Medicine
Tulsa, Oklahoma

Erin Corella, Pharm.D., BCPS, BCOP
Oncology Clinical Pharmacist
Oregon Health & Science University
Portland, Oregon

Jason M. Cota, Pharm.D., M.S., BCPS
Assistant Professor of Pharmacy Practice
University of the Incarnate Word Feik School of Pharmacy
San Antonio, Texas

Caitlin Curtis, Pharm.D.
Nutrition Support Pharmacist
University of Wisconsin Hospital and Clinics
Madison, Wisconsin

Michelle Shah, Pharm.D.
Clinical Staff Pharmacist
University of Illinois Medical Center
Chicago, Illinois

Ellen R. DeGrasse, Pharm.D.
Clinical Assistant Professor of Pharmacy Practice
University of Washington
Seattle, Washington

Andrew J. Donnelly, Pharm.D., MBA, FASHP
Director, Pharmacy Services
Clinical Professor of Pharmacy Practice
University of Illinois Medical Center at Chicago
Chicago, Illinois

Robert Dupuis, Pharm.D., FCCP
Clinical Associate Professor of Pharmacy
UNC Eshelman School of Pharmacy
University of North Carolina at Chapel Hill
Chapel Hill, North Carolina

Lea S. Eiland, Pharm.D., BCPS
Associate Clinical Professor
Associate Department Head
Department of Pharmacy Practice
Auburn University, Harrison School of Pharmacy
Huntsville, Alabama

Edward H. Eiland III, Pharm.D., MBA, BCPS (AQ-ID)
Clinical Practice and Business Supervisor
Huntsville Hospital System
Huntsville, Alabama

Sharon M. Erdman, Pharm.D.
Clinical Professor, Infectious Diseases, Clinical
Pharmacist
Purdue University College of Pharmacy
Wishard Health Service
Indianapolis, Indiana

Emily K. Flores, Pharm.D., BCPS
Assistant Professor of Pharmacy Practice
Bill Gatton College of Pharmacy, East Tennessee State University
Johnson City, Tennessee

Steven Gianakopoulos, Pharm.D.
Clinical Staff Pharmacist
University of Illinois Medical Center at Chicago
Chicago, Illinois

Belinda (Kay) Green, R.Ph., BCPS
Clinical Pharmacist, Neonatal Intensive Care Unit
Residency Coordinator
University Health System
San Antonio, Texas

Myke R. Green, B.S., Pharm.D., BCOP
Oncology Clinical Pharmacy Specialist
University Medical Center/Arizona Cancer Center
Tucson, Arizona

Sharlyn Guillema Vera, Pharm.D., BCPS
Assistant Professor, Pharmacotherapy and Outcomes Science
Loma Linda University School of Pharmacy
Loma Linda, California

Contributors

Kathleen M. Gura, Pharm.D., BCNSP, FASHP, FPPAG
Clinical Pharmacist Gastroenterology and Nutrition
Children's Hospital, Boston
Boston, Massachusetts

Lori B. Hornsby, Pharm.D.
Assistant Clinical Professor of Pharmacy Practice
Auburn University
Huntsville, Alabama

Jeffrey Josephs, M.D.
Senior Staff Psychiatrist
Austin Travis County Integral Care
Austin, Texas

Sharon Jung Tschirhart, Pharm.D., BCPS
Residency Coordinator
Geriatrics Clinical Pharmacy Specialist
PGY2 Geriatric Pharmacy Residency Program Director
South Texas Veterans Health Care System
San Antonio, Texas

Pramodini Kale-Pradhan, Pharm.D.
Associate Professor
Department of Pharmacy Practice
Eugene Applebaum College of Pharmacy and Health Sciences
Wayne State University
Detroit, Michigan

Nancy Kang, Pharm.D.
Pharmacy Practice Resident
Loma Linda University
Loma Linda, California

James A. Karboski, Pharm.D.
Clinical Associate Professor
University of Texas at Austin
College of Pharmacy
Austin, Texas

Catherine Kline, Pharm.D.
Pharmacist
Advocate Lutheran General Hospital
Park Ridge, Illinois

Eric C. Kutscher, Pharm.D., BCPP
Associate Professor of Pharmacy Practice
South Dakota State University College of Pharmacy
Adjunct Associate Professor of Psychiatry
Sanford School of Medicine, University of South Dakota
Director
Psychiatry Pharmacy Practice Residency Program (PGY-II)
Avera Behavioral Health Center
Clinical Pharmacy Specialist, Psychiatry
Avera Behavioral Health Center
Sioux Falls, South Dakota

Greg Laine
Clinical Coordinator, Pulmonary/Critical Care
Department of Pharmacy
St. Luke's Episcopal Health System
Houston, Texas

Nancy A. Letassy, Pharm.D., CDE
Associate Professor
University of Oklahoma Health Science Center
College of Pharmacy

Director of Pharmacotherapy Service
Family Medicine Center
University of Oklahoma Health Sciences Center
Oklahoma City, Oklahoma

Anne Marie Liles, Pharm.D., BCPS
Assistant Clinical Professor
Auburn University Harrison School of Pharmacy
Auburn, Alabama

Katheleen Louis-Pinto, Pharm.D.
Medical Science Liaison
Bristol-Myers Squibb
Houston, Texas

Lisa Lubsch, Pharm.D., AE-C
Clinical Associate Professor, Department of Pharmacy Practice
Southern Illinois University Edwardsville School of Pharmacy
Edwardsville, Illinois

Pediatric Clinical Pharmacy Specialist
Cardinal Glennon Children's Medical Center
Saint Louis, Missouri

Robert MacLaren, Pharm.D.
Associate Professor
University of Colorado School of Pharmacy
Aurora, Colorado

Karl Madaras-Kelly, Pharm.D., M.P.H.
Professor
Dept. of Pharmacy Practice
Idaho State University
Meridian, Idaho

Pamela R. Maxwell, Pharm.D., BCPS
Clinical Pharmacy Manager, University Transplant Center
University Health System
San Antonio, Texas

Patrick Murray, Pharm.D.
Assistant Professor
Irma Lerma Rangel College of Pharmacy
Texas A&M Health Science Center
Department of Pharmacy Practice
Temple, Texas

Kevin O'Donnell, B.S. Neurobiology
Graduate Research Assistant
The University of Texas at Austin
Austin, Texas

Catherine M. Oliphant, Pharm.D.
Associate Professor of Pharmacy Practice
College of Pharmacy
Idaho State University
Meridian, Idaho

Kathryn N. Pidcock, Pharm.D., BCPS
Clinical Specialist in Internal Medicine
The Methodist Hospital
Houston, Texas

Celtina K. Reinert, Pharm.D.
Integrative Pharmacist
Sastun Center of Integrative Health Care
Overland Park, Kansas

Contributors

Treavor T. Riley, Pharm.D., BCPS
Clinical Assistant Professor
University of Mississippi School of Pharmacy
Jackson, Mississippi

Rebecca A. Rottman-Sagebiel, Pharm D, BCPS, CGP
Geriatrics Clinical Pharmacy Specialist
PGY1 Pharmacy Residency Program Director
South Texas Veterans Health Care System
San Antonio, Texas

Amista L. Salcido, Pharm.D.
Director of Pharmacy
El Paso State Supported Living Center
El Paso, Texas

Colleen Shipman, Pharm.D., MPH
Clinical Pharmacist
OHSU Hospital and Clinics
Portland, Oregon

Chris Terpening, Ph.D., Pharm.D.
Clinical Associate Professor
West Virginia University School of Pharmacy
Charleston, West Virginia

Nancy Toedter Williams, Pharm.D., FASHP, BCPS, BCNSP
Professor of Pharmacy Practice
Southwestern Oklahoma State University
College of Pharmacy
Weatherford, Oklahoma

Candy Tsourounis, Pharm.D.
Professor of Clinical Pharmacy
UCSF School of Pharmacy
San Francisco, California

Jason M. Vaughn, Ph.D.
Director of Research
Enavail LLC
Austin, Texas

Jesse Vivian, R.Ph., JD
Professor of Pharmacy Practice
Wayne State University
Detroit, Michigan

Nicholas A. Votolato, R.Ph., BCPP
Clinical Assistant Professor
College of Pharmacy
Clinical Assistant Professor
College of Medicine
Ohio State University
Columbus, Ohio

Tara Whetsel, Pharm.D.
Clinical Assistant Professor
West Virginia University School of Pharmacy
Morgantown, West Virginia

Sheila M. Wilhelm, Pharm.D., BCPS
Clinical Assistant Professor
Wayne State University Eugene Applebaum College of Pharmacy and
Health Sciences
Harper University Hospital
Detroit, Michigan

Robert O. (Bill) Williams III, Ph.D., R.Ph.
Johnson & Johnson Centennial Professor, Pharmaceutics
College of Pharmacy
University of Texas at Austin
Austin, Texas

Alexandria Garavaglia Wilson, Pharm.D., BCPS
Assistant Professor, Pharmacy Practice
St. Louis College of Pharmacy
St. Louis, Missouri

C. Brock Woodis, Pharm.D., BCPS, CPP
Assistant Professor of Pharmacy Practice
Campbell University College of Pharmacy and Health Sciences
Clinical Pharmacy Specialist in Family Medicine
Assistant Professor
Duke Family Medicine
Durham, North Carolina

John L. Woon, Pharm.D., FASHP
Manager, Pharmacy Informatics
Providence Sacred Heart Medical Center & Children's Hospital
Providence Holy Family Hospital
Spokane, Washington

Clinton Wright, Pharm.D., BCPP
San Antonio, Texas

Contributors

Reviewers

Justine S. Gortney, Pharm.D., BCPS
Assistant Professor (Clinical) of Pharmacy Practice
Eugene Applebaum College of Pharmacy and Health Sciences
Detroit, Michigan

Robert E. Smith, Pharm.D.
Professor and Assistant to the Dean for Professional Affairs
Department of Pharmacy Practice
Harrison School of Pharmacy
Auburn University, Alabama

Paul M. Dombrower, R.Ph.
Pharmacy Clinical Specialist: Nephrology, General Medicine
UNC Hospitals
Chapel Hill, North Carolina

Jill A. Morgan, Pharm.D., BCPS
Associate Dean Student Affairs
University of Maryland School of Pharmacy
Baltimore, Maryland

Jill T. Johnson, Pharm.D., BCPS
Associate Professor
Department of Pharmacy Practice
University of Arkansas for Medical Sciences
College of Pharmacy
Little Rock, Arkansas

Jolene Bostwick, Pharm.D., BCPS, BCPP
Clinical Pharmacist, Adult Psychiatry
Clinical Assistant Professor
University of Michigan Health System and College of Pharmacy
Ann Arbor, Michigan

Jeong Mi Park, M.S., Pharm.D., BCPS
Clinical Associate Professor of Pharmacy
Clinical Pharmacist, Solid Organ Transplantation
University of Michigan
Ann Arbor, MI

Colleen Catalano, Pharm.D., CGP, FASCP
Clinical Assistant Professor
Clinical Pharmacist
University of Washington School of Pharmacy & Dept of Family Medicine
Seattle, Washington

Michael Steinberg, Pharm.D., BCOP
Associate Professor of Pharmacy Practice
Massachusetts College of Pharmacy and Health Sciences
Worcester, Massachusetts

Joseph Saseen, Pharm.D., FCCP, BCPS
Professor
University of Colorado
Schools of Pharmacy and Medicine
Aurora, Colorado

PharmPrep: ASHP's NAPLEX® Review, fourth edition is a multidisciplinary review guide that will provide a comprehensive review of disease states that are covered on the NAPLEX® through a review of real patient cases accompanied by questions that address all of the NAPLEX® competency statements (Appendix A). *PharmPrep Online* allows the student to review information by specific disease state or simulate the examination with a computer-adapted format similar to that seen on the NAPLEX®.

The layout of each case is presented like a medical chart with subjective patient information and objective data to give a clear depiction of the patient. The physician's assessment of the patient is included, when available, to assist the student in making a decision on the best course of treatment, proper drug therapy, and construction of a plan for the patient. Each case includes a profile similar to those seen in on the NAPLEX® and is followed by 10 questions with the NAPLEX® competency statement designated in the answer section. Explanations for all answers, correct and incorrect, are included.

Format of ASHP's PharmPrep Cases

The patient cases in this review guide are intended to be used as a review of common disease states that are likely to be seen by general pharmacy practitioners as well as several clinical specialties. The format and organization of the cases are meant to mirror what is usually seen in practice in a clinical setting. When using *PharmPrep,* it is recommended that additional resources be accessible to facilitate study, including a comprehensive drug information text (e.g., *AHFS*), medical dictionary, therapeutics text (e.g., *Pharmacotherapy*), and laboratory data reference.

Patient Demographics

The patient's demographical information will include (if known) his or her name (a fictional name to ensure patient confidentiality), address/location, age, height and weight, race, sex, and any known allergies.

Chief Complaint

The Chief Complaint is a brief statement that describes the reason the patient sought medical treatment and presents symptoms in his or her own words.

History of Present Illness

This is a complete chronology and description of the events and symptoms that led up to the patient seeking medical care. Included in this section are:

> Date of onset
> Type of condition, severity, and duration
> Status of any disease state (acute exacerbation or remission)
> Treatments/modalities attempted and their effect
> Impact on system function (e.g., increase/decrease urinary
>   function, etc.)
> Impact on activities of daily living

Past Medical History

Includes all pertinent information related to conditions for which the patient is currently being treated or has been treated for or sought medical care.

Social History

The social history includes the characteristics and habits of the patient that may or may not have contributed to his or her condition. Included in this section are the patient's marital status, drug and alcohol abuse, caffeine intake, and the use of tobacco, among other lifestyle information.

Family History

The family history includes status of the patient's family members, medical conditions, etc., that may provide useful hereditary information (e.g., diabetes, cancer, heart disease).

Review of Systems

This section includes information from the patient describing his or her symptoms with positive and negative findings noted.

Physical Examination

This section denotes the information found on physical examination of the patient. This section usually includes the following information:

GEN: General appearance

VS: Vital signs (including height, weight, blood pressure, heart rate, respiratory rate, and temperature)

HEENT: Head, eyes, ears, nose, and throat status

CHEST: Pulmonary status

CV: Cardiovascular status

ABD: Abdominal status

RECTAL: Rectal area status

GU: Genitourinary systems status

NEURO: Neurologic status

MS: Musculoskeletal status

EXT: Extremities status

Laboratory and Diagnostic Tests

The results of all laboratory and diagnostic tests are included in this section. Normal ranges vary from lab to lab and within different institutions. For information on normal values, consult a laboratory value text.

Diagnosis

All diagnoses for the patient are presented in this section.

Medication Record (Prescription and OTC)

This section includes all prescription and over-the-counter medications the patient is currently taking and/or received in the past. Prescribing physician, prescription number (Rx only), date filled, drug name, strength and quantity, directions for use, and refill information are provided. Medications are presented in a list for hospitalized patients.

Pharmacist Notes and Other Patient Information

Information documented in the patient's record, provided either by the pharmacist of another health care provider, is included in this section.

PharmPrep Online duplicates the environment of the NAPLEX® and will allow the student to simulate taking the NAPLEX® or will allow the student to review a specific disease state. The more practice the student has in the actual test environment, the more the student will relax and feel comfortable during actual testing.

PharmPrep: ASHP's NAPLEX® Review, fourth edition is a tool to assist with preparation for the NAPLEX® and for pharmacy practice. I hope this text will be a useful addition to your professional library and representative of the patients that you may see in practice.

Nancy F. Fjortoft, Ph.D.

Introduction

After years of preparation, you are ready to begin your career as a pharmacist. Congratulations! To practice pharmacy, individuals must be licensed by the state in which they wish to practice. Licensure ensures a minimum level of competence. Licensure by examination is the method by which new graduates achieve licensure. All state boards of pharmacy require individuals to take and pass the North American Pharmacy Licensure Examination (NAPLEX®) to be licensed.[1] The goal of the NAPLEX® is to ensure that you are competent to safely and effectively provide pharmacy practice services at the entry level. Your state board of pharmacy will use the NAPLEX® score as part of their determination if you are eligible for a license to practice pharmacy. This chapter will describe the NAPLEX® and assist you in preparing for the NAPLEX® and provide basic test-taking strategies. The objectives of this chapter are to:

1. describe the NAPLEX® and computer-adaptive testing;
2. describe types of questions on the NAPLEX®;
3. review test preparation strategies;
4. describe test-taking strategies; and
5. recognize test-taking anxiety and define how to cope with it.

Description of the NAPLEX® CAT

The NAPLEX® is a 4-hour and 15-minute computer adaptive test (CAT). The exam is based on the NAPLEX® Blueprint, which is revised regularly to assure that the examination evaluates current pharmacy practice. The Blueprint was revised in 2010, and as a result of the revision, the NAPLEX® now includes questions on pharmacoeconomics. There are three broad areas or content domains that the NAPLEX® evaluates: 1) assess pharmacotherapy to assure safe and effective therapeutic outcomes (approximately 56% of the test); 2) assess safe and accurate preparations and dispensing of medications (approximately 33% of the test); and 3) assess, recommend, and provide health care information that promotes public health (approximately 11% of the exam).[2]

The exam consists of 185 questions. 150 of those questions are used to calculate your score, and the remaining 35 are test questions. You will not know which are "real" questions and which are "test" questions. Computer-adaptive test simply means that you take the test on a computer, and the computer selects questions based on your level of ability. CAT is a relatively new method of testing. The questions are the same as they would be on a paper and pencil test; however, the computer "selects" questions for you based on whether you answered the previous question correctly. The computer "grades" your answer before presenting the next question. If you answered the question correctly, the computer will then select a more difficult question. If you answered the question incorrectly, the computer will select an easier question for your next question. Because of this format, taking a CAT is different from standard paper-and-pencil tests.

Special Considerations in Taking CAT

CATs are distinct from paper-and-pencil tests in a number of ways. Because of the adaptive nature of the test, you cannot go back and change an answer. In other words, you have one opportunity to answer the question. You may not go back and review your answer.

You may not skip questions. Again, because of the adaptive nature of the test, the computer selects your next question based on your answer to the current question. Therefore, you cannot skip questions. You must answer all questions, even if you need to guess (more on guessing later).

The disadvantage then of CATs is that your practice of answering all the easy questions first to build confidence and ensure that you answer as many questions as possible simply does not work. You need to answer one question at a time, and then leave that question permanently and move on. The questions are all independent and do not build on one another.

Types of Questions on the NAPLEX®

The NAPLEX® is a multiple-choice test. It consists of 185 questions that are either "scenario-based format" or "stand-alone" questions.[2] Scenario-based format questions present you with a patient profile or brief information regarding a specific situation (typically about a patient). Then you are asked a specific question. You answer the question using the data or case presented immediately above the question. The majority of NAPLEX® questions are scenario-based format questions.

The other type of question on the NAPLEX® is the stand-alone question. This is simply a question with a series of potential responses.

These are the types of questions you will see on the NAPLEX®. The responses may either be single-answer or combination. The question that has single-answer responses (probably the most familiar) looks like this:

1. CC's physician discusses initiating Risperdal therapy with you. What is your most appropriate response?
   A. Risperdal is an antipsychotic and should be used in this patient.
   B. CC's symptoms of disorientation and confusion are likely to improve with Risperdal therapy.
   C. CC's symptoms of memory loss and tremor are unlikely to improve with Risperdal therapy.
   D. Risperdal has been found to be safe in the elderly population.
   E. A baseline ECG is required before initiation of Risperdal.

   The combined-response question (Type K) looks like this:

2. Which of CC's medications may be contributing to his disorientation?
   I. Aricept
   II. Vitamin E
   III. Temazepam

   A. I only
   B. III only
   C. I and II only
   D. II and III only
   E. I, II, and III

Many pharmacy faculty use combined response questions in their examinations partly to give you practice opportunities in answering these kinds of questions.

Preparation for Success

Keep in mind that the NAPLEX® assesses years of education both in the classroom and on rotation. You cannot cram for the NAPLEX®; you must plan a review schedule. This review schedule should cover several months, not just several days.

Establish a schedule, with several hours a day set aside for review. Make an outline of topics to be reviewed. Use the NAPLEX® competency statements (Appendix A) to assist you in preparation for the exam. Keep in mind that you need to spend more time on areas in which you are weak. For example, if cardiovascular topics were difficult for you, plan to spend more time studying and reviewing cardiovascular topics. Do not spend large amounts of time on material that you already know.

Establish a study routine and set goals for each study period. Be realistic in setting your study goals. Most people are not effective when they set aside large blocks of time to study. Set aside 3–4 hours a day. Find your best time of day. After years of going to school, you probably have a pretty good idea whether you are a morning person or a night person. Use your best time of day for NAPLEX® study.

Be selective in the books and notes you use. Choose a good review book that is comprehensive and is easy for you to read. A number of review books are available. This book is unique in that it follows a case-based approach and provides plenty of sample questions with in-depth discussion explaining the correct answers.

By now you should also have developed a large library of reference books that will help as you begin your review process. Some suggestions include:

1. McEvoy, GK, ed. *AHFS Drug Information, 2011.* Bethesda, MD: American Society of Health-System Pharmacists; 2011.
2. MedOutcomes Inc. *Ambulatory Care Clinical Skills Program, Core Module.* Bethesda, MD: American Society of Health-System Pharmacists; 1998.
3. Koda-Kimble, MA et al. ed. *Applied Therapeutics: The Clinical Use of Drugs.* 9th ed. Philadelphia: Lippincott Williams & Wilkins; 2008.
4. Lee, M, ed. *Basic Skills in Interpreting Laboratory Values.* 4th ed. Bethesda, MD: American Society of Health-System Pharmacists; 2009.
5. Facts and Comparisons. *Drug Facts and Comparisons 2010.* Philadelphia: Lippincott Williams & Wilkins; 2010.
6. Trissel, LA. *Handbook on Injectable Drugs.* 16th ed. Bethesda, MD: American Society of Health-System Pharmacists; 2010.
7. Ansel HC. *Pharmaceutical Calculations.* 13th ed. Philadelphia: Lippincott Williams & Wilkins; 2009.
8. DiPiro JT et al., ed. *Pharmacotherapy: A Pathophysiologic Approach.* 8th ed. Stamford, CT: Appleton & Lange; 2011.
9. Fauci, A et al., ed. *Harrison's Principles of Internal Medicine.* 17th ed. New York: McGraw Hill Text; 2008.
10. *Stedman's Medical Dictionary,* 28th ed. Philadelphia: Lippincott Williams & Wilkins; 2006.
11. Brunton, LL et al., ed. *Goodman & Gilman's The Pharmacological Basis of Therapeutics.* 12th ed. New York: McGraw Hill Professional; 2011.

The National Association of Boards of Pharmacy (NABP) prepares extensive information and practice test questions available in the Registration Bulletin.[2] Review all of this information so that you thoroughly understand the NAPLEX®. Make sure you understand and are versatile with the CAT format. Make sure you are absolutely confident in using the mouse, the computer keyboard, and the screen. You do not want to waste any precious time while taking the examination figuring out computer logistics. Above all, practice answering sample questions. Practice test questions are available in the NABP Pre-NAPLEX® exam.[2] This exam uses questions developed by NABP staff and the same CAT format as the NAPLEX®. This is particularly important for the CAT.

Taking the NAPLEX®

You have been preparing and studying for the NAPLEX® for weeks, you are familiar with the NAPLEX® competency statements, and have spent hours answering practice questions and using the CAT format. You are ready for the examination.

Be Prepared

Your first step in achieving success on the NAPLEX® is to arrive for the test well prepared. Arrive at your testing center 30–40 minutes early. This will allow you time to find the rest rooms and get comfortable. If any distracting noises exist, ask for a new seat. You may find that a ticking clock or a neighbor with an annoying cough may distract you from concentrating. Also be aware of blowing air vents and any glare from overhead lights on your computer screen. You do not want any environmental distracters. People have various tolerance levels, so do not hesitate to ask to be moved if you are bothered. This is your test. Please keep in mind that if you arrive at the test center 30 minutes after your scheduled appointment time you may be required to forfeit your appointment time and your fee! It is essential to read the NABP Registration Bulletin very carefully. There are strict rules and procedures that must be followed.

Monitor Your Time

You have 4 hours and 15 minutes to complete the examination and the examination consists of 185 questions. Therefore, at about the 2-hour mark you should be at the halfway point or have about 90 questions completed. Make yourself a schedule in 15-minute increments. Every 15 minutes you should answer at least 11 questions. You may want to pace yourself during the first 30 minutes of the examination to make sure you are on target for completion.

Read Carefully

Read directions carefully and read each question carefully. Do not rush through the question. You have made yourself a time schedule; now, simply monitor the schedule and do not rush. Do not make assumptions or jump to conclusions. Do not look for answers you have memorized. Read the question and think about the correct answer. Use your mouse to highlight key words in the question. Look for common question words such as how, which, define, and when. Answer the question. Do not assume trick questions. This may sound obvious to you but many careless errors are made because the question was not read carefully.

Guessing

In computer adaptive testing, you must answer the question before you proceed to the next question. Therefore, at times you must guess. Everyone has to guess occasionally. Do not panic. Use the following strategies for intelligent guessing:

1) The most general option is often the correct one because it allows for exception. If four of the five options are specific in nature and one is more general, choose the more general option.

2) The correct choice is often a middle value. If the options range in value from high to low, then eliminate the extreme values and choose from the middle values.

3) The longest option is most often the correct one. If three options are much shorter than the fourth, then choose the longest answer.

4) When two options have opposite meanings, then the correct answer is usually one of these.

5) Look for grammatical agreement between the question and the answer. For example, if the question uses a singular verb tense, then the answer should also be singular. Eliminate the answers that do not produce a grammatically correct sentence.[3]

6) Use your medical terminology. You have learned a whole new language of prefixes and suffixes. You may not recall the exact details of osteoarthritis, but you do know that the prefix "ost" denotes bone. Use that knowledge to help you eliminate responses and increase your chances of guessing the correct response.

7) Use your logic. Think in terms of time sequence, priorities, and severity. Select an appropriate framework, and review the responses in terms of that framework. Then make a logical guess.

The Princeton Review has coined the term process of elimination, or POE.[4] This strategy focuses on eliminating responses to improve your chances of guessing the correct answer. Keep in mind at all times the NAPLEX® competencies (Appendix A).

The NAPLEX® is testing only those competencies. In other words, each question and each answer supports and assesses a competency. If a response has nothing to do with a competency area, eliminate it as a choice. By eliminating responses, you increase your chance of guessing the correct response.

Trouble Areas in Objective Tests

There are two trouble areas for people taking objective tests. The first factor to be aware of is specific determiners. These are words that give statements an absolute sense, and, as we know, there are few absolutes in the world. For example, positive specific determiners are words like all, every, everybody, everyone, always, all of the time, invariably, will certainly, will definitely, will absolutely, and the best. Negative specific determiners include the words none, not one, nobody, no one, never, at no time, will certainly not, will definitely not, will absolutely not, the worst, and impossible. When these words are included in an option, that option is usually incorrect.

For example:

Which of the thyroid function tests listed below will always accurately assess euthyroidism?
A.   Free thyroxine
B.   Total triiodothyronine
C.   Free thyroxine index
D.   Free triiodothyronine
E.   Thyroid-stimulating hormone

An example of specific determiners in the responses or answers follows:

When should KL expect most of her symptoms of hypothyroidism to improve after starting the levothyroxine?
A.   Always after 1 week of therapy
B.   Never before the third day of therapy
C.   After 3 days of therapy
D.   After 21 days of therapy
E.   After the first dose

Again, you can probably eliminate Response A, always after 1 week of therapy, and B, never before the third day of therapy, because there are no definite guarantees in pharmacotherapeutic treatments. However, some specific determiners are associated with correct statements. Look for more general terms such as often, perhaps, seldom, generally, may, and usually. When you are reading the questions, use your mouse to highlight specific determiners so that you are aware of them. Do not ignore them when answering the question.

The second area to be aware of is negative terms. Statements that contain negatives are more difficult to interpret than those statements without negatives. Here is an example of a double negative statement:

Which of the following are not potential reasons for patients to not adhere to the prescribed anticoagulant regimen?

Strike out the negatives, and read the question again.

Which of the following are not potential reasons for patients to not adhere to the prescribed anticoagulant regimen?

The question is now easier to read, understand, and interpret.

Coping with Test Anxiety

In spite of the fact that you have been taking examinations for years to obtain your pharmacy degree, you may be anxious about the NAPLEX®. You are not alone. Graduates from pharmacy schools, medical schools, nursing programs, and other professional programs are all preparing to take their licensure examination. It is an exciting and stressful time for graduates all over the country! But do not let the excitement and the stress get the best of you. It has been estimated that half of the nation's students suffer test anxiety and one quarter of them are significantly hampered by it.[5] Test anxiety may manifest itself both mentally and physically. You may experience mental black-outs, difficulty concentrating or negative thoughts. You may also feel faint, nauseous, sweaty with tense muscles or increased breathing rate. Some students even have heart palpitations.[6] Some amount of test anxiety is normal. Performers all feel nervous before they go on stage. It is your body preparing you. Make that anxiety work for you.

To make anxiety work for you, you need to understand it.

There are several possible causes of test anxiety. The first one is not being familiar with the test. Read the Registration Bulletin and make sure you understand the content domains, the process and the procedures. The second one is concern over the test content. By now you know where to find the NAPLEX® content domains, you have developed a study schedule, and you have selected review books. The rest is up to you. A third component of test anxiety is negative thoughts. We all have them occasionally, however, now is not the time! You have successfully completed the pharmacy curriculum, which has prepared you for the NAPLEX® There is no reason to believe you will fail, however if you do fail, keep in mind that you always have the opportunity to retake it. Nationally, the success rate on the NAPLEX® is more than 90%. That means that less than 1 in 10 students fail the exam on the first attempt. With proper preparation you will not be one of the failures! Another component of text anxiety is that you do not know the facts about the test, rather you are believing rumors and test-myths. Read the Registration Bulletin and go into the test understanding the facts. Know how much time you have for the test and how many questions to expect.[6]

As discussed earlier, some amount of test anxiety is normal. You may find relaxation techniques helpful in assisting you in focusing on the exam. There are two kinds of relaxation techniques: physical and mental. For physical relaxation, first sit comfortably with both feet on the floor and your hands resting on your thighs. Release all your body tension and close your eyes and count backward from 10 to 1. Count only on each exhalation and breathe very deeply from the abdomen. Alternatively, clench your hands tightly for 5–10 seconds and then slowly relax your hands. Repeat this process using muscles throughout your entire body. Complete the relaxation exercise by taking a deep breath and tensing the entire body, then relaxing it. You may find the first exercise to be particularly helpful during the exam. Mental relaxation techniques include techniques as mental imaging.[7] Picture yourself in a peaceful setting, one that pleases you. For example, picture yourself by the ocean or taking a walk in the woods. Avoid negative thoughts and consequences. Focus your thoughts on the positive outcomes of the NAPLEX®.

Conclusion

The NAPLEX® represents years of education and is the final step before embarking on your career. The success rate of pharmacy students taking the NAPLEX® is very good. Do not think about failure. Think about success. You have had years of excellent education and weeks of review and preparation for the NAPLEX®. You are familiar with the CAT and test-taking strategies. You are ready to be a pharmacist. Congratulations!

References

1. National Association of Boards of Pharmacy. Survey of Pharmacy Law. Mount Prospect, IL: National Association of Boards of Pharmacy; 2011.
2. National Association of Boards of Pharmacy. NAPLEX®/MPJE® Registration Bulletin. Mount Prospect, IL: National Association of Boards of Pharmacy; 2011
3. Pauk W. How to Study in College. 5th ed. Boston: Houghton Mifflin; 1993.
4. Meyers JA. Cracking the NCLEX-RN. New York: Random House; 2000.
5. Hill KT. Interfering effects of test anxiety on test performance: A growing educational problem and solutions to it. Ill Sch Res Dev. 1983; 20:8-19.
6. Educational Testing Service. Reducing Test Anxiety. Princeton, NJ: Educational Testing Service; 2005.
7. Heiman M, Slomianko J. Success in College and Beyond. Allston, MA: Learning to Learn Inc.; 1992.

Cardiac and Vascular Diseases

Section Editor: James A. Karboski

Patient Name: Winnie King
Address: 5000 State Street
Age: 59   **Sex:** Female
Height: 5′ 6″   **Weight:** 112 kg
Race: African American
Allergies: Penicillin (hives, itching), codeine (nausea)

Chief Complaint

WK is a 59-yo African American female who was directly admitted to the coronary care unit (CCU) with chest pressure and numbness in the fingers of her left hand.

History of Present Illness

WK stated that she was vacuuming her home this morning when she developed dyspnea and chest pressure that radiated to the left side of her neck and the fingers of her left hand, which later became numb. She took two nitroglycerin tablets with some relief of pressure and pain in her chest, but she remained short of breath and nauseous. WK reported that she had been noticing chest pressure and shortness of breath for the past 6 weeks during activities such as walking up the driveway and vacuuming her house. She admitted that she has experienced similar symptoms at rest on occasion. After limited relief following administration of sublingual nitroglycerin, WK went immediately to her physician's office and was subsequently transported to the hospital and admitted directly to the CCU. EMS personnel initiated oxygen via nasal cannula and administered morphine 3 mg IV. Following the morphine, she reported her pain was 5 on a scale of 1-10 with no shortness of breath. An EKG was obtained immediately on arrival at the CCU, which showed 2-mm T wave inversion with sinus bradycardia and first-degree AV block. The cardiology fellow made a preliminary diagnosis of unstable angina and ordered a troponin-I level, digoxin level, serial CPK isoenzymes, chemistry profile, and CBC. An early, noninterventional approach to therapy was planned. A nitroglycerin IV infusion was initiated at 10 μg/min along with enoxaparin 110 mg SC q 12 h. WK's medications prior to admission were also ordered to be continued while in the hospital.

Past Medical History

CHF, type 2 DM, HTN, CAD, obstructive sleep apnea, mild renal insufficiency, PTCA performed in 1998

Social History

Tobacco use: 20 pack-year history of smoking, quit in 1990

Alcohol use: none

Family History

Father died of an MI at age 66. Mother died of CHF at age 75.

Review of Systems

Noncontributory

Physical Examination

GEN: Obese, anxious female with chest pain and SOB

VS: BP 120/63 mmHg, HR 56 bpm, RR 20 rpm, T 98.5°F, Wt 112 kg

CV: Regular rhythm, no murmurs

LUNGS: CTA bilaterally

ABD: NT/ND, (+) bowel sounds

EXT: (1+) Edema; pulses 2+/4

CXR: Cardiomegaly, mild blunting of angles

Laboratory and Diagnostic Tests

Sodium 141 mEq/L	Potassium 5.6 mEq/L
Chloride 110 mEq/L	CO_2 content 29 mEq/L
BUN 45 mg/dL	Serum creatinine 4.2 mg/dL
Glucose 175 mg/dL	Magnesium 2.3 mg/dL
Hgb 11.8 g/dL	Hct 36.8%
Platelets 285,000 cells/mm³	WBC 9,400 cells/mm³
Troponin-I <0.4 ng/mL	CPK 60 U/L
CPK-MB 0.8 U/L	MB relative index 1.3%
Total cholesterol 225 mg/dL	LDL 106 mg/dL
PT 12.0 sec	INR 1.0
Digoxin 3.4 ng/mL (last dose 21 hours ago)	

Diagnosis

Primary:

1) Unstable angina

Secondary:

1) Congestive heart failure
2) Type 2 diabetes mellitus
3) Coronary artery disease
4) Renal insufficiency
5) Obstructive sleep apnea
6) Hypertension

Medication Record

(on admission)

1/24, K-Dur 20 mEq

1/24, Lipitor 20 mg

1/24, Furosemide 40 mg

1/24, Metoprolol 50 mg

1/24, Glyburide 5 mg

1/24, Digoxin 0.25 mg

1/24, Lisinopril 20 mg

1/24, Nitroglycerin 0.4 mg

1/24, Alprazolam 0.5 mg

1/24, Nitroglycerin 50 mg/D₅W 250 mL

1/24, Enoxaparin 110 mg

Pharmacist Notes and Other Patient Information

None available.

Questions

1. Drug therapy of unstable angina differs from chronic stable angina in which of the following respects?

   A. Lipid-lowering agents are only indicated in patients with stable angina.

   B. Beta-adrenergic blockers should never be utilized in patients with unstable angina.

   C. Antiplatelet therapy and anticoagulation with unfractionated heparin or LMWH are the cornerstones of treatment for unstable angina.

   D. Organic nitrates should only be utilized in patients with unstable angina.

   E. Aspirin should be continued indefinitely only in patients with unstable angina.

2. In addition to enoxaparin and nitroglycerin, the cardiology fellow orders aspirin 325 mg PO daily and morphine 2-3 mg IV q 2 h PRN chest pain. An additional medication that should be considered for WK is:

   A. clopidogrel.

   B. dopamine 2 mcg/kg/min IV infusion.

   C. reteplase.

   D. dobutamine 5 mcg/kg/min IV infusion.

   E. diltiazem 0.25 mg/kg IV bolus.

3. Which of the following medication(s) should the pharmacist recommend to hold or discontinue based on information provided in the case?

   I. Digoxin, because of elevated serum level and possible toxicity

   II. Scheduled doses of potassium chloride, because of risk for accumulation and cardiac toxicity secondary to marked renal impairment

   III. Enoxaparin, because of risk for accumulation and bleeding secondary to marked renal impairment

   A. I only

   B. III only

   C. I and II only

   D. II and III only

   E. I, II, and III

4. What is a likely reason to explain WK's elevated serum digoxin level based on information provided in the case?

   A. Concurrent glyburide therapy

   B. Serum digoxin level obtained too soon after the previous dose

   C. Renal insufficiency

   D. Concurrent lisinopril therapy

   E. Exercise (housework) prior to admittance

5. Which of the following tests should be performed as soon as possible to facilitate early risk stratification for patients who present with chest discomfort consistent with acute coronary syndrome?

   A. Liver function tests and troponin-I and/or CPK-MB

   B. Troponin-I and/or CPK-MB and fasting lipid panel

   C. 12-lead EKG and liver function tests

   D. Troponin-I and/or CPK-MB and 12-lead EKG

   E. Liver function tests and fasting lipid panel

6. Which of the following statements regarding the use of low-molecular-weight heparin (LMWH) in unstable angina are true?

   I. LMWH is more predictably absorbed from the subcutaneous route than unfractionated heparin.

   II. Enoxaparin is now preferable to unfractionated heparin in patients with unstable angina unless CABG is planned within 24 hours.

   III. LMWH dosage should be adjusted based on aPTT results.

Case 1

A. I only
B. III only
C. I and II only
D. II and III only
E. I, II, and III

7. The efficacy of aspirin therapy in unstable angina is secondary to its:

   A. analgesic effect.
   B. uricosuric effect.
   C. antiplatelet effect.
   D. vasodilatory effect.
   E. antipyretic effect.

8. WK reports continuing episodes of chest pain. A repeat EKG shows 2-mm ST segment depression. The cardiology fellow consults you regarding the suitability of a GP IIb/IIIa inhibitor for WK. You are asked to explain the differences between abciximab, eptifibatide, and tirofiban in the treatment of unstable angina. Which of the following statements is TRUE?

   A. Abciximab should only be administered to patients in whom PCI is not planned.
   B. Eptifibatide or tirofiban should be added because of signs of continuing ischemia and presence of new onset ST depression on the EKG.
   C. Eptifibatide and tirofiban dosage should be reduced in cases of significant hepatic impairment.
   D. Abciximab dosing should be adjusted in patients with renal impairment.
   E. A common adverse reaction associated with eptifibatide is back pain.

9. WK subsequently underwent a successful balloon angioplasty procedure and was discharged from the hospital 3 days later. One of WK's discharge prescriptions includes clopidogrel 75 mg daily. The prescription could be appropriately filled with:

   A. Persantine.
   B. Aggrenox.
   C. Pletal.
   D. Ticlid.
   E. Plavix.

10. WK asks you to recommend an OTC analgesic product. Which of the following could you recommend given her history of CHF and renal insufficiency?

    A. Ibuprofen
    B. Naproxen
    C. Acetaminophen
    D. Ketoprofen
    E. Diphenhydramine

Patient Name: Paul Gold
Address: 4301 Rossiter Street
Age: 79   **Sex:** Male
Height: 5' 9"   **Weight:** 95.4 kg
Race: White
Allergies: NKDA

Chief Complaint

PG is 79-yo white male seen in the ED with respiratory distress with severe dyspnea and wheezing.

History of Present Illness

PG was coming home from the grocery store when he became short of breath and started wheezing while carrying in his groceries. He could only say a couple words between breaths. His neighbor noticed him in distress and called 911. PG experienced severe shortness of breath 6 months ago and was hospitalized for acute severe asthma.

Past Medical History

PG was diagnosed with asthma approximately 20 years ago, rheumatoid arthritis about 5 years ago, and benign prostatic hyperplasia last year. PG has been using an herbal product to treat his benign prostatic hyperplasia. He was admitted to the hospital three times in the past 2 years for exacerbation of asthma. At a previous office visit 5 weeks ago, a blood pressure reading of 150/95 mmHg was documented.

Social History

Tobacco use: 1/2 pack per week

Alcohol use: six-pack of beer per week

Caffeine use: 2 cups of coffee every morning

Family History

Mother died of an MI at age 68. Father died of lung cancer at age 75.

Review of Systems

Wheezing and coughing

Physical Examination

VS: BP 160/100 mmHg, HR 120 bpm, RR 31 rpm, T 38.5°C, Ht 5' 9", Wt 95.4 kg

CHEST: Expiratory wheezes

Laboratory and Diagnostic Tests

Potassium 3.8 mEq/L	Sodium 145 mEq/L
Serum creatinine 1.5 mg/dL	FBG 100 mg/dL
Total cholesterol 200 mg/dL	HDL 35 mg/dL
RBC 4.7 cells/mm^3	Hgb 15 g/dL
Hct 44%	pH 7.40
PaO$_2$ 55 mmHg	PaCO$_2$ 40 mmHg

Diagnosis

Primary:

1) Hypertension

Secondary:

1) Asthma

2) Rheumatoid arthritis

3) BPH

Medication Record

Furosemide 40 mg po q am

Albuterol inhaler 2 puffs qid prn

Beclomethasone inhaler 1 puff qid

Ibuprofen 800 mg po tid

Herbal product with licorice po qd

Acetaminophen po prn

Pharmacist Notes and Other Patient Information

None available.

Questions

1. Which medications/OTC product(s) that PG was taking prior to admission may be the cause of an inadequate response to his current treatment for HTN?

   A. Ibuprofen and furosemide

   B. Beclomethasone and acetaminophen

   C. Ibuprofen and licorice

Case 2

D. Licorice only

E. Acetaminophen only

2. Which of the following statement(s) is TRUE?

   I. Oral albuterol can cause a problem with HTN control, but inhaled albuterol is of less concern if used appropriately.

   II. Oral corticosteroids can cause a problem with HTN control, but inhaled corticosteroids are of more concern because of the solubility of steroids in the lungs.

   III. Low-dose furosemide can cause a problem with HTN control, but high-dose furosemide is of less concern if used appropriately.

   A. I only

   B. III only

   C. I and II only

   D. II and III only

   E. I, II, and III

3. Which information present in PG's medical record is NOT a major cardiovascular risk factor?

   A. History of hypertension

   B. Body weight

   C. Age

   D. Renal function

   E. Family history

4. What is the patient's estimated GFR using the MDRD formula?

   A. 31 mL/min

   B. 41 mL/min

   C. 48 mL/min

   D. 55 mL/min

   E. 62 mL/min

5. Which antihypertensive medication is contraindicated in this patient?

   A. Hydrochlorothiazide

   B. Propranolol

   C. Captopril

   D. Diltiazem

   E. Valsartan

6. What compelling indications would you discuss with the physician regarding this patient's hypertensive treatment?

   A. Chronic kidney disease

   B. Benign prostatic hyperplasia

   C. Rheumatoid arthritis

D. Asthma

E. This patient has no compelling indications

7. PG's physician is interested in starting him on a combination antihypertensive product. Which of the following contains two different medications in a single dosage form?

   A. Kerlone

   B. Lotrel

   C. Coreg

   D. Altace

   E. Norvasc

8. In this patient with Stage 2 hypertension and a compelling indication of renal insufficiency, JNC 7 recommends a thiazide-type diuretic and ACEI. Which combination medication meets this requirement?

   A. Candesartan-hydrochlorothiazide

   B. Enalapril-hydrochlorothiazide

   C. Amlodipine-benazepril hydrochloride

   D. Reserpine-hydrochlorothiazide

   E. Amiloride-hydrochlorothiazide

9. A physician asks if an alpha-1-blocker may have a favorable effect on any comorbid condition present in this patient. Which of the following would you report to the physician?

   I. Prostatism

   II. Dyslipidemia

   III. Chronic kidney disease

   A. I only

   B. III only

   C. I and II only

   D. II and III only

   E. I, II, and III

10. According to JNC 7 guidelines, what is the proper classification in a patient with a sustained blood pressure of 160/100 mmHg?

    A. Normal

    B. Prehypertension

    C. Stage 1 hypertension

    D. Stage 2 hypertension

    E. Stage 3 hypertension

Patient Name: Kenneth Morris
Address: 27 Catfish Lane
Age: 38   **Sex:** Male
Height: 6′ 3″   **Weight:** 150 kg
Race: White
Allergies: NKDA

Chief Complaint

KM is a 38-yo white male who presents to the ED with chest pain.

History of Present Illness

KM stated a sudden onset of burning chest pain approximately 1 hour ago while watching television, which was not relieved by three nitroglycerin tablets taken 5 minutes apart. The pain spread over the entire pericardium area, radiating to the left shoulder. Other symptoms reported by KM included nausea, shortness of breath, and diaphoresis. There was no dizziness reported. The pain was initially rated at 3, on a scale of 1-10, and progressed to 10 by the time EMS arrived to transport KM to the hospital. EMS personnel initiated oxygen via nasal cannula and a nitroglycerin IV infusion and administered two doses of morphine 2 mg IV. Pain was now 5/10 with no shortness of breath reported. A stat EKG was obtained immediately on arrival at the ED, which showed 3 mm ST segment elevation and Q waves in leads I and V2-V4, consistent with an acute transmural myocardial infarction. The ED physician ordered alteplase 15 mg IV bolus, followed by 50 mg IV infusion over 30 minutes, followed by 35 mg IV infusion over 60 minutes.

Past Medical History

KM was diagnosed with HTN and hypercholesterolemia approximately 10 years ago. About 2 years ago, KM began to experience isolated episodes of chest pain when performing activities such as mowing the lawn or raking leaves and was subsequently diagnosed with CAD. He also had surgery performed on his left knee about 1 year ago.

Social History

Tobacco use: about 2 ppd

Alcohol use: occasional

Family History

Father died of an MI at age 52. Mother is 60 years old and in relatively good health.

Review of Systems

Noncontributory

Physical Examination

GEN: Obese, pale, anxious diaphoretic male with chest pain

VS: BP 141/83 mmHg, HR 83 bpm, RR 18 rpm, T 98.7°F, Wt 150 kg

CV: RRR, no murmurs

LUNGS: CTA bilaterally

ABD: NT/ND, (+) bowel sounds

EXT: No edema; pulses 2+/4

Laboratory and Diagnostic Tests

Sodium 138 mEq/L	Potassium 4.0 mEq/L
Chloride 105 mEq/L	CO_2 content 29 mEq/L
BUN 20 mg/dL	Serum creatinine 1.5 mg/dL
Glucose 105 mg/dL	Magnesium 1.9 mg/dL
Hgb 13.9 g/dL	Hct 40.6%
Platelets 207,000 cells/mm³	WBC 13,700 cells/mm³
Troponin-I 5.8 ng/mL	CPK 218 U/L
CPK-MB 25.5 U/L	MB Relative Index 11.7%
Total cholesterol 270 mg/dL	LDL 165 mg/dL
PT 11.5 sec	INR 0.9

Diagnosis

Primary:
1) Acute myocardial infarction
2) HTN
3) Hypercholesterolemia

Medication Record

Hydrochlorothiazide 25 mg po qd

Pravastatin 20 mg po qd

Pharmacist Notes and Other Patient Information

None available.

Case 3

Questions

1. What relative contraindication to thrombolytic therapy must be ruled out prior to administration of alteplase to KM?

   A. Active internal bleeding
   B. History of hemorrhagic stroke
   C. Severe uncontrolled hypertension
   D. Significant closed head trauma within past 3 months
   E. Intracranial neoplasm

2. Which fibrinolytic agent is the drug of choice for the treatment of acute myocardial infarction?

   A. Tissue plasminogen activator (tPA, alteplase, Activase)
   B. Streptokinase
   C. Anistreplase (APSAC, Eminase)
   D. Reteplase (rPA, Retavase)
   E. No specific thrombolytic is the clear drug of choice

3. Thrombolytics have demonstrated proven benefit in the treatment of acute MI if administered within how many hours following onset of symptoms?

   A. 6 hours
   B. 12 hours
   C. 24 hours
   D. 48 hours
   E. Time from onset of symptoms is not important

4. Heparin dosage for KM should be adjusted based on which of the following lab test(s)?

   A. Prothrombin time (PT)
   B. International Normalized Ratio (INR)
   C. Partial thromboplastin time (PTT)
   D. Bleeding time
   E. Platelet aggregation time

5. Which of the following test results for KM is relatively specific for and consistent with myocardial injury?

   I. Troponin-I
   II. CPK-MB
   III. ST segment elevation greater than or equal to 1 mm on EKG

   A. I only
   B. III only
   C. I and II only
   D. II and III only
   E. I, II, and III

6. Which of the following medications can be given to KM at discharge to reduce his risk of having a second myocardial infarction?

   I. Beta-blocker
   II. ACE inhibitor
   III. Statin

   A. I only
   B. III only
   C. I and II only
   D. II and III only
   E. I, II, and III

7. Which of the following antiplatelet agents would you recommend for KM for long-term therapy in the event that he is intolerant of aspirin therapy?

   A. Nifedipine
   B. Clopidogrel
   C. Abciximab
   D. Acetaminophen
   E. Enoxaparin

8. On the basis of information provided in the case, KM's risk factor(s) for MI includes all of the following EXCEPT:

   A. obesity.
   B. HTN.
   C. tobacco use.
   D. age.
   E. hypercholesterolemia.

9. One of KM's discharge prescriptions includes simvastatin 40 mg qd. The prescription could be appropriately filled with:

   A. Lipitor.
   B. Mevacor.
   C. Zocor.
   D. Pravachol.
   E. Lopid.

10. KM wants to stop smoking and asks about nicotine replacement options. All of the following dosage forms are available EXCEPT:

    A. transdermal patch.
    B. oral tablets.
    C. gum.
    D. oral inhaler.
    E. nasal spray.

Patient Name: Sharon Jordan
Address: 5879 Rough Rides Trail
Age: 40   **Sex:** Female
Height: 5′ 5″   **Weight:** 220 lb
Race: African American
Allergies: PCN

Chief Complaint

SJ is a 40-yo African American female who presents to her primary care provider with complaints of intermittent, brief periods of diplopia, left-sided weakness and numbness, and tingling of the left hand that last about 20 minutes at a time. She denies loss of consciousness or changes in her speech or swallowing. She has a past medical history of an ischemic stroke 2 years ago. Patient states that she has been trying to lose weight but denies using any diet aids. She is anxious and concerned that she is having another stroke.

History of Present Illness

The patient was brought to the doctor's office by her husband, who appears equally concerned about his wife's health. The patient's mother confirmed at least two occasions in the past 2 months that she noticed her daughter's speech was slurred and appeared sluggish but assumed her to be tired. The patient was scheduled to be admitted to the hospital for a full neurologic assessment.

Past Medical History

SJ has a past medical history of lupus, controlled HTN, and MVR with a St. Jude 35-mm mechanical valve 5 years ago, and an ischemic stroke 1 year after the heart prosthesis.

Social History

SJ is 40-year-old, G_0P_0, recently married female who denies use of tobacco, alcohol, or coffee. She states that she has been trying to lose weight and has stopped drinking sodas but now drinks green tea with ginko biloba. She admits that she intentionally lowered her dose of coumadin in the past month because she read that ginko may increase the risk of bleeding in patients taking blood thinners. The patient denies use of other herbals or illicit drugs.

Family History

SJ lives with her husband and mother. Her mother has HTN and DM, and her father died in a MVA. Her father's PMH is remarkable for CAD, HTN, and CVA, which occurred at 49

years of age. She has four siblings: one sister has HTN, one brother has DM and HTN, and the two other siblings are in good health.

Review of Systems

SJ is an obese, pleasant young woman who appears moderately distressed. She has a slight gait abnormality consistent with the prior CVA but has no other complaints. She states that she had been having headaches with visual changes, but attributes it to her not eating as much in an effort control her weight. Her speech is not normal and has a significant lisp. She has a blunted response to pin prick on her left lower extremity.

Physical Examination

GEN: Moderately obese female in moderate distress; appears anxious; A&O x 3

VS: BP 140/100 mmHg, HR 90 bpm, RR 20 breaths/min, T 98.5°F, Wt 100 kg, Ht 5′ 5″

HEENT: PERRL without accommodation; EOMI, fundoscopic exam reveals mild AV nicking, sclera and conjunctiva pink and mucous membranes moist

CHEST: Lungs CTA bilaterally, audible mechanical valve prosthesis in the mitral position, tachycardic with normal S_1 and S_2 heart sounds

NEURO: Altered gait

NECK: Supple, mild JVD, left-sided carotid bruit, no lymphadenopathy

ABD: Obese, nontender with (+) BS, no hepatosplenomegaly

EXT: Shows 1-2+ pitting edema bilaterally; diminished sensations of lower extremities on left side

Laboratory and Diagnostic Tests

Nonfasting levels:

Sodium 143 mEq/L	Potassium 5.1 mEq/L
Chloride 106 mEq/L	CO_2 content 23 mEq/L
BUN 28 mg/dL	$Cr_{(s)}$ 1.5 mg/dL
Glucose 220 mg/dL	Hgb_{A1C} 8%
$Chol_{total}$ 210 mg/dL	HDL 28 mg/dL
LDL 120 mg/dL	Triglycerides 300 mg/dL
RBCs 3.59 cells/mm³	WBCs 14.1 cells/mm³
Platelets 403 cells/mm³	Hgb 10.4 g/dL

Case 4

HCT 23%   ANA titer 1:320

PT/INR 14.7 sec/1.6   PTT 32.4 sec

Urine analysis: Cloudy and straw colored, casts, proteinuria 3+, many RBCs, WBCs >10,000 cells/mm^3

 ## Diagnosis

TIA   r/o impending stroke

HTN   DM

Acidosis   Obesity

Hyperlipidemia   SLE

Inadequate anticoagulation

 ## Medication Record

MEDS PTA:

Hydroxychloroquine 200 mg tablet po bid

Warfarin 5 mg tablet po daily (previously prescribed 7.5 mg daily)

Metformin 500 mg po bid

Acetaminophen 500 mg 1-2 tablets po q6h prn

Prednisone 5 mg 1 tablet po q day

 ## Pharmacist Notes and Other Patient Information

None available

Questions

1. Which of the following is not a contraindication for the administration of rt-PA to treat acute ischemic stroke?

    A. Evidence of intracranial hemorrhage
    B. Active internal bleeding
    C. Serious non-head trauma within the past 30 days
    D. Serious head trauma within the past 3 months
    E. Known cerebral aneurysm

2. What are SJ's risk factors for acute ischemic stroke?

    A. Systemic lupus erythromatosus
    B. Cardiac mechanical prosthesis in the mitral position
    C. Diabetes mellitus
    D. Age
    E. TIA

3. The attending physician diagnosed SJ with a transient ischemic attack but doesn't feel surgery is an appropriate option for her. He requests a discussion with the neuropharmacist, who suggests the patient has a number of medication-related issues that must be focused on and correctly recommends the following:

    A. adjustment in the patient's pharmacologic therapy is unnecessary at this time.
    B. the patient requires antihypertensive therapy and adjustment of oral anticoagulation therapy.
    C. that she be started on antiplatelet therapy with aspirin, her hypertension be controlled with an angiotensin receptor antagonist, she be initiated on an HMG CoA reductase inhibitor, there be an adjustment of the warfarin intensity, and metformin should be discontinued and another oral hypoglycemic agent started.
    D. the patient should receive antihypertensive management only.
    E. the patient's home meds should be resumed without adjustment.

4. Which of the following is true regarding mechanical valves and stroke prevention?

    A. Patients with mechanical valves in the aortic position have a greater thrombogenic potential than those with valves in the mitral position.
    B. The patient requires no anticoagulation therapy and should proceed to rehabilitation.
    C. It would be beneficial for the patient to have a repeat CT scan of the brain before receiving anticoagulation therapy no less than 48 hours after management of the acute stroke.
    D. Aspirin and warfarin are equally effective in preventing systemic embolization.
    E. All mechanical and bioprosthetic valves are treated with the same intensity of anticoagulation.

5. Other therapies that should be employed in this patient to prevent recurrent stroke include:

    I. antihyperlipidemic therapy.
    II. oral antidiabetic therapy plus insulin during the acute phase of recovery from the stroke.
    III. prophylactic treatment with lorazepam 1-4 mg IV push over 10 minutes.

    A. I only
    B. III only
    C. I and II only
    D. II and III only
    E. I, II, and III

6. What level of monitoring should be performed on patients who have suffered an acute ischemic cerebral event?

   I. Patients should be hospitalized in the ICU or specialized stroke unit for frequent assessments for the first 24-36 hours.
   II. Frequent neurologic assessments should occur every 15 minutes during the infusion of the thrombolytic, then every 30 minutes for the next 6 hours, then every hour for the next 16 hours.
   III. Blood pressure measurements should occur every 15 minutes for 2 hours, then every 30 minutes for the next 6 hours, then every hour for the next 16 hours.

   A. I only
   B. III only
   C. I and II only
   D. II and III only
   E. I, II, and III

7. All of the following conditions/signs are associated with increased risk of death in patients who have suffered a stroke EXCEPT:

   A. pneumonia.
   B. sepsis.
   C. cerebral edema.
   D. fever.
   E. dysphagia.

8. Choose the best statement that describes the use of aspirin in the treatment of stroke.

   I. Aspirin is the only antiplatelet agent that has been evaluated for the treatment of acute ischemic stroke.
   II. The use of aspirin in the treatment of acute ischemic stroke is safe and produces a small but significant benefit.
   III. Early death, recurrent stroke, or late death can be prevented in patients with acute ischemic stroke when treated with aspirin in doses of 160 mg to 325 mg.

   A. I only
   B. III only
   C. I and II only
   D. II and III only
   E. I, II, and III

9. SJ is relieved that she did not need surgery and is being discharged from the hospital on warfarin 5 mg 1 tablet qd, Plaquenil 200 mg 1 tablet bid, Actos 15 mg 1 tablet qd, and Tylenol 325 mg 1-2 tablets q6 hours prn pain. The pharmacist is asked to perform discharge counseling. Which of the following counseling points is FALSE?

   A. Actos can cause swelling of the feet and difficulty breathing. These should be reported to your physician.
   B. You are taking the Plaquenil for your SLE.
   C. Do not make major changes in your diet and exercise without consulting with your physician.
   D. Another name for Plaquenil is hydroxychloroquine sulfate.
   E. If aspirin does not upset your stomach, you may use it instead of Tylenol.

10. Which of the following is a modifiable risk for recurrent stroke in this patient?

   A. Systemic lupus erythromatosus
   B. Cardiac mechanical prosthesis in the mitral position
   C. Diabetes mellitus
   D. Age
   E. History of a CVA in the patient's father

Respiratory and Pulmonary Diseases

Section Editor: Michelle Condren

Patient Name: Sarah Lucas
Address: 368 Bayberry Drive
Age: 68   **Sex:** Female
Height: 5'4"   **Weight:** 76 kg
Race: Caucasian
Allergies: Codeine

Chief Complaint

SL is a 68-yo white female who was seen this afternoon in her family medicine physician's office for an exacerbation of asthma. SL was outside tending her flowers when she noticed tightness in her chest. She complained of difficulty catching her breath. On arriving at the office she was audibly wheezing and had a peak flow of 240 L/min. (Personal best for SL is 400 L/min.)

History of Present Illness

SL has been in good control of her asthma over the last several years. Her health overall has been good until today.

Past Medical History

SL has a long-standing history of mild persistent asthma with no identifiable triggers. She has been maintained on theophylline for at least 5 years without any reports of exacerbations. Her family physician has tried to change her to an inhaled corticosteroid, but she refuses because she has done well on the theophylline. She has moderate to severe osteoarthritis in her hands. She had a right hip replacement 6 years ago. She has a history of hypercholesterolemia, but no reports of angina or HTN. She has recently been diagnosed with glaucoma and started on Betagan®. Other health information is noncontributory.

Social History

Tobacco use: None   Alcohol: 1 martini a day

Caffeine use: 1 cup of coffee in the morning; occasional iced tea

Family History

Father and brother died from MI in their mid-sixties

Mother died in her eighties from Alzheimer's disease

Review of Systems

No URI symptoms, audible wheezes bilaterally

Physical Examination

GEN: Tanned, anxious woman in moderate respiratory distress VS: On presentation to the office: BP 160/90 mmHg, HR 120 bpm, RR 28 rpm, T 38.5°C, Wt 76 kg; post-nebulizer treatment: BP 135/85 mmHg, HR 120 bpm, RR 22 rpm

HEENT: PERRLA, full set of dentures present, oral cavity without lesions, nasal passages not inflamed

CHEST: Bilateral wheezes

NEURO: Alert and oriented

Laboratory and Diagnostic Tests

Theophylline 10 mcg/mL

Diagnosis

Asthma exacerbation

Medication Record

Lipitor® 10 mg 1 tablet q HS

Theo-Dur® 300 mg 1 tablet BID

Betagan® 0.5% 1 drop in each eye BID

Acetaminophen 500 mg 2 tablets q 6 h prn

Pharmacist Notes and Other Patient Information

None available

Questions

1. Of the scenarios listed below, the most likely contributor to SL's current exacerbation is:

   A. acetaminophen interfering with theophylline clearance.
   B. the addition of Betagan® ophthalmic drops.
   C. subtherapeutic theophylline levels.
   D. Betagan® interfering with theophylline clearance.
   E. nonadherence to theophylline therapy.

2. Which of the following therapies would also be appropriate for a patient with mild persistent asthma?

Case 5

   A. Albuterol inhaler 1 puff QID
   B. Singulair® 10 mg QD
   C. Serevent® Diskus 1 puff prn
   D. Prednisone 15 mg BID
   E. Nothing; no daily medications are necessary

3. You are working in the clinic pharmacy and the physician orders a STAT Xopenex 1.25 mg nebulizer treatment for SL. The pharmacy only carries albuterol for nebulization. You call the physician and tell her which of the following?

   A. Use 5 mg of albuterol
   B. Use 2.5 mg of albuterol
   C. Use 0.63 mg of albuterol
   D. Use 0.31 mg of albuterol
   E. You do not have to call the physician; use the same dose and substitute albuterol

4. Physical symptoms of an asthma exacerbation could include:

   I. coughing.
   II. tightness in chest.
   III. fever.

   A. I only
   B. III only
   C. I and II only
   D. II and III only
   E. I, II, and III

5. Peak flow meters measure:

   A. the rate at which air is taken into the lungs.
   B. total lung capacity.
   C. the rate at which air is forced out of the lungs.
   D. the rate of air exchange.
   E. respiratory rate.

6. SL's physician decides to change her from oral theophylline to a Pulmicort® inhaler. In counseling the patient, which of the following points are important to cover?

   A. The physician will need to follow renal function periodically
   B. The medication should be taken for relief from an acute exacerbation
   C. The patient should gargle water and spit it out after using the inhaler
   D. The patient should begin feeling better within 3 days of starting the Pulmicort®
   E. Pulmicort® should be used with a spacer device

7. SL's response to albuterol can best be evaluated by:

   I. more comfortable breathing.
   II. decreased respiratory rate.
   III. heart rate.

   A. I only
   B. III only
   C. I and II only
   D. II and III only
   E. I, II, and III

8. SL is given an albuterol inhaler to use at home in the case of worsening symptoms. Which of the following is NOT something that should be reviewed as you counsel the patient on the appropriate use of this medication?

   A. Shake container
   B. Prime the inhaler (if inhaler has not been used for 4 days or more)
   C. Breathe in as rapidly as possible after depressing the canister
   D. Before starting, breathe out fully, emptying air from the lungs
   E. Keep canister upright and place either in a spacer device or loosely between open lips

9. The physician would like SL to use a peak flow meter for the next 2 months. When you counsel her you include the following points:

   A. She should breathe out slowly into the device
   B. If possible, stand up to perform the test
   C. Twice a day, blow into the meter once and record the result
   D. Twice a day, blow into the meter three times and record the average of the three results
   E. It will take 2 days to determine her personal best

10. If SL were experiencing more frequent symptoms and her status was moderate persistent asthma, a reasonable treatment choice for her would be:

   A. Use albuterol on a scheduled basis
   B. Begin prednisone 30 mg once daily
   C. Begin cromolyn 2 puffs QID
   D. Add fluticasone 110 mcg (1 puff) BID
   E. Add Foradil inhaler 12 mcg BID

Patient Name: William Heckford
Address: 2111 Cherry Hill Lane
Age: 73   **Sex:** Male
Height: 5'10"   **Weight:** 84 kg
Race: African American
Allergies: Penicillin (hives)

Chief Complaint

WH is a 73-yo African American male who was seen this morning in his internal medicine physician's office for asthma. WH was gardening with his grandchildren in the backyard. He stated that his heart was pounding. WH complained of feeling anxious all the time and a slight tremor in his hands. WH admits that he began feeling these symptoms right around the time his doctor changed his asthma medication.

History of Present Illness

WH gardens with his grandchildren often during the mornings. He is usually able to play games and run around the yard with his 2-year-old grandson. This morning WH complained of slight hand tremors, headache, and a rapid heartbeat.

Past Medical History

WH has a long history of moderate persistent asthma. His physician has tried different inhalers throughout the years. WH has been well controlled on fluticasone and salmeterol therapy for several months. Two months ago, his physician recommended changing therapy to Advair® because WH was forgetting which inhaler to take. WH admits to having difficulty sleeping since he began his Advair® therapy. WH also has a history of HTN and angina.

Social History

Tobacco use: None   Alcohol: None

Caffeine use: 1 cup of tea every morning

Family History

Father died of an MI at age 60. Mother died of lung cancer at age 58. Brother is reported to be without health problems.

Review of Systems

No URI symptoms, wheezing, or shortness of breath

Physical Examination

GEN: Well-nourished anxious male in some degree of discomfort

VS: On presentation to the office: BP 175/90 mmHg, HR 145 bpm, RR 38 rpm, T 37.5°F, Wt 84 kg

HEENT: PERRLA

CHEST: RRR, no murmurs, no wheezes

NEURO: Alert and oriented

Laboratory and Diagnostic Tests

None available

Diagnosis

Asthma

Medication Record

Lasix® 80 mg 1 tablet once daily

Advair® Diskus 250/50 mcg 2 puffs BID

Albuterol inhaler 1 puff every 4 hours prn

Nitroglycerin SL 0.4 mg use as directed

Altace® 5 mg 1 tablet by mouth once daily

Flovent® 110 mcg 2 puffs BID

Pharmacist Notes and Other Patient Information

None available

Questions

1. Possible causes of WH's recent heart palpitations and tremors since he began Advair® therapy include which of the following?

    A. Drug interaction between Advair® and Lasix®
    B. Drug interaction between Advair® and Flovent®
    C. Advair® prescribed above the maximum recommended dose
    D. Noncompliance with albuterol inhaler regimen
    E. Advair® contraindicated in patients with hypertension

Case 6

2. Advair® is a combination product of which two medications?
    A. Fluticasone and albuterol
    B. Triamcinolone and albuterol
    C. Fluticasone and levalbuterol
    D. Fluticasone and salmeterol
    E. Levalbuterol and salmeterol

3. WH needs to be counseled:
    A. to use the Advair® only as needed for serious asthma exacerbations.
    B. to use the albuterol inhaler daily to maintain asthma control.
    C. to discontinue using the Flovent® and use the Advair® only one puff twice daily.
    D. to discontinue the use of the albuterol inhaler.
    E. to continue to use both the Flovent® and Advair® inhalers.

4. When using a peak flow meter at home, when should WH proceed to the emergency department?
    A. When PEF is 80% predicted or personal best
    B. When PEF is <70% predicted or personal best
    C. When PEF is 50%-80% predicted or personal best
    D. When PEF is <50% predicted or personal best
    E. When PEF is 70%-80% predicted or personal best

5. According to NHLBI guidelines, which of the following is true regarding intermittent asthma therapy?
    A. Controller medications should be used daily
    B. Short-acting beta2-agonists should be used greater than three times per day to treat symptoms
    C. Short-acting beta2-agonists should be required less than three times per week to treat symptoms
    D. A combination of short- and long-acting beta2-agonists should be used to treat daily symptoms
    E. Controller medications and long-acting beta2-agonists should be used daily

6. Advair® should be used:
    A. for relief of acute exacerbations.
    B. only in combination with salmeterol.
    C. for severe asthma only.
    D. as a controller medication.
    E. for intermittent asthma only.

7. Which of the following is true?
    I.   Hepatic enzyme inducers may enhance corticosteroid metabolism.
    II. Rifampin may reduce corticosteroid efficacy.
    III. Hepatic enzyme inhibitors may enhance corticosteroid metabolism.
    A. I only
    B. III only
    C. I and II only
    D. II and III only
    E. I, II, and III

8. All of the following are true regarding leukotriene modifiers EXCEPT:
    A. These medications should be used daily for prevention or chronic treatment of asthma
    B. Patients should take these medications only when symptomatic
    C. Headache is a potential side effect of agents in this class
    D. Leukotriene modifiers may be useful for prevention of exercise-induced bronchospasm
    E. These agents may be used in combination with an inhaled corticosteroid

9. If WH was previously taking fluticasone propionate 110 mcg, 2 puffs BID, what initial Advair® strength and dosing schedule is recommended?
    A. 100/50 twice daily
    B. 250/50 once daily
    C. 250/50 twice daily
    D. 500/50 twice daily
    E. 500/50 once daily

10. Which of the following should have been discussed with WH when he first began using Advair®?
    A. Advair® will stop an asthma attack once it has started
    B. This medication should be used together with the salmeterol inhaler
    C. Rapid heartbeat may be associated with Advair® and you should report it to your doctor
    D. You will never need to use your albuterol inhaler once you have started Advair® therapy
    E. If you feel any shortness of breath or increased wheezing, increase your number of puffs

Patient Name: Emily Fitch
Address: 65 N. Roses Boulevard
Age: 6 years   **Sex:** Female
Height: 107.9 cm, 5-10% of growth percentile
Weight: 17.7 kg, 10-25% of growth percentile
Race: Caucasian
Allergies: NKDA, sensitive to vancomycin (reaction: Redman's syndrome)

Chief Complaint

Emily is at the pediatric cystic fibrosis ambulatory care clinic for a hospital follow-up visit. She has no chief complaint.

History of Present Illness

Emily has done well since her hospitalization 5 weeks prior for a pulmonary exacerbation. Cough has been rare and productive of no significant sputum. Her bowel movements are reported as normal.

She was hospitalized for 2 weeks due to complaints of daily yellow-green sputum production and post-tussive emesis. Prior to admission, mother reported decreased appetite and vomiting more with tube feeds. Emily's weight declined 2.8 kg since the previous clinic visit. Her SpO2 was 86% on admission and she was managed with oxygen via face mask. Emily was treated with airway clearance 4 times per day and intravenous antibiotics of oxacillin for 3 days, then tobramycin plus ceftazidime for 11 days.

Past Medical History

Cystic fibrosis diagnosed by sweat chloride at 2 weeks of age, homozygous for deltaF508 genotype, hospitalized 4 times for pulmonary exacerbations. Pancreatic insufficiency and vitamin D deficiency. Acute bronchiolitis due to respiratory syncytial virus requiring intubation at 2 weeks of age.

Surgical history: gastrostomy-tube placement at 2 years

Immunization history: up-to-date, received seasonal influenza and H1N1 vaccinations last fall

Social History

Emily lives with mother, father, and 2 sisters. She will be starting the 1st grade this fall. Positive smoke exposure in the home from both parents.

Nutrition: high-fat, high-calorie diet of 3 meals and 1 snack each day. She also supplements with Peptamen Jr 1.5, 2 cans at night and 3 cans during the day with meals.

Family History

2 sisters with cystic fibrosis (both currently mild in severity)

Review of Systems

CHEST: airway clearance with vest TID

Physical Examination

GEN: healthy, alert, and no distress

VS: BP 90/54 mmHg, HR 86 bpm, RR 20 rpm, SpO2 96% on room air

HEENT: ear canals clear, tympanic membranes normal, no visible nasal polyps or discharge, oral mucosa not inflamed, no adenopathy, neck supple, trachea midline

Lungs: breath sounds symmetrical without rales or wheezes but some barrel chesting

Heart: regular rate and rhythm, normal S1 and S2, no murmurs

Abdomen: soft without mass or tenderness, no hepatosplenomegaly

Extremities: no clubbing, cyanosis, or edema

Laboratory and Diagnostic Tests

Today

Pulmonary function test: There is scooping of the expiratory limb of the flow volume loop. Bronchodilator response was not performed. Findings are consistent with moderate obstruction.

	FVC	FEV1	FEV1/FVC
Actual	0.87 L	0.66 L	75.9%
% Predicted	78%	66%	

5 weeks prior (hospitalization)

Sputum culture: heavy growth of 1) Pseudomonas aeruginosa which is sensitive to aztreonam, cefepime, ceftazidime, ciprofloxacin, imipenem, levofloxacin, meropenem, ticarcillin/clavulanate, tobramycin and intermediate to amikacin and 2) Staphylococcus aureus which is sensitive to cefazolin, ceftriaxone, clindamycin, erythromycin, linezolid, oxacillin, trimeth/sulfa, vancomycin

Vitamin D, 25-OH 23.15 ng/mL (30-100)

3 months prior (routine clinic visit)

Pulmonary function test

	FVC	FEV1	FEV1/FVC
Actual	0.84 L	0.6 L	71.4%
% Predicted	74%	59%	

Sputum culture: heavy growth of Staphylococcus aureus which is sensitive to cefazolin, ceftriaxone, clindamycin, erythromycin, linezolid, oxacillin, trimeth/sulfa, vancomycin

Case 7

6 months prior (routine clinic visit)

Vitamin D, 25-OH 30.12 ng/mL (30-100)

9 months prior (annual clinic visit)

All labs WNL except vitamin D, 25-OH 24.18 ng/mL (30-100)

 Diagnosis

Cystic fibrosis

Pancreatic insufficiency

 Medication Record

Dornase alfa (Pulmozyme®) 1 mg/mL	Inhale 2.5 mg via nebulizer daily
Albuterol 2.5 mg/3 mL	Inhale 2.5 mg via nebulizer TID
ADEKs	1 tablet PO daily
Vitamin D (Cholecalciferol) 1,000 unit	2 tablets PO BID
Pancrelipase (Creon®) 12,000 unit	3 capsules PO TID with meals, 2 capsules PO with snacks or supplements
Lansoprazole (Prevacid®) 15 mg	1 capsule PO daily
Polyethylene glycol (Miralax®) 3350 g	Dissolve 17 g (1 capful) in 8 oz liquid daily

 Pharmacist Notes and Other Patient Information

Medication adherence: caregiver reported good adherence to therapy

Questions

1. According to national CHF data, which is the correct order from the most prevalent to the least prevalent pathogen likely to cause a cystic fibrosis pulmonary exacerbation in EF?

   A. Haemophilus influenza > Pseudomonas aeruginosa > Burkholderia cepacia
   B. Burkholderia cepacia> Staphylococcus aureus > Pseudomonas aeruginosa
   C. Staphylococcus aureus > Pseudomonas aeruginosa > Haemophilus influenza
   D. Pseudomonas aeruginosa > Haemophilus influenza > Stenotrophomonas maltophilia
   E. Pseudomonas aeruginosa > Staphylococcus aureus > Stenotrophomonas maltophilia

2. When EF has another exacerbation, which is the most appropriate intravenous antibiotic regimen for empiric management (based on her most recent sputum culture)?

   A. Tobramycin
   B. Tobramycin and ticarcillin/clavulanate
   C. Meropenem and ceftazidime
   D. Oxacillin
   E. Vancomycin

3. How many pancrelipase (Creon®) capsules should be dispensed to EF, based on the current prescription, for a 30 day supply?

   A. 260
   B. 290
   C. 320
   D. 350
   E. 390

4. When educating EF on administration of pancrelipase (Creon®), which statement is correct?

   A. Take on an empty stomach
   B. Separate from calcium/aluminum-containing products
   C. Capsule contents may be sprinkled on small amount of acidic food
   D. Capsule contents may be crushed or chewed
   E. Hold capsule in mouth with first bite of food

5. EF suffers from vitamin D deficiency without adequate supplementation. What is another recommendation for EF to help correct her vitamin D status?

   A. Decrease dietary intake of green vegetables
   B. Increase dietary intake of organ meats (liver)
   C. Increase dietary intake of citrus fruits
   D. Increase exposure to ultraviolet-B rays
   E. Decrease carbonated beverage consumption

6. What are the correct storage conditions for Pulmozyme® (dornase alfa)?

   A. Refrigeration
   B. Refrigeration, protect from light
   C. Room temperature, until the expiration date
   D. Room temperature, protect from light
   E. Room temperature for up to 28 days

7. EF continues to culture Pseudomonas aeruginosa on subsequent sputum cultures. What maintenance therapy may be initiated in EF that acts as an anti-inflammatory and may decrease the virulence of Pseudomonas aeruginosa?

   A. Azithromycin
   B. Hypertonic saline
   C. Inhaled fluticasone
   D. Prednisone
   E. Tobramycin inhaled (TOBI)

8. EF is given a prescription for tobramycin inhaled BID alternating months. Which product should be dispensed?

    A. Tobramycin injection 40 mg/mL, 30-mL vial, #4
    B. Tobramycin injection 40 mg/mL, 2-mL vials, #56
    C. Tobramycin injection 80 mg/mL, 2-mL vials, #28
    D. Tobramycin inhalation solution 160 mg/2 mL, #56
    E. Tobramycin inhalation solution 300 mg/5 mL, #56

9. EF now takes albuterol, dornase alfa (Pulmozyme®), and tobramycin inhaled (TOBI®). All three inhaled medications require a nebulizer for administration. Which statement is true regarding the nebulizer or nebulized therapy for cystic fibrosis?

    A. EF's inhaled medications may be mixed together in the nebulizer cup
    B. EF may administer the inhaled medications in any order/sequence
    C. Sharing of nebulizers between patients is acceptable
    D. Regular disinfection of nebulizer parts using vinegar and water is recommended
    E. Regular disinfection of nebulizer parts using bleach, isopropyl alcohol or hydrogen peroxide is recommended

10. CF is a disease affecting many organ systems; but primarily the lungs and gastro-intestinal tract. Which are other common comorbidities that occur in CF to monitor for in EF?

    I.   Obesity
    II.   Diabetes
    III. Coronary heart disease
    IV.   Depression
    V.   Osteoporosis
    VI.   Liver disease

    A. I, II, IV, VI
    B. I, III, IV, V
    C. II, III, V, VI
    D. II, IV, V, VI
    E. III, IV, V, VI

Case 8   Rhinitis (Seasonal) and Rhinitis (Perennial)

Patient Name: John Mason Olsen
Address: 2120 Windfair Drive
Age: 42   **Sex:** Male
Height: 5'8"   **Weight:** 233 lb
Race: Caucasian
Allergies: NKDA

Chief Complaint

JMO is a 42-year old white male who was referred to the allergy clinic for his ongoing nasal and eye symptoms as well as episodes of cough and wheezing.

History of Present Illness

JMO has rhinitis symptoms that have been present for about the last 10 years. This past year has been worse for him. His symptoms occur from spring through fall. In addition to rhinorrhea, nasal congestion, and itching, he also notes that his eyes are frequently itchy, red, and tearing. Along with the nasal and eye symptoms, he has a cough that is particularly troublesome in the morning, with chest tightness, dyspnea on exertion, and wheezing.

Past Medical History

Over the past several years, the patient has been diagnosed by his primary care physician with acute sinusitis. He has about one episode, generally in the fall of each year. No other remarkable history.

Social History

JMO is married with two children: a son who is 10 years old and a daughter who is 7 years old. He does not smoke and has about one or two beers a day. He drinks two or three cups of coffee a day. There are no pets in the home.

Family History

Mother is alive and has allergic rhinitis. A brother has both allergic rhinitis and asthma. His son may also have allergic rhinitis. Father is alive and has mild hypertension.

Review of Systems

Occasional sinus pressure and tension headaches

Physical Examination

VS: BP 114/82 mmHg, HR 72 bpm, RR 16 rpm

HEENT: Pale, boggy nasal turbinates, inflamed conjunctiva

CHEST: Lungs clear to auscultation; heart: regular rate and rhythm

Laboratory and Diagnostic Tests

Allergy skin testing revealed positive reactions to trees, grasses, and ragweed pollen. He also had decreased pulmonary function. His forced expiratory volume after 1 second (FEV1) was at 84% of predicted. His pulmonary function improved by 13% after two puffs of albuterol.

Diagnosis

Rhinitis

Medication Record

Patient is taking loratadine 10 mg daily as needed. He occasionally uses an albuterol inhaler that his family practice physician prescribed for him about 2 years ago when he had difficulty breathing during an episode of acute sinusitis.

Pharmacist Notes and Other Patient Information

He buys generic loratadine from his local pharmacy.

Questions

1. This patient has a supply of Contact® capsules that he bought from your pharmacy a while ago. It has not yet reached its expiration date. The patient asks you if he can still take it for his allergy symptoms. You see that this product contains phenylpropanolamine. What would you advise?

   A. Because it was properly stored, you recommend that the patient can take it.

   B. Because you do not believe that OTC medications are appropriate for the treatment of allergy symptoms, you recommend that the patient not take it.

   C. Because it contains phenylpropanolamine, you recommend that the patient not take it.

   D. Because you do not believe it will help his allergy symptoms, you do not recommend that the patient take it.

   E. Because the product contains phenylpropanolamine, you recommend that the patient take it.

2. Which of the following would be a risk factor for this patient to have developed allergic rhinitis?

   A. The fact that his mother has allergic rhinitis.
   B. The fact that his son has allergic rhinitis.
   C. The fact that his father has hypertension.
   D. The fact that he has frequent sinus infections.
   E. The fact that he has a history of asthma symptoms.

3. The patient's physician has prescribed intranasal fluticasone. How soon can the patient expect to see some relief?

   A. Onset of action can occur within the first hour
   B. Onset of action can occur after 4 hours
   C. Onset of action can occur within 8 hours
   D. Onset of action can occur within 12 hours
   E. Onset of action can occur after 24 hours

4. How would you instruct this patient in administering fluticasone nasal spray? Please order the following steps:

   I. Spray in each nostril, alternating sides
   II. Blow nose
   III. Tilt head forward
   IV. Direct spray away from the nasal septum

   A. II, III, IV, I
   B. III, II, IV, I
   C. IV, I, III, II
   D. III, IV, I, II
   E. IV, I, II, III

5. Which of the following is NOT a potential adverse effect of intranasal corticosteroids?

   A. Epistaxis
   B. Nasal septal perforation
   C. Cataracts
   D. Decreased intraocular pressure
   E. Nasal sores

6. The patient notices a slight improvement in his symptoms after he has been on fluticasone two sprays in each nostril once a day for about 1.5 months and loratadine every day. He is still not satisfied and would like to know what else he could do to improve his symptoms. Which of the following is NOT an appropriate course of therapy?

   A. Increase fluticasone to two sprays each nostril BID
   B. Discontinue the loratadine and add a combination antihistamine/decongestant product
   C. Continue fluticasone at the same dose and add an intranasal antihistamine
   D. Consider starting immunotherapy
   E. Add an ophthalmic antihistamine eye drop

7. During the winter, this patient was able to remain symptom-free and did not require any allergy medications. In anticipation of the upcoming spring allergy season, JMO restarted his intranasal corticosteroid. He also has a supply of fexofenadine and pseudoephedrine combination to use if his symptoms are not controlled by the intranasal corticosteroid. So far this spring, his congestion, rhinorrhea, sneezing, and nasal itching are fairly well controlled. However, his eyes remain red, itchy, and watery. How should this patient be managed?

   A. Begin on OTC decongestant eye drop
   B. Begin using a corticosteroid eye ointment
   C. Begin using an artificial-tear eye drop
   D. Begin using an antihistamine eye drop
   E. Begin using a mast cell stabilizer eye drop

8. A family member of JMO was alarmed to find out that he uses an antihistamine combination. The family member had been told several years ago that antihistamines could not be taken by those patients with asthma. JMO wants to know if he should continue to use his antihistamine. What is your reply?

   A. Antihistamines are safe to take by those with asthma
   B. Antihistamine use is contraindicated in those with asthma
   C. Antihistamine use is safe in those with asthma if the dose is decreased by 50%
   D. Antihistamines should only be used in combination with other medications to treat allergic rhinitis
   E. Antihistamines should only be used intranasally by those with asthma

9. Although JMO was receiving good relief from his intranasal corticosteroid and his antihistamine/decongestant combination, he did not want the bother and expense of a prescription medication. On his own, he started using oxymetazoline. He now complains that his symptoms are much worse, especially the congestion. What is the most likely reason for the congestion?

   A. The pollen season is worse than previous seasons
   B. The oxymetazoline is effective for rhinorrhea but ineffective for congestion
   C. He is experiencing rhinitis medicamentosa
   D. He is administering the nasal spray improperly
   E. There is a drug interaction between the oxymetazoline and the antihistamine which decreases their efficacy

10. Outdoor pollen is best avoided by which of the following?

    A. Sleeping with the bedroom windows opened
    B. Replacing central air filters every month
    C. When driving, opening the car windows
    D. Avoiding being outside on windy days
    E. Mowing the lawn in the early afternoon rather than the early morning

Gastrointestinal Disorders

Section Editors: Pramodini Kale-Pradhan and Sheila M. Wilhelm

Patient Name: Mary Johnson
Address: 631 Rosemont Circle
Age: 65   **Sex:** Female
Height: 5' 5"   **Weight:** 215 lb
Race: African American
Allergies: NKDA

Chief Complaint

MJ is a 65-yo African American woman who presents to her primary care provider with complaints of an "upset stomach" for about 2 weeks. During this time she noted several days of "black stools," which has since "cleared up."

History of Present Illness

Worsening epigastric pain for 2 weeks accompanied by several days of black-colored stools. Patient states that about 3 weeks ago she started self-treatment with nonprescription naproxen in addition to her prescription medication (ibuprofen) because it was not providing adequate relief of her arthritic knee pain. She states that she also started taking Famotidine (Pepcid AC) for "upset stomach" but it has provided very little relief of her symptoms.

Past Medical History

Osteoarthritis of both knees x 10 yr treated with various NSAIDs including naproxen, diclofenac, piroxicam, and nabumetone; switched to ibuprofen 1 month ago.

Hypertension x 7 yr   Diabetes type 2 x 3 yr

Social History

Retired registered nurse

Tobacco use: Used to smoke 1PPD cigarettes for 20 yr, but quit 10 years ago

Alcohol use: Denies ETOH use

Caffeine use: 1 to 2 cups of coffee a day

Exercise is limited because of chronic knee pain

Family History

Married with no children. Lives with husband.

Father: Died at 49 in MVA

Mother: Died at 70 from DM-related complications

Review of Systems

Positive for bilateral knee pain. Negative for joint swelling, headache, nausea, chest pain, increased fatigue, weight gain, diarrhea, or constipation. No polyphagia, polydipsia; occasional polyuria.

Physical Examination

GEN: Well-developed, obese African American woman in moderate distress

VS: BP 140/82 mmHg, HR 82 bpm, RR 18 rpm, T 98.8°F, Wt 215 lb

HEENT: PERRLA

CV: NL S_1 and S_2; no m/r/g

CHEST: Lungs clear to A/P

ABD: Obese, moderate epigastric pain on palpation, normal BS; no guarding, masses, hepatomegaly or splenomegaly

GU: Deferred

RECTAL: Normal rectum; guaiac-positive stool

MS/EXT: Pulses equal and bilateral, no edema or erythema; normal ROM; no evidence of cyanosis

NEURO: A&O x 3; CN intact; normal DTR

SKIN: Warm and dry

Laboratory and Diagnostic Tests

Sodium 140 mEq/L	Potassium 4.2 mEq/L
Chloride 100 mEq/L	CO_2 28 mEq/L
BUN 20 mg/dL	Serum creatinine 1.2 mg/dL
Glucose 160 mg/dL	HbA 1C 6.4%
Hemoglobin 11.0 g/dL	Hematocrit 33.5%
Platelets 230,000/mm³	WBC 6500/mm³
MCH 29.4 pg	MCHC 34.5 g/dL
MCV 85.3 mm³	

EGD: 7 mm GU in antrum along the lesser curvature. No visible evidence of active bleeding at this time. Biopsy negative for Helicobacter pylori.

X-rays: Moderate degenerative changes in both knees.

Case 9

Diagnosis

Primary:
1. Gastric ulcer (Helicobacter pylori-negative)

Secondary:
1. Osteoarthritis
2. Hypertension
3. Diabetes - type 2
4. Overweight

Medication Record

Ibuprofen 600 mg po tid with food

Lisinopril 10 mg po daily

Hydroclorothiazide/triamterene 25 mg/37.5 mg po in the AM

Glyburide 5 mg po daily

Naproxen 200 mg po bid for knee pain

Famotidine (Pepcid AC) 1 tablet po bid upset stomach

Pharmacist Notes and Other Patient Information

None available.

Questions

1. Which of the following describes the PRIMARY mechanism of how nonselective NSAIDs cause peptic ulcers?

    A. Gastric acid hypersecretion
    B. Topical damage of gastrointestinal (GI) mucosa
    C. Stimulation of mucosal prostaglandins
    D. Inhibition of cyclooxygenase (COX)-1
    E. Inhibition of cyclooxygenase (COX)-2

2. Which of the following is NOT a well-established risk factor for NSAID-induced ulcers and related GI complications?

    A. Age >65 years
    B. History of peptic ulcer disease (PUD)
    C. Psychological stress
    D. Concomitant anticoagulation use
    E. Concomitant use of multiple NSAIDs

3. Which of the following MOST accurately describes the information you should convey to this patient about aspirin and PUD?

    A. Enteric-coated aspirin does not cause peptic ulcers.
    B. Buffered aspirin may cause peptic ulcers.
    C. Low-dose aspirin, e.g., 81 mg/day, does not cause peptic ulcers.
    D. Taking food or milk with aspirin prevents peptic ulcers.
    E. Taking an antacid with aspirin prevents peptic ulcers.

4. Which of the following NSAIDs, when used in recommended arthritic dosages, is associated with the LOWEST ulcer risk?

    A. Ibuprofen
    B. Naproxen
    C. Diclofenac
    D. Nabumetone
    E. Aspirin

5. Which of the following is the MOST frequent serious GI complication associated with nonselective NSAIDs?

    A. Gastric outlet obstruction
    B. Gastric cancer
    C. Ulcer perforation
    D. Ulcer bleeding
    E. Ulcer penetration into an adjacent organ

6. What is the RECOMMENDED ulcer healing regimen if this woman were unable to discontinue the NSAID?

    A. Misoprostol 200 mcg qid
    B. Pantoprazole 40 mg qd
    C. Famotidine 20 mg bid
    D. Famotidine 10 mg bid
    E. Sucralfate 1 g qid

7. What is the PREFERRED regimen for reducing the risk of NSAID-induced ulcer in this patient once the ulcer is healed and the patient continues to take the NSAID?

    A. Cotherapy with standard-dose H 2 RA, e.g., ranitidine 150 mg bid
    B. Cotherapy with high-dose H 2 RA, e.g., famotidine 40 mg bid
    C. Cotherapy with standard-dose PPI, e.g., rabeprazole 20 mg qd
    D. Cotherapy with low-dose misoprostol, e.g., 100 mcg bid
    E. Cotherapy with standard-dose sucralfate, e.g., 1 g qid

8. When misoprostol is used as cotherapy to reduce the risk of NSAID-related ulcers, what are the MOST important potential side effects you should discuss with the patient?

A. Abdominal cramping and diarrhea
B. Nausea and vomiting
C. Headache and dizziness
D. Drowsiness and fatigue
E. Bloating and constipation

9. What is the MOST important clinical dilemma the clinician faces if this patient was taking low-dose (81 mg) aspirin and celecoxib?

A. Low-dose aspirin may negate the anti-inflammatory effects of celecoxib.
B. Celecoxib may negate the antiplatelet effects of low-dose aspirin.
C. Combining low-dose aspirin and celecoxib causes nephrotoxicity.
D. Combining low-dose aspirin and celecoxib increases the chance for cardiac toxicity.
E. Low-dose aspirin may negate the ulcer-sparing effects of celecoxib.

10. Which of the following is a contraindication for patients on misoprostol?

A. Liver disease
B. Asthma
C. Pregnancy
D. Diabetes
E. Systemic lupus erythematous (SLE)

Patient Name: Jessica Coleman
Address: 426 Meadowbrook Lane
Age: 32   **Sex:** Female
Height: 5′ 6″   **Weight:** 161 lb
Race: White
Allergies: NKDA

Chief Complaint

JC is a 32-yo white woman who visits your pharmacy with complaints of "heartburn" and an occasional sour taste in her mouth for about 1 month.

History of Present Illness

JC states that she first noticed these symptoms about 1 month ago when she got promoted to a more stressful job. In response to your questions, she indicates that she has heartburn about 3 to 4 days a week and that is not adequately relieved by Zantac 75 or Mylanta Maximum Strength when taken prn. She rates her heartburn severity as about a 4 or 5 on a scale of 1-10 (1 = very mild and 10 = very severe). She describes a "sour" taste in her mouth especially when she bends over after eating. She asks you if it is okay for her to take Prilosec OTC.

Past Medical History

JC is in generally good health and is not being treated for any chronic conditions

Social History

Accountant with high-stress job

Tobacco use: 1 PPD x 10 yr

Alcohol use: None. It causes her heartburn to worsen.

Caffeine use: About 2-3 diet colas/day (caffeinated)

Loves to go out for dinner; tends to eat dinner late at night.

Family History

Father seemed to have "same" problem for a long time.

Review of Systems

Negative except as previously noted.

Physical Examination

GEN: Well-developed woman in NAD with complaints of heartburn and occasional "sour" taste in her mouth

VS: None available

Laboratory and Diagnostic Tests

None available

Diagnosis

Primary:
1. Frequent heartburn

Medication Record

Zantac 75 po prn heartburn

Mylanta Maximum Strength 15 mL po prn heartburn

Advil 1 tablet po prn menstrual cramps once a month

Multivitamins 1 tablet po daily

Pharmacist Notes and Other Patient Information

None available.

Questions

1. Heartburn is a burning sensation that arises from the:
   A. epigastrium and moves up toward the chest.
   B. epigastrium and radiates to the back.
   C. chest and moves up toward the neck.
   D. chest and moves down toward the stomach.
   E. umbilicus and moves up toward the sternum.

2. Which of the following is considered to be an EXCLUSION to the self-treatment of heartburn?
   A. Heartburn occurring 3-4 days a week
   B. Heartburn accompanied by a sour taste
   C. Heartburn unresponsive to nonprescription H 2 RAs
   D. Heartburn of mild-to-moderate severity
   E. Heartburn occurring 3-4 days a week that persists for 3 months or longer

3. JC notices that Prilosec OTC is indicated for "frequent" heartburn. She asks you, "What is meant by frequent heartburn?"

   A. Heartburn that occurs daily
   B. Heartburn that occurs two or more times a day
   C. Heartburn that occurs two or more days a week
   D. Heartburn that occurs two or more days a month
   E. Heartburn that occurs two or more months a year

4. All of the following are recommended nonpharmacologic modifications for JC with regard to her heartburn EXCEPT:

   A. elevate the foot of the bed by 6 inches, using blocks.
   B. reduce weight, if possible.
   C. stop or reduce cigarette smoking.
   D. reduce stress.
   E. eat at least 2-3 hours before bedtime.

5. In addition to nonpharmacologic measures, what is the PREFERRED pharmacologic management of this woman's heartburn?

   A. Do not recommend pharmacologic self-treatment; refer to primary care provider
   B. Prilosec OTC 20 mg daily for 14 days
   C. Zantac 150 twice daily for 14 day
   D. Zantac 75 twice daily for 14 days
   E. Mylanta Maximum Strength 30 mL before meals and at bedtime

6. What is the BEST advice to give JC if her heartburn returns 5 days after completion of a 14-day Prilosec OTC regimen?

   A. Take an additional 14-day regimen of Prilosec OTC 20 mg/day
   B. Increase Prilosec OTC dose to 20 mg twice daily for 14 additional days
   C. Take Prilosec OTC 20 mg only when you have heartburn symptoms
   D. Continue taking Prilosec OTC 20 mg/day for 14 days; add Pepcid 40 mg at bedtime
   E. Contact your primary care provider and he/she will determine whether you should continue taking Prilosec OTC

7. What are the MOST common side effects associated with the short-term use of nonprescription omeprazole?

   A. Headache and diarrhea
   B. Constipation and intestinal gas
   C. Nausea and vomiting
   D. Dry mouth and cough
   E. Itching and skin rash

8. What is the PREFERRED management of a person who anticipates that he/she is most likely to have heartburn after eating a spicy dinner meal?

   A. Take H 2 RA immediately after eating spicy dinner
   B. Take H 2 RA immediately prior to eating spicy dinner
   C. Take H 2 RA 1 hour prior to eating spicy dinner
   D. Take H 2 RA twice daily in AM and PM day of spicy dinner
   E. Take H 2 RA at bedtime the night before spicy dinner

9. Why should magnesium-containing antacids be AVOIDED if JC had renal failure?

   A. Increased renal elimination of magnesium in renal failure leads to toxicity
   B. Increased magnesium absorption in renal failure leads to toxicity
   C. Increased distribution of magnesium in renal failure leads to toxicity
   D. Decreased renal elimination of magnesium in renal failure leads to toxicity
   E. Decreased magnesium absorption in renal failure leads to toxicity

10. What is the preferred INITIAL management of a pregnant woman who has mild and infrequent heartburn after eating large meals and when lying down?

    A. Take no action as heartburn is mild and infrequent
    B. Dietary and lifestyle modifications
    C. Antacid 1 and 3 hours after meals and at bedtime
    D. Nonprescription H 2 RA
    E. Nonprescription omeprazole

Case 11

Patient Name: Amy Wu
Address: 214 Bright Avenue
Age: 29   **Sex:** Female
Height: 5' 2''   **Weight:** 120 lb
Race: Asian
Allergies: NKDA

Chief Complaint

AW is a 29-yo Asian woman who visits your pharmacy with complaints of "hard pellet-like" stools and "bloating" and requests your assistance in selecting a laxative that will help relieve her constipation quickly.

History of Present Illness

AW states that she first noticed these symptoms about 1 week ago when she returned from a business trip to Toronto. She indicates that she usually has a bowel movement every day, but during the last week or so she has only moved her bowels 3 to 4 times. She describes straining with each bowel movement and complains of feeling bloated and uncomfortable. When questioned, AW recalls having similar symptoms several years ago.

Past Medical History

AW is an otherwise healthy young woman who is not being treated for any chronic conditions.

Social History

Works full time as a computer programmer

Tobacco use: None

Alcohol use: None

Caffeine use: 1 to 2 cups of tea (decaffeinated)

Usually runs 2 miles a day when not traveling

Usually drinks 1 to 2 glass of water/day and eats a well-balanced diet

Family History

Both parents are alive and well.

Review of Systems

Negative except as previously noted.

Physical Examination

GEN: Healthy appearing young woman in no apparent distress with complaints of hard stools and abdominal bloating

VS: None available

Laboratory and Diagnostic Tests

Not available

Diagnosis

Primary:
1. Acute (temporary or occasional) constipation

Medication Record

Acetaminophen 500 mg po prn headache

Diphenhydramine 25 mg po for seasonal allergies

Pharmacist Notes and Other Patient Information

Patient complains of hard stools and bloating for about 1 week. Indicates that she usually has daily bowel movements but that during the past week she has only moved her bowels about 3 to 4 times. She wants a laxative that provides "quick" relief.

Questions

1. Which of the following does NOT reflect how patients typically describe their perception of "constipation"?
   A. "Hard" stools
   B. "Black-colored" stools
   C. "Straining" when passing stool
   D. "Incomplete" evacuation
   E. "Infrequent" bowel movements

2. Constipation is particularly prevalent in which of the following groups of people?
   A. Women and the elderly
   B. Women and patients with IBD
   C. Men and patients with IBS
   D. Children under 18 years of age and the elderly
   E. Pregnant women and children under 18 years of age

3. In what situation is it appropriate to self-treat constipation?

    A. Changes in stool caliber, e.g., pencil-thin
    B. Marked abdominal pain
    C. Blood in the stool
    D. Constipation that persists for 1 week
    E. Constipation that persists after 1 week of self-treatment

4. All of the following nonpharmacologic measures may be useful in minimizing the risk of constipation in this patient EXCEPT:

    A. increasing dietary fiber.
    B. increasing fluid intake.
    C. increasing physical activity.
    D. increasing ambulation during travel.
    E. increasing sleep time.

5. Which of the following foods is low in fiber?

    A. Bran muffins
    B. Prunes
    C. White pasta
    D. Legumes (e.g., kidney beans)
    E. Broccoli

6. In addition to nonpharmacologic measures, what is the PREFERRED pharmacologic management of this woman's symptoms?

    A. No need for pharmacologic therapy because symptoms are mild and will resolve on their own
    B. Fiber supplement daily for 14 days
    C. Docusate sodium 100 mg daily for 7 days
    D. Milk of Magnesia 15-30 mL at bedtime or on arising
    E. Do not recommend pharmacologic self-treatment; refer to primary care provider

7. AW wants to know how long it will take for Milk of Magnesia to work. What is the usual onset of action of a recommended oral dose of magnesium hydroxide when used as a laxative to treat constipation?

    A. 15-30 minutes
    B. 1-2 hours
    C. 6-8 hours
    D. 12-24 hours
    E. 1-2 days

8. Which of the following agents work by facilitating the mixture of water with stool?

    A. Fiber supplements
    B. Docusate sodium
    C. Bisacodyl
    D. Magnesium hydroxide
    E. Polyethylene glycol (PEG) 3350

9. Which of the following statements about senna is INCORRECT when it is used orally to treat constipation?

    A. Acts by exerting an osmotic effect on the colon
    B. May cause discoloration of the urine
    C. May cause mild abdominal cramping
    D. Onset of action is between 6 and 12 hours
    E. May develop a dark brown/black pigmentation of the colonic mucosa

10. Which of the following medications is NOT associated with an increased risk of constipation?

    A. Amitriptyline
    B. Sucralfate
    C. Hydrochlorothiazide
    D. Misoprostol
    E. Verapamil

Patient Name: Sally Quinn
Address: 555 Buena Vista Circle
Age: 44   **Sex:** Female
Height: 5′ 7″   **Weight:** 182 lb
Race: White
Allergies: None

Chief Complaint

SQ is a 44-yo white woman who visits your pharmacy and asks you, "What can I take for motion sickness?"

History of Present Illness

SQ states that she is going on an ocean cruise in a few weeks with her husband to celebrate their wedding anniversary and doesn't want to get seasick. She relates that she has trouble flying on a plane and gets sick when riding in a car, especially when she sits in the back seat. On further questioning, she tells you that she does not tolerate amusement park rides and has difficulty when she goes to the movies and sits too close to the screen. She recalls taking Bonine 25-mg tablets when she got sick, but it did not seem to help.

Past Medical History

Motor vehicle accident 10 years ago, injured left hip and knee. Most symptoms resolved with physical therapy. Otherwise unremarkable.

Social History

Works at home to care for children and husband

Tobacco use: None

Alcohol use: One glass of wine with dinner sometimes

Caffeine use: Herbal tea

Family History

Married and lives at home with her husband and four children. Otherwise not relevant.

Review of Systems

Apprehensive about going on a cruise. Occasional hip and knee pain. No other pertinent findings.

Physical Examination

GEN: Very pleasant women, somewhat anxious

VS: Information not available

Laboratory and Diagnostic Tests

None available

Diagnosis

Primary:
1. Motion sickness
Secondary:
1. Joint pain secondary to MVA

Medication Record

Advil 200 mg po prn joint pain

Tums Extra Strength 1 po tid

Glucosamine 750 mg/Chondroitin 600 mg 2 tabs po qd

Centrum 1 po qd

Pharmacist Notes and Other Patient Information

None available.

Questions

1. Which of the following are the CLASSIC symptoms of motion sickness?

    A. Headache and loss of appetite
    B. Pallor and difficulty in breathing
    C. Nausea and vomiting
    D. Belching and flatulence
    E. Cold sweat and increased heart rate

2. All of the following factors contribute to motion sickness EXCEPT:

    A. fear, stress, and anxiety.
    B. smoking or being in close proximity to smokers.
    C. duration or length of trip.
    D. reading or playing hand-held games during travel.
    E. looking outside the window of a car.

3. Which of the following helpful "tips" is INCORRECT regarding the nondrug measures SQ should use to prevent motion sickness?

    A. Avoid strong odors and aromas
    B. Get up and move around when possible
    C. Sit facing forward in a slightly reclined position

D. Avoid excess food or alcohol before and during travel

E. Sit over the wing in an airplane and in the front seat of a car

4. Which of the following drug classes is considered FIRST-LINE therapy for motion sickness?

A. Corticosteroids

B. Phenothiazines

C. Proton-pump inhibitors

D. Antihistamines

E. Butyrophenones

5. What is the MOST likely reason why Bonine did "not work" to prevent this individual's motion sickness?

A. Incorrect indication

B. Incorrect dosage form

C. Dose was too low

D. Dose given too early

E. Drug given too late

6. SQ would require a prescription for which of the following anti-motion sickness medications?

A. Dramamine

B. Phenergan

C. Bonine

D. Antivert

E. Marezine

7. Which of the following are the most common side effects associated with nonprescription motion sickness medications?

A. Dry mouth and drowsiness

B. Dizziness and drowsiness

C. Dry mouth and blurred vision

D. Drowsiness and fatigue

E. Dry mouth and diarrhea

8. Which of the following BEST describes oral scopolamine tablets when used for motion sickness?

A. One dose prevents motion sickness for up to 72 hours

B. Only effective for motion sickness associated with sea travel

C. Better suited than transdermal scopolamine for travel of short duration

D. Must be taken 8 hours before exposure to travel

E. More costly than transdermal scopolamine

9. All of the following instructions are correct when teaching a patient how to apply transdermal scopolamine EXCEPT:

A. wash and dry hands immediately after handling the patch.

B. use only one patch at a time.

C. apply at least 4 hours before traveling.

D. apply to hairless skin on the upper arm or chest.

E. remove the clear plastic backing from the patch prior to application.

10. SQ asks you about Sea-Bands and how they work. Which of the following BEST describes how Sea-Bands theoretically work to prevent motion sickness?

A. Acupressure

B. Acupuncture

C. Acustimulation

D. Acupoint

E. Acutherm

Hepatic and Pancreatic Disorders

Section Editor: Robert MacLaren

Patient Name: John Graham
Address: 2913 Yellowhammer Road H-1
Age: 70   **Sex:** Male
Height: 5' 9"   **Weight:** 160 lb
Race: African American
Allergies: Penicillin (rash)

Chief Complaint

JG presents to the emergency department complaining of SOB, fatigue, and nausea. JG said that he had lost weight over the past 1–2 months although his pants seem tighter around the waist. He also states that he has "fatty looking stools." He is subsequently admitted for evaluation.

History of Present Illness

JG has experienced increasing malaise and nausea over the past month with weight loss but increased abdominal girth. JG had an MI and CABG 18 months ago, subsequently developing atrial fibrillation and heart failure (ejection fraction = 34%). Patient has been in normal sinus rhythm most of the time since the sotalol he had been taking post-MI was discontinued and amiodarone was started. Patient's heart failure has also been well controlled over the past year.

Patient's symptoms could be related to decompensated heart failure, possibly triggered by worsening atrial fibrillation, or to some other etiology.

Past Medical History

HTN x20 years (generally well controlled)

S/P MI 18 months ago

S/P CABG 18 months ago

Atrial fibrillation x18 months

Heart Failure x1 year (EF = 34%)

Gout

Social History

JG is married with a son 45 years old and a daughter 42 years old, both in good health. He is retired from a job in retail sales. He denies alcohol and illegal drug use and has not smoked since high school.

Family History

Father died at age 64 of an MI, and his mother died at age 75 from an unknown cause. JG has one brother, 62 years old, who has recently been diagnosed with small-cell lung cancer.

Review of Systems

Patient is somewhat short of breath and complaining of nausea. He denies chest pain, but has been experiencing slight tingling and burning of his lower extremities for several months.

Physical Examination

GEN: Well-nourished, alert and pleasant male in mild-to-moderate distress

VS: BP 150/90 mmHg, HR 82 bpm, RR 22 rpm, T 98.1°F, Wt 160 lb, Ht 69 inches

HEENT: PERRLA, EOMI, corneal microdeposits present (do not appear to interfere with vision), oropharynx unremarkable, neck shows slight JVD, no bruit, no LAD, no thyromegaly

CV: RRR, normal S_1, S_2, + S_3, displaced PMI

CHEST: Slight rales bilaterally in lung bases

ABD: NT but distended, +BS, +ascites, liver edge palpable 3 cm below right costal margin, no splenomegaly

GU: Deferred

EXT: 1+ LE edema, peripheral neuropathy, skin has grayish cast

NEURO: A&O x3

Laboratory and Diagnostic Tests

Sodium 134 mEq/L	Potassium 3.9 mEq/L
Chloride 98 mEq/L	CO_2 25 mEq/L
BUN 18 mg/dL	Serum creatinine 1.4 mg/dL
Glucose 71 mg/dL	Albumin 3.5 g/dL
Total cholesterol 255 mg/dL	HDL-C 38 mg/dL
Triglycerides 180 mg/dL	LDL-C (calculated) 166 mg/dL
Uric acid 5.2 mg/dL	T. bili 0.8 mg/dL
AST 135 U/L	ALT 160 U/L
ALP 110 U/L	CBC w/ diff WNL
PT 20 seconds	INR 2.5
Digoxin 1.6 µg/L	Thyroid function test WNL

Liver biopsy consistent with pseudoalcoholic liver disease: evidence of cirrhosis, macrovesicular steatosis, Mallory bodies

Case 13

Diagnosis

Primary: Presumed drug-induced hepatotoxicity

Secondary:

1) HTN   2) Afib   3) Heart Failure   4) s/p MI & CABG   5) Gout   6) Peripheral neuropathy

Medication Record

Date	Rx No	Physician	Drug/Strength	Quantity	Sig	Refills
2/4	009	Mitchell	KCL 30 mEq		IV infusion	
2/2	008	Watkins	ECASA 325 mg		1 po qd	
2/2	007	Watkins	KCL 10 mEq		1 po qd	
2/2	006	Watkins	Lisinopril 10 mg		1 po bid	
2/2	007	Watkins	Digoxin 0.125 mg		1 po qd	
2/2	006	Watkins	Warfarin 3 mg		1 po qhs	
2/2	005	Watkins	Allopurinol 300 mg		1 po qd	
2/2	004	Watkins	Amiodarone 400 mg		1 po qd	
2/2	003	Watkins	Furosemide 40 mg		1 po qam	

Pharmacist Notes and Other Patient Information

None available.

Questions

1. JG is presumed to have drug-induced hepatotoxicity. The medical resident wants to know which of the following medications on JG's profile has been documented to cause hepatotoxicity in a manner that is dependent on cumulative dose.

   A. Amiodarone
   B. Lisinopril
   C. Allopurinol
   D. Furosemide
   E. Warfarin

2. Hepatotoxicity from which of the following medications is consistent with JG's clinical presentation, laboratory values, and liver biopsy results?

   A. Amiodarone
   B. Lisinopril
   C. Allopurinol
   D. Furosemide
   E. Warfarin

3. JG's daughter read a recent report that milk thistle is good for the liver. The physicians ask you to conduct a literature search and make an assessment of whether it might be of value to JG. You find one recently published pilot study that randomized 60 patients with chronic liver disease (mostly due to past alcohol use or chronic viral hepatitis) to milk thistle or placebo for 6 months. The results show that compared to baseline, ALT values were statistically lower at the end of the 6 month study period with milk thistle but not placebo. No other benefits were apparent and the only common side effect was nausea, which was found at equal rates in both study groups. Which of the following is the best recommendation for the consideration of using milk thistle in JG?

   A. Milk thistle should be tried because JG likely has chronic liver disease.
   B. Milk thistle should be tried because it may help improve JG's liver function.
   C. Milk thistle should not be tried because it's only going to cause JG to be nauseated.
   D. Milk thistle should not be tried because it lacks evidence of clinical benefits in patients like JG.
   E. Milk thistle should not be tried because this is a pilot study.

4. Drug interactions are a significant concern with warfarin. Which of the following agents may alter the metabolism of warfarin and necessitate additional anticoagulation monitoring?

   A. Amiodarone
   B. Lisinopril
   C. ECASA
   D. Furosemide
   E. Digoxin

5. When sotalol was discontinued and amiodarone added to JG's regimen, which of the following dosage changes should have been implemented empirically?

   A. Increase lisinopril dose by 40%–50%
   B. Increase warfarin dose by 40%–50%
   C. Increase ECASA dose by 40%–50%
   D. Decrease digoxin dose by 40%–50%
   E. Decrease KCL dose by 40%–50%

6. All of the following should be routinely monitored for a patient taking amiodarone **EXCEPT**:

   A. vital signs.
   B. liver function.
   C. pulmonary function.
   D. thyroid function.
   E. renal function.

7. JG has been in the hospital for 3 days and develops atrial fibrillation while not receiving his amiodarone. The physician orders an intravenous infusion of 0.5 mg/minute for 12 hours to be followed tomorrow with his home regimen. What diluent provides optimal stability of the solution when compounding the intravenous infusion?

   A. Saline 0.45%
   B. Saline 0.9%
   C. Dextrose 5% water
   D. Ringer's lactate
   E. Sterile water

8. JG asks you if his hypercholesterolemia may have predisposed him to hepatotoxicity. Which of the following types of liver injury is hypercholesterolemia a risk factor for?

   A. Steatotic liver injury
   B. Cytotoxic hepatocellular injury
   C. Cholestatic liver injury
   D. Vascular liver injury
   E. Neoplastic liver injury

9. During hospitalization JG's serum potassium concentration dropped to 3.2 mmol/L and the physician decided to administer IV KCl. A bag was sent to the floor containing 40 mEq KCl in 500 mL of 0.9% NaCl. In order to deliver a dose of 15 mEq KCl per hour, what should the infusion rate be in mL/min (rounded to the nearest mL/min)?

   A. 1 mL/min
   B. 2 mL/min
   C. 3 mL/min
   D. 4 mL/min
   E. 5 mL/min

10. The physician asks you for a recommendation to treat JG's hypercholesterolemia. Given JG's liver injury, which of the following statins is the most appropriate agent to initiate as therapy for his hypercholesterolemia?

    A. Lovastatin
    B. Atorvastatin
    C. Pravastatin
    D. Simvastatin
    E. Rosuvastatin

Patient Name: Earl Kent
Address: 201 Chestnut Road
Age: 52   **Sex:** Male
Height: 6' 0"   **Weight:** 77 kg
Race: Black
Allergies: Penicillin (anaphylaxis) and sulfa (maculopapular rash)

Chief Complaint

EK is a 52-yo black male who is brought to the emergency room overnight by his wife because he had two episodes of vomiting bright red blood within the past 6 hours. He is admitted to the ICU and placed on a mechanical ventilator for airway protection.

History of Present Illness

EK has never vomited blood in the past. Over the course of the night, EK receives 4 L normal saline and 2 U packed red blood cells and is started on octreotide 50 U/hr and esomeprazole 8 mg/hr. The gastroenterologist performed an endoscopy this morning and banded four bleeding esophageal varices. A nasogastric tube is left in place after the endoscopy.

Past Medical History

EK has a lengthy history of admissions for alcohol withdrawal tremors and seizures and one admission approximately 2 months ago for dyspnea secondary to ascites.

Social History

Tobacco use: 1 ppd for 40 years

Alcohol use: his wife states EK drinks 1 pint of whiskey/day plus 1 6-pack/day of beer over past 30 years

Illicit drug use: none

Family History

Father died at age 65 of lung cancer; mother died at age 69 of breast cancer. Mother had diabetes. One sister has asthma. He has been married to his second wife for 25 years. He has two grown children. He is a retired contractor for air conditioning and heating systems.

Review of Systems

Esophageal varices

Physical Examination

GEN: BM who is lethargic and disoriented; several spider angioma

VS: BP 110/50 mmHg, HR 140 bpm, RR 24 rpm, T 39.2°C, Wt 77 kg

HEENT: Scleral icterus present

CHEST: Bilateral crackles; decreased breath sounds over all lung fields

GI: Abdomen is grossly distended, fluid wave present, tympanitic in the upper abdomen; superficial abdominal veins prominent; unable to palpate liver due to ascites and distension; stool is heme-positive

Laboratory and Diagnostic Tests

Sodium 126 mEq/L	Potassium 4.7 mEq/L
Chloride 101 mEq/L	CO_2 content 25 mEq/L
BUN 30 mg/dL	Serum creatinine 1.9 mg/dL
Glucose 92 mg/dL	Albumin 2.0 g/dL
T. bili 9.4 mg/dL	D. bili 7.0 mg/dL
ALP 56 U/L	AST 272 U/L
ALT 362 U/L	PT 30.7 sec
INR 2.11	Hemoglobin 9.0 g/dL
Hematocrit 27%	Platelets 88,000/mm³

WBC 5400/mm³ with 55% PMN, 37% bands, 7% lymphocytes, 1% monocytes

CXR reveals flattened diaphragm and changes consistent with emphysema; in addition, there appears to be diffuse bilateral haziness suggestive of hypervolemia.

Peritoneal fluid reveals 280 x 10³ WBC/mm³, albumin 0.7 g/dL, Gram negative bacilli

Diagnosis

No information available.

Medication Record

Thiamine 100 mg IV qd	Folate 1 mg IV qd
Levofloxacin 250 mg IV qd	Albuterol MDI 2 puffs qid
Ipratropium Br MDI 2 puffs qid	

Octreotide 50 U bolus, then 50 U/hour

Esomeprazole 80 mg bolus, then 8 mg/hour

Lorazepam 2 mg IV q 2 hours PRN agitation

Furosemide 40 mg IV x 1 dose

Pharmacist Notes and Other Patient Information

None available.

Questions

1. It is determined that the cause of EK's hematemesis is bleeding esophageal varices. EK remains critically ill. Which of the following interventions to EK's medication profile should occur as a result of this information?

    A. Discontinue octreotide and start propranolol for long-term variceal bleeding prevention
    B. Discontinue PRN lorazepam and start scheduled lorazepam to better treat alcohol withdrawal
    C. Discontinue IV levofloxacin and start enteral levofloxacin for long-term prevention of spontaneous bacterial peritonitis
    D. Discontinue esomeprazole infusion and start scheduled IV ranitidine for stress ulcer prophylaxis
    E. Discontinue thiamine and folate and start enteral dietary intake for nutrition support

2. EK's Child-Pugh classification system is calculated to be 10 (grade C). Which of the following variables is not included in the calculation of the Child-Pugh score?

    A. Albumin
    B. Creatinine
    C. Total bilirubin
    D. Presence of ascites
    E. Presence of encephalopathy

3. If octreotide is compounded by placing 400 U in 200 mL of D_5W, at what rate should EK's octreotide be administered?

    A. 2.5 mL/hour
    B. 12.5 mL/hour
    C. 25 mL/hour
    D. 50 mL/hour
    E. 100 mL/hour

4. EK is diagnosed with spontaneous bacterial peritonitis. The hepatologist orders albumin 125 g IV now and 75 g IV in 3 days. Which of the following best explains the reason for using albumin in EK?

    A. To reverse hypoalbuminemia
    B. To reduce the volume of ascitic fluid
    C. To prevent pleural fluid collection
    D. To reduce the likelihood of renal dysfunction
    E. As a nutritional supplement

5. The hepatologist would like to use recombinant factor VIIa (rFVIIa) to treat EK's variceal bleed. The results of the only study conducted to date in patients with varices suggest that rFVIIa may reduce the need for additional blood products that cost the institution about $1000. The cumulative dose of rFVIIa used in the study was 800 mcg/kg. The cost of rFVIIa is approximately $1000/mg. Which of the following best describes the use of rFVIIa for this indication?

    A. It is likely not cost-effective due to its high drug cost.
    B. It is likely cost-neutral since its high drug cost is offset by the savings of blood product usage.
    C. It is likely cost-effective since it reduces the costs associated with blood product usage.
    D. It is impossible to assess costs without knowing precise values.
    E. It is impossible to assess effectiveness without knowing quality-of-life variables.

6. The coagulopathy exhibited by EK is best treated with which of the following products?

    A. Desmopressin
    B. Vitamin K
    C. Fresh frozen plasma
    D. Cryoprecipitate
    E. Amicar

7. The medical team asks you for a recommendation to treat EK's hyponatremia. Which of the following is the best recommendation?

    A. Normal saline at 150 mL/hour
    B. Hypertonic saline 3% at 35 mL/hour
    C. Hydrochlorothiazide 50 mg po qd
    D. Daily fluid restriction to 1000 mL/day
    E. Demeclocycline 300 mg po tid

8. Vasopressin 0.04 U/hr is initiated for suspected hepatorenal syndrome. The dose is to be titrated by 0.04 U/hr every 12 hours as tolerated. In addition to renal function, what parameter should be monitored as a possible adverse event that may prevent dose escalation of vasopressin?

    A. Worsening encephalopathy
    B. Occurrence of DVT
    C. Occurrence of cardiac ischemia
    D. Hypernatremia
    E. Hypotension

9. Two days later EK is to begin enteral feeding with Nutren 2.0. Nutren 2.0 contains 2.0 kcal/mL and 80 g/L of protein. The team would like to provide 25 kcal/kg/day. Assuming the tube feed is not stopped, how much protein will EK receive daily?

   A. 0.5 g/kg
   B. 0.75 g/kg
   C. 1 g/kg
   D. 1.25 g/kg
   E. 1.5 g/kg

10. It is now 10 days later and EK is stable for discharge. He is still receiving levofloxacin 250 mg po daily. The team would like to know what to do with EK's antibiotic therapy upon discharge. Which of the following is the best recommendation?

   A. Discontinue levofloxacin and do not restart another antibiotic

   B. Complete a 14-day course of therapy for spontaneous bacterial peritonitis

   C. Complete a 14-day course of therapy for presumed community-acquired pneumonia

   D. Switch to Augmentin to complete a 14-day course of therapy for spontaneous bacterial peritonitis

   E. Switch the levofloxacin regimen to twice weekly for lifelong prevention of spontaneous bacterial peritonitis

Patient Name: Bob Wood
Address: 2690 Ocean Drive
Age: 52 **Sex:** Male
Height: 5′ 10″ **Weight:** 150 lb
Race: White
Allergies: NKDA

Chief Complaint

BW is a 52-yo male who presents to the ED on 2/28 with a chief complaint of abdominal pain, nausea, and vomiting. BW has a 10-year history of alcohol abuse, and his current symptoms began approximately 24 hours prior to presentation, following a weekend of heavy drinking. BW reports that he has continued to drink alcohol during this time to avoid the "shakes."

History of Present Illness

BW's abdominal pain began on the Sunday evening prior to his arrival at the ED. His upper abdominal pain was acute in onset and increased in intensity over 30 minutes. He describes the pain as a steady, dull ache that moves to his back, and he rates its severity as 8 out of 10. He cannot identify any alleviating factors for his pain. BW developed severe, persistent nausea approximately 2 hours after the onset of his abdominal pain and reports three episodes of emesis during the 24 hours prior to presentation. BW consumed "a gallon" of liquor and "several" six-packs of beer during the 2 days prior to the onset of his symptoms. He reports no loss of consciousness during his 2-day drinking binge but admits to having little memory of the specific events of the weekend. Despite his nausea and vomiting, BW has attempted to consume alcohol to prevent the shakes. He relates that the alcohol only worsens his symptoms.

Past Medical History

BW has abused alcohol for approximately 10 years. He currently consumes two six-packs of beer every day but admits to occasional binge drinking on the weekends. He has been admitted to the hospital on several occasions for the management of alcohol withdrawal. His past medical history also includes hypertension, osteoarthritis, and GERD. His medications prior to admission include amlodipine, hydrochlorothiazide, PRN lansoprazole, PRN ranitidine, PRN ibuprofen, and PRN acetaminophen.

Social History

BW divorced 7 years ago and currently resides with his mother. He works as a security guard at a local warehouse.

Tobacco use: 25 pack-year history

Alcohol use: as stated in Past Medical History

Illicit drug use: none

Family History

BW's father was an alcoholic who died of an MI at age 55. His mother is alive and well at age 73. He has no siblings. His family history is negative for type 2 DM and cancer.

Review of Systems

BW does not report fever, chills, hematemesis, melena, hematochezia, chest pain, shortness of breath, or cough. He denies recent weight loss.

Physical Examination

GEN: Ill-appearing, diaphoretic, tremulous man in moderate distress

VS: On presentation to the ED, BP 160/95 mmHg, HR 120 bpm, RR 20 rpm, T 101.2°F

HEENT: NCAT, PERRLA, EOMI, mild scleral icterus, funduscopic exam without hemorrhages or exudates; oropharynx clear without exudates

NECK: Supple, no lymphadenopathy or thyromegaly, no bruits

CV: RRR without m/r/g

CHEST: CTA bilaterally

NEURO: A & O x 4, CN II-XII intact, 2+ DTRs

ABD: Diminished bowel sounds in all quadrants; mild abdominal distention with diffuse tenderness on palpation; liver span is 10 cm; no splenomegaly or fluid wave

GU: Normal circumcised male

RECTAL: Heme (-), normal prostate

EXT: No CCE; normal pulses throughout

Laboratory and Diagnostic Tests

Sodium 133 mEq/L	Chloride 96 mEq/L
BUN 30 mg/dL	Potassium 3.0 mEq/L
CO_2 28 mEq/L	Serum creatinine 1.4 mg/dL
Glucose 210 mg/dL	Magnesium 1.2 mg/dL
Serum amylase 400 U/L	Serum lipase 800 U/L
AST 150 U/L	ALT 70 U/L
T. bili 1.3 mg/dL	Alkaline phosphatase 130 U/L

Case 15

Lactate (venous) 3.5 mmol/L

WBC 17 x 10^3/L with 70% polys, 8% bands, 20% lymphs, 2% monos

Hemoglobin 100 g/L (10.0 g/dL)

Hematocrit 30.0%   MCV 110 fL

MCHC 350 g/L (35 g/dL)   Platelets 100 x 10^3/μL

pH 7.45 $PaCO_2$ 35 mm Hg

PaO_2 88 mm Hg SaO_2 98%

Blood alcohol level 30 mg/dL

CXR: no active disease

ECG: Sinus tachycardia with a rate of 120 bpm. No ST-segment or T-wave abnormalities.

Abdominal ultrasound: normal biliary tree

 Diagnosis

Primary:

1) Acute pancreatitis

2) Alcohol withdrawal

3) Acute alcoholic hepatitis

Secondary:

1) Hypertension

2) Osteoarthritis

3) GERD

 Medication Record

D_5 1/2NS infuse at 150 mL/h

Thiamine 100 mg; folic acid 1 mg; MVI 1 vial IVPB qd

Diazepam 10 mg IV q 4 h

Promethazine 25 mg 25 mg IV q 4 h prn

 Pharmacist Notes and Other Patient Information

D_5 1/2NS infuse at 150 mL/h

Thiamine 100 mg; folic acid 1 mg; MVI 1 vial IVPB qd

Diazepam 10 mg IV q 4 h

Promethazine 25 mg IV q 4 h prn

Questions

1. Which of BW's home medications is the most likely medicinal cause of his acute pancreatitis?

    A. Acetaminophen
    B. Amlodipine
    C. Hydrochlorothiazide
    D. Ibuprofen
    E. Lansoprazole

2. What analgesic is considered the agent of first choice for the management of pain in acute pancreatitis?

    A. Meperidine
    B. Morphine
    C. Hydromorphone
    D. Codeine
    E. Fentanyl

3. Which laboratory test would be preferred to assess the presence of acute pancreatitis in BW?

    A. Serum amylase
    B. Serum lipase
    C. Blood alcohol content
    D. C-reactive protein
    E. Lactate

4. If BW is too sedated due to too much diazepam, which of the following agents could be used with caution to reverse the effects of diazepam in BW?

    A. Naloxone
    B. Physostigmine
    C. Acetylcysteine
    D. Naltrexone
    E. Flumazenil

5. Compared with enteral nutrition, the use of parenteral nutrition support in patients with acute pancreatitis has been shown to result in which of the following outcomes?

    A. Significantly increases the risk of infection
    B. Significantly reduces the length of stay
    C. Increases abdominal pain and nausea
    D. Decreases the requirements for pain medications
    E. Significantly reduces mortality

6. Which of the following best describes BW's red blood cell indices upon admission?

    A. Normochromic, macrocytic anemia

    B. Normochromic, microcytic anemia

    C. Hypochromic, macrocytic anemia

    D. Hypochromic, microcytic anemia

    E. BW is not anemic and has normal red blood cell indices

7. The physician requests your assistance in designing a parenteral nutrition regimen for BW. Using the Harris-Benedict equation, calculate the basal energy expenditure (BEE) for BW:

    Men (kcal/day): 66.47 + (13.75 X W) + (5.0 X H) - (6.76 X A)

    W = weight (Kg); H = height (cm); A = age (years)

    A. 1236 kcal/day

    B. 1305 kcal/day

    C. 1420 kcal/day

    D. 1542 kcal/day

    E. 2205 kcal/day

8. BW requires a parenteral nutrition formulation that delivers 1500 kcal daily from the dextrose component. If parenteral nutrition formulations are compounded from 70% dextrose, what volume of 70% dextrose should be included in BW's daily parenteral nutrition formulation?

    A. 420 mL

    B. 580 mL

    C. 630 mL

    D. 710 mL

    E. 770 mL

9. The physician requests your assistance regarding the selection of empiric antibiotic therapy for BW? Which of the following antibiotics is the best choice for empiric management if BW had infected pancreatic necrosis?

    A. Aztreonam

    B. Gentamicin

    C. Vancomycin

    D. Cefazolin

    E. Imipenem-cilastatin

10. BW's mother brings to the hospital a non-FDA approved prescription pancreatic enzyme product called *Superzyme* that reads "Superzyme MS 12 Capsules." How would you interpret this labeling?

    A. 12,000 units of lipase per capsule encased in microspheres

    B. 12,000 units of amylase per capsule encased in microspheres

    C. 12,000 units of protease per capsule encased in microspheres

    D. 12 maximum strength enzyme capsules per bottle

    E. 12,000 units of lipase, amylase, and protease per capsule encased in microspheres

Rheumatic Disorders

Patient Name: Francis Grant
Address: 1018 N. Plainfield Street
Age: 64   **Sex:** Male
Height: 5' 11"   **Weight:** 225 lb
Race: White
Allergies: NKDA

Chief Complaint

FG is a 64-yo male seen in the ED on September 21 who states that he awoke 24 hours ago with pain and swelling of his right great toe.

History of Present Illness

The toe pain has increased since its onset, and the swelling and redness of the first MTP joint have spread across the dorsum of the foot. He is unable to wear a shoe on his right foot and presents to the clinic with only a white sock on that foot. He reports no injury to the foot and has had no previous history of gout or other forms of arthritis.

Past Medical History

HTN

Hypercholesterolemia

CAD, MI 2 years ago

Social History

Patient is a widower who lives alone. Works for a construction firm but is considering retirement soon. Has smoked 1 ppd for the past 40 years. Drinks alcohol, about 1 L of whiskey per week.

Family History

Mother died at age 54 of an MI. Father died at age 72 of unknown causes. Patient has no siblings.

Review of Systems

No fever or chills. All other systems are negative.

Physical Examination

GEN: The patient is an obese man who appears to be in moderate discomfort

VS: BP 154/86 mmHg, HR 82 bpm, RR 18 rpm, T 37.2°C

SKIN: Warm and dry

NECK: No lymphadenopathy, thyromegaly, or JVD

HEENT: PERRLA; EOMI; sclerae anicteric; the oropharynx is clear

CHEST: CTA bilaterally; no CVA tenderness or spinal tenderness

CV: RRR with a II/VI SEM; normal S_1 and S_2; no S_3 or S_4

ABD: Soft, obese, NT/ND, no masses. Normo-active bowel sounds. No guarding or rebound tenderness.

GU/RECT: Normal rectal tone; stool heme negative

MS/EXT: The first MTP joint of the right foot is acutely swollen, erythematous, warm, and exquisitely tender to the touch. There is a blush of redness spreading to a 2 x 2-cm area across the dorsum of the foot adjacent to the first MTP joint. There is no tenderness over this adjacent area. The remaining joints and extremities are without abnormality. No CCE.

NEURO: A&O x3; CN II-XII intact; no focal neurologic findings

Laboratory and Diagnostic Tests

Sodium 138 mEq/L	Potassium 3.8 mEq/L
Chloride 105 mEq/L	CO_2 25 mEq/L
BUN 14 mg/dL	Serum creatinine 1.2 mg/dL
Glucose 118 mg/dL	AST 17 IU/L
ALT 10 IU/L	Uric acid 9.9 mg/dL
Total cholesterol 266 mg/dL	HDL cholesterol 64 mg/dL
Triglycerides 245 mg/dL	Hemoglobin 12.6 g/dL
Hematocrit 39%	Platelets 246,000/mm³

WBC 6500/mm³ with 65% PMN, 3% bands, 1% eosinophils, 28% lymphocytes, 3% monocytes

Diagnosis

Primary:

1. Acute gouty arthritis

Secondary:

1. Hypertension

2. Hypercholesterolemia

3. CAD

4. Alcohol abuse

5. Tobacco abuse

Case 16

Medication Record

Date	Rx No	Physician	Drug/Strength	Quantity	Sig	Refills
3/15			Aspirin 81 mg	100	1 po qd	
3/15	688795	Potter	Hydrochlorothiazide 25 mg	30	1 po qd	6
3/15	688796	Potter	Metoprolol 25 mg	60	1 po bid	6
3/15	688797	Potter	Lisinopril 20 mg	30	1 po qd	6
6/19	723501	Potter	Simvastatin 10 mg	30	1 po qd	3
9/20			Acetaminophen 500 mg	100	1-2 tid prn pain	
9/21	857410	Hall	Naproxen 500 mg	10	1 po bid	0

Pharmacist Notes and Other Patient Information

3/15 Patient requested "baby aspirin" on the recommendation of his doctor for prevention of another MI. Advised him to take it daily with food.

9/21 Advised patient to take naproxen on a regular basis with food for 5 days to resolve his attack of gout. Cautioned on possible adverse GI effects.

Questions

1. Uric acid in the body results from:
   A. breakdown of old red blood cells by the reticuloendothelial system.
   B. degradation of dietary and tissue purines.
   C. enhanced anaerobic metabolism.
   D. synthesis in the liver by hepatocytes.
   E. resorption of bone due to increased parathyroid hormone activity.

2. Which of the following non-drug measures would NOT be effective for management of acute or chronic gout in this patient?
   A. Weight loss
   B. Alcohol cessation
   C. Smoking cessation
   D. Apply ice to affected joint during acute attack
   E. Immobilize affected joint during acute attack

3. Which of the patient's medications increases the risk of hyperuricemia and gout?
   A. Lisinopril
   B. Hydrochlorothiazide
   C. Simvastatin
   D. Metoprolol
   E. Acetaminophen

4. Janssens and colleagues conducted a randomized clinical trial comparing prednisolone 35 mg daily and naproxen 500 mg twice daily for the treatment of monoarticular gout. The primary outcome was pain measured on a 100 mm visual analogue scale. The reduction in pain score was 44.7 mm and 46.0 mm for prednisolone and naproxen, respectively (difference 1.3 mm; 95% CI -9.8 to 7.1). Adverse effects were similar between groups and minor. Which of the following statements is an accurate interpretation of study results?
   A. Naproxen is more effective than prednisolone for treatment of acute gout.
   B. Prednisolone is more effective than naproxen for treatment of acute gout.
   C. Neither naproxen nor prednisolone is effective for treatment of acute gout.
   D. Prednisolone and naproxen are equally effective for treatment of acute gout.
   E. Results cannot be interpreted because a p value is not provided.

5. Other treatments effective for acute gouty arthritis include:
   I. allopurinol.
   II. colchicine.
   III. corticosteroids.

   A. I only
   B. III only
   C. I and II only
   D. II and III only
   E. I, II, and III

6. Alternatives to NSAIDs for treatment of acute gouty arthritis would need to be considered if this patient had which of the following medical conditions?
   A. Chronic heart failure
   B. Chronic obstructive pulmonary disease
   C. Hyperlipidemia
   D. Gastroesophageal reflux disease
   E. Parkinson's disease

7. Which of the following statements about the signs and symptoms of gout is true?

   A. Increased serum uric acid levels are always present.
   B. There is gradual onset of joint pain.
   C. The first metatarsophalangeal joint is most commonly affected.
   D. Joint involvement is typically symmetrical.
   E. A definitive diagnosis can be made by x-ray of involved joints.

8. Which of the following statements about colchicine is true?

   A. It is effective in relieving an acute attack of gout because it enhances renal elimination of uric acid.
   B. When used for the treatment of an acute attack of gout, it should be administered every hour until the joint symptoms subside.
   C. It is a useful alternative to other drugs in situations where fluid retention might be detrimental (e.g., CHF and HTN).
   D. It is very effective in relieving inflammation, even if the patient has had symptoms for 3 or 4 days before seeking treatment.
   E. Colchicine should be administered intravenously to achieve a safe and rapid reduction in uric acid levels.

9. Which of the following medications does NOT interact with colchicine?

   A. Clarithromycin
   B. Diltiazem
   C. Cyclosporine
   D. Atorvastatin
   E. Losartan

10. Which of the following naproxen formulations would be suitable for treatment of this patient's acute gouty arthritis?

   I. Immediate release
   II. Enteric coated
   III. Delayed release

   A. I only
   B. III only
   C. I and II only
   D. II and III only
   E. I, II, and III

Patient Name: Samuel Taylor
Address: 531 S. Washington Street
Age: 56   **Sex:** Male
Height: 5' 10"   **Weight:** 225 lb
Race: African American
Allergies: Penicillin (rash)

Chief Complaint

ST is a 56-yo man who presents to the clinic complaining of the gradual worsening of joint pain over the past 4-6 months.

History of Present Illness

The patient states that aspirin is not helping his arthritis pain. The pain is most noticeable in his right knee and hip. The onset of pain has been gradual over the past 4-6 months. He has attempted to treat the pain with aspirin up to 18 tablets per day and has gained some relief from this treatment. He is unsure of the current dosage of aspirin that he is taking. The patient states that he has pain in the morning that improves within about 15 minutes but that the pain worsens with increased use of the affected joints during the day. He also states that he sometimes feels like his knee is going to give out when he is walking, especially when going down stairs.

Past Medical History

Hypertension

S/P appendectomy approximately 30 years ago

Social History

Married and lives with his wife of 30 years; has three grown children who are all healthy. Employed as a carpenter. Quit smoking cigarettes 25 years ago; currently smokes one or two cigars per day. Heavy alcohol intake in the past but claims to have cut back in the past 5 years. Currently drinks two to three alcoholic beverages per day, 4 to 6 days per week.

Family History

Father died at age 72 of a CVA; mother alive at age 88 with RA. Patient has no siblings. Family history is otherwise unremarkable.

Review of Systems

Denies shortness of breath, chest pain, fever, chills, or night sweats. No complaints of nausea, diarrhea, constipation, abdominal pain, vomiting, melena, or bloody stools. No dysuria, urgency, or frequency. No skin rashes or changes, intolerance to heat or cold, and no history of any STD. Appetite has been normal.

Physical Examination

GEN: The patient is a W/D African American male in NAD

VS: BP 144/88 mmHg, HR 96 bpm and regular, RR 16 rpm, T 36.9°C, Wt 225 lb, Ht 5' 10"

SKIN: Warm and dry

HEENT: NC/AT, PERRLA; sclerae are anicteric; EOMI; oropharyngeal mucosa is pink, moist, and without lesions. There are multiple dental caries throughout.

NECK: Supple with full ROM. No thyromegaly, lymphadenopathy, or JVD.

CHEST: CTA bilaterally with no wheezes or crackles

CV: Slightly tachycardic with no m/r/g appreciated

ABD: Soft, NT/ND, normo-active bowel sounds

GU/RECT: Deferred

MS/EXT: Full ROM of all extremities. Local tenderness and crepitus noted on right knee. Strength is +4/5 in both UE and +4/5 in both LE. There is no CCE.

NEURO: A&O x3; DTRs 2+ bilaterally

Laboratory and Diagnostic Tests

Sodium 139 mEq/L	Potassium 3.9 mEq/L
Chloride 101 mEq/L	CO_2 26 mEq/L
BUN 19 mg/dL	Serum creatinine 1.1 mg/dL
Glucose 99 mg/dL	AST 26 IU/L
ALT 29 IU/L	ANA titer negative
RA titer negative	Hemoglobin 13.3 g/dL
Hematocrit 39.4%	Platelets 327,000/mm³

WBC 5400/mm³ with 57% PMNs, 3% bands, 1% eosinophils, 36% lymphocytes, 3% monocytes

Hip x-ray: No fractures or dislocations. There is minimal joint space narrowing. Small osteophyte formation at femoral joint margin. No osteopenia or joint erosions are observed.

Knee x-ray: No fractures or dislocations. There is moderate joint space narrowing and osteophyte formation at the joint margins. No osteopenia or joint erosions are observed.

Diagnosis

Osteoarthritis of hip and knee

Hypertension

 Medication Record

Date	Rx No	Physician	Drug/Strength	Quantity	Sig	Refills
10/15	593848	Williams	Lisinopril 40 mg	90	1 po qd	0
10/15	593847	Williams	Hydrochlorothiazide 25 mg	90	1 po qd	0
11/5			Aspirin 325 mg	100		
11/29		Williams	Glucosamine 500 mg	100	1 po tid	
11/29		Williams	Acetaminophen 325 mg	200	2 qid	
12/28		Williams	Acetaminophen 500 mg	200	2 qid	
1/14	594003	Williams	Lisinopril 40 mg	90	1 po qd	3
1/14	594002	Williams	Hydrochlorothiazide 25 mg	90	1 po qd	3
1/14	594001	Williams	Ibuprofen 600 mg	90	1 po tid prn	3

 Pharmacist Notes and Other Patient Information

10/15: Patient 10 days late for refill of hypertension meds. Discussed importance of compliance with regimen. Recommended a pill box as patient sometimes forgets to take medicine.

11/29: Counseled patient on dosage of acetaminophen. Cautioned patient to avoid alcohol or at least limit to no more than 2 drinks per day while taking acetaminophen. If unable/unwilling to decrease alcohol intake, advised to speak with PCP about decreasing dose to max of 2.5 gm daily or using a different medication.

12/28: Patient has decreased alcohol intake to one or two drinks on the weekend.

1/14: Counseled on adverse effects of ibuprofen. Advised to check blood pressure at home regularly and inform his physician if it increases. Hypertension medications refilled on time. Patient states the pill box helped him remember to take his medication daily.

Questions

1. The drug of choice for initial treatment of OA is:

    A. acetaminophen.

    B. tramadol.

    C. oxycodone.

    D. an NSAID.

    E. intra-articular hyaluronate injections.

2. ST's acetaminophen dose was increased to 1000 mg QID but failed to provide adequate pain relief. The acetaminophen was discontinued and ST was started on ibuprofen. What monitoring parameters should be assessed periodically to ensure safety?

    I. Hepatic enzymes

    II. CBC

    III. Serum creatinine

    A. I only

    B. III only

    C. I and II only

    D. II and III only

    E. I, II, and III

3. How many mg of ibuprofen would it take to compound 50 grams of 5% ibuprofen cream?

    A. 1000 mg

    B. 2500 mg

    C. 5000 mg

    D. 400 mg

    E. 200 mg

4. Which brand/generic pair is correctly matched?

    A. Celebrex/piroxicam

    B. Daypro/oxaprozin

    C. Lodine/meloxicam

    D. Relafen/naproxen

    E. Voltaren/nabumetone

5. NSAIDs have the potential to cause clinically significant drug-drug interactions with each of the following medications EXCEPT:

Case 17

A. warfarin.
B. lithium.
C. phenytoin.
D. lisinopril.
E. ranitidine.

A. I only
B. III only
C. I and II only
D. II and III only
E. I, II, and III

6. Crepitus was noted during this patient's physical exam. What does crepitus mean?

   A. Crackling noise
   B. Swelling
   C. Bruise
   D. Thickened cartilage
   E. Joint enlargement

7. Which of the following NSAIDs are available on a nonprescription basis?

   A. Ibuprofen 400 mg and meloxicam 7.5 mg
   B. Naproxen 220 mg and piroxicam 20 mg
   C. Ibuprofen 200 mg and naproxen 220 mg
   D. Naproxen 500 mg and ketoprofen 75 mg
   E. Ibuprofen 200 mg and diclofenac 75 mg

8. This patient returns to his physician for follow-up at 6 weeks. He has been taking ibuprofen 600 mg tid but is not experiencing adequate pain relief. Which of the following would be the most appropriate medication to try next?

   A. Intra-articular hyaluronic acid injection
   B. Intra-articular glucocorticoid injection
   C. Naproxen
   D. Tramadol
   E. Oxycodone/acetaminophen

9. This patient's physician recommended glucosamine for treatment of his OA. Which of the following statements is true regarding glucosamine use for OA?

   A. Onset of pain relief can be expected within a few hours.
   B. It is not effective for OA.
   C. The main adverse effect is GI discomfort.
   D. It should be avoided in this patient because of his penicillin allergy.
   E. It should be avoided in this patient because he has hypertension.

10. Which of the following non-drug measures could be recommended to this patient for his OA?

    I. Rest
    II. Weight loss
    III. Exercise

Patient Name: Margaret Harrison
Address: 1415 Main Street
Age: 52   **Sex:** Female
Height: 5′ 2″   **Weight:** 200 lb
Race: African American
Allergies: NKDA

Chief Complaint

MH is a 52-yo female with rheumatoid arthritis and osteoporosis who returns to the clinic on August 7 for follow-up of elevated liver enzymes.

History of Present Illness

The patient had RA diagnosed 5 years ago and was much improved since starting once-weekly methotrexate approximately 4 years ago. She has had regular blood tests for hepatic enzymes, and all of these were normal until 6 weeks ago. At that time AST was 64 and ALT was 59. Methotrexate was continued and ALT and AST were repeated 2 weeks later and found to be 86 and 98, respectively. The methotrexate dose was reduced to 10 mg weekly. Two weeks later, ALT was 97 and AST, 110. Patient returns today for repeat labs. MH has had no recent flare-ups of her disease but does continue to have mild swelling in her joints. She has good ROM and states that the swelling has been a lot worse in the past and is actually quite good. She had bilateral knee replacements 3 years ago for RA. She was treated with oral corticosteroids in the past, which were discontinued when she developed osteoporosis. A DXA scan at that time (exact date unclear) showed her femur to be 2.7 standard deviations below the norm and her lumbar spine to be 2.4 standard deviations below the norm. She is presently receiving alendronate for osteoporosis. She states that she is adherent to her medication regimen.

Past Medical History

RA x5 years

S/P bilateral knee replacements 3 years ago

Corticosteroid-induced osteoporosis

Social History

MH is a retired seamstress. She is no longer able to sew because of the extent of the arthritis in her hands. She is married and has two grown children. She drinks 3-4 cups of coffee per day. She also smokes two ppd, which she enjoys and does not intend to quit. She does not drink EtOH. She states that she is not sexually active.

Family History

Mother and sister both had MIs in their sixties. Her father died at age 59 in an industrial accident. There is no family history of DM, cancer, or rheumatologic diseases.

Review of Systems

No fever, chills, night sweats, chest pain, shortness of breath, nausea, vomiting, diarrhea, constipation, bright-red blood from her rectum, or melena. The patient states that she moves her bowels approximately one or two times per day. She denies any heat or cold intolerance.

Physical Examination

GEN: The patient is an African American woman in NAD

VS: BP 144/86 mmHg, HR 76 bpm, RR 16 rpm, T 37.2°C, Wt 200 lb (stable), Ht 5' 2"

SKIN: No rashes

HEENT: PERRLA, EOMI, sclerae anicteric, oropharynx clear without lesions

NECK: Supple without JVD, lymphadenopathy, or thyromegaly

CHEST: CTA bilaterally

CV: RRR with no m/r/g

ABD: Soft, NT/ND, normal bowel sounds, no hepatosplenomegaly

GU/RECT: Deferred

MS/EXT: Positive for bilateral swelling of the proximal interphalangeal and DIP joints without pain. There is ulnar deviation of her fingers and swan neck deformities of both hands; knees show healed surgical incisions from bilateral knee replacements in the past. She has good ROM in the knees. She has very little ROM of the left or right ankle.

NEURO: A&O x 3; CN II-XII intact; normal sensory function; DTRs 2+; Babinski's negative bilaterally

Laboratory and Diagnostic Tests

Sodium 137 mEq/L	Potassium 3.9 mEq/L
Chloride 97 mEq/L	CO_2 24 mEq/L
BUN 21 mg/dL	Serum creatinine 1.0 mg/dL
Glucose 112 mg/dL	AST 101 IU/L
ALT 122 IU/L	Albumin 3.5 g/dL

Case 18

Hemoglobin 12.2 g/dL   Hematocrit 36.1%

Platelets 272,000/mm³

WBC 5300/mm³ with 54% PMN, 2% bands, 1% eosinophils, 40% lymphocytes, 3% monocytes

Chest x-ray: Normal; no infiltrates or effusions observed

ECG: Normal sinus rhythm; no significant change from previous tracing done 6 months ago

 ## Diagnosis

Rheumatoid arthritis

Corticosteroid-induced osteoporosis

 ## Medication Record

Date	Rx No	Physician	Drug/Strength	Quantity	Sig	Refills
2/1		Harris	Vitamin D 400 IU	100	1 po qd	prn
2/1	48594	Harris	Nabumetone 750 mg	60	2 po qd	12
2/1	521783	Harris	Methotrexate 2.5 mg	24	6 tabs po q week	6
2/1		Harris	Calcium carbonate 500 mg	100	1 po tid with meals	prn
2/1	48595	Harris	Alendronate 70 mg	4	1 po q week	3
2/1	521784	Harris	Folic acid 1 mg	30	1 po qd	6
8/7	89013	Harris	Adalimumab 40 mg Pen	2	SC injection every other week	2

 ## Pharmacist Notes and Other Patient Information

2/1: Patient has been receiving methotrexate for over 4 years and is currently taking 15 mg once weekly. She has no complaints related to this or her other medications. I wrote down all of the patient's medications for her and reviewed how to take each one. I reminded her to take her calcium with meals for maximum absorption. I reviewed proper administration of alendronate; patient is taking it correctly.

8/7: Patient voiced concern over having to discontinue methotrexate. I explained how adalimumab differs from methotrexate, advised her on proper administration and disposal of the pen, and reviewed possible adverse effects.

Questions

1. Because this patient responded well to the first DMARD (methotrexate) selected for treatment of RA but subsequently developed intolerable toxicity, the proper course of action is to:

    A. add a systemic corticosteroid to mask the side effects of the DMARD and provide additional anti-inflammatory activity.

    B. discontinue the DMARD and substitute an immunosuppressive agent.

    C. discontinue the DMARD and begin treatment with a different DMARD.

    D. refer the patient for surgical joint replacement.

    E. maintain the present DMARD dose and ask the patient to comply with the regimen until tolerance to the toxicity develops.

2. All of the following should be recommended to this patient to help reduce her risk of comorbidities EXCEPT:

    A. stop smoking.

    B. adopt DASH diet.

    C. reduce dietary fat and cholesterol intake.

    D. reduce carbohydrate intake.

    E. engage in routine physical activity.

3. All of the following measures are beneficial in assessing an RA patient's clinical response to therapy EXCEPT:

    A. evaluating the degree of reduction in joint swelling, warmth, and tenderness on physical exam.

    B. performing periodic laboratory monitoring of ANA and rheumatoid factor.

    C. asking the patient about changes in time to onset of afternoon fatigue.

D. administering standardized tests that measure quality of life.

E. asking the patient about his or her perception of the degree of pain and morning stiffness.

4. Which vaccinations should this patient receive?

A. FluMist (intranasal influenza vaccine)
B. Zostavax (herpes zoster vaccine)
C. Pneumovax (pneumococcal vaccine) and influenza vaccine injection
D. Pneumovax (pneumococcal vaccine), influenza vaccine injection, and Recombivax HB (hepatitis B vaccine)
E. Zostavax (herpes zoster vaccine), Pneumovax (pneumococcal vaccine), and influenza vaccine injection

5. All of the following should be communicated to the patient regarding storage, administration, and disposal of adalimumab EXCEPT:

A. inject into a different site each time.
B. never inject into areas where the skin is tender, bruised, red, or hard.
C. do not freeze.
D. store at room temperature.
E. dispose of used syringes in a puncture-resistant container.

6. The mechanism of action of adalimumab is:

A. antagonism of interleukin-1 receptors.
B. inhibition of cyclooxygenase.
C. inhibition of pyrimidine synthesis.
D. inhibition of cytokine production.
E. binding tumor necrosis factor.

7. Which drug/potential adverse effect pair is correctly matched?

A. Etanercept/pulmonary fibrosis
B. Leflunomide/hepatotoxicity
C. Sulfasalazine/lymphoma
D. Hydroxychloroquine/infection
E. Methotrexate/retinal toxicity

8. Which of the following DMARDs requires taking cholestyramine to eliminate the drug in females and males wanting to conceive?

A. Azathioprine
B. Methotrexate
C. Etanercept
D. Leflunomide
E. Sulfasalazine

9. The recommended dose of infliximab for treatment of rheumatoid arthritis is 3 mg/kg. If this drug were to be given to this patient, how many 100-mg vials would need to be reconstituted to provide the correct dose?

A. 2 vials
B. 3 vials
C. 4 vials
D. 5 vials
E. 6 vials

10. Reconstituted infliximab should be diluted in 0.9% sodium chloride injection to provide a total volume of 250 mL. If the patient's dose is 273 mg, what is the final concentration of the infliximab solution?

A. 0.50 mg/mL
B. 0.98 mg/mL
C. 1.09 mg/mL
D. 1.92 mg/mL
E. 2.46 mg/mL

Patient Name: Ann Smith
Address: 126 W. 51st Street
Age: 24   **Sex:** Female
Height: 64″   **Weight:** 136 lb
Race: African American
Allergies: NKDA

Chief Complaint

AS is a 24-yo female who was referred to the rheumatology clinic after she presented to the university health service complaining of joint pain, a skin rash, and hair loss.

History of Present Illness

The patient first noticed the skin rash about 4 weeks ago while on vacation in North Carolina. The rash gets worse if she is outdoors exposed to the sun for prolonged periods. The pain in her hand joints began approximately 3 weeks ago. She has noted the alopecia for the past 2 weeks and states that she pulls out clumps of hair with each brushing.

Past Medical History

The patient states that she had an episode of sinusitis 4-5 months ago that was treated with an antibiotic. She denies any recent illnesses. She had a tonsillectomy at age 8 and chicken pox at about age 12.

Social History

Patient is a graduate student in anthropology at the local university. She has never been married, and she lives in an apartment with two other women. She smokes a half pack or whole pack of cigarettes per day and drinks wine only occasionally (two or three glasses per week).

Family History

The patient has an older sister who has SLE. Her mother is alive with DM and HTN; her father died at age 47 in an MVA.

Review of Systems

Negative except for the complaints noted above. The patient reports no history of fatigue, weight loss, mouth ulcers, chest pain, nausea, abdominal pain, fever, seizures, or mental status changes.

Physical Examination

GEN: The patient is a WD/WN African American woman in NAD

VS: BP 110/70 mmHg, HR 72 bpm, RR 16 rpm, T 37.1°C, Wt 62 kg

SKIN: A diffuse maculopapular rash is present on sun-exposed areas of the arms and legs. A facial rash is apparent over the bridge of the nose and the malar eminences.

HEENT: NC/AT, some diffuse thinning of hair noted on scalp, PERRLA, EOMI, disks flat, no hemorrhages or exudates, oropharynx clear with no oral ulcers

CHEST: CTA

CV: RRR; no m/r/g

ABD: Soft, NT/ND, no hepatosplenomegaly

GU/RECT: Normal female genitalia, stool guaiac negative

MS/EXT: Joint examination reveals tender, swollen joints of the MCP and proximal interphalangeal joints of both hands. Grip strength is +4/5 bilaterally. Wrist and knee joints also tender bilaterally. Peripheral pulses 2+; no CCE.

NEURO: A&O x3; CN II-XII intact; sensory and motor function normal; DTRs 2+ throughout; negative Babinski's

Laboratory and Diagnostic Tests

Sodium 141 mEq/L	Potassium 4.2 mEq/L
Chloride 104 mEq/L	CO_2 content 24 mEq/L
BUN 32 mg/dL	Serum creatinine 1.6 mg/dL
Glucose 110 mg/dL	ANA 1:1280
ESR 45 mm/h	C4 14 mg/dL
C3 65 mg/dL	Anti-ds DNA antibody 1:90
Sm antigen positive	Hemoglobin 11.0 g/dL
Hematocrit 34.4%	Platelets 115,000/mm³

WBC 4500/mm³ with 62% PMN, 2% bands, 1% eosinophils, 29% lymphocytes, 6% monocytes

ECG NSR

CXR Lungs clear; heart size is WNL

UA Color yellow, specific gravity 1.014, pH 6.0, blood +1, protein +1

Diagnosis

Probable systemic lupus erythematosus (SLE)

Medication Record

Date	Rx No	Physician	Drug/Strength	Quantity	Sig	Refills
6/2	129533	Nichols	Amoxicillin 250 mg	30	1 po tid	0
7/16	134498	Samuels	Ortho-Novum 1/35-28	1 pack	1 po qd	5
9/22	155493		Acetaminophen 500 mg	100		
10/14	155492	Hayes	Naproxen 500 mg	60	1 po bid	2
10/14	155492	Hayes	Hydroxychloroquine 200 mg	30	1 po qd	2

Pharmacist Notes and Other Patient Information

None available.

Questions

1. SLE is a disease characterized by:

    I. excessive or abnormal autoantibody production.
    II. constitutional, dermatologic, and rheumatologic manifestations.
    III. kidney, bone marrow, pulmonary, cardiac, and/or CNS manifestations.

    A. I only
    B. III only
    C. I and II only
    D. II and III only
    E. I, II, and III

2. Which of the following demographic groups are NOT at increased risk of developing SLE?

    A. History of frequent UV light exposure
    B. Age 15-45
    C. African American race
    D. Male gender
    E. Family history of SLE

3. Which of the following tests need to be performed on a scheduled basis in monitoring the use of hydroxychloroquine?

    A. Ophthalmic exam
    B. Serum creatinine and BUN
    C. Potassium
    D. Liver function tests
    E. Hemoglobin A1c

4. This patient brings you some information printed off from a website advertising a product called "Lupus Bane." In this advertisement, it states, "In a clinical trial, 15 of 17 patients receiving "Lupus Bane" reported more energy and less pain after only two weeks of treatment." Based on the information provided, what type of clinical trial design best describes this report?

    A. Randomized controlled trial
    B. Retrospective cohort
    C. Meta-analysis
    D. Case series
    E. Case-control

5. A renal biopsy is ordered based on the serum creatinine and urinalysis, which reveals a mild focal proliferative lupus nephritis (WHO Class III). Based on these results, which of the following would be the best therapeutic recommendation to facilitate maintenance of renal function in the long term?

    A. Continue current regimen
    B. Discontinue naproxen
    C. Increase dose of hydroxychloroquine
    D. Add a low-dose steroid
    E. Add a high-dose steroid and cyclophosphamide

6. While commonly utilized in tablet form, prednisone is also available in which of the following dosage forms?

    A. Reconstitutable powder for injection
    B. Oral solution
    C. Ophthalmic suspension
    D. Topical cream
    E. Dry powder for inhalation

7. Appropriate nonpharmacologic therapy that may help to control SLE symptoms in this patient include all of the following EXCEPT:

Case 19

    A.   a balanced regimen of rest and reasonable exercise.

    B.   avoidance of smoking.

    C.   limitation of exposure to sunlight when outdoors.

    D.   consumption of omega-3 fatty acids.

    E.   consumption of a dietary supplement containing copper.

8. The FDA has determined that all NSAIDs should carry which of the following warnings regarding increased risk?

    I.   Hepatotoxicity

    II.   Cardiovascular events

    III. GI bleeds

    A.   I only

    B.   III only

    C.   I and II only

    D.   II and III only

    E.   I, II, and III

9. Which of the following strengths of naproxen, as its sodium salt, are available over the counter?

    A.   220 mg

    B.   275 mg

    C.   375 mg

    D.   500 mg

    E.   550 mg

10. While all of the following agents have been implicated in case reports to cause drug-induced lupus, which has the greatest likelihood of causing that condition?

    A.   Captopril

    B.   Hydrochlorothiazide

    C.   Ciprofloxacin

    D.   Procainamide

    E.   Valproic acid

Fluids, Electrolytes, and Nutrition

Section Editor: Charles W. Jastram, Jr.

Patient Name: Sam Goldberg
Address: 1431 Hunt Drive
Age: 63   **Sex:** Male
Height: 5'9"   **Weight:** 60 kg
Race: White
Allergies: NKDA

Chief Complaint

Weakness, vomiting, and 8-lb weight loss for 6 weeks

History of Present Illness

SG is a 63-yo male previously in excellent health who was admitted to the hospital for evaluation of a 6-week history of lethargy, early satiety, postprandial vomiting, and 8-lb weight loss.

Past Medical History

Mild HTN x10 years, osteoarthritis x5 years, benign prostatic hypertrophy x3 years; transurethral resection of prostate 1 year ago.

Social History

Ethanol intake of 3 beers/day, denies illicit drug abuse, no history of sexually transmitted diseases, smoked 2 packs/day for 20 years but stopped 5 years ago.

Family History

Automobile mechanic for 35 years, plans to retire at age 65. Married with two children. Mother and father both deceased (mother died of breast cancer at age 79, and father died of heart failure at age 77). One brother, age 60, is in good health.

Review of Systems

Prior to 6 weeks ago, ate three meals a day with an occasional snack of ice cream before bedtime. Moderately active, walking and climbing stairs without difficulty.

Physical Examination

GEN: Well-nourished, healthy male in NAD or pain at present. Appears tired.

VS: BP 90/60 mmHg, HR 100 bpm, RR 16 rpm, T 38°C

HEENT: Head normocephalic, PERRLA

CHEST: Normal chest, no wheezes, rales, or rhonchi

CV: No murmurs/gallops/arrhythmias

ABD: Mild tenderness in right upper quadrant on palpation, no abdominal distention present, bowel sounds present in all quadrants

RECTAL: No masses, hemorrhoids present, prostate large and soft to digital palpation

NEURO: Grossly intact. Appears oriented to time and place, apathetic, and depressed.

MS: No definitive musculoskeletal abnormalities present except slightly decreased ROM in lower and upper limbs

SKIN: No abnormalities noted

Laboratory and Diagnostic Tests

Sodium 149 mEq/L	Potassium 3.4 mEq/L
Chloride 92 mEq/L	CO_2 content 36 mEq/L
BUN 30 mg/dL	Serum creatinine 0.8 mg/dL
Glucose 88 mg/dL	Amylase 150 U/L
Lipase 240 U/L	Calcium 8.0 mg/dL
Magnesium 1.9 mg/dL	Phosphorus 2.8 mg/dL
Total protein 8.0 g/dL	Albumin 4.5 g/dL
WBC 4600 cell/mm³	Hemoglobin 15 g/dL
Hematocrit 48%	

Results of upper gastrointestinal endoscopy:

Esophagus: Normal

Stomach: 3-cm lesion with bleeding in pyloric channel with no sign of active bleeding, biopsy was positive for adenocarcinoma of stomach and negative for Helicobacter jejuni

Duodenum: Normal

Diagnosis

Primary:

Adenocarcinoma of stomach

Medication Record

Prazosin 5 mg po daily at 8 p.m.

Ibuprofen 800 mg po qid prn arthritis pain

Pharmacist Notes and Other Patient Information

None available

Questions

1. SG's total body water represents how many kilograms of his total body weight of 60 kg?

   A. 15 kg
   B. 25 kg
   C. 36 kg
   D. 48 kg
   E. 60 kg

2. SG's intravascular fluid compartment represents how many kilograms of his total body weight of 60 kg?

   A. 3 kg
   B. 5 kg
   C. 8 kg
   D. 10 kg
   E. 24 kg

3. What percentage of total weight loss as pure extracellular fluid loss would induce tachycardia and orthostatic hypotension?

   A. 4%
   B. 8%
   C. 12%
   D. 18%
   E. 24%

4. The medical impression is that SG has extracellular fluid deficit based on which of the following parameters listed below:

   A. Hypertension
   B. Bradycardia
   C. Hyponatremia
   D. Hypocalcemia
   E. Hypotension

5. Calculate SG's fluid deficit based on the information provided.

   A. 0.6 L
   B. 1.3 L
   C. 2.3 L
   D. 4.6 L
   E. 6.0 L

6. SG's initial fluid requirement is approximately how many L/day (requirement + deficit)?

   A. 2.5 L
   B. 3.0 L
   C. 3.5 L
   D. 4.0 L
   E. 8.0 L

7. All the general statements concerning potassium are true EXCEPT:

   A. Highest concentration of potassium is in the intracellular compartment
   B. 2% of total body potassium is contained in the extracellular fluid compartment
   C. Highest concentration of potassium is in the interstitial fluid compartment
   D. Potassium shifts from the intracellular to extracellular compartment in metabolic acidosis
   E. Insulin causes a shift of potassium into the intracellular compartment

8. SG should be counseled that the following medication may precipitate depression:

   A. Prazosin
   B. Potassium chloride
   C. Sodium bicarbonate
   D. Ibuprofen
   E. Prazosin, potassium chloride, and ibuprofen can precipitate depression

9. Which of the following precautions should be considered when taking alpha blockers?

   A. Alpha blockers commonly cause first dose syncope.
   B. Common side effects include palpitations, headache, and drowsiness.
   C. NSAIDs may increase the effectiveness of alpha blockers.
   D. A and B are correct
   E. B and C are correct

10. The etiology of SG's hypochloremia includes which of the following?

   A. Metabolic acidosis
   B. Diuretic therapy
   C. Vomiting
   D. Excessive use of saline-containing intravenous solutions
   E. Hypoaldosteronism

Chief Complaint

HP is a 27-yo female complaining of the common cold. She would like to take zinc lozenges to treat her symptoms. She is also complaining of insomnia and is considering taking melatonin again.

History of Present Illness

HP's cold symptoms began last night. She reports nasal symptoms (runny nose), watery eyes, and sneezing. She denies any allergies or any other symptoms.

Past Medical History

HP is being treated for ovulatory failure with Clomid (clomiphene) to increase her chances of conceiving. She occasionally complains of insomnia (trouble falling asleep). She has tried OTC hypnotics like Sominex (diphenhydramine). Although these products help her fall asleep, she complains of feeling groggy the next day and being unable to concentrate at work.

Social History

Tobacco use: None

Alcohol use: Occasional glass of wine with dinner

Caffeine use: Drinks 1 cup of coffee daily

Drugs of abuse: Denied

Family History

Mother and father alive and well

Medication Record

Date	Rx No	Physician	Drug/Strength	Quantity	Sig	Refills
12/01			Melatonin 1 mg	30	1 po q h s prn insomnia	
2/02	024217	Conway	Clomid 50 mg	10	2 po qd	0
2/02			Ovulation predictor	1		
1/02			Ovulation predictor	1		
1/02	023001	Conway	Clomid 50 mg	5	1 po qd	0
12/01			Ovulation predictor	1		
8/01			Sominex 10 mg	30	1 po q h s prn insomnia	

Review of Systems

Negative except as noted previously

Physical Examination

GEN: Well-developed female in NAD

VS: BP 110/78 mmHg, HR 60 bpm, RR 28 rpm, T 37.0°C, Ht 5' 4", Wt 54 kg

HEENT: PERRLA, EOMI

CHEST: CTA

NEURO: A & O x3

Laboratory and Diagnostic Tests

Sodium 138 mEq/L	Potassium 3.6 mEq/L
Chloride 108 mEq/L	CO_2 content 24 mEq/L
BUN 10 mg/dL	Serum creatinine 1.0 mg/dL
Glucose 90 mg/dL	Hemoglobin 13 g/dL
Hematocrit 36%	Platelets 204/mm^3
WBC 4 x 109/L	

Pregnancy test (ELISA) negative

Diagnosis

Primary:

1) Common cold

2) Insomnia

Secondary:

1) Ovulation failure

Pharmacist Notes and Other Patient Information

None available.

Patient Name: Holly Potter
Address: 654 Main Street
Age: 27   **Sex:** Female
Height: 5'4"   **Weight:** 119 lb
Race: White
Allergies: NKDA

Questions

1. Melatonin is most effective in treating which of the following conditions?

   A. Generalized anxiety disorder
   B. Sleep onset insomnia
   C. Early morning awakenings
   D. Narcolepsy
   E. Jet lag symptoms

2. Which of the following melatonin consequences is NOT likely to occur with routine use?

   A. Daytime drowsiness
   B. Tachycardia
   C. Depressed mood
   D. Inhibition of ovulation
   E. Hyperpigmentation

3. Which of the following statements regarding melatonin is FALSE?

   A. Initial melatonin starting doses for insomnia range between 0.3 and 5 mg of the immediate-release formulation.
   B. Melatonin should be taken just prior to bedtime, and reading lights should be turned off to help trigger endogenous melatonin release.
   C. Following a dose of melatonin, sleep onset occurs between 30 and 45 minutes.
   D. Endogenous melatonin is released between 4 and 6 p.m.
   E. Exogenous melatonin is less potent than benzodiazepines for inducing sleep.

4. Which of the following statements regarding melatonin is FALSE?

   A. Melatonin supplements have been studied as an adjunct to chemotherapy in patients with cancer.
   B. Taking melatonin for jet lag may help trigger somnolence at the new bedtime hour.
   C. Melatonin supplements should probably be avoided in patients with depression or mania.
   D. Taking fluvoxamine with melatonin supplements may increase the effects of melatonin.
   E. Taking melatonin with zolpidem will decrease the effects of zolpidem.

5. Melatonin:

   A. does not affect prolactin levels.
   B. is effective in treating insomnia in children.
   C. has been studied for chronic insomnia.
   D. should be combined with alcohol.
   E. may worsen depression.

6. Which of the following statements regarding zinc lozenges is FALSE?

   A. Zinc gluconate, zinc acetate, and zinc gluconate-glycine have all been shown to reduce the symptoms of the common cold.
   B. Zinc lozenges should be started within 24-48 hours of the first cold symptom.
   C. Zinc lozenges may shorten the duration of the common cold by 1-2 days.
   D. Multivitamins containing zinc can be used as lozenges to prevent the common cold.
   E. Zinc lozenges should be taken every 2 hours while awake.

7. Zinc lozenges:

   A. have been proven effective in children.
   B. have been studied during pregnancy.
   C. may be used to supplement dietary zinc requirements.
   D. are effective in treating influenza.
   E. should not be chewed or crushed.

8. Which of the following zinc lozenge side effects has NOT been reported in clinical trials?

   A. Nausea
   B. Mouth sores
   C. Taste disturbances
   D. Numbness
   E. Astringency in the mouth

9. Which of the following statements regarding the zinc lozenge clinical trials is FALSE?

   A. The zinc lozenge clinical trials involved patients with naturally acquired colds and healthy volunteers who agreed to be inoculated with the rhinovirus.
   B. Some of the zinc lozenge clinical trials used formulations that inactivated the release of Zn++ from the lozenge.
   C. The zinc lozenge clinical trials used varying doses of zinc.
   D. Some of the zinc lozenge clinical trials used lozenges that had a distinctive taste compared to placebo, and this compromised study blinding.
   E. The zinc lozenge clinical trials all show a reduction in symptom severity and symptom duration.

10. The common cold is usually associated with all of the following symptoms EXCEPT:

    A. watery eyes.
    B. sneezing.
    C. fever.
    D. nasal stuffiness.
    E. runny nose.

Patient Name: Janet Jackson
Address: 1210 Down Valley Court
Age: 41   **Sex:** Female
Height: 5'2"   **Weight:** 70 kg
Race: Caucasian
Allergies: Allopurinol

Chief Complaint

Diarrhea

History of Present Illness

JJ is a 41-year-old Caucasian female presenting with complaints of chronic diarrhea with an acute exacerbation over the preceding week. She has experienced 8-10 episodes of watery diarrhea daily without any blood or significant crampy abdominal pain. She denies any nausea or vomiting and has decreased oral intake. She has undergone evaluation with colonoscopy and biopsy.

Past Medical History

Crohn's disease and dyslipidemia that has been treated for a number of years.

Social History

Patient denies any tobacco, alcohol, or IV drug usage. The patient is under the care of her mother and attended special education school during her high school years.

Family History

No history of inflammatory bowel disease

Review of Systems

Unremarkable for any fever or chills, chest pain, shortness of breath, or productive cough. She denies any significant abdominal pain or focal abdominal pain. The patient reports chronic diarrhea, watery in nature, containing food particles. She denied any hematuria or dysuria.

Physical Examination

GEN: The patient is awake, alert and oriented. No acute distress apparent.

VS: BP 120/70 mmHg, HR 68 bpm, RR 20 rpm, T 38°C, Ht 6'2", Wt 70 kg

HEENT: Head normocephalic, sclerae are anicteric. Mucous membranes were dry.

CV: RRR; no murmurs, gallops, or rubs

LUNGS: Clear to auscultation

ABD: Soft, nontender, nondistended, normoactive bowel sounds present

RECTAL: Slight perianal fistula which was draining. Rectal exam deferred by patient.

EXT: Pulses 2+ and equal with no clubbing, cyanosis, edema or rash

Laboratory and Diagnostic Tests

Sodium 129 mg/dL	Potassium 2.6 mEq/L
Chloride 96 mg/dL	CO_2 29 mEq/L
BUN 15 mg/dL	Serum creatinine 1.2 mg/dL
Glucose 109 mg/dL	Calcium 8.8 mg/dL
Magnesium 1.1 mg/dL	Phosphorus 3 mg/dL
Total protein 8.1 g/dL	Albumin 3.2 g/dL
WBC 10.6	Hemoglobin 12.4 g/dL
Hematocrit 38.3%	Platelets 216

Diagnosis

Crohn's exacerbation

Medication Record

Asacol dose unknown

Pravachol 20 mg po at bedtime

Flagyl 500 mg 3 times po daily

Potassium chloride 40 mEq po daily

Ferrous sulfate 325 mg po daily

Protonix 40 mg po daily

Pharmacist Notes and Other Patient Information

None available.

Questions

1. Which of the following sign or symptom is NOT consistent with hypomagnesemia?

    A. Positive Chvostek's and Trousseau's signs
    B. Tremor
    C. Generalized convulsions
    D. Refractory hyperkalemia
    E. Prolonged QRS complex

2. What is the etiology of JJ's hyponatremia?

    A. Hypovolemic hyponatremia
    B. Euvolemic hyponatremia
    C. Hypervolemic hyponatremia
    D. Hypervolemic hypernatremia
    E. Euvolemic hypernatremia

3. Which of the following is the most likely sodium deficit in mEq/L for JJ?

    A. 100
    B. 200
    C. 385
    D. 500
    E. 750

4. What is JJ's maintenance fluid need in mL based on her weight of 70 kg?

    A. 1000
    B. 1500
    C. 2000
    D. 2500
    E. 3000

5. Which of the following conditions is the most likely cause of hypokalemia in JJ?

    A. Metabolic acidosis
    B. Use of potassium-sparing diuretics
    C. Chronic diarrhea
    D. Sickle cell disease
    E. Chronic renal disease

6. Which of the following pharmacologic therapies should be considered to treat hypokalemia in JJ?

    A. Sodium polystyrene sulfonate
    B. Sodium bicarbonate
    C. Insulin and dextrose 50%
    D. Parenteral potassium replacement
    E. Furosemide

7. Cardiovascular signs and symptoms of hypokalemia include which of the following?

    A. ST segment elevations
    B. Hypotension
    C. Atrial flutter
    D. Absence of U-waves
    E. Elevated T-waves

8. JJ has concomitant hypomagnesemia and hypokalemia. How should treatment be initiated to correct the disorders?

    A. Treat hypokalemia only
    B. Treat hypomagnesemia only
    C. Treat hypomagnesemia first, then treat hypokalemia
    D. Treat hypokalemia first, then treat hypomagnesemia
    E. No treatment needed

9. JJ's physician has decided to increase her potassium supplementation. What counseling information should be provided to the patient?

    A. An oral liquid preparation should be diluted first then used in patients with esophageal compression or delayed gastric emptying.
    B. Chronic potassium supplementation is not of concern in patients taking ACEIs.
    C. Wax matrix tablets and sustained-release products must be cut prior to administration.
    D. If you forget to take a dose, just double up with the next dose.
    E. Take this medication on an empty stomach.

10. Which of the following should be considered when taking magnesium supplements?

    I. Serum magnesium levels will correct immediately.
    II. Use with caution in renally impaired patients.
    III. Use with caution in digitalized patients.

    A. I only
    B. III only
    C. I and II only
    D. II and III only
    E. I, II, and III

Patient Name: Janice Carlson
Address: 503 Independence Avenue
Age: 63   **Sex:** Female
Height: 5'4"   **Weight:** 82 kg
Race: White
Allergies: NKDA; sensitive to morphine sulfate, hydromorphone

Chief Complaint

"I feel OK but the skin around the stoma is sore, my stomach hurts, I'm dizzy, and I have diarrhea all the time."

History of Present Illness

JC is a 63-yo female who had a recent surgery (21 days PTA) for metastatic ovarian cancer with intra-abdominal carcinomatosis approximately 2 months ago at a local hospital. A diverting ileostomy performed with the stoma placement in the lower left abdomen quadrant during that hospitalization. Her appetite has been poor and she is experiencing early satiety (despite wanting to eat more) since surgery. Her ileostomy output has increased over the past 2 weeks and is progressively more watery, with increasing stool frequency over the last week. With these changes, the area around the stoma became more irritated. She has had minor complaints of fatigue and stomach ache and has experienced a sudden weight loss (estimated at 20-25 lb in 3-4 weeks). JC had increased complaints of vertigo (a chronic problem that increased with current medical condition changes).

Past Medical History

JC had a recent surgery (21 days ago) for metastatic ovarian cancer. She is S/P ileostomy placement (LLQ). She had her left ovary removed in 1957 and a hysterectomy in 1967 (right ovary retained). Her past medical history also included an appendectomy at age 17 and a gall bladder stone removal in 1982.

JC has not had major medical problems. She has had a history of minor procedures for accidental injuries and gynecological problems in her twenties and thirties (as related to the above surgeries). She is gravida 1.

Social History

JC recently retired from the telephone company where she worked for 45 years. She has never smoked and does not drink alcohol. She is married and has one living daughter. She is heterosexual and lives with her husband. Both her daughter and husband provide her with an excellent social support system.

Family History

JC's family history is significant for cancer (maternal grandmother, mother, and father), heart disease (father, AMI; brother, AMI), and type 2 diabetes mellitus (mother, sister, and brother).

Review of Systems

Moderately obese, pale, anxious female in NAD, complains of pain at the stoma site, episodes of dizziness of increasing frequency, episodes of severe and frequent diarrhea (>8 loose stools per 24 hours), is easily fatigued with light exertion, and food consumption has diminished greatly over the past 10 days. Sudden weight loss coinciding with the increasing diarrhea; she complains of increasing pain, irritation, and excoriation of the skin around the stoma; readily admits to depression since her surgery but denies any suicidal ideations; acted appropriate during the examination but was very anxious and complained of vertigo during the exam.

Physical Examination

GEN: Pale, weak, woman complaining of pain around the site of the ileostomy; the area was very red with areas of skin loss

VS: BP 125/84 mmHg, HR 70 bpm, T 99.6°F; Wt 82 kg; Ht 6'4", lost a total of 12 kg the last 2 weeks

HEENT: WNL

CHEST: Lungs clear to auscultation and percussion

ABD: Hyperactive bowel sounds, demonstrates no tenderness and guarding over the abdomen; no hepatomegaly was noted; recently stapled surgical scar in the midline and upper part of the epigastric region was noted; stoma was about 1" long, of good quality, but associated with irritation and excoriation

BREAST/GU: Deferred; reports menstrual periods stopped at age 56 (on no medications)

RECTAL: Stools were hemoccult negative; external hemorrhoids were noted

NEURO: All reflexes equal and reactive, normal response to stimuli, memory normal

Laboratory and Diagnostic Tests

Sodium 128 mEq/L	Potassium 3.3 mEq/L
Chloride 94 mEq/L	BUN 6 mg/dL
Serum creatinine 1.6 mg/dL	Amylase WNL
Lipase WNL	Calcium 7.5 mg/dL

Magnesium 1.5 mg/dL

Albumin 3.1 g/dL

Hematocrit 33.3%

MCV WNL

RBC 3.9

pO$_2$ WNL

Total protein 5.8 g/dL

Hemoglobin 11 g/dL

Platelets WNL

WBC 5.5

pH WNL

pCO$_2$ 46 mmHg

CT of abdomen and pelvis: WNL

CXR: WNL

ECG: WNL

Diagnosis

1) Unusable (per admitting MD) stoma secondary to the state of the tissue surrounding the opening

2) Severe diarrhea

3) Sudden weight loss

4) Chronic vertigo

5) Mild dehydration

6) Pain at the site of the stoma

7) Normochromic and normocytic anemia

Pharmacist Notes and Other Patient Information

None available.

Medication Record

Date	Rx No	Physician	Drug/Strength	Quantity	Sig	Refills
1/16		Lyle	Antivert 12.5 mg		1 tab tid	
1/25		Jacob	Iron 325 mg		1 tab bid	
1/25		Jacob	Darvocet-N 100		2 tabs q 4 h prn	
2/24		Jacob	Compazine 10 mg		1 po q 8 prn	

Questions

1. All of the conditions listed below are absolute contraindications to enteral feedings EXCEPT:

   A. diffuse peritonitis.
   B. complete bowel obstruction.
   C. mild to moderate diarrhea.
   D. paralytic ileus.
   E. hemodynamically unstable.

2. All the statements listed below regarding indications for enteral nutrition are true EXCEPT:

   A. patient must have a functioning gastrointestinal tract.
   B. enteral feeding is indicated in patients that cannot eat.
   C. enteral feeding is indicated in patients that should not eat because it may worsen overall medical condition.
   D. enteral feeding is indicated in patients that refuse to eat or will not give consent to the feedings.
   E. enteral feedings can help prevent infections originating in the gut.

3. JC is a candidate for enteral nutrition because she:

   A. has diarrhea, sudden weight loss, and cancer.
   B. has diarrhea and greater than 10% weight loss in 2 weeks.
   C. is unable to eat due to nausea and vomiting.
   D. has irritation around her stoma.
   E. is not a candidate for enteral nutrition.

Case 23

4. Assuming JC will require short-term enteral feeding (7 to 14 days), which of the following enteral access devices would be most appropriate?
   A. Surgically placed gastrostomy (g-tube)
   B. Nasogastric tube
   C. Percutaneous endoscopic gastrostomy (peg tube)
   D. Surgically placed jejunostomy (j-tube)
   E. The choice of access device does not matter

5. Fiber content in enteral feeding formulas is an important factor when considering which formula to use. Some formulas are fiber-free. However, JC may benefit from a fiber-containing formula because of all the following EXCEPT:
   A. increased fecal bulk is desired, as in cases of severe diarrhea.
   B. lowering cholesterol is desired, due to family history of AMI.
   C. reduced intestinal transit times are desirable, as in the case of constipation.
   D. assistance in controlling blood glucose levels.
   E. assistance with maintenance of the gut mucosal lining.

6. JC displays all of the following factors indicative of malnutrition EXCEPT:
   A. involuntary loss of 10% or more of usual body weight within 6 months.
   B. involuntary loss of 5% of more of usual body weight within 1 month.
   C. current weight of 20% or more greater than ideal body weight
   D. inadequate nutrient intake.
   E. history of ovarian cancer.

7. The choice of an enteral formula is based on all of the following EXCEPT:
   A. total nutrient requirements of the patient.
   B. the extent of normal digestive ability of the patient.
   C. the amount of bacterial translocation the patient has experienced.
   D. the extent of normal absorption of the patient's gastrointestinal tract.
   E. size of the tubing and the placement of the tube in the gastrointestinal tract.

8. Specialized formulas are available for patients with renal and hepatic dysfunction, diabetes, pulmonary disease, and the critically ill (in the ICU). JC may benefit from such a formula because:
   A. she requires lower than normal potassium, magnesium, and phosphorous, such as in the commercially available renal formulas.

B. she cannot tolerate a high carbohydrate load because of her pulmonary function.
   C. she will have difficulty metabolizing the aromatic amino acids in the standard formulas because of her hepatic dysfunction.
   D. she will not require one of the specialized formulas for these disease states unless her condition worsens.
   E. she cannot tolerate a hyperosmolar feeding because of her diarrhea.

9. Complications of enteral feedings include which of the following?
   I. Severe sepsis
   II. Metabolic complications such as fluid/electrolyte imbalances, hyperglycemia, hyponatremia, or hypokalemia
   III. Mechanical complications such as GI perforation, peritonitis, sinusitis, tube dislodging, tube clogging, or aspiration
   A. I only
   B. III only
   C. I and II only
   D. II and III only
   E. I, II, and III

10. JC will initially benefit from continuous enteral feedings for all the following reasons EXCEPT:
   A. initially this method is better tolerated in the metabolically unstable patient.
   B. it will not interfere with her daily activities.
   C. it will lower her risk of aspiration as she is slowly able to tolerate enteral and oral feedings.
   D. the chance of gastric distention and discomfort are much lower.
   E. there is less chance of developing nausea and vomiting, bloating, and flatulence.

Blood Disorders

Section Editors: Lori B. Hornsby, Anne Marie Liles

Patient Name: Gary Hanes
Address: 7758 W. Queen Road
Age: 66 **Sex:** Male
Height: 5'9" **Weight:** 95.7 kg
Race: Caucasian
Allergies: NKA

Chief Complaint

GH is a 66-yo man seen in the clinic with general complaints of fatigue. He states that he has not been able to participate in his ballroom dancing classes for the past 2 months because he becomes progressively weak and short of breath. Over the past 2 weeks he states that his fatigue has prevented him from leaving his home except for church on Sundays.

History of Present Illness

For the last year GH has had occasional tinnitus. For 5 years he has had one to two dizzy spells per month, lasting approximately 15 minutes each.

Past Medical History

GH was diagnosed with depression approximately 9 months ago. Although treatment with citalopram as been successful in improving his mood, his appetite remains poor and he has lost 9 kgs over the last 3 months. Osteoarthritis complaints have been ongoing for about 3 months. Six years ago he was discovered to have arteriovenous malformations (AVMs) between arteries and veins located in his spinal cord; these were determined to be diffuse and did not require surgery or treatment.

Social History

Tobacco use: none

Alcohol use: none

Caffeine use: 2 cups of coffee per day

Family History

Father died of CVA at age 55. Mother is alive at age 86 with DM.

Review of Systems

(+) fatigue daily, (+) headache, (+) pallor, (-) anorexia, (-) chest pain, (+) shortness of breath only upon exercise

Physical Examination

GEN: Obese man in NAD

VS: BP 148/84 mmHg, HR 96 bpm, RR 15 rpm, T 38.5°C, Wt 95.7 kg

HEENT: PERRLA, neck supple no adenopathy, thyroid WNL

CHEST: Clear to A-&-P

CV: RRR, no murmurs

NEURO: A-&-O x3

ABD: Liver WNL, no masses, bruits, or tenderness

RECTAL: No masses, guaiac negative

Laboratory and Diagnostic Tests

Sodium 140 mEq/L	Potassium 3.9 mEq/L
Chloride 107 mEq/L	CO_2 28 mEq/L
BUN 21 mg/dL	Serum creatinine 0.9 mg/dL
Glucose 116 mg/dL	TSH 4.56 IU/mL
Albumin 4.2 g/dL	MCV 68 fL
Hemoglobin 10.4 g/dL	Hematocrit 31.2%
Platelets 180,000/mm³	RDW 19%
Serum iron 18 mcg/dL	TSAT 4%
TIBC 440 mcg/dL	Ferritin 8 ng/mL
RBC folate 390 ng/mL	Vitamin B_{12} 153 pg/mL

Diagnosis

Iron deficiency anemia likely due to AVMs and nutritional deficiency.

Medication Record

Date	Rx No	Physician	Drug/Strength	Quantity	Sig	Refills
3/1	29384	Lone	Citalopram 20 mg	30	1 po daily	3
3/1	29385	Dane	Naproxen 250 mg	60	1 po BID prn	1
3/1	OTC	Dane	Acetaminophen 500mg	100	1po QID prn	0
3/1	29382	Hind	Ferrous sulfate 324 mg	90	1 po TID	1
3/1	OTC	Hind	Docusate 100mg	90	1 po BID prn	0
3/1	OTC	Hind	Vitamin C	90	1 po daily	0

Questions

1. Which one of the following is NOT true regarding oral iron products?

    A. Iron decreases the absorption of fluoroquinolones.
    B. H_2 blockers may decrease the absorption of iron.
    C. Administering with food increases the bioavailability of iron.
    D. Antacids may decrease the absorption of iron.
    E. Iron decreases the efficacy of levothyroxine.

2. Laboratory findings present in GH that may be associated with iron deficiency anemia include:

    I. decreased MCV.
    II. increased TIBC-.
    III. decreased ferritin.

    A. I only
    B. III only
    C. I and II only
    D. II and III only
    E. I, II, and III

3. Which of GH's medications may have contributed to the development of his iron deficiency anemia?

    A. Citalopram
    B. Docusate
    C. Acetaminophen
    D. Naproxen
    E. Vitamin C

4. Which of the following statements is true regarding the duration of treatment with oral iron for iron deficiency anemia?

    A. Iron supplementation should continue for lifetime.
    B. Once hemoglobin/hematocrit levels return to normal, iron supplementation may be discontinued.
    C. Once ferritin levels return to normal, iron supplementation may be discontinued.
    D. All patients with iron deficiency anemia require at least 12 months of iron supplementation.
    E. Once iron deficiency is resolved, all patients should be continued on a decreased dose of 30 mg to 60 mg elemental iron daily.

5. Which of the following is NOT a cause of iron deficiency anemia?

    A. Inadequate intake
    B. Blood loss
    C. Administration of erythropoiesis-stimulating agents
    D. Malabsorptive syndrome
    E. Pica

6. Which one of the following is most appropriate to monitor for chronic iron overload?

    A. MCV
    B. Transferrin
    C. Ferritin
    D. RDW
    E. Serum iron

7. Ferrous sulfate is available as:

    I. over-the counter tablets.
    II. over-the-counter oral drops.
    III. prescription only oral drops.

    A. I only
    B. III only
    C. I and II only
    D. II and III only
    E. I, II, and III

8. If GH is intolerant to all oral iron products and requires IV iron, which of the following is the most appropriate recommendation?

    A. Iron dextran, because it has the safest toxicity profile and does not require a test dose.
    B. Iron sucrose, because it is less likely than iron dextran to cause the fatal reactions seen with iron dextran.
    C. Ferric gluconate, because it does not cause the hypotensive reactions associated with "free iron" seen with the other preparations.
    D. Iron sucrose, because it may be given as an IM injection.
    E. Ferric gluconate, because a 1000 mg dose may be given in 1 infusion.

9. Five new oral iron products have been compared to placebo to determine their ability to increase ferritin levels in patients with iron deficiency anemia. Administration of which of the following products did NOT result in a statistically significant increase in ferritin levels?

    A. Iron A increased ferritin an average of 35 ng/mL ($p = 0.01$)
    B. Iron B increased ferritin an average of 9 ng/mL ($p = 0.04$)
    C. Iron C increased ferritin an average of 18 ng/mL ($p = 0.06$)
    D. Iron D increased ferritin an average of 18 ng/mL (95% confidence interval, 0.5 to 22 ng/mL)
    E. Iron E increase ferritin an average of 9 ng/mL (95% confidence interval, 4 to 15 ng/mL)

Case 24

10. Patients on oral iron products should be provided information on which of the following?

   A. Immediately discontinue oral iron if stools become dark.
   B. Taking larger amounts of oral iron for fewer doses will help to decrease side effects.
   C. Oral iron should not be taken with food because food may increase gastrointestinal side effects.
   D. Constipation may worsen as the dose of oral iron increases.
   E. All oral iron products contain the same amount of iron.

Patient Name: Alleen Brock
Address: 3904 Brie Lane
Age: 81   **Sex:** Female
Height: 5' 4''   **Weight:** 60.4 kg
Race: Caucasian
Allergies: Morphine (confusion), alprazolam (confusion)

Chief Complaint

AB is a 81-yo white female who has been discharged from the hospital with a long history of multiple cardiovascular problems.

History of Present Illness

AB was admitted to the hospital with chest pain. She was diagnosed with CAD with occlusion of bypass grafts with 2 MIs. Patient is refusing further cardiovascular surgery and cardiac catheter interventions.

Past Medical History

AB had cardiovascular bypass surgery in 1998. She also has a history of HF, chronic atrial fibrillation, ischemic cardiomyopathy, HTN, T2DM, and DJD.

Social History

Tobacco use: none   Alcohol use: none

Caffeine use: 1 cup of coffee per day

Patient lives alone; refuses home health aide services at this time; has sister that visits patient 3 or more times per week. Sister provides assistance with activities for daily living and environmental support.

Family History

Father was diabetic with history of HTN; died in MVA at age 63. Mother died of MI at age 78.

Review of Systems

CV: Patient reports angina 3-4 times weekly with midsubsternal sharp pain lasting approximately 10 minutes and relieved with one sublingual nitroglycerin tablet.

Physical Examination

GEN: Patient presents as thin and frail. Poor endurance, psychosocial behavior appropriate.

VS: BP 120/60 mmHg, RR 22 rpm, HR 80 bpm, T 97.2°F oral, O_2 sat 98% (room air), Ht 5' 4", Wt 60.4 kg, Blood glucose 264 (1.5 hours postprandial)

CHEST: Lung: CTA

CV: RRR, systolic murmur, no JVD

NEURO: Oriented to person, place, time, and situation. Patient cooperative. Gait steady.

ABD: Soft, nondistended, no ascites, no tenderness, bowel sounds present

Laboratory and Diagnostic Tests

Sodium 138 mEq/L	Potassium 3.8 mEq/L
Chloride 105 mEq/L	CO_2 25 mEq/L
BUN 15 mg/dL	Serum creatinine 1.1 mg/dL
Glucose 285 mg/dL	PT 23
INR 2.8	Hemoglobin 12.2 g/dL
Hematocrit 35.1%	Platelets 185,000/mm³
WBC 4.9 k/mm³	RBC 3.78 m/mm³

Diagnosis

CAD, HF, chronic atrial fibrillation, HTN, T2DM, and DJD.

Medication Record

Date	Rx No	Physician	Drug/Strength	Quantity	Sig	Refills
4/22	56914	Inhorn	Omeprazole 20 mg	90	1 po daily	3
4/22	56915	Inhorn	Clopidogrel 75 mg	90	1 po daily	3
4/22	56908	Inhorn	Furosemide 40 mg	60	1 po bid	3
4/22	56910	Inhorn	Glipizide XL 10 mg	90	1 po a.m.	3
4/22	56913	Inhorn	Potassium Cl SR 20 mEq	60	1 po bid	5
4/22	56905	Inhorn	Nitroglycerin 0.4 mg	25	1 SL prn	prn
4/22	56907	Inhorn	Warfarin 4 mg	30	1 po daily	3
4/22	56912	Inhorn	Metoprolol 75 mg	90	1 po daily	3
4/22	56906	Inhorn	Isosorbide mononitrate 60 mg	90	1 po daily	4
4/22	56909	Inhorn	Quinapril 30 mg	90	1 po bid	3
4/22			Ibuprofen 200 mg	100	3 po tid	

Case 25

Questions

1. The mechanism(s) by which NSAID therapy may increase the risk of bleeding with warfarin when used in combination include(s):

   I. pharmacokinetic interactions.
   II. harmful effects to the GI mucosa.
   III. inhibition of platelet function.

   A. I only
   B. III only
   C. I and II only
   D. II and III only
   E. I, II, and III

2. Which of the following would likely result in an elevated INR?

   A. Patient starting carbamazepine.
   B. Patient changed dietary habits by increasing consumption of green leafy vegetables.
   C. Patient nonadherent to medication regimen.
   D. Patient starting amiodarone.
   E. Patient previously euthyroid, develops hypothyroidism.

3. When monitoring a patient receiving warfarin for atrial fibrillation, which of the following is a sign or symptom of a supratherapeutic INR?

   A. Sudden vision changes
   B. Hemoptysis
   C. Word finding difficulties
   D. Dysphagia
   E. Unilateral extremity weakness

4. AB has been taking warfarin 4 mg po daily x several months with monthly INRs within goal. Her INR is checked by the home health nurse with a result of 1.6. The patient denies any missed doses as well as changes in her diet or medications. The nurse calls for new orders. Which of the following is the most appropriate?

   A. Decrease the weekly dose by 5% and repeat INR in 1 week.
   B. Increase the weekly dose by 25% and repeat the INR in 4 weeks.
   C. Hold the dose for 24 hours and repeat the INR in 24 hours.
   D. Make no adjustment in the dose and repeat INR in 1 month.
   E. Increase the weekly dose by 5% and repeat INR in 1 week.

5. AB has her INR repeated in 2 weeks and the result is an INR of 5.8. On interview you find that she inadvertently wrote down the wrong directions and is taking more warfarin than previously instructed. Which of the following is the most appropriate plan?

   A. Decrease the weekly dose by 10% and recheck the INR in 1 week.
   B. Hold one dose and instruct the patient to decrease her intake of green vegetables.
   C. Hold the next 2 doses, recheck the INR in 48 hours, and have the patient restart at the previously prescribed dose once her INR is within the goal range.
   D. Hold one dose, administer one aspirin tablet, and recheck INR in 48 hours.
   E. Increase the weekly dose by 10% and recheck INR in 1 week.

6. The preferred route of vitamin K administration for warfarin reversal in a patient with an INR of 9.5 in the absence of bleeding is:

   A. oral.
   B. subcutaneous.
   C. intramuscular.
   D. intravenous.
   E. sublingual.

7. Which of the following foods has the highest amount of vitamin K in a typical serving?

   A. Tomatoes
   B. Mayonnaise
   C. Roasted turkey
   D. Green beans
   E. Broccoli

8. AB comes into your pharmacy after a recent appointment with her physician. She reports that her cholesterol is high and she is tired of taking medications. Her neighbor told her about garlic and wants more information. Why should she avoid garlic supplementation while on warfarin therapy?

   A. Garlic contains high amounts of vitamin K.
   B. Garlic can decrease platelet aggregation.
   C. Garlic has hypotensive effects.
   D. Garlic extract contains high amounts of alcohol.
   E. Garlic is an antipyretic.

9. Three weeks later, AB was seen by her PCP for dysuria. She was diagnosed with a UTI and prescribed Bactrim DS 1 tab BID x 14 days. What change would you expect in the patient's INR?

A.   An increase in the INR requiring a decrease in the
     warfarin dose
B.   No change in the INR or the warfarin dose
C.   A decrease in the INR requiring an increase in the
     warfarin dose
D.   No change in the INR, but a decrease in the
     effectiveness of the Bactrim
E.   A minimal increase in the INR requiring no change
     in the warfarin dose

10. The color of a Coumadin 4-mg tablet is:

   A.   pink.
   B.   green.
   C.   blue.
   D.   tan.
   E.   yellow.

Patient Name: Edward Heller
Address: 329 Lincoln Avenue
Age: 42   **Sex:** Male
Height: 6' 0"   **Weight:** 198 lb
Race: Caucasian
Allergies: NKDA

Chief Complaint

EH is a 42-year-old male who presents to the Clozapine Treatment Team to have his blood counts monitored for continued clozapine use. He presents to the clinic every 4 weeks for monitoring of CBC and a physician visit. He is without complaints today except that he continues to experience sialorrhea. EH denies hallucinations as well as suicidal or homicidal thoughts.

History of Present Illness

EH is a well-known patient to the mental health clinic. He has a history of paranoid schizophrenia but has not been hospitalized in the last 2 years. Several years ago, he reported having some homicidal ideations, although they were not directed towards any particular person. He also reported auditory hallucinations of others laughing and talking about him. He was socially and emotionally withdrawn. Due to his hallucinations, he could not maintain a job for any extended period of time and was homeless for long periods of time. EH had tried several antipsychotics in the past, including haloperidol, which caused akathisia. Other medications that did not result in clinically significant improvement with an adequate trial included fluphenazine, risperidone, and quetiapine. EH was started on clozapine about 2 years ago and has generally been stable since the initiation of clozapine. Based on patient report and refill history, EH has been compliant with his clozapine. Since using the clozapine, he has been able to live in a group home and maintain employment. His auditory hallucinations and homicidal ideations have resolved and he is much less withdrawn. He also has mild osteoarthritis of his knees bilaterally and hypertension controlled with 25 mg of hydrochlorothiazide.

Past Medical History

Diagnosed with schizophrenia, paranoid type, 18 years ago

Hypertension

Osteoarthritis

Social History

EH is employed part-time through a temporary agency and is currently living in a group home.

(+) tobacco use: 2 ppd x 26 years

(-) alcohol

(-) illicit drug use

(+) caffeine: 2-3 cups of coffee per day

Family History

Significant for alcohol abuse in his older brother. He stated his younger brother was treated for depression and that his father was hospitalized once because of a nervous condition. Mother is alive and well.

Review of Systems

Negative except as noted previously

Physical Examination

(Patient is seen in primary care clinic for treatment of hypertension and osteoarthritis. Complete physical exam and blood pressure evaluation referred to primary care clinic).

VS: Ht 5' 10, Wt 90 kg, HR 82 bpm, RR 16 rpm, T 97.9° F, BP 132/80 mmHg

Mental Status Exam

General: EH is neatly dressed and groomed. He is pleasant and cooperative with the interview. He has good eye contact.

Mood: Euthymic affect: mood-congruent

Speech: Normal rate, rhythm, and volume

Thought processes: Logical with no looseness of associations or flight of ideas

Thought content: Denies suicidal or homicidal ideation, auditory or visual hallucinations, obsessions or compulsions

Sensorium and cognition: A&O x 3

Insight and judgment: Insight into his illness is good, and he has good judgment with continued compliance with his medications and appointments

Laboratory and Diagnostic Tests

WBC 8400/mm³, absolute neutrophils 5500/mm³

Diagnosis

Schizophrenia, paranoid type; hypertension; osteoarthritis

Case 26

Medication Record

Date	Rx No	Physician	Drug/Strength	Quantity	Sig	Refills
6/24	6731	Bruce	Tylenol 500 mg	240	2 tab po qid	0
6/24	7118	Meyers	Clozapine 100 mg	112	2 tabs po qam and 2 tabs qhs	0
6/24	6732	Bruce	HCTZ 25 mg	30	1 tab po qam	5
7/22	7564	Meyers	Clozapine 100 mg	112	2 tabs po qam and 2 tabs qhs	0

Pharmacist Notes and Other Patient Information

Patient was reminded to maintain physician visits and lab monitoring every 4weeks.

Questions

1. Which of the following statements is true regarding the occurrence of agranulocytosis with clozapine?

   A. Of all the antipsychotics, clozapine has the highest rate of agranulocytosis.
   B. White blood cell counts should be monitored monthly for the first 6 months of therapy.
   C. Longer treatment with clozapine results in higher risk of developing agranulocytosis.
   D. The dose of clozapine should be reduced if white blood cell count is < 2000/mm³ or absolute neutrophil count is < 1000/mm³.
   E. Monitoring of white blood cell counts may stop immediately upon discontinuation of clozapine due to agranulocytosis.

2. Which of the following statements should you make when counseling a patient who has just been initiated on clozapine?

   I. Report fever, sore throat, or flulike symptoms.
   II. Clozapine may cause drowsiness.
   III. Do not stop clozapine abruptly as adverse effects may occur.

   A. I only
   B. III only
   C. I and II only
   D. II and III only
   E. I, II, and III

3. The Clozapine Treatment Team provides patient information handouts on clozapine annually to their patients for educational purposes. Which one of the following would be the best source for patient information regarding clozapine?

   A. Drug Facts and Comparisons
   B. Physician's Desk Reference
   C. Merck Manual
   D. USP DI
   E. The Red Book

4. Which one of the following choices is NOT a black-box warning for clozapine?

   A. Risk of agranulocytosis
   B. Risk of osteoporosis
   C. Risk of seizures
   D. Risk of myocarditis
   E. Risk of other cardiovascular and respiratory effects

5. The medical resident in your clinic inquires about the management of drug-induced agranulocytosis. Your response includes the following statement(s):

   I. removal of the offending agent generally results in resolution of the neutropenia.
   II. antimicrobials are utilized for any infections that may have resulted secondary to the neutropenia.
   III. granulocyte colony-stimulating factors can shorten the recovery time.

   A. I only
   B. III only
   C. I and II only
   D. II and III only
   E. I, II, and III

6. Which of the following drugs/drug classes have NOT been associated with agranulocytosis?

   A. Anti-thyroid medications (e.g., methimazole or propylthiouracil)
   B. Ticlopidine
   C. Metformin
   D. Sulfasalazine
   E. Dapsone

7. Which of the following metabolic or endocrinologic adverse effects have NOT been reported to occur with the use of clozapine?

    A.   Weight gain

    B.   Hyperglycemia

    C.   Hypertriglyceridemia

    D.   Hypothyroidism

    E.   Hypercholesterolemia

8.   Which of the following statements is true regarding the discontinuation of clozapine?

    A.   Discontinue clozapine immediately if white blood cell count is < 2000/mm^3 and/or absolute neutrophil count is < 1000/mm^3; may re-challenge once white blood cell count is > 3500/mm^3 and absolute neutrophil count is > 2000/mm^3.

    B.   If discontinuation of clozapine is planned, gradually decrease dose over 1 to 2 weeks.

    C.   Discontinue clozapine immediately if white blood cell count is < 3500/mm^3 and/or absolute neutrophil count is < 2000/mm^3; do not re-challenge.

    D.   If therapy with clozapine is interrupted for e" 48 hours, therapy can be reinitiated at the same dose.

    E.   Abrupt discontinuation of clozapine can lead to development of extrapyramidal symptoms.

9.   The new technician goes to pull clozapine off the shelf to refill EH's prescription. Which one of the following is the correct medication?

    A.   Clinoril

    B.   Klonopin

    C.   Catapres

    D.   Clozaril

    E.   Cogentin

10. When asking EH about common dose-related side effects to his clozapine, you should inquire about all of the following EXCEPT:

    A.   weight gain.

    B.   drowsiness.

    C.   bradycardia.

    D.   hypersalivation.

    E.   constipation.

Endocrine and Metabolic Disorders

Section Editor: Dannielle O'Donnell

Patient Name: Joshua Walkingstick
Address: 123 Main Street
Age: 26   **Sex:** Male
Height: 72 in   **Weight:** 170 lb
BMI: 23
Race: Native American
Allergies: NKDA

 ## Chief Complaint

JW is a 26-yo Native American male who is seen by his primary care provider complaining of nausea and abdominal pain. He has had high blood sugars and ketones in his urine for the past 2 days.

 ## History of Present Illness

JW reports blood glucose values greater than 300 mg/dL for the past 2 days. Several days ago he was seen at an urgent care clinic for a widespread poison ivy rash. He was given 4 mg of dexamethasone sodium phosphate IM injection and a prescription for Medrol dosepack to be administered over 6 days. The first 2 days of the methylprednisolone made him nauseated so he skipped several doses of his NovoLog and one dose of Lantus. His glucometer reading this morning was 560 mg/dL and his urine ketones measured positive. His nausea is worse this morning with some mild abdominal pain.

 ## Past Medical History

JW was diagnosed with type 1 diabetes mellitus 12 years ago. He is currently treated with Lantus 28 units at bedtime and NovoLog 1 unit for every 10 grams of carbohydrate in his meal (usual dose is 6 to 8 units/meal). His blood sugars are usually 130 to 180 mg/dL before meals. His last HbA$_{1c}$ 2 months ago was 7.6%. His last retinopathy screen was 6 months ago and was negative for glaucoma, cataracts, or evidence of retinopathy. At the same time the A1c was drawn, he had a lipid profile that was normal and a microalbumin screening that was negative. His blood pressure average over the past 6 months was 118/75 mmHg. He is up to date on his immunizations. His past medical history is positive for hypothyroidism treated with levothyroxine 150 mcg daily. He also has allergic rhinitis treated with loratadine 10 mg QD and Singulair 10 mg QD during the spring and fall months.

 ## Social History

He is married, teaches math, and coaches the girls' golf team at the local high school. He does not smoke and drinks two bottles of beer a month. He likes to play golf once or twice a week.

 ## Family History

HTN, type 2 diabetes in grandmother, who also has CHF. He has a younger sister who also has type 1 diabetes. No heart disease, HTN, lipid disorders in the rest of his first-degree relatives. His father and one brother have asthma.

 ## Review of Systems

Negative other than as noted previously

 ## Physical Examination

GEN: Athletic-appearing man in moderate distress and somewhat drowsy

VS: BP 90/55 mmHg with pulse 110. Ht 72 inches

 ## Laboratory and Diagnostic Tests

(nonfasting, in emergency department)

Sodium 132 mEq/L	Potassium 3.2 mEq/L
Chloride 108 mEq/L	CO_2 12 mEq/L
BUN 25 mg/dL	Serum creatinine 1.0 mg/dL
Glucose 600 mg/dL	

 ## Medication Record

Loratadine 10 mg QD

Date	Rx No	Physician	Drug/Strength	Quantity	Sig	Refills
10/1	10005679	Couch	NovoLog FlexPen U-100	5 pens	Inject 1 unit for every 10 g of carbohydrate per meal	9
10/1	10005678	Couch	Lantus U-100	1	Vial, inject 28 units of insulin subcutaneously at 9 PM every evening	6
7/15	1004493	Kincaid	levothyroxine 150 mcg	90	Take one tablet daily	1
8/24	10005017	Kincaid	Singulair 10 mg QD	90	Take one tablet every evening	1
10/25	10006891	Dooley	Medrol dosepak	1	Take tablets as directed for 6 days	

Effective serum osmolality 297 mOsm/kg

Anion gap 12

Arterial blood gases on room air

pH 7.1   pO$_2$ 100 mmHg

pCO$_2$ 25 mmHg   Bicarbonate 12 mEq/L

Serum ketones 1:16   Urine ketones large

ALT 20 mg/dL   HbA$_{1c}$ 7.6%

 ## Diagnosis

Diabetic ketoacidosis

 ## Pharmacist Notes and Other Patient Information

Lantus 28 units at bedtime, NovoLog 1 unit for every 10 g of carbohydrate per meal; patient reports that he averages about 20 to 25 units of NovoLog per day, Loratadine 10 mg QD, Singulair 10 mg QD, Medrol dosepak (2 days remaining)

Questions

1. JW is admitted to the hospital and started on IV fluids. An insulin infusion to be given as an IV piggyback via a pump is ordered. Which of the following insulins should be used to prepare this order?
   A. Levemir
   B. Regular
   C. Humalog 75/25
   D. Humalog
   E. NovoLog

2. JW's lab results reveal hypokalemia. The physician orders 40 mEq of potassium to be given as 2/3 potassium chloride and 1/3 potassium phosphate added to the second liter of fluid once adequate renal output is established. It is. You have in stock a bottle of potassium chloride 20 mEq/10 mL. How many milliliters of the potassium chloride solution will you add to the IV bag?
   A. 7
   B. 13
   C. 27
   D. 32
   E. 40

3. Identifying precipitating factors for the development of DKA is important to prevent future events. What is the MOST important education that needs to be reviewed with JW to enable him to manage sick days more effectively?
   A. Stress the importance of continuing to take insulin during illness. Do not stop taking insulin without contacting diabetes care team.
   B. Review blood glucose goals and the use of supplemental rapid-acting insulin.
   C. Intake of easily digested liquids containing carbohydrates and salt when ill.
   D. Instruct patient to purchase a home blood ketone monitoring device.
   E. Keep medications readily available to treat fever and nausea.

4. What is the generic name of Levemir?
   A. insulin glargine (rDNA)
   B. insulin glulisine (rDNA origin)
   C. human insulin lispro (rDNA)
   D. human insulin aspart (rDNA)
   E. insulin detemir (rDNA origin)

5. JW's insulin regimen is Lantus 28 units at bedtime and he usually takes between 6 to 8 units of NovoLog before meals (breakfast, lunch, and supper) based on one unit of insulin for every 10 grams of carbohydrates that he eats. His mealtimes are at 7 a.m., noon, and 6 p.m. JW reports that once or twice a week he experiences shakiness, sweating, and weakness around 1:30 p.m. Which insulin is most likely the cause of his symptoms?
   A. Prebreakfast NovoLog
   B. Prelunch NovoLog
   C. Presupper NovoLog
   D. Bedtime Lantus
   E. Symptoms not due to insulin

6. According to the American Diabetes Association Standards of Care, what is the HbA$_{1c}$ goal for JW?
   A. 5%
   B. 6.5%
   C. 7%
   D. 8%
   E. 9%

7. JW reports that he gets five NovoLog FlexPens each time he picks up his prescription. He wants to verify that he is storing them correctly. Which of the following statements is true regarding the storage of the NovoLog FlexPen?

Case 27

A. Opened FlexPens should be stored in the refrigerator until their expiration date.

B. Once FlexPens have been used they should be discarded after 14 days.

C. Opened FlexPens (in use) can be stored at room temperature for up to 28 days.

D. Since JW uses 2 to 3 pens monthly the quantity dispensed should be decreased since the pens expire 30 days after they leave the pharmacy.

E. JW may be advised to freeze the FlexPens that will not be used in the next 30 days to prolong their shelf life.

A. ASA 81 mg QD

B. Retinopathy screening

C. Microalbumin screening

D. Lipid panel

E. Foot examination for pulses, sensation, and vascular changes

8. JW has been reading about vitamin D deficiency and wants to know how much he should take. Which of the following information is the BEST advice for JW?

A. It is best to get vitamin D through the diet and sun exposure, not by taking supplements.

B. He should take 400 IU of vitamin D daily.

C. He should take 2,000 IU of vitamin D daily.

D. A serum 25-hydroxyvitamin D level should be obtained first to determine if he is deficient, then a replenish dose can be recommended.

E. Vitamin D supplements can adversely affect diabetes control and should not be taken.

9. JW's physician wants to place him on Symlin to improve his glycemic control. What is this drug's mechanism of action?

A. It is a glucagon-like peptide-1 agonist. It causes a glucose-dependent enhancement of insulin secretion to lower blood sugar after a meal.

B. Its primary effect is on the liver to decrease hepatic glucose production from gluconeogenesis and glycogenolysis.

C. It is a synthetic analog of amylin. It decreases glucagon production, hepatic glucose production, and postprandial glucose levels.

D. It binds to the SU receptor on a subunit of the ATP-dependent K+ channels located on the beta cells to increase insulin release.

E. Its interactions with a nuclear receptor known as peroxisome-proliferator-activated receptor gamma results in an increase in glucose transporter molecules on the cell membrane to eventually reduce insulin resistance.

10. Which of the following preventative interventions for diabetic complications should be recommended to JW at this time?

Patient Name: L. Bradley Jr.
Address: 8539 Francek Avenue
Age: 61   **Sex:** Male
Height: 5' 8"   **Weight:** 91 kg
Race: African American
Allergies: ACEI (cough)

Chief Complaint

LBJ is a 61-yo African American man who went in for his annual exam on October 22. Labs performed a week prior revealed an elevated triglyceride concentration. Endocrinology is consulted regarding therapeutic options for this patient.

History of Present Illness

LBJ went in for his annual visit with his primary care provider. Labs were ordered the week prior, which revealed a triglyceride concentration of 899 mg/dL. His PCP decided to start LBJ on simvastatin 80 mg daily and gemfibrozil 600 mg BID. A consult was sent to endocrinology and LBJ was seen in their clinic later that week.

Past Medical History

Hypertriglyceridemia	Diabetes mellitus
Obesity	Hypertension
Chronic kidney disease	Gout
Erectile dsfunction	

Social History

LBJ is currently retired on medical disability secondary to health problems. Prior to that, he worked as a forklift operator for 22 years. Patient has no history of smoking or IV drug abuse. Patient reports to drinking 4 to 6 shots of alcohol daily. He is married with 4 children.

Family History

LBJ's father and older brother both had hypertension and diabetes. No knowledge of any heart problems within his family. He also had a brother who died from lung cancer.

Review of Systems

Unremarkable

Physical Examination

GEN: pleasant, overweight man in no apparent distress

VS: BP 142/92 mmHg, HR 88 bpm, RR 16 rpm, T 98.4°F, Ht 5' 8", Wt 200 lb

CHEST: lungs CTA, heart RRR

EXT: pedal pulses present, no edema, cuts, or bruises

Laboratory and Diagnostic Tests

(Measured October 15, fasting)

TC = 337, TG = 899, HDL = 18, LDL = unable to calculate

Sodium 140 mEq/L	Potassium 4.2 mEq/L
CO_2 22 mEq/L	Chloride 101 mEq/L
Glucose 136 mg/dL	BUN 8 mg/dL
Serum creatinine 1.4 mg/dL	
AST 20 IU/L	ALT 24 IU/L
Uric acid 6.8 mg/dL	TSH 1.8 IU/L

Diagnosis

Hypertriglyceridemia

Medication Record

Date	Rx No	Provider	Drug/Strength	Quantity	Sig	Refills
10/22	946	Hague	Zocor 80 mg	30	1 po qhs	7
9/18	763	Hague	Toprol 75 mg	30	1 po daily	3
10/25	1093	Steins	Actos 7.5 mg	30	1 po daily	3
10/1	762	Friemoth	Neurontin 100 mg	30	1 po BID	8
9/18	764	Hague	Glucotrol 10 mg	100	1 po BID	3
10/22	947	Hague	Lopid 600 mg	60	1 po BID	4

Case 28

Questions

1. With a triglyceride (TG) concentration of 899 mg/dL, LBJ asks you if he is at risk for anything. Your response to his question is which of the following?

    A. Gouty attack
    B. Kidney failure
    C. Pancreatitis
    D. Heart failure
    E. Hepatitis

2. Which of the following medications could be added to further reduce this patient's TG concentration if his TG remains significantly elevated on his current regimen?

    A. Zetia
    B. Lovaza
    C. Cholestyramine
    D. Metformin
    E. Welchol

3. Which of the following medications by itself would be expected to lower triglycerides to the greatest extent?

    A. Lipitor
    B. Niacin
    C. Lovaza
    D. Lopid
    E. Glucotrol

4. LBJ read on the Internet that fish oil may help lower his cholesterol. The most appropriate response to his statement would be which of the following?

    A. Fish oil is an alternative therapy that has been shown to be beneficial in lowering LDL cholesterol concentrations but does not lower triglycerides.
    B. Fish oil cannot be used in this patient because he has diabetes mellitus.
    C. The article the patient read was incorrect because fish oil can help with erectile dysfunction.
    D. Fish oil supplementation can lower triglyceride concentrations if used with appropriate doses.
    E. Fish oil may decrease the frequency and severity of gouty attacks.

5. Which of the following statements is true?

    A. Diabetes mellitus does not have any effect on triglyceride concentrations.
    B. Hyperthyroidism can contribute to elevated triglyceride concentrations.
    C. Triglyceride concentrations can be elevated due to excessive alcohol consumption.
    D. Genetics has nothing to do with hypertriglyceridemia.
    E. Elevated uric acid in patients with a history of gout leads to elevated triglyceride levels.

6. Given the patients lipid profile, the endocrinologist has decided to add on Niaspan. Which of the following statements is most appropriate?

    A. Niaspan may cause flushing as a potential side effect.
    B. Niaspan does not affect triglyceride concentrations.
    C. Niaspan does not affect HDL concentrations.
    D. Niaspan added to a statin does not increase the risk of myalgias.
    E. Niaspan is more hepatotoxic than the IR or ER formulations.

7. Advicor is the trade name for which two products?

    A. Atorvastatin and amlodipine
    B. Niacin and lovastatin
    C. Simvastatin and fenofibrate
    D. Pravastatin and aspirin
    E. Simvastatin and ezetimibe

8. Which of LBJ's medical conditions may be worsened by using Niaspan for his cholesterol treatment plan?

    I. Obesity
    II. Gout
    III. Diabetes mellitus

    A. I only
    B. III only
    C. I and II only
    D. II and III only
    E. I, II, and III

9. When you initially fill the 10/22 prescriptions for simvastatin 80 mg daily plus Lopid 600 mg BID, what, if any, potential adverse effects will the patient be at risk for with this combination that you should counsel about?

    A. Depression
    B. Low HDL concentrations
    C. Hypertension
    D. Rhabdomyolysis
    E. No significantly increased risk for adverse effects with this combination

10. The endocrinologist has decided to switch the patient from simvastatin 80 mg po daily to another statin. The patient needs a drug that would be at least equivalent in LDL-C lowering as his simvastatin regimen. Your response is:

    A. atorvastatin 10 mg q hs would be equivalent.
    B. lovastatin 40 mg q hs would be equivalent.
    C. pravastatin 80 mg q hs would be equivalent.
    D. rosuvastatin 10 mg q hs would be equivalent.
    E. there is no equivalent because simvastatin is the most potent statin currently available.

Patient Name: Kent Sleep
Address: 971 Dream Street
Age: 41   **Height:** 6' 0"
Sex: M   **Race:** Caucasian
Weight: 350 lb
Allergies: NKA

Chief Complaint

KS is a 41-yo white male referred by his primary care physician to the weight management clinic for weight loss. This is his first visit to the clinic.

History of Present Illness

KS initially went to see his primary care physician for worsening of fatigue during the day. He had fallen asleep while driving, resulting in an accident in which his car ran into the ditch alongside the interstate. He feels tired during the day even though he goes to bed at 10 p.m. and wakes up at 6 a.m. His wife recently moved out of the bedroom because his snoring is so loud she could not sleep. He was diagnosed with obstructive sleep apnea 2 months ago and prescribed orlistat to lose weight and a BiPAP machine to help breathing at night. He has had a gradual weight gain over the years. He admits he has occasional dietary indiscretions while taking orlistat resulting in diarrhea, and he reports mild gastrointestinal side effects such as oily spotting and oily stool. He denies fecal urgency or increased flatulence.

Past Medical History

Obstructive sleep apnea (OSA) diagnosed 2 months ago, HTN x2 years, dyslipidemia

Social History

Married for 20 years, 3 children all alive and well. Does not smoke, drinks occasional alcohol. Employed as sales representative, covers a large territory requiring long distance driving.

Medication Record

Date	Rx No	Physician	Drug and Strength	Quantity	Sig	Refills
04/02	95	Smith	Amlodipine 10 mg	30	1 po qd	6
04/02	96	Smith	HCTZ 25 mg	30	1 po qd	6
04/02	97	Smith	Quinapril 20 mg	30	1 po qd	6
06/02	98	Smith	Orlistat 120 mg	90	1 po tid	2
06/02	99	Smith	Pravastatin 40 mg	30	1 po qhs	3

Multivitamin at bedtime

Nasal biPAP

Family History

Father died in his sleep. Mother and four siblings alive. Describes his family as large and heavy.

Review of Systems

None available

Physical Examination

GEN: BP: 140/90 mmHg, heart rate 75, morbidly obese middle-aged male with thick and short neck

ENT: Neck circumference 21 inches, thyroid not enlarged; mouth shows large tongue and swollen uvula, baldness, 2+ edema in lower extremities, RR 14

CV: Sounds are distant; RRR: No murmur; ABD: Obese

Labs and Diagnostic Tests

Hgb 13.5 g/dL

Thyroid studies normal

Bicarbonate 28 mEq/L

Total cholesterol (fasting) 262 mg/dL

LDL (fasting) 192 mg/dL

HDL (fasting) 52 mg/dL

TG (fasting) 90 mg/dL

Diagnosis

Primary:

Obesity, obstructive sleep apnea, dyslipidemia, hypertension

Pharmacist Notes and Other Patient Information

None available

Questions

1. Based on the NHLBI Clinical Guidelines, what is the recommended nutrient content for a weight reduction diet?

    A. 55% carbohydrate, 30% Fat, 15% protein.

    B. 3% carbohydrates, 34% fat, 63% protein.

    C. 5% CHO, 67% fat, 28% protein.

    D. 37% carbohydrates, 30% fat, 33% protein.

    E. The nutrient content varies on the body type. NHLBI recommends a very low carbohydrate, high fat content if most of the body fat is abdominal while it recommends a low fat content for others.

2. The package insert for Xenical encourages the use of a multivitamin because:

    A. long-term use of orlistat results in mild hypomagnesemia.

    B. orlistat use decreases absorption of calcium and vitamin D and may result in increase risk of osteoporosis in middle-aged women.

    C. orlistat may cause reduced levels of vitamins A, D, E, and K and beta-carotene.

    D. the vitamin B6 included in a multivitamin can treat hyperhomocysteinemia associated with obesity.

    E. orlistat short-term can cause hypokalemia which left untreated may result in arrhythmias.

3. When dispensing orlistat, KS should be instructed to:

    A. follow a low-fat diet (<30% fat intake) to minimize the occurrence of the GI effects. Recommend a three-meals-a-day program where fat content is as much as possible, is equally distributed across the three meals. Adhere to a diet rich in fiber (as it may decrease the risk for GI events with orlistat).

    B. buy adult diapers (Attends) to prevent soiling his clothes. The oily spotting effect of orlistat is unrelated to diet and may occur at any time.

    C. follow a low-fat, low-calorie diet to maximize efficacy and minimize adverse events. Because of the possible drug interaction with pravastatin (decreased absorption with orlistat), you recommend to KS not to take orlistat with pravastatin.

    D. follow a low-fat, low-calorie diet to maximize efficacy and minimize adverse events. Emphasize the importance of taking orlistat three times a day with a meal regardless of the fat content.

    E. follow a regular diet. There is no need to alter his diet because orlistat dissolves the fat in the gut and has not been associated with increased GI adverse events.

4. KS is concerned about his son (13 years old) also suffering of obesity (211 pounds) and sleep apnea. He asks you whether weight loss drugs are safe in adolescents. Which weight loss drug therapy is FDA approved for use in adolescents aged 12 to 16 years old?

    A. Phentermine

    B. Orlistat

    C. Bupropion

    D. Sibutramine

    E. Phenylpropanolamine

5. Which of the following drugs should not be taken within 2 hours of orlistat?

    A. Cyclosporine

    B. Phenytoin

    C. Digoxin

    D. Pravastatin

    E. Nifedipine

6. The weight loss medication orlistat works by which of the following mechanisms?

    A. Orlistat reduces hunger and is a dopamine reuptake inhibitor

    B. Orlistat increases levels of serotonin and dopamine

    C. Orlistat is an appetite suppressant and decreases CNS levels of leptin

    D. Orlistat inhibits gastric and pancreatic lipases

    E. Orlistat decreases ghrelin levels

7. All of the following statements about diethylpropion are correct EXCEPT:

    A. Diethylpropion is an appetite suppressant and stimulates norepinephrine release.

    B. Diethylpropion is generally prescribed as 75 mg, extended release, once per day.

    C. Diethylpropion is associated with insomnia if taken in the late afternoon.

    D. Diethylpropion is indicated for long-term weight loss (studied for more than 2 years).

    E. Diethylpropion should not be prescribed in obese patients with severe hypertension or cardiovascular disease.

8. Which of the following statements about obesity is FALSE:

    A. Obesity is a chronic condition just like hypertension. For that reason, pharmacotherapy should be continued long term.

    B. Almost all weight loss clinical trials found that a weight loss plateau is reached after 6 months of therapy, if pharmacotherapy is discontinued the weight loss is likely to be regained.

Case 29

C. The newer antiobesity agents allow short-term treatment (approximately 6 months) after which the drug(s) should be discontinued.

D. Drug therapy for obesity should always be added to diet, exercise and behavioral therapy to maximize its efficacy.

E. Only Xenical has been approved by FDA for long-term use.

9. KS has read about chitosan and asks you if it could replace orlistat, since it is less expensive. All of the following statements are true EXCEPT which one?

A. Compared to orlistat, chitosan did not show significant reduction in fat absorption.

B. The FDA does not regulate labeling of chitosan and content is not guaranteed.

C. Chitosan is a polysaccharide that exhibits similar activity to cellulose.

D. Chitosan when combined with caffeine achieved better short-term weight loss than low-calorie, low-fat diets in a few randomized, controlled trials.

E. Chitosan is one of the ingredients of several OTC weight-loss agents.

10. Match the following weight loss agents with their respective brand name:

I.   Sibutramine-Meridia, Orlistat-Xenical, Phentermine-Ionamin

II.   Diethylpropion-Tenuate, Phentermine-Fastin, Mazindol-Sanorex

III. Phentermine-FenFen, Mazindol-Mazorex, Orlistat-Xenical

A. I only
B. III only
C. I and II only
D. II and III only
E. I, II, and III

Renal Disorders

Section Editor: Holli Temple

Patient Name: J.D. Carver
Address: 1138 Gettysburg Pike
Age: 40   **Sex:** Male
Height: 6' 3"   **Weight:** 185 lb
Race: African American
Allergies: NKDA

Chief Complaint

JC is a 40-yo male who presents to the ED with a cloudy dialysate bag, abdominal pain, and low-grade fever. He has vomited twice.

History of Present Illness

JC has been on continuous ambulatory peritoneal dialysis (CAPD) for 2 months.

Past Medical History

JC has had type 1 DM since age 16. Diabetic complications include retinopathy, neuropathy, and nephropathy. JC has been hypertensive for 8 years. Approximately 1 year ago, JC's renal function declined to ESRD and subsequently required hemodialysis. Two months ago, JC was converted to CAPD. JC has also been diagnosed with hyperlipidemia, restless leg syndrome, and has a remote history of PUD. JC's past surgical history is significant for peritoneal catheter placed 1 year ago. Multiple laser surgeries for diabetic retinopathy.

Social History

JC is a real estate broker. JC denies tobacco, alcohol, and illicit drug use.

Family History

(+) diabetes on maternal side of family

Review of Systems

As above. Patient denies chest pain, shortness of breath, and diarrhea.

Physical Examination

GEN: WD/WN male in mild distress; A&O x 3

VS: BP 136/85 mmHg, HR 110 bpm, RR 20 rpm, T 100.3°F, Wt 84 kg

HEENT: NC/AT, PERRLA, EOMI, TM intact

LUNGS: CTA bilaterally

CV: RRR

ABD: Soft, diffusely tender, catheter site clean and does not appear infected, fluid wave consistent with CAPD, no focal tenderness or mass

EXT: No CCE

Laboratory and Diagnostic Tests

Sodium 138 mEq/L	Potassium 4.0 mEq/L
Chloride 99 mEq/L	CO_2 content 25 mEq/L
BUN 78 mg/dL	Serum creatinine 6.4 mg/dL
Glucose 98 mg/dL	Calcium 10.2 mg/dL
Phosphorus 3.9 mg/dL	Albumin 2.7 g/dL
Magnesium 2.7 mg/dL	Hgb 9.3 g/dL
Hct 29.4%	Platelets 195,000/mm³

WBC 12,000/mm³ with 95.5% PMNs, 3.4% lymphocytes, 0.7% monocytes, 0.7% eosinophils

Lipid panel:

TC 94	HDL 34
LDL 28	VLDL 32
TG 163	%HDL 36

CrCl 10 mL/min

Microbiology: Peritoneal fluid, gram stain, few gram-positive cocci

Dialysate cell count:

WBC 10,200/mm³	RBC 650/mm³
Neutrophils 90%	Lymphocytes 10%

Diagnosis

No information available.

Medication Record

9/19, Medicated dialysate bags per protocol; number of exchanges per day: 4

9/19, Catapres-TTS-3 patch TOP, change weekly

9/19, Nexium 20 mg po daily

9/19, Cardizem CD 240 mg po bid

9/19, Lipitor 20 mg po daily

9/19, Humulin N insulin 30 units SQ q AM

9/19, Humulin N insulin 10 units SQ q hs

9/19, Accuchecks ac hs

9/19, Humalog sliding scale SQ ac hs

9/19, Tums 500 mg chewable, 4 tid ac

9/19, Neurontin 300 mg prn

9/19, Klonopin 0.5 mg po hs

9/19, Niferex 150 mg po bid

9/19, Renagel 403 mg, 2 po tid ac

9/19, EPO 4000 units IV twice weekly

Pharmacist Notes and Other Patient Information

9/19, Dextrose 50% IV 25 mL STAT

9/19, Medicated dialysate bags per protocol; number of exchanges per day: 4

9/19, Catapres-TTS-3 patch TOP, change weekly

9/19, Nexium 20 mg po daily

9/19, Cardizem CD 240 mg po bid

9/19, Lipitor 20 mg po daily

9/19, Humulin N insulin 30 units SQ q AM

9/19, Humulin N insulin 10 units SQ q hs

9/19, Accuchecks ac hs

9/19, Humalog sliding scale SQ ac hs

9/19, Tums 500 mg chewable, 4 tid ac

9/19, Neurontin 300 mg prn

9/19, Klonopin 0.5 mg po hs

9/19, Niferex 150 mg po bid

9/19, Renagel 403 mg, 2 po tid ac

9/19, EPO 4000 units IV twice weekly

Questions

1. Gentamicin was ordered as empiric antibiotic coverage for peritonitis. What other antibiotics could be used as an alternative to gentamicin?

   A. Ampicillin
   B. Cefoxatin
   C. Ceftazidime
   D. Linezolid
   E. Azithromycin

2. The peritoneal culture comes back and is positive for MRSA. The MD wants to start vancomycin in place of cefazolin. You recommend:

   A. vancomycin IP every 6 hours.
   B. vancomycin IP every 12 hours.
   C. vancomycin IP every 5 days.
   D. vancomycin IV every 12 hours.
   E. vancomycin po every 6 hours.

3. JC recovered from his peritonitis. Towards the end of his hospital stay, a urine culture was positive for a gram-negative bacteria which was sensitive to ciprofloxacin. The plan is to send him home on oral Cipro 250 mg daily. JC wants to know if he can take Cipro at same time as his Tums, Niferex, and Nexium. You recommend that JC:

   A. take Cipro with Tums.
   B. take Cipro with Niferex.
   C. take Cipro with Nexium.
   D. take Cipro with Renagel.
   E. take Cipro separately from all other medications.

4. Cefazolin was chosen as part of the initial empiric antibiotic therapy because the most common pathogen associated with CAPD-related peritonitis is:

   A. *Candida*
   B. *Klebsiella*
   C. *Pseudomonas*
   D. *Staphylococcus* (coagulase-negative)
   E. Culture negative

5. JC has an order for EPO 4000 units IV twice a week. JC does not have IV access. Which route of administration do you recommend?

   A. Give EPO IM
   B. Give EPO IP
   C. Give EPO SQ
   D. Give Aranesp IM
   E. Give EPO SQ

6. In the past, JC had an anaphylactic reaction to iron dextran. He has a significant iron deficit and needs iron replacement, particularly since he is receiving EPO therapy. What would you recommend?

A. Give iron dextran at a slower rate with next dose
B. Desensitize him to iron dextran
C. Give a test dose first
D. Double the dose of his oral iron therapy
E. Give him iron sucrose

7. Just before discharge you note that JC's hemoglobin is 9.3 g/dL (14-18) and his hematocrit is 29.4% (42-52). Three weeks ago his Hgb was 8.2 g/dl and Hct was 27.2 %. What would you recommend doing with his EPO dose?

A. Keep EPO dose the same
B. Increase EPO dose by 25%
C. Increase EPO dose by 50%
D. Increase EPO dose by 100%
E. Decrease EPO dose by 25%

8. Which parameters must be evaluated before initiating and during therapy with epoetin alfa?

A. PT/INR
B. Transferrin saturation and serum ferritin
C. Blood urea nitrogen and serum creatinine
D. AST and total bilirubin
E. RBC and platelets

9. Aranesp (darbepoetin alfa) is also an approved erythropoietin product. Which of the following statements are incorrect when comparing Aranesp to Epogen (epoetin alfa)?

A. Doses used for Aranesp are much higher numerically
B. The dosing interval is more frequent with Epogen
C. The half-life of Aranesp is longer
D. Side effect profile is similar
E. Target goals are similar

10. The resident indicates that JC's restless leg syndrome, which is more of a problem at night, and his peripheral neuropathy have not been well controlled. What would you recommend for JC?

A. Change Neurontin to scheduled dosing
B. Increase clonazepam dose
C. Change to phenytoin
D. Add ropinirole
E. Start quinine

Case 31

Dosing of Drugs in Renal Failure

Patient Name: Jay Marcus
Address: 146 Rossiter Street
Age: 61 **Sex:** Male
Height: 5′ 11″ **Weight:** 165 lb
Race: Caucasian
Allergies: Codeine, levofloxacin

Chief Complaint

JM is a 61-yo male who came to the ED complaining of intermittent chest pain for the past 2 days. An EKG revealed an acute inferolateral infarction.

History of Present Illness

None available

Past Medical History

JM was diagnosed with HTN in his 30's. He began antihypertensive therapy and initially responded well. A few years later, JM had financial problems and stopped filling his prescriptions. At the age of 45, JM was diagnosed with ESRD due to uncontrolled hypertension. He has been maintained on hemodialysis three times a week for the past 10 years. JM also has a history of generalized tonic-clonic seizures and anemia of chronic disease.

Social History

JM lives alone. Wife died last year.

Tobacco use: 1/2 ppd

Alcohol use: occasional beer

Drug use: denies

Caffeine use: two cups of coffee/day

Family History

Significant for ESRD in maternal aunt; father died at age 65 of heart attack.

Review of Systems

Negative except as noted previously

Physical Examination

GEN: Alert, cooperative male in obvious discomfort

VS: BP 150/90 mmHg, HR 110 bpm, afebrile

LUNGS: Clear to A&P

CV: Irregular rhythm, no murmurs

GU: Very little urine output

Laboratory and Diagnostic Tests

Sodium 140 mEq/L	Potassium 4.6 mEq/L
Chloride 105 mEq/L	CO_2 content 26 mEq/L
BUN 55 mg/dL	Serum creatinine 6.6 mg/dL
Glucose 109 mg/dL	Albumin 3.1 g/dL
Phenytoin 6.4 mg/L	Hgb 10.5 g/dL
Hct 31.5%	CK 101 IU/L
CKMB index 3.3%	Troponin-I 4.02 ng/mL

Urinalysis: 2+ protein, (-) glucose, specific gravity 1.025

Diagnosis

No information available.

Medication Record

Calcium acetate 667 mg 2 tabs po with each meal

Amlodipine 10 mg po daily

Plavix 75 mg po daily

Vital-D RX 1 tab po daily

Lovenox 1 mg/kg SQ Q24H

Phenytoin 200 mg po nightly at bedtime

Epoetin alfa 50 units/kg IV three times weekly with HD

Atenolol 50 mg po daily

Integrilin 1 mcg/kg/min continuous IV infusion

Pharmacist Notes and Other Patient Information

None available.

Case 31

Questions

1. Which of the following medications should be adjusted in ESRD?
   I. Amlodipine
   II. Atenolol
   III. Enoxaparin

   A. I only
   B. III only
   C. I and II only
   D. II and III only
   E. I, II, and III

2. The cardiologist calls the pharmacy to ask for the recommended dose of Integrilin in a dialysis patient. As the pharmacist, you reply:

   A. No adjustment is needed in dialysis patients (180 mcg/kg bolus, then 2 mcg/kg/min).
   B. Decrease infusion time in dialysis patients (180 mcg/kg bolus, then 2 mcg/kg/min x 4 hours).
   C. Decrease dose by one half in dialysis patients (90 mcg/kg bolus, then 1 mcg/kg/min).
   D. Integrilin is contraindicated; recommend Aggrastat. Renal dosing of Aggrastat: 0.2 mcg/kg/min for 30 minutes, followed by continuous infusion of 0.05 mcg/kg/min.
   E. No bolus needed. Begin with continuous infusion rate of 1 mcg/kg/min.

3. According to JNC VII, the recommended goal blood pressure for patients with renal failure and proteinuria >1 g/24 hrs is a SBP <130 and DBP <80. Since JM's HTN is not being adequately controlled on non-dialysis days, which class of agents may be added to his current therapy?

   A. ACE inhibitors
   B. Change angiotensin-receptor blockers to clonidine
   C. Thiazide diuretics
   D. Hydralazine
   E. Minoxidil

4. Which of the following statements are TRUE for treating hypertensive patients with ESRD?

   A. Lisinopril dose should be adjusted in patients with renal failure.
   B. Spironolactone is preferred over furosemide in patients with renal failure.
   C. Metoprolol dose should be adjusted in patients with renal failure.
   D. Clonidine dose should be adjusted in patients with renal failure.
   E. Angiotensin-receptor blockers should not be used in patients with renal failure.

5. The physician calls concerned about JM's low phenytoin level (6.4 mg/L). You assure him that you will follow up. What other information is needed to appropriately evaluate the phenytoin level?

   A. Type of dialysis
   B. PT/INR
   C. Albumin level
   D. Calcium level
   E. Phosphorus level

6. On rounds there is some discussion about whether JM has evidence of congestive heart failure. As part of the discussion, the use of digoxin comes up and the question is asked as how to appropriately dose digoxin in patients with renal failure and on dialysis? Which is a TRUE statement regarding digoxin in HD patients?

   A. Digoxin loading dose doesn't need to be adjusted in HD patients.
   B. Digoxin is mostly metabolized by the liver and does not need to be adjusted in HD patients.
   C. Digoxin is removed by HD and a supplemental dose should be given after each HD.
   D. Digoxin loading dose and maintenance dose must be adjusted in HD patients.
   E. Digoxin is removed by peritoneal dialysis to a greater extent than hemodialysis.

7. JM begins to complain of diffuse abdominal pain and spikes a fever. Cultures are obtained but are not available at this time. The physician wants to begin an antibiotic. Which of the following needs to be adjusted in renal failure?

   A. Piperacillin/tazobactam
   B. Metronidazole
   C. Clindamycin
   D. Linezolid
   E. Oxacillin

8. After receiving a tirofiban drip, the nurse calls the pharmacy because the physician ordered 0.05 mcg/kg/min and the nurse needs help calculating the drip rate. The label reads tirofiban 25 mg in NS 500 mL. Patient's weight = 75.3 kg. The correct rate is:

   A. 4.5 mcg/h.
   B. 4.5 mL/h.
   C. 45 mL/h.
   D. 2.5 mcg/h.
   E. 2.5 mL/h.

9. Which factors determine a drug's dialyzability?

    I.   Molecular weight
    II. Protein binding
    III. Clearance

    A. I only
    B. III only
    C. I and II only
    D. II and III only
    E. I, II, and III

10. Since JM had an acute myocardial infarction, what other agents should be considered for use in preventing future cardiovascular events?

    A. Digoxin
    B. Vitamin E
    C. Aspirin
    D. Vitamin D
    E. Folic acid

Patient Name: Don White
Address: 939 Field Drive
Age: 43 **Sex:** Male
Height: 5' 8'' **Weight:** 140 lb
Race: Caucasian
Allergies: NKDA

Chief Complaint

DW, a 43-yo male, presents to the diabetes clinic for a follow-up outpatient appointment.

History of Present Illness

Eight weeks ago, DW was discharged from the hospital with diagnoses of MI (NSTEMI), pulmonary edema (resolved), severe HTN, and renal insufficiency. Before this hospitalization, DW had not seen a physician in a year. A cardiac catheterization was postponed until renal function stabilized.

Past Medical History

DW has had type 1 DM for 30 years and has been hospitalized approximately 10 times for DKA. Diabetic complications include diabetic retinopathy, nephropathy, gastroparesis, and mild peripheral neuropathy. DW states that he does have a blood glucose meter, but that "it has been broken for awhile." Also, DW has been hypertensive for approximately 5 years. DW's past surgical history is significant for retinal laser photocoagulation 2 weeks ago.

Social History

Remote smoking history 1 ppd x 2 years, but has not smoked in 10 years. DW is a salesman. He drinks alcohol socially. He denies any illicit drug use.

Family History

Father: Alive age 65. MI at age 49, (+) hypercholesterolemia, (-) diabetes, (+) renal insufficiency

Mother: Alive age 63. (+) diabetes, (+) hypercholesterolemia

Review of Systems

DW has noted some lower extremity edema. He denies orthopnea, palpitations, syncope, angina, or dyspnea on exertion.

Physical Examination

GEN: Pleasant Caucasian man in NAD who is A&O x 3.

VS: BP 155/95 mmHg, HR 70 bpm, RR 12 rpm, T 98.8°F, Wt 64 kg

HEENT: NC/AT, moist oral mucosa with poor dentition, thyroid WNL, no carotid bruits detected

CHEST: Clear to auscultation

CV: RRR, no murmurs/rubs/gallops

ABD: Positive BS, no hepatosplenomegaly

EXT: 2+ pretibial edema on lower extremities, calluses on bottom of both feet, decreased sensation bilaterally to 10 gm monofilament (5.07 Semmes-Weinstein (10-g) nylon filament test)

Laboratory and Diagnostic Tests

Sodium 133 mEq/L	Potassium 5.4 mEq/L
Chloride 105 mEq/L	CO_2 22 mEq/L
BUN 58 mg/dL	Serum creatinine 3.7 mg/dL
Glucose 456 mg/dL	Calcium 8.5 mg/dL
Phosphorus 4.7 mg/dL	Albumin 2.2 g/dL
HgbA$_{1c}$ 12.0	TSH 3.05
Hgb 12.2 g/dL	Hct 36.1%
Platelets 223,000/mm^3	WBC 6900/mm^3

Urine analysis:

Color yellow	Specific gravity 1.015
Blood 3+	Protein 3+
pH 5.0	Glucose trace

Urine collection 24 hours:

Urine creatinine clearance 25 mL/min

Urine total protein 17.7 g/24 h

Lipid panel (fasting):

TChol 336	HDL 30
LDL 221	TG 348

Renal ultrasound:

Small kidneys bilaterally consistent with chronic renal disease, no mass or hydronephrosis

2-D echocardiogram:

EF 44%

Diagnosis

DM-1, CKD, Hypertension, Hyperlipidemia

 Medication Record

Vaccinations: Received Pneumovax and hepatitis B vaccine before discharge from the hospital on the prior admission.

Outpatient medication record

Date	Physician	Drug/Strength	Quantity	Sig	Refills
5/22	Vincent	Aspirin EC 325 mg	100	1 po daily	prn
5/22	Vincent	Lipitor 80 mg	30	1 po hs	3
5/22	Vincent	Toprol XL 100 mg	30	1 po daily	2
5/29	Sergeant	Zestril 20 mg	30	1 po daily	3
5/29	Sergeant	Diovan 80 mg	30	2 po daily	3
5/29	Sergeant	Norvasc 5 mg	30	2 po daily	3
6/10	Moore	Insulin aspart SQ		5 units ac& hs	3
6/18	Sergeant	Furosemide 80 mg	60	1 po bid	3
6/22	Vincent	Toprol XL 100 mg	30	1 po daily	3
6/29	Moore	Accucheck test strips	100	ac hs	3
6/29	Moore	Lantus	15 units SQ	q AM	3

Questions

1. Which of the following factors would NOT be contributing to the progression of renal disease for DW?

    A. Diabetes
    B. Hypertension
    C. Hyperlipidemia
    D. Hyperkalemia
    E. Family history of CKD

2. Which combination of medications may be responsible for DW's increase in potassium?

    A. Furosemide + valsartan
    B. Lisinopril + valsartan
    C. Valsartan + atorvastatin
    D. Amlodipine + lisinopril
    E. Metoprolol + amlodipine

3. If the patient's potassium increases, it might be necessary to give him oral/rectal Kayexalate. Which phrase best describes Kayexalate?

    A. Sequestration agent
    B. Water in oil emulsion
    C. Oil in water emulsion
    D. Anion exchange resin
    E. Cation exchange resin

4. Since DW travels for his job, he often carries his insulin on the road with him. He is not sure how long an insulin pen is "good for" once it has been used. How long is a Lantus SoloStar pen stable once punctured?

    A. 7 days
    B. 28 days
    C. 3 months
    D. 6 months
    E. 1 year

5. Using the MDRD equation (for labs who are using a standardized serum creatinine assay), which stage of chronic kidney disease does DW have?

    A. Stage 1
    B. Stage 2
    C. Stage 3
    D. Stage 4
    E. Stage 5

6. Which of the following sources can help identify medications?

    I. Identidex
    II. Goodman and Gillman's The Pharmacological Basis of Therapeutics
    III. Applied Therapeutics

    A. I only
    B. III only
    C. I and II only
    D. II and III only
    E. I, II, and III

Case 32

7. Which of the following is NOT a typical, common complication of chronic renal disease?

   A. Osteodystrophy
   B. Hyperparathyroidism secondary to hyperphosphatemia
   C. Anemia
   D. Hypokalemia
   E. Hypertension

8. The attending physician has suggested using both an ACEI and an ARB in this patient. You are not familiar with any advantage of using both together. Which of the following would be the best source to explore the value of this combination?

   A. Drug Interaction Facts
   B. Handbook of Nonprescription Drugs
   C. Bruce's guide to combination therapies
   D. UpToDate
   E. Lexi-Comp Drug Information on your hand-held device

9. The patient presents a prescription for furosemide, but mentions to you that in the hospital they had to use two "water pills" to keep the edema at bay. What diuretic would most likely be synergistic when used in combination with furosemide?

   A. HCTZ 25 mg po
   B. Diamox 250 mg IV
   C. Bumex 2 mg po
   D. Zaroxolyn 5 mg po
   E. Demadex 20 mg po

10. Which medication(s) have been demonstrated to improve patients' outcomes post-MI?

    I.   ACE inhibitors
    II. Calcium channel blockers
    III. Beta blockers

    A. I only
    B. III only
    C. I and II only
    D. I and III only
    E. I, II, and III

Psychiatric Disorders

Section Editor: Lawrence J. Cohen

Patient Name: John Deer
Address: 1234 Corn Row Lane
Age: 30 **Sex:** Male
Height: 6' 2'' **Weight:** 187 lb
Race: Caucasian
Allergies: Salicylates with skin rash, hives, and swelling

Chief Complaint

JD is a 30-yo man who presents to his PCP with complaints of occasional racing heartbeat, dizziness, shortness of breath, irritable bowels, and trouble sleeping. He is agitated and tense and admits to trying to ignore these symptoms because they have been present most of the time for the past year. JD tearfully states that his father has recently suffered a massive heart attack and he is very concerned that he might be following in his father's footsteps. He's even started aspirin therapy in hopes of preventing a heart attack.

History of Present Illness

JD was referred from the ED for follow up. In the ED, he presented with symptoms of chest pain, shortness of breath, restlessness, and sweating. Full cardiac workup at ED was WNL. He admits to constantly worrying about his health and whether he will physically be around to see his kids grow up. He realizes that there is no basis for many of these feelings because all physical exams in the past have revealed him as healthy. JD is very restless throughout the interview with significant mood lability. Given JD's physical symptoms and emotional distress, he is now walking a fine line at work. He constantly battles with staying awake during the day and finds it incredibly difficult to concentrate on most tasks.

Past Medical History

JD was diagnosed with adjustment disorder with anxiety (acute anxiety lasting <6 months) approximately 10 months ago when his father's health started to decline. He was prescribed lorazepam but admits to never taking more than 1-2 tablets of his prescription because he read about all the potential adverse events.

Social History

Tobacco use: Nicorette chewing gum 4-mg strength (10-15 pieces/day) for the past couple of years

Alcohol use: 2 beers with dinner

Caffeine use: 1/2 pot of coffee and 4 cans of Mountain Dew/day

Family History

Father had an MI at age 52. Mother diagnosed with major depression with a comorbid panic disorder at age 30. Brother diagnosed with social phobia (social anxiety disorder) at age 25.

Review of Systems

Shortness of breath; dry cough; nonproductive, unrealistic, and excessive worry; autonomic hyperactivity; insomnia

Physical Examination

GEN: Patient is a WD/WN white male who appears restless with significant mood lability

VS: BP 132/84 mmHg, HR 123 bpm, RR 20 rpm, T 38.4°C, Wt 85 kg

HEENT: PERRLA, nasal congestion, neck supple, no lymphadenopathy, no thyromegaly

CHEST: CTA bilaterally

CV: Normal S_1, S_2, no m/r/g

ABD: Soft NT/ND, no HSM, (+) BS

EXT: No C/C/E, good pedal pulses bilaterally

NEURO: Tense but cooperative, thought coherent, A&O x3

Laboratory and Diagnostic Tests

Sodium 141 mEq/L	Potassium 4.6 mEq/L
Chloride 107 mEq/L	CO_2 content 27 mEq/L
BUN 16 mg/dL	SCr 0.8 mg/dL
Glucose 90 mg/dL	Hgb 12.2 g/dL
Hct 32%	Platelets 320,000/mm³
WBC 6700/mm³	Total calcium 9.7 mg/dL
Folate 2.5 ng/mL	Vitamin B_{12} 200 pg/mL

ECG: Sinus tachycardia otherwise NL ECG

Serial cardiac enzymes: WNL

Diagnosis

General anxiety disorder (GAD)

Medication Record

Date	Rx No	Physician	Drug/Strength	Quantity	Sig	Refills
5/21	678988	Stone	Claritin-D 24 Hour	30	1 po qd	prn
3/14			Sudafed 30 mg	100		
3/14	899754	Puckett	BuSpar Dividose 30 mg	30	1/2 po bid	3
5/99			St. Joseph's Aspirin			
3/14	899756	Puckett	Anaprox 550 mg	30	1 po qd	1
5/21	678987	Stone	Ativan 1 mg	30	1-2 po bid prn	1
3/14	899755	Puckett	Ambien 10 mg	30	1 po q hs prn	1

 Pharmacist Notes and Other Patient Information

Not available.

Questions

1. Which of the following compounds have FDA indications for the treatment of GAD?

    A. Venlafaxine
    B. Gabapentin
    C. Desipramine
    D. Propranolol
    E. Sertraline

2. Which of the following disease states have symptoms that mimic generalized anxiety disorder?

    I. Pheochromocytoma
    II. Myocardial infarction
    III. Panic disorder

    A. I only
    B. III only
    C. I and II only
    D. II and III only
    E. I, II, and III

3. The pharmacologic mechanism of benzodiazepines is best described as:

    A. facilitating influx of chloride ions into the cell.
    B. inhibiting influx of chloride ions into the cell.
    C. facilitating influx of sodium ions into the cell.
    D. inhibiting influx of sodium ions into the cell.
    E. inhibiting influx of potassium ions into the cell.

4. JD's nurse asks you about nonpharmacologic treatment options to treat his GAD. Which of the following has clinical evidence of efficacy to treat GAD?

    A. Individual psychotherapy (IPT)
    B. Cognitive behavioral therapy (CBT)
    C. Dialectical behavior therapy (DBT)
    D. Family-focused therapy (FFT)
    E. Psychodynamic therapy (PDT)

5. Based on his medication profile, JD is most likely to have sensitivity to which of the following?

    A. Claritin-D 24 Hour
    B. St. Joseph's aspirin 162 mg
    C. Venlafaxine 75 mg
    D. Ambien
    E. Sudafed

6. On the basis of his laboratory profile, JD should be ruled out for what type of anemia(s)?

    I. Pernicious anemia
    II. Folate deficiency megaloblastic anemia
    III. Vitamin B_{12} deficiency anemia

    A. I only
    B. III only
    C. I and II only
    D. II and III only
    E. I, II, and III

7. You receive a prescription for Effexor XR DAW 225 mg daily x 30 days. How do you dispense this medication?

    A. 30 225 mg capsules
    B. 60 100 mg capsules and 30 25 mg capsules
    C. 30 75 mg capsules and 30 150 mg capsules
    D. 30 200 mg capsules and 30 25 mg capsules
    E. 30 100 mg capsules and 60 62.5 mg capsules

8. The DSM-IV diagnostic criteria for GAD require that a patient's symptoms occur more days than NOT for a period of at least:

    A. 2 weeks.
    B. 1 month.
    C. 6 months.
    D. 9 months.
    E. 1 year.

Case 33

9. JD's mother responded to an SSRI in the past for her GAD, but the patient cannot remember which one. He states that "it was a small blue tablet and was oblong in shape." Which antidepressant do you recommend?

   A. Venlafaxine
   B. Fluoxetine
   C. Citalopram
   D. Sertraline
   E. Mirtazapine

10. The patient would like to learn more about treatment options for his sleep disorders. What would be the best source for information?

   A. NIMH website
   B. Library book
   C. DSM-IV-TR
   D. Wikipedia
   E. Support group

Patient Name: Antonio Valdez
Address: 815 Sixth Street
Age: 7   **Sex:** Male
Height: 4′ 2″   **Weight:** 55 lb
Race: Hispanic
Allergies: NKDA
Practice Setting: Public child and adolescent mental health outpatient clinic

Chief Complaint

He was referred to the clinic due to problems with his very short attention span and inability to sit still in class. Patient's mother reports she is concerned about the patient's motor hyperactivity and seeming not to listen when spoken to directly.

History of Present Illness

When AV started kindergarten at age 5, it was noticed that he had difficulty staying seated, paying attention or concentrating, following directions, getting organized, and finishing assigned work. He was frequently daydreaming, easily distracted, and distracting others from their classwork. He was impatient, impulsive, and intrusive and exhibited motor restlessness and excessive activity—not waiting his turn and making inappropriate noises in class. About 2 years ago, shortly after his symptoms were noticed, his mother took him to his pediatrician who diagnosed ADHD and had him start methylphenidate 5 mg morning and noon. His target symptoms were well controlled; but his mother noticed his significant decline in appetite. A medication change was tried to dextroamphetamine, then to mixed amphetamine salts; but again his appetite was severely decreased. His regimen was then changed to atomoxetine with good symptom control and no noted side effects. He has no oppositional or defiant behavior, no physical or verbal aggression, and no problems with conduct.

Past Medical History

In infancy he had a benign heart murmur, which has since resolved. All immunizations are current. Last year he had a simple fracture of his left radius from jumping out of a tree. No other significant current or past medical or surgical history.

Social History

He lives with both biological parents and his 9-yo sister in a well-kept three-bedroom house in a quiet neighborhood. He is in second grade in regular classes, makes good grades, and shows no learning disability. No particular stressors, trauma, or abuse.

Family History

Father's older brother has bipolar disorder; and a 10-yo male first cousin has ADHD. Father reports having similar problems in school as patient has now, but was never brought to medical attention. Father admits to several years of heavy alcohol abuse as a young adult, but he quit when he got married.

Review of Systems

Occasional mild-to-moderate frontal headache, and decreased appetite as side effects when he was on stimulant medication. Height and weight between 50th and 75th percentile of growth chart.

Physical Examination

Patient appears stated age and was neatly dressed, with good grooming and hygiene. He remained quiet and his mother did all the talking for him; he did not intrude or interrupt. He was attentive off and on, but after 10-15 minutes, he became restless and impatient. He got up from his seat and wandered around the office examining, touching, and occasionally picking up objects from the desk and bookshelves. His mood was euthymic and his affect showed a broad range but rapidly appeared bored. Remainder of exam WNL for age and grade level.

Laboratory and Diagnostic Tests

ECG: Normal sinus rhythm   CBC: WNL

Chem 14: WNL except alk phos 433

UA: WNL   TSH: 0.82

T_4: 10.9 T_3: uptake 23

FTI: 2.5

Diagnosis

Axis I: Attention deficit hyperactivity disorder, combined type

Medication Record

Atomoxetine 60 mg q AM

Pharmacist Notes and Other Patient Information

ADHD target symptoms apparently well controlled on current medication regimen with no noted medication side effects.

Case 34

Questions

1. Effective medication treatments for ADHD are thought to improve attention span and decrease motor hyperactivity by modulating which neurotransmitters?

   A. GABA and serotonin
   B. Epinephrine and glutamate
   C. Norepinephrine and dopamine
   D. Histamine and acetylcholine
   E. Serotonin and acetylcholine

2. Commercially available forms of methylphenidate are known by the following proprietary names EXCEPT:

   A. Methylin.
   B. Ritalin.
   C. Concerta.
   D. Adderall.
   E. Metadate.

3. Patients and parents should be counseled about potential side effects of psychostimulant medications including:

   I. headache and decreased appetite.
   II. stomachache and insomnia.
   III. nervousness, rebound hyperactivity, and dysphoria.

   A. I only
   B. III only
   C. I and II only
   D. II and III only
   E. I, II, and III

4. Common comorbid conditions associated with ADHD that benefit from nondrug measures include:

   I. learning disorders.
   II. serious conduct problems and defiance of authority.
   III. abuse of tobacco, alcohol, and/or other illicit or prescription drugs.

   A. I only
   B. III only
   C. I and II only
   D. II and III only
   E. I, II, and III

5. The use of pemoline for ADHD is no longer considered first-line treatment because of the risk of:

   A. renal toxicity.
   B. agranulocytosis.
   C. hepatic toxicity.
   D. development of type II diabetes.
   E. cardiac toxicity.

6. Adequate treatment of ADHD can prevent or reduce morbidity from all the following medical conditions that are significantly more common if ADHD is untreated EXCEPT:

   A. precocious sexual activity, STDs, and early pregnancy.
   B. benign and malignant neoplasms of the central nervous system.
   C. tobacco, alcohol, and prescription and illegal drug abuse.
   D. reckless driving and injury from motor vehicle accidents.
   E. injury from pedestrian, bicycle, and motorcycle accidents.

7. A prescription for Concerta could be filled for which one of the following dosages?

   A. 10 mg
   B. 20 mg
   C. 25 mg
   D. 36 mg
   E. 42 mg

8. Which of the following is a nonstimulant proven to be effective in treating ADHD?

   A. Strattera
   B. Vyvanse
   C. Daytrana
   D. Focalin
   E. Dextrostat

9. Which one of the following is the most commonly abused drug in adolescents and adults with ADHD?

   A. Dextroamphetamine
   B. Methylphenidate
   C. Benzodiazepines
   D. Marijuana
   E. Cocaine

10. Which of the following drug products commercially available to treat ADHD is NOT in capsule form?

    A. Adderall XR
    B. Provigil
    C. Metadate CD
    D. Ritalin LA
    E. Strattera

Patient Name: Joseph Mayburn
Address: 8103 Echo Valley Drive
Age: 78 **Sex:** Male
Height: 6′ 1″ **Weight:** 257 lb
Race: Caucasian
Allergies: Codeine (nausea)

Chief Complaint

JM is a 78-yo white man who was admitted 4 weeks ago to a skilled nursing facility after suffering a myocardial infarction. Since that time, he has become increasingly withdrawn. He will not participate in any group activities and no longer is interested in his usual hobbies such as watching TV. JM's daughter is concerned and has asked for a psychiatric consultation for her father.

History of Present Illness

JM was living independently until 5 weeks ago when his daughter found him unconscious in his house. He was admitted to the hospital, after experiencing an MI, with left ventricular dysfunction with an ejection fraction of 30%. With his difficulty with ambulation, a significant decrease in his level of functioning, and difficulty with his complicated medication regimen, JM was admitted to a skilled nursing facility.

Past Medical History

JM has no known past psychiatric history. His medical history includes CAD, HTN, hypercholesterolemia, type 2 DM, chronic back pain, and BPH.

Social History

Tobacco use: 2 ppd for 55 years; quit smoking 5 years ago

Alcohol use: six-pack of beer/week until admitted to the skilled nursing facility

Caffeine use: 2 cups of coffee every morning

Widowed 4 years ago

Family History

JM's parents died of unknown causes, but his father was known to have HTN. JM has one son with HTN and hypercholesterolemia and one daughter who is currently being treated for HTN and depression.

Review of Systems

Negative except as noted previously

Physical Examination

Old chart is reviewed. During patient's last clinic visit to his PCP, an abnormal EKG was noted with changes in the QRS interval. A cardiologist was following with serial EKGs. Complete physical exam is deferred because patient has routine care from a PCP.

Mental status examination: The patient is a moderately obese white male in no acute distress. He is oriented x 4. He is fairly cooperative, although he is often hesitant to answer. He avoids sustained eye contact. There is some psychomotor retardation. Speech is somewhat slow with normal tone and low volume.

Thought content contains no homicidal ideation; patient does admit to thinking about death a lot and has considered stopping his medication to increase the likelihood of death. He has no auditory or visual hallucinations.

Patient describes his mood as "sad and down" and displays a somewhat blunted affect. Patient displays fairly good judgment with moderate insight displayed in that he has not refused his medications but reports that he does not feel he is acting any differently than usual.

Patient does express difficulty in adjusting to the skilled nursing facility. When asked about pleasurable activities, patient reports he used to enjoy TV but now it just does not seem entertaining anymore.

Laboratory and Diagnostic Tests

No current labs available

Diagnosis

Major depression

Case 35

 Medication Record

Date	Rx No	Physician	Drug/Strength	Quantity	Sig	Refills
6/2	1295	Garner	Lisinopril 20 mg	30	1 qd	5
6/2	1297	Garner	ASA EC 325 mg	30	1 qd	5
6/2	1300	Garner	Acetaminophen 500 mg	30	1-2 q 4-6 h prn	5
6/2	1304	Garner	Doxazosin 4 mg	30	1 qd	5
6/2	1299	Garner	Lovastatin 40 mg	30	1 qd	5
6/2	1301	Garner	MOM 30 cc	4	oz prn	2
6/2	1305	Garner	Amitriptyline 50 mg	60	bid	2
6/2	1298	Garner	Alprazolam 0.25 mg	30	1 tid prn	2
6/2	1302	Garner	Glyburide 5 mg	60	1 bid	5
6/2	1296	Garner	Furosemide 40 mg	60	1 bid	5
6/2	1306	Garner	Metoprolol tartrate 25 mg	60	1 bid	5
6/2	1303	Garner	Metformin 500 mg	60	1 bid	5

 Pharmacist Notes and Other Patient Information

None available.

Questions

1. Which of the following is a reason(s) for the pharmacist to recommend discontinuation of amitriptyline for JM?

   I. Antidepressants are not indicated.

   II Amitriptyline can worsen glucose control and widen the QRS interval.

   III. Anticholinergic effects of amitriptyline can worsen symptoms associated with BPH.

   A. I only
   B. III only
   C. I and II only
   D. II and III only
   E. I, II, and III

2. Which of the medications on JM's profile is associated with greatest potential for increased falls and morbidity in elderly patients?

   A. Lisinopril
   B. Furosemide
   C. Alprazolam
   D. Lovastatin
   E. Acetaminophen

3. Which of the following is a TRUE statement(s) regarding the use of antidepressants in patients experiencing depression and comorbid cardiac disease?

A. The Class IA/IC antiarrhythmic effects of tricyclic antidepressants make them the antidepressant drugs of choice in patients with cardiac disease.
B. Comorbid depression has been associated with an increase in post-myocardial infarction mortality.
C. Antidepressants are ineffective in the treatment of depression with comorbid cardiac disease.
D. Amitriptyline is without a risk for postural hypotension.
E. Mirtazapine has an FDA approval for depression in heart disease.

4. Compared to younger patients with depression, the response to antidepressants seen in elderly patients is characterized as being associated with:

   A. decreased time to response with a lower rate of remission.
   B. increased time to response with a lower rate of remission.
   C. decreased time to response with a higher rate of remission.
   D. increased time to response with a higher rate or remission.
   E. increased time to response but no difference in the rate of remission.

5. Selective serotonin antidepressants exhibit a sigmoidal dose-response curve. This means that:

   A. increases in efficacy (i.e., percentage of responders/percent remitters) would be expected as the dose of sertraline is increased from 25 mg to above 200 mg.
   B. increases in efficacy can be expected as the dose of sertraline is increased from 25 mg to 100 mg, but further increases in doses up to 200 mg and above would be associated with much smaller incremental increases in response.

C. increases in a dose of sertraline from 25 mg to 100 mg would result in incremental increases in efficacy but higher doses would lead to a worsening of symptoms of depression.

D. increases in a dose of sertraline from 25 mg to 100 mg result in a worsening of depression with higher doses of up to 200 mg in incremental increases in efficacy.

E. the incidence of side effects is not dependent on dose but the response to therapy is dose-dependent.

6. JM is changed to Zoloft but is having trouble swallowing tablets and needs a liquid preparation. Which of the following would be most appropriate?

A. Change the same 25-mg dose of sertraline to a liquid.

B. Have patient chew tablets.

C. A switch to fluoxetine 10 mg is necessary since it is the only liquid SSRI available.

D. Change to the same dose of sertraline in a disinte-grating tablet formulation.

E. Change the patient to 5 mg of aripiprazole in a liquid or M (dissolvable) formulation as it is an FDA-approved augmentation strategy.

7. The pharmacist reviews a study comparing venlafaxine to amitriptyline for the treatment of depression. The mean dose of venlafaxine in the study was 158.6 mg daily while the mode was 150 mg/d. This means that:

I. the average dose per patient was 158.6 mg/d.

II. the most common dose per patient was 150 mg/d.

III. JM should be taking 158.6 mg/d to get maximum effect

A. I only

B. III only

C. I and II only

D. II and III only

E. I, II, and III

8. Phenelzine is an irreversible, nonselective monoamine oxidase inhibitor. If a patient were to be switched from phenelzine 60 mg to venlafaxine XR, the appropriate strategy would be to:

A. discontinue phenelzine immediately, wait 2 weeks, and then start venlafaxine XR 37.5 mg qd

B. cross-titrate phenelzine and venlafaxine (i.e., simultaneously decrease phenelzine while increasing venlafaxine) over a 2-week period.

C. start venlafaxine 37.5 mg and keep dose the same while slowly tapering phenelzine over a 2-week period.

D. taper phenelzine completely off over 1-2 weeks, wait 2 weeks, then start venlafaxine XR 37.5 mg qd.

E. discontinue phenelzine immediately and start venlafaxine XR 37.5 mg qd.

9. JM's only partial improvement to sertraline 50 mg qd leads the physician to change to venlafaxine 75 mg bid. His depressive symptoms start to improve, but he has complaints of GI discomfort when he takes this medica-tion. Which of the following would be an appropriate management strategy?

A. Change back to Zoloft at a higher 200 mg dose

B. Change to venlafaxine XR starting at 150 mg daily, which was the improving dose.

C. Change from 75 mg bid to 150 mg of once-daily dosing of immediate-release venlafaxine as once-daily dosing has less side effects

D. Switch sertraline CR

E. Add prochlorperazine to sertraline as it will improve the nausea and be an augmentation strategy in depression

10. JM's daughter would like some information about venlafaxine to take home and read. Which of the following would be the best source for patient/family educational materials about this medication?

A. AHFS

B. Pharmacotherapy, 4th edition

C. USP DI

D. Merck Manual

E. Physicians' Desk Reference

Patient Name: Aaron Hobson
Address: 316 E. Hudson Avenue
Age: 36   **Sex:** Male
Height: 5' 10''   **Weight:** 170 lb
Race: Caucasian
Allergies: NKDA

Chief Complaint

AH is a 36-yo married white man who was brought into the ER 1 week ago when he was found staggering outside a bar on Main Street. He was treated for alcohol detoxification and was discharged to an intensive day-treatment program for substance abuse the next day. Today AH is reporting to your pharmacy requesting medication refills.

History of Present Illness

While being brought by the police to the ER, AH vomited once and then appeared to pass out. He was unconscious on arrival (at midnight) but still breathing with a respiratory rate of 15 breaths/minute. His breath and clothes smelled of alcohol and he was very disheveled. He woke up feeling restless and staff reported that he became agitated at 3:30 a.m. Subsequently, he was given a dose of lorazepam 1 mg po. He fell back asleep within 30 minutes and slept through the night. The next morning he was alert and oriented and was discharged to an intensive day-program for substance abuse the next day. From your patient interview you find that he has a history of heart failure, which was diagnosed about 8 years ago. He reports an 8-lb weight loss over the past 2 months and feels like life is just not worth it any more. He complains of not having any energy but also has trouble falling asleep. He states that he recently stopped going to play cards with his poker club because "it just isn't any fun anymore." His wife reports that he is not able to complete normal daily tasks as of late and he often "only finishes jobs and chores about half way then just walks away from them."

Past Medical History

AH has had two admissions for alcohol detoxification, and this is his second outpatient treatment. He has been smoking for 20 years with a 40 pack-year history. He reports he has been treated for depression in the past and was diagnosed with heart failure for 8 years. He reports he does not take any medications currently.

Social History

AH is currently employed and has had four jobs in the past 2 years. His wife moved out 3 months ago, and he reports he drinks 6-8 beers and 1/2 pint of "hard liquor" daily. He denies illicit drug use.

Tobacco use: 40 pack-year history

Alcohol use: heavy (6-8 beers and 1/2 pint of "hard liquor" daily)

Illicit drug use: denied

Family History

AH has two brothers whom he has not spoken to in more than 10 years. His parents are deceased, and his father reportedly had a "problem with the bottle."

Review of Systems

Negative

Physical Examination

(From ER records)

GEN: Obese WM, odor of alcohol, pt was coherent

VS: BP 143/122 mmHg, HR 115 bpm, RR 20 rpm, T 99.0°F

SKIN: Moist secondary to diaphoresis

MS/EXT: Tremor in both hands (R > L), pulses 1+ dorsalis pedis, none in posterior tibial

NEURO: A&O x3, (+) tremors in both hands, CN II-XII intact; DTRs are exaggerated

Laboratory and Diagnostic Tests

(From ER Records)

Sodium 139 mEq/L	Potassium 3.7 mEq/L
Chloride 108 mEq/L	CO_2 content 25.5 mEq/L
BUN 9 mg/dL	Serum creatinine 1.4 mg/dL
Glucose 136 mg/dL	Magnesium 1.2 mg/dL
Calcium 9.8 mg/dL	Phosphorous 2.5 mg/dL
WBC 700/m³	Hgb 13.8 g/dL
Hct 40%	Platelets 240,000/mm³
AST 254 IU/L	GGT 265 IU/L
ALT 113 IU/L	Alb 4.3 g/dL
T. bili 1.1 mg/dL	D. bili 0.4 mg/dL
Alk phos 41 IU/L	LDH 321 IU/L
UA 10.8 mg/dL	PT 12.2 sec
INR 1.03	

Toxicology screen: (-) illicit drugs, (+) alcohol

Diagnosis

Hypertension

Seasonal allergies

Nicotine dependence

Heart failure

Medication Record

Currently does not report taking any medications, but your prescription records show the following.

Date	Rx No	Physician	Drug/Strength	Quantity	Sig	Refills
11/1	782452	Johnson	Digoxin 0.5 mg	30	1 q am	4
11/1	782453	Johnson	Enalapril 10 mg	60	1 bid	4
11/1	782456	Johnson	Fexofenadine 60 mg		1 bid	2
11/1	782455	Johnson	Nicotine patch 21 mg	28	apply 1 qd	0
11/1	782451	Johnson	Naltrexone 50 mg	30	1 qd	2
11/1	782455	Johnson	Bupropion SR 150 mg	60	1 qd x 3 d then bid	1

Pharmacist Notes and Other Patient Information

Not seen by pharmacy in the ER

Questions

1. AH questions you about using naltrexone to help him stop drinking. Which of the following is an absolute contraindication to naltrexone use?

    A. Depression
    B. Heart failure
    C. Liver failure
    D. Renal failure
    E. Uncontrolled hypertension

2. Which of the following is NOT FDA-approved for the treatment of alcoholism?

    A. Acamprosate
    B. Disulfiram
    C. Naltrexone
    D. Topiramate
    E. Buprenorphine

3. Naltrexone should not be initiated in a patient taking which of the following?

    I.   Antabuse
    II. Campral
    III. Suboxone

    A. I only
    B. III only
    C. I and II only
    D. II and III only
    E. I, II, and III

4. AH reports that he was given a medication to help him sleep in the hospital that made him feel "unusual." His records indicate that the only medication used was lorazepam. Which of the adverse effects would you not expect with the use of benzodiazepines?

    A. Anterograde amnesia
    B. Bradycardia
    C. Lightheadedness
    D. Disinhibition
    E. Somnolence

5. Which of the following is an assessment tool used to screen for alcohol use disorders?

Case 36

A. SF-36
B. BPRS
C. GAF
D. CAGE
E. Beck-A

6. Which of the following is true regarding smoking cessation treatment?

   A. Smoking cessation treatments should be offered to all smokers at every intervention.
   B. Patient-specific health problems will always be linked to cigarette smoking.
   C. The concomitant use of Zyban and nicotine replacement therapy is contraindicated.
   D. Smoking cessation therapy should only be offered if concurrent health problems exist.
   E. If a patient has a psychiatric diagnosis, smoking cessation therapy should not be offered.

7. AH reports his physician is considering a medication to help treat his alcoholism. He cannot remember the name but remembers the physician stating that he should avoid the use of Listerine and other mouthwash products. What medication is AH's physician referring to?

   I. Antabuse
   II. Campral
   III. Revia

   A. I only
   B. III only
   C. I and II only
   D. II and III only
   E. I, II, and III

8. Which of the following medications is commercially available as an OTC for smoking cessation?

   A. Nicoderm CQ 21 mg
   B. Nicorette 10 mg
   C. Zyban 150 mg
   D. Chantix 1 mg
   E. Nicotrol 10 mg

9. If you were to recommend starting smoking cessation for AH with bupropion, which of the following is an adverse events would you include in your counseling?

   A. Sexual dysfunction
   B. Arthralgias
   C. Xerostomia
   D. Sedation
   E. Hypertension

10. AH reports many symptoms when he presented to your pharmacy, of which some appear they could be either related to depression or a substance use disorder. Which of the following symptoms are more indicative of a substance use disorder than depression?

    A. Anhedonia and insomnia
    B. Avolition and weight loss
    C. Poor concentration and hypersomnia
    D. Confusion and dysphoria
    E. Mood reactivity and amotivation

Patient Name: Delma Lane
Address: 1417 Rose Lane
Age: 38 **Sex:** Female
Height: 5′ 7″ **Weight:** 135 lb
Race: Hispanic
Allergies: NKDA

Chief Complaint

DL is a 38-yo Hispanic woman with a history of bipolar I disorder in a current episode of depression who comes to the mental health clinic reporting that she feels "more depressed and I'm thinking of harming myself." Her mother accompanied her to the clinic.

History of Present Illness

During the past month, DL has become increasingly depressed. She has been trying to get custody of her daughter, but her ex-husband is trying to prevent it. Although DL reports having suicidal thoughts on and off for years, thoughts of harming herself have increased recently. Her mother is concerned that DL has not been taking her medication for several weeks. She reports that she has experienced "stomach burning" most often after taking Depakene. DL has been living alone and admits to partial inadherence with her medication.

Past Medical History

DL has received treatment for depression from her PCP starting at age 26. She was first diagnosed with major depressive disorder 6 years ago. Since then, she has experienced a manic episode for which she was hospitalized. However, the majority of time spent ill in the last 6 years has been in the depressed phase. DL has been treated with some success after several short trials of antidepressants in the past, although she is unable to name them. DL's past medical history is also significant for a hysterectomy 1 year ago, episodic tachycardia, and indigestion.

Social History

Tobacco use: 1/2 ppd for 5 years
Alcohol use: "occasional use"

Family History

DL was married for approximately 10 years but was divorced 8 years ago. She has one daughter and is trying to obtain custody of her. Her mother is alive and has a history of depression and alcohol abuse. DL's sister carries a diagnosis of bipolar disorder.

Review of Systems

None available.

Physical Examination

Unremarkable except for a report of gastrointestinal symptoms.

Mental status examination:

The patient is a neatly dressed 38-yo female, alert and oriented x4 and is cooperative with the examination. Her speech is clear with a normal rate. She has a depressed mood with a blunted affect and psychomotor retardation. DL reports intermittent suicidal thoughts but denies hallucinations, delusions, or homicidal ideation.

Laboratory and Diagnostic Tests

None available

Diagnosis

Bipolar disorder, depressed

Pharmacist Notes and Other Patient Information

None available.

Medication Record

Date	Rx No	Physician	Drug/Strength	Quantity	Sig	Refills
6/4	7892	Young	Clonazepam 1 mg	60	1 bid	4
6/4	7894	Green	Propranolol 40 mg	90	1 tid	4
6/10			Acetaminophen 500 mg	100	1-2 prn ha	
6/5	7496	Nelms	Conjugated estrogens 0.625 mg	30	1 qd	3
6/4	7893	Young	Depakene 250 mg	60	1 bid	4

Case 37

Questions

1. Which of the following are likely to contribute to this episode of major depression in DL?

   I. Inadherence to her medication regimen
   II. Stress from family and financial problems
   III. Alcohol use

   A. I only
   B. III only
   C. I and II only
   D. II and III only
   E. I, II, and III

2. Which of the following would be the most appropriate strategy to decrease the indigestion and GI burning DL experiences after taking Depakene?

   A. Change to Depakote ER tablets
   B. Change to sodium valproate liquid
   C. Increase the dose of Depakene
   D. Take the entire dose of Depakene at bedtime
   E. Switch to generic valproic acid capsules

3. DL's dysphoric mood and history of some benefit to antidepressants leads Dr. Young to consider adding citalopram to her current regimen. Which statement(s) most accurately describes the risks associated with destabilization of the patient's mood?

   A. Citalopram may increase the risk for cycling.
   B. Citalopram may increase the risk for an acute switch into a manic episode.
   C. Citalopram may increase the potential for switching into a manic episode within the year following its initiation.
   D. Citalopram increases the risk of switching even with concurrent use of mood stabilizers.
   E. Each of the above statements represents a potential risk associated with using citalopram in DL.

4. Which of the following tests is necessary for monitoring therapy with valproic acid?

   I. Serum drug concentration
   II. Liver enzymes
   III. Serial chest roentgenograms

   A. I only
   B. III only
   C. I and II only
   D. II and III only
   E. I, II, and III

5. DL reports increased somnolence over the past month. All of the following provide possible explanations for this problem EXCEPT:

   A. depressed mood.
   B. clonazepam.
   C. hypomanic episode.
   D. valproic acid.
   E. propranolol.

6. An alternative medication(s) that could be used if DL has a suboptimal response to Depakene is:

   A. olanzapine.
   B. lamotrigine.
   C. lithium.
   D. lithium plus risperidone.
   E. all of the above.

7. A decision is made to add lamotrigine to DL's regimen in order to improve the treatment of the depressed phase of her bipolar disorder. The manufacturer's recommended titration schedule is provided below.

   > Weeks 1 and 2: 25 mg/day
   > Weeks 3 and 4: 50 mg/day
   > Week 5: 100 mg/day
   > Week 6: 200 mg/day
   > Week 7: 200 mg/day (target dose)

   Given that DL is also on valproic acid, which of the following would be the recommended dose titration strategy?

   A. No special strategy needed. Use the manufacturer's recommended titration schedule.
   B. Start lamotrigine at twice the recommended starting dose and increase at twice the recommended rate since valproic acid is a CYP450 enzyme inducer.
   C. Start lamotrigine at half the recommended dose and titrate at half the recommended rate.
   D. The use of valproic acid and lamotrigine in combination is contraindicated.
   E. Reduce the dose of valproic acid by 50% and use the manufacturer's recommended starting dose and titration schedule.

8. Despite improvements in GI side effects following a change from Depakene, DL continues to be partially inadherent to her regimen. What would be the most appropriate strategy (or strategies) for the pharmacist to recommend in order to improve DL's compliance?

A. Insist that DL take all doses of each medication every day.
B. Assess DL's daily routine and assist her in figuring out how to take her medications in conjunction with other routine activities such as meals or brushing her teeth, capitalizing on a regular schedule.
C. Decrease DL's regimen to two medications to decrease the number of daily doses.
D. Have DL come to the clinic each day to have the medication administered to her.
E. Arrange for a social worker to visit DL daily to witness DL taking each dose of medication.

9. A serum drug concentration for valproic acid is ordered for DL. When should the blood be drawn for this?

A. 2-4 hours after any dose
B. 2-4 hours before any dose
C. Immediately before the next dose the following day
D. Immediately following any dose
E. Plasma levels and response have not been established in acute mania

10. Which of the following medications used in bipolar disorder is associated with the lowest incidence of clinically significant weight gain?

A. Valproic acid
B. Lamotrigine
C. Lithium carbonate
D. Olanzapine
E. Risperidone

Patient Name: Danny Caldwell
Address: 365 Lincoln Avenue
Age: 25   **Sex:** Male
Height: 6' 1''   **Weight:** 210 lb
Race: Caucasian
Allergies: Sulfa antibiotics
Practice Setting: Veteran's Administration psychiatric outpatient clinic

Chief Complaint

The patient comes to the Veteran's Administration psychiatric outpatient clinic today and reports that his current medication is maintaining his target symptoms under good control, but complains of decreased libido as a side effect.

History of Present Illness

The patient experienced onset of symptoms at age 19 after 1 year of active duty in the U.S. Army. He had not been stationed outside the continental U.S., had no history for physical or emotional trauma, and was not known to abuse drugs or alcohol, except occasionally going out drinking with his buddies on weekend pass. He had been promoted to corporal and squad leader. He showed a gradual prodrome for a few months when he had progressive difficulty concentrating and making decisions, and developed an excessive interest in Buddhist religion and literature. He began having a firm belief that his thoughts were being controlled by a computer chip in his brain, that people were sending their thoughts into his head, that there was an underground plot to capture and torture him, and he heard someone calling his name when no one was there. He was found late one night cringing in fear in the corner of a warehouse on base mumbling incoherently and trembling uncontrollably. He was taken by ambulance to the psychiatric unit of a nearby military hospital. He was given Zyprexa Zydis 20 mg sublingual and started calming down within 30 minutes. His toxicology screen was negative, and he denied any precipitating factor.

Past Medical History

A sulfa antibiotic in childhood caused him to break out in a rash. Tonsillectomy at age 7. No history of head injury, seizure, migraine, poisoning, or exposure to toxins.

Social History

Born and raised in eastern Colorado, intact family, one older sister, younger brother and sister. He was in regular classes, maintained B average, fairly popular with peers, and had no symptoms of learning disability, conduct problems, or ADHD. Joined the Army right after high school graduation, had no problem in basic training. Heterosexual orientation, has a current girlfriend, employed full time doing custodial work at the VA hospital where he receives outpatient psychiatric and medical treatment, lives independently in his own apartment. Never married or fathered any children, never had any legal involvement.

Family History

Both parents have hypertension and osteoarthritis, all three siblings are alive and well. Father has a first cousin with schizophrenia, maternal grandfather was alcoholic.

Review of Systems

Mildly to moderately overweight, recent complaint of decreased libido, otherwise unremarkable. He has a consistent history of treatment adherence.

Physical Examination

Mental Status Examination:

The patient was a casually dressed white male, appearing his stated age, who was alert and oriented to person, place, and time. Mood, euthymic; Affect, cheerful, friendly. He was calm and cooperative. Speech was clear and direct; normal rate and tone of voice. Thought process coherent and goal directed, denies hallucinations or delusions, average cognition and intellectual function, good eye contact, normal psychomotor activity.

Laboratory and Diagnostic Tests

CBC, Chem 14, Lipid Panel, Thyroid function tests, ECG all WNL. Urine drug screen negative. Due to patient's chief complaint a serum prolactin level was obtained, which was elevated at 125 ng/mL.

Diagnosis

Axis I Schizophrenia, chronic undifferentiated type
Axis III Iatrogenic hyperprolacinemia

Medication Record

Patient has been maintained as an outpatient on risperidone 3 mg p.o.q HS over past 5 to 6 years.

Pharmacist Notes and Other Patient Information

Due to elevated serum prolactin level and clinically significant sexual dysfunction side effect, risperidone was discontinued, and patient was started on aripiprazole 10 mg q AM

Questions

1. The cause of cogwheel rigidity and psychomotor retardation in patients treated with first generation antipsychotic medication is attributable to:
   A. blockade of dopamine D_2 receptors.
   B. blockade of histamine H_1 receptors.
   C. blockade of alpha-1 adrenergic receptors.
   D. blockade of muscarinic acetylcholine receptors.
   E. blockade of serotonin $5HT_{2a}$ receptors.

2. Which of the following are available as orally disintegrating tablets?
   A. Abilify, Geodon, Seroquel
   B. Haldol, Prolixin, Thorazine
   C. Loxitane, Stelazine, Trilafon
   D. Risperdal, Zyprexa, Saphris
   E. Mellaril, Fanapt, Invega

3. For a patient who is being prescribed a first-generation antipsychotic medication, what precautions and warnings should the patient be counseled about prior to giving informed consent for treatment?
   A. Risk for autoimmune disorder
   B. Risk for potentially irreversible movement disorder
   C. Risk for weight loss
   D. Risk for chronic diarrhea
   E. Risk for alopecia

4. A delusion whose theme is that events, persons, or objects in one's environment have a particular and unusual significance is known as:
   A. thought insertion.
   B. thought broadcasting.
   C. ideas of reference.
   D. delusions of being controlled.
   E. erotomanic delusion.

5. Potential advantages of second-generation antipsychotic medications over first-generation antipsychotic medications include which of the following?
   I. Less severe side effect profile
   II. Improved medication adherence
   III. More effective for negative and cognitive symptoms

   A. I only
   B. III only
   C. I and II only
   D. II and III only
   E. I, II, and III

6. Which of the following best describes the mechanism by which antipsychotic medications cause movement disorders?
   A. Postsynaptic blockade of dopamine receptors in the CNS
   B. Presynaptic blockade of dopamine receptors in the periphery
   C. Decreased synthesis of dopamine in the CNS
   D. Increased synthesis of dopamine in the periphery
   E. Imbalance between dopamine and serotonin in the CNS

7. When counseling a patient or patient's family about the symptoms that comprise schizophrenia, which of the following would be included?
   I. For most of a 1-month period the patient has had at least two of the following symptoms: delusions, hallucinations, disorganized speech or behavior, or negative symptoms.
   II. Signs of the disturbance persist at least 6 months and a significant deterioration in one or more major areas of functioning occurs.
   III. There has been a serious disturbance of mood (e.g., mania, depression, or mixture of both) for the duration of the psychotic symptoms.

   A. I only
   B. III only
   C. I and II only
   D. II and III only
   E. I, II, and III

8. One of the most important non-drug measures to promote health and minimize the impact of schizophrenia symptoms is a comprehensive psychosocial program aimed at improving the level of patients' adaptive functioning and can include all of the following EXCEPT:
   A. training and practice in appropriate social skills.
   B. regular monitoring of vital signs including weight and blood pressure.
   C. teaching basic independent living skills and self-care.
   D. education and training in employment skills.
   E. provision of supported housing including budgeting, laundry, and housekeeping.

9. Which of the following medications require routine monitoring of WBC counts because of the potential for bone marrow suppression?

A. Clozapine
B. Thiothixene
C. Risperidone
D. Quetiapine
E. Olanzapine

10. Of the new-generation antipsychotics, which is associated with sustained hyperprolactinemia at practically any dose?

A. Risperidone
B. Quetiapine
C. Olanzapine
D. Ziprasidone
E. Clozapine

Neurological Disorders

Section Editor: Jack J. Chen

Patient Name: Carol Galt
Address: 136 Avenue F
Age: 48   Sex: Female
Height: 5' 3"   Weight: 82 kg
Race: Caucasian
Allergies: Penicillin (rash)

Chief Complaint

CG, a 48-yo female, presents to your clinic for routine follow-up of her migraine headaches. Additionally, she was seen last night in the urgent care center for a severe migraine headache, her second one in the past 2 weeks.

History of Present Illness

Last evening, CG developed a severe pulsating headache on the right side that eventually spread throughout her head. After taking 800 mg of ibuprofen, she rested in a darkened bedroom. The pain continued to increase in severity. Two hours later she was driven to the urgent care center by her husband where she was treated with sumatriptan, with significant relief.

Past Medical History

CG has had migraine headaches since menarche (age 12). After initial diagnosis, CG has averaged 1-2 migraines per year. During college, her frequency of migraines increased to 1-2 per month. After graduation, her migraines decreased to 1-2 per year. However, in the past 2 months, CG has had 4 migraines.

Two years ago, CG was diagnosed with type 2 DM and currently takes metformin 500 mg bid. At the same time, her cholesterol and triglycerides were significantly elevated. After failing 6 months of diet therapy, CG was prescribed atorvastatin 10 mg daily.

Social History

Tobacco use: occasional

Alcohol use: none

Caffeine use: 4-5 cups of coffee per day

Family History

Father is 78 yo with type 2 DM, hypercholesterolemia, and HTN

Mother is 69 yo and healthy

Review of Systems

Negative except as noted previously

Physical Examination

GEN: Obese WF in NAD
VS: BP 140/85 mmHg, HR 72 bpm, RR 16 rpm, T 38.5°C
HEENT: WNL
CHEST: Clear to A&P
CV: NSR without murmurs
NEURO: WNL
EXT: Diabetic foot exam NL

Laboratory and Diagnostic Tests

Sodium 140 mEq/L	Potassium 4.6 mEq/L
Chloride 101 mEq/L	CO_2 content 27 mEq/L
BUN 12 mg/dL	Serum creatinine 1.0 mg/dL
FBG 184 mg/dL	Total cholesterol 224 mg/dL
Triglycerides 298 mg/dL	LDL 120 mg/dL
HDL 48 mg/dL	HbA_{1c} 7.4%

Diagnosis

Migraine headaches

Pharmacist Notes and Other Patient Information

None available.

Medication Record

Date	Rx No	Physician	Drug/Strength	Quantity	Sig	Refills
8/4	72458	Jones	Metformin 500 mg	60	1 bid	3
8/4	72457	Adams	Atorvastatin 10 mg	30	1 q hs	3
8/4	72456	Adams	HCTZ 25 mg	30	1 q am	2
7/20	68834	Adams	Ibuprofen 800 mg	100	1 q 4-6 h prn	3
7/4	62456	Adams	HCTZ 25 mg	30	1 q am	3
7/3	62124	Adams	Atorvastatin 10 mg	30	1 q hs	4
7/3	62123	Adams	Metformin 500 mg	60	1 bid	4

Questions

1. Which of the following symptoms is not typically associated with migraines?

   A. Pain
   B. Photophobia
   C. Nausea
   D. Vomiting
   E. Diarrhea

2. Upon arrival to urgent care, CG was given sumatriptan. Randomized controlled trials suggest that triptans are most effective for acute treatment of migraines when taken:

   A. daily as prophylaxis.
   B. after other agents have failed.
   C. immediately at the onset of symptoms.
   D. if pain is at its most severe.
   E. 1 hour after symptoms present.

3. Which of the following statements is true regarding the availability of triptans in the U.S.?

   A. Sumatriptan is available as a rapidly disintegrating oral tablet.
   B. Naratriptan is available as a nasal inhalation.
   C. Rizatriptan is available as a subcutaneous injection.
   D. Almotriptan is available as a rapidly disintegrating oral tablet.
   E. Zolmitriptan is available as a nasal inhalation.

4. Triptans work by which of the following mechanisms?

   A. Triptans have nonselective serotonergic effects leading to central vasodilation.
   B. Triptans inhibit prostaglandin synthesis in the CNS.
   C. Triptans act peripherally by blocking pain-impulse generation.
   D. Triptans have dopaminergic activity that affects cerebral blood flow.
   E. Triptans stimulate 5-HT 1B/1D receptors, causing vasoconstriction of the intracranial blood vessels.

5. The following are possible side effects of Migranal except:

   A. rhinitis.
   B. diarrhea.
   C. rash.
   D. dizziness.
   E. hypotension.

6. Melatonin has been shown in limited studies to be useful in the prophylaxis of certain types of headaches. Melatonin is also commonly used to treat:

   I. liver toxicity.
   II. depression.
   III. circadian rhythm disorders.

   A. I only
   B. III only
   C. I and II only
   D. II and III only
   E. I, II, and III

7. Which of the following has been shown to be effective in the prophylaxis of migraine headaches and should be recommended to CG if prophylaxis is indicated?

   A. Atenolol
   B. Calcium carbonate
   C. Dexamethasone
   D. Fentanyl transdermal patch
   E. Vitamin E

8. What nonpharmacologic recommendations would be least appropriate for CG in the setting of migraine prevention?

   A. Avoid alcohol
   B. Smoking cessation
   C. Stop drinking coffee immediately
   D. Maintain a headache diary to track precipitating factors
   E. Avoid foods with high amounts of monosodium glutamate

9. What is the trade name of sumatriptan?

   A. Amerge
   B. Axert
   C. Imitrex
   D. Maxalt
   E. Migranal

10. Which of the following is FDA pregnancy category X?

    A. Aspirin
    B. Butorphanol
    C. Dihydroergotamine
    D. Midrin
    E. Naratriptan

Patient Name: Taylor Swift
Address: 12747 Cernelu Court
Age: 52 **Sex:** Male
Height: 5' 10" **Weight:** 182 lb
Race: White, Non-Hispanic
Allergies: Morphine (nausea, vomiting)

Chief Complaint

TS is a 52-yo male who is currently in the postoperative recovery room following surgical fixation of multiple fractures. He is complaining of pain (intensity score of 8-10 out of 10 on a numeric pain scale) postoperatively.

History of Present Illness

He was involved in a recreational vehicle ("three-wheeler") accident from which he sustained multiple fractures (right tibia, right femur, and right ulna).

Past Medical History

His PMH is significant for anxiety (diagnosed approximately 5 years ago), controlled with pharmacotherapy. He also has a history of chronic kidney disease from long-standing uncontrolled hypertension and diabetes.

Social History

Tobacco use: occasional, social

Alcohol use: social, approximately 3 servings of beer/week

Caffeine use: 1-2 cups of coffee daily, occasional soft drinks

Family History

Father: hypertension, diabetes, hyperlipidemia

Mother: anemia

Review of Systems

Complaining of severe right upper and lower extremity pain

Physical Examination

GEN: WD male, slightly sedated but agitated

VS: BP 135/80 mmHg, HR 100 bpm, RR 30 rpm, T 99.0°F

HEENT: PERRLA, multiple minor lacerations on several areas of the face

CHEST: Clear to auscultation and percussion

ABD: Soft, ND, incision tender to touch

EXT: Grade II fractures of R ulna, R tibia, and R femur

NEURO: Alert and oriented x3

Laboratory and Diagnostic Tests

Sodium 135 mEq/L	Potassium 4.5 mEq/L
Chloride 101 mEq/L	CO_2 content 25 mEq/L
BUN 41 mg/dL	Serum creatinine 2.4 mg/dL
Glucose 170 mg/dL	WBC 8,000 cells/mm³
Platelets 353,000 cells/mm³	Hgb 14.1 g/dL
Hct 31.1%	PT 1.2 sec
INR 1.1	Hgb A_{1c} 8.4

CXR: Fractured collar bone, no puncture to the lung

UE XR: Grade II fracture R ulna

LE XR: Grade II fracture R tibia, R femur

Diagnosis

Primary:

Trauma with multiple fractures

Medication Record

Prior to Admission

Fluoxetine 20 mg PO Qam

Lisinopril 20 mg PO Qday

Insulin glargine 45 units SQ QHS

Regular insulin 10 units SQ with each meal

Emergency Department

Morphine 15 mg IVP x1

Metronidazole 500 mg IVPB x1

Cefazolin 1 gm IVPB x1

Operating Room

Fentanyl continuous IV infusion

Propofol IV infusion

Recovery Room

Morphine 5 mg IVP x1

Questions

1. Which of the following is most appropriate initial analgesic therapy for TS?

   A. Intermittent IM morphine q 6 h prn
   B. Fentanyl 25 mcg/hour patch applied every 72 hours
   C. Intravenous morphine patient-controlled analgesia
   D. Darvocet N-100 2 tablets q 6 h prn
   E. Meperidine IV q 6 h prn

2. What parameter should be considered when placing TS on morphine PCA?

   A. His weight since morphine doses are calculated on mg/kg basis
   B. The maximum daily morphine dose recommended by the manufacturer
   C. PCA dosing regimen, which includes the self-administered dose, lock-out interval, and hourly dose limit
   D. His drug allergy
   E. C & D

3. Given TS' medical history, which of the following medications should not be used for analgesia long term?

   A. Meperidine
   B. Tramadol
   C. Morphine
   D. Hydromorphone
   E. Acetaminophen as an adjunct to opioids

4. Two weeks after his accident and continuous analgesic therapy, TS is ready for discharge. His physician would like to convert his pain medications to an oral regimen. The total daily dose of morphine 60 mg IV has been sufficient in controlling his pain. What is the equivalent conversion from IV morphine to an oral regimen?

   A. Morphine 15 mg po q 6 h prn
   B. Oxycodone 20 mg po q 4 h prn
   C. Morphine 30 mg po q 4 h prn
   D. Hydromorphone 2 mg po q 6 h prn
   E. Hydromorphone 4 mg po q 4 h prn

5. TS' physician would like to transition him to a sustained-release product in which the total daily dose can be administered once or twice daily. The total daily dose of which listed regimen may be converted to a sustained-release product (of the same opioid) to be given once or twice daily?

   I. Morphine 15 mg po q 6 h prn
   II. Oxycodone 5 mg po q 6 h prn
   III. Morphine 30 mg po q 6 h prn

   A. I only
   B. III only
   C. I and II only
   D. II and III only
   E. I, II, and III

6. What is important to discuss with TS regarding sustained-release morphine prior to his discharge?

   A. It is important to take a laxative with this pain medication because it may cause constipation.
   B. Acetaminophen cannot be used with this opioid analgesic.
   C. Promethazine will help the nausea and potentiates the analgesic effects this medication.
   D. If a dose is missed close to the next scheduled dose, an additional dose may be taken.
   E. Take this pain medication only as needed, at the onset of pain.

7. The mechanism by which opioid analgesics are believed to provide analgesic activity is:

   I. via opioid receptors in the brain.
   II. via opioid receptors in the spinal column.
   III. via opioid receptors in gastrointestinal tract.

   A. I only
   B. III only
   C. I and II only
   D. II and III only
   E. I, II, and III

8. Morphine PCA was ordered at your pharmacy. The PCA was compounded by taking 0.6 mL of a 50 mg/mL morphine solution and diluted it with normal saline to total volume of 30 mL. What is the final concentration of the morphine PCA prepared?

   A. 1 mg/mL
   B. 2 mg/mL
   C. 3 mg/mL
   D. 5 mg/mL
   E. 10 mg/mL

9. TS' wife is concerned about TS becoming addicted to his opioid analgesic. You assure her that when opioid analgesics are used correctly for pain, the addiction rate is:

   A. 50 percent.
   B. 40 percent.
   C. 25 percent.
   D. 10 percent.
   E. <1 percent.

Case 40

10. After poor control of TS' pain, a pain consultant initiates him on a continuous IV infusion of hydromorphone with as needed hydromorphone boluses based on TS' verbal pain score. Two hours after receiving the continuous IV hydromorphone, TS fell asleep. His nurse is concerned and contacts the physician responsible for his care. What should be done at this point?

   A. Switch to another opioid
   B. Administer naloxone
   C. Examine TS, check vital signs, confirm proper dose is administered, and monitor
   D. Administer a stimulant
   E. Discontinue therapy immediately

Patient Name: Monroe Fjord
Address: 11205 Loma Avenue
Age: 72   **Sex:** Male
Height: 5' 10"   **Weight:** 180 lb
Race: Caucasian
Allergies: Bromocriptine (rash)

Chief Complaint

MF comes into the pharmacy to pick up his prescriptions. He is accompanied by his wife, who states that MF has been "behaving strange lately" and is "imagining little children in the house." In addition, the wife states that over the past month, MF's urine appears to be darker than usual.

History of Present Illness

MF has advanced Parkinson's disease and requires assistance to perform his activities of daily living. Several years ago, MF began to experience worsening "wearing off" (end-of-dose failure) while on carbidopa/levodopa. His wife reports that the carbidopa/levodopa "just wore off after a couple of hours." However, after modifications to the carbidopa/levodopa dose and the eventual addition of pramipexole, entacapone, and apomorphine over the years, the problem improved. In addition to wearing off, MF also developed moderate dyskinesias. However, after several medication adjustments, such as variations in carbidopa/levodopa dosage reduction, the dyskinesias also improved. His wife states that although MF requires assistance with his activities of daily living, he had remained "sharp as a whistle" until recently. Within the past 3 months, MF has begun to experience visual hallucinations consisting of images of young children appearing in the living room. MF does not realize the children are hallucinations and is often startled by them. On other occasions he tries to talk to them. This is complicated by the fact that MF has begun to exhibit uncooperative behavior toward his wife and is accusing her of having an extramarital affair with his brother (who is deceased). Although MF has not made any gestures or threats of harm, his wife is having great difficulty looking after him and is feeling helpless.

Medication Record

Past Medical History

1) Parkinson's disease

2) Depression

3) Benign prostatic hypertrophy

4) Chronic hepatitis C

Social History

Occupation: retired, formerly a mechanic

Martial status: married; one son; one daughter

Tobacco use: quit 20 years ago

Alcohol use: none

Caffeine use: none

Family History

Father had "tremor"

Review of System

GEN: Well-developed, well-nourished white male

Neurologic exam: Findings as noted

Physical Examination

Neurologic: Moderate bilateral rigidity in all extremities, mild bilateral rest and postural tremor in upper extremities, slow finger taps, bradykinetic ambulation, postural instability. Remainder of examination unremarkable.

Laboratory and Diagnostic Tests

ALT 88 U/L

AST 69 U/L

Date	Rx No	Physician	Drug/Strength	Quantity	Sig	Refills
6/27	56018	Coutet	Finasteride 5 mg	30	1 po qd	1
6/27	56015	Suduiraut	Entacapone 200 mg	120	1 po qid	2
6/27	56016	Suduiraut	Rasagiline 1 mg	30	1 po qd	1
6/27	56013	Suduiraut	Carbidopa/levodopa 25/100 mg	120	1 po qid	2
6/27	56017	Coutet	Sertraline 50 mg	30	1 po qd	2
6/27	56014	Suduiraut	Pramipexole 1 mg	90	1 po tid	2

Case 41

 Diagnosis

1) Parkinson's disease

2) Depression

3) Benign prostatic hypertrophy

4) Chronic hepatitis C

 Pharmacist Notes and Other Patient Information

None available.

Questions

1. When educating MF on his pramipexole (Mirapex) prescription, which of the following statements would be appropriate?
   I. May cause nausea
   II. May cause drowsiness
   III. Do not take dairy products, antacids, or iron preparations within 1 hour of this medication

   A. I only
   B. III only
   C. I and II only
   D. II and III only
   E. I, II, and III

2. Given MF's concurrent benign prostatic hypertrophy, which of the following should be avoided or used with caution?
   A. Pramipexole
   B. Rasagiline
   C. Ropinirole
   D. Selegiline
   E. Trihexyphenidyl

3. In general, if the frequency of administration of MF's carbidopa/levodopa is increased to 5 times per day, his entacapone frequency of administration should be:
   A. unchanged.
   B. changed to qd.
   C. changed to bid.
   D. changed to tid.
   E. changed to 5 times per day.

4. The prescribing clinician believes that some medications may be causing MF's hallucinations and delusions. You agree. He would like to adjust the antiparkinsonian medications and asks for your advice. You recommend to:
   A. add selegiline.
   B. increase rasagiline dose.
   C. reduce the pramipexole dose.
   D. increase the pramipexole dose.
   E. increase carbidopa/levodopa dose.

5. If MF requires therapy for the hallucinations/psychosis, which of the following is an antipsychotic and can be recommended?
   A. Amitriptyline
   B. Chlorpromazine
   C. Citalopram
   D. Haloperidol
   E. Quetiapine

6. Which of the following will result in plasma accumulation of pramipexole?
   A. Renal impairment
   B. Hepatic impairment
   C. Inhibition of dopa decarboxylase
   D. Inhibition of monoamine oxidase type B
   E. Inhibition of catechol-O-methyltransferase

7. Which of the following medications is most commonly associated with urine discoloration?
   A. Benztropine
   B. Carbidopa/levodopa
   C. Entacapone
   D. Pramipexole
   E. Rasagiline

8. Which of the following statements regarding Stalevo is FALSE?
   A. It should be administered together with Comtan.
   B. Only one Stalevo tablet should be administered at each dosing interval.
   C. It bears FDA-approved labeling for the management of end-of-dose wearing-off.
   D. Product formulation contains a 1:4 ratio of carbidopa/levodopa + 200 mg of entacapone.
   E. It contains drugs that block both major enzymes involved in levodopa metabolism.

9. Which of the following regarding levodopa-induced dyskinesias is true?

    A. Can be exacerbated by the addition of entacapone
    B. Commonly associated with trough levels of levodopa
    C. Management may consist of increasing the levodopa dose
    D. Management may consist of adding an anticholinergic agent
    E. Management may consist of adding an atypical antipsychotic

10. Instead of sertraline, which of the following antidepressant agents also would be appropriate for MF given his medical and medication history as documented on 6/27?

    I.   Citalopram
    II.   Phenelzine
    III. Amitriptyline

    A. I only
    B. III only
    C. I and II only
    D. II and III only

Patient Name: Steven Booker
Address: 1485 Hampton Place
Age: 12   **Sex:** Male
Height: 4' 8"   **Weight:** 42 kg
Race: Caucasian
Allergies: Sulfa (hives)

Chief Complaint

SB is a 12-yo WM who was brought to the emergency room for a seizure that lasted 3-5 minutes while playing in a soccer game.

History of Present Illness

During the second half of the soccer game, SB fell to the ground, was stiff at first, and then began having rhythmic contractions of his arms and legs. EMS was called to the scene. The mother reports that the seizure only lasted about 3-5 minutes. She was not able to get his attention during the seizure and he would not look at her when she called his name. After the seizure stopped, SB was very confused and wanted to go to sleep.

In the ER 2 hours later, SB has another witnessed seizure involving both arms and legs that lasted 2 minutes. SB again lost consciousness. No medication was needed to stop the seizure.

His mother reports SB had 1 seizure about 4 months ago. It occurred one morning and he was rushed to the ER. Test results were fine and he was released without any medication the next day.

Mom reports no sick contacts recently and that SB has been feeling fine and eating like normal.

He is a very active boy and loves soccer. The pediatric emergency department physician believes SB is having generalized tonic-clonic seizures and admits the child for observation and neurology consult.

Past Medical History

Chicken pox at 7 years old, mild persistent asthma diagnosed at age 8, ADHD diagnosed at age 10, one seizure 4 months ago

Immunizations: UTD

Social History

SB lives with both parents in a single-story home along with 3 brothers and sisters. He rides his bike to school daily and enjoys playing soccer on the weekends.

Family History

Father has diabetes mellitus type 2. Brother had febrile seizures growing up but none since age 5.

Review of Systems

Negative except as noted previously

Physical Examination

GEN: Well-appearing male, sleepy but arousable, no acute distress

VS: T 97.3°F, HR 72 bpm, RR 22 rpm, BP 99/65 mmHg, O_2 sat. 99% room air, Wt. 42 kg

HEENT: PERRLA, EOMA, moist membranes, oral mucosa clear, no hemorrhages, exudates, or papilledema

CHEST: Lungs clear to auscultation & percussion bilaterally

CV: RRR, NL heart sounds, no murmur

ABD: Positive bowel sounds, no masses, soft

GU: WNL

NEURO: Symmetric, positive reflexes

Laboratory and Diagnostic Tests

(In ER)

Sodium 136 mEq/L	Potassium 4.1 mEq/L
Chloride 101 mEq/L	CO_2 content 25 mEq/L
BUN 14 mg/dL	Creatinine 0.5 mg/dL
Calcium 10.1 mEq/L	Glucose 94 mg/dL
WBC 9.4 mm³	RBC 4.8 mm³
HCT 38.5%	Hgb 13.7g/dL
Platelet 305 mm³	Neutrophils 54%
Eosinophils 3%	Lymphocytes 38%
Monocytes 4%	Basophils 1%

CT scan: no affirmative focal lesions identified

EEG: slow, generalized pattern

Tox screen: negative

U/A: clear

Diagnosis

Primary: Probable generalized tonic-clonic seizures

Secondary: ADHD, asthma

 Medication Record

(Home Medication)

Albuterol MDI 2 puffs q4h PRN wheeze/cough

Flovent 110 mcg MDI 1 puff BID

Adderall XR 20 mg PO daily

(On Admission)

Lorazepam 2 mg IV PRN seizure lasting > 5 minutes

Albuterol MDI 2 puffs q4h PRN wheeze/cough

Flovent 110 mcg MDI 1 puff BID

 Pharmacist Notes and Other Patient Information

None available.

Questions

1. SB is started on carbamazepine 100 mg chew tabs and complains that the chew tab does not taste good. His mother asks if there is another form of carbamazepine that SB could try. Which of the following is true regarding carbamazepine formulations?

    A. There is an extended-release tablet or capsule that SB could take, but swallow whole.
    B. There is a citrus-vanilla–flavored suspension but SB will have to take this three or four times a day.
    C. There is an extended-release capsule that can be opened and placed on applesauce.
    D. The extended-release tablets should be dosed twice daily.
    E. All of the above.

2. The nurse asks if the generic carbamazepine that she is administering to SB is equivalent to the brand name Tegretol. She asks where you can find this information to determine generic equivalence. Which of the following sources do you recommend?

    A. Package insert
    B. Lexi-Comp Drug Information Handbook

    C. AHFS Drug Information
    D. FDA's Orange Book
    E. Neofax

3. The nurse then asks you how much she should give the patient. Lorazepam is available in a 2 mg/mL and 4 mg/mL vials. The nurse has the 4 mg/mL vial in her hand. How many mL do you tell her to administer to the patient?

    A. 0.5 mL
    B. 1 mL
    C. 1.5 mL
    D. 2 mL
    E. 2.5 mL

4. SB tolerates his carbamazepine therapy in the hospital and the neurologist decides to place him on chronic therapy. When would you have SB return to clinic to have a carbamazepine level obtained?

    A. 3 days
    B. 7 days
    C. 14 days
    D. 28 days
    E. 2 months

5. SB and his family need to be counseled on carbamazepine use. Which of the following adverse effects do you NOT include in your counseling session to the family?

    A. Carbamazepine may cause a rash. If he develops one, stop the medication and call the neurologist.
    B. SB may experience some dizziness and drowsiness on initiation and at times of dose increases.
    C. Carbamazepine may cause an increase in kidney stone formation. SB should stay well hydrated, especially when playing soccer.
    D. SB can take his carbamazepine with food if it upsets his stomach.
    E. If he starts any other medication, his neurologist and pharmacist need to be notified.

6. SB returns to clinic and has his carbamazepine level drawn. What is the therapeutic concentration range for carbamazepine?

    A. 1-5 mcg/mL
    B. 4-12 mcg/mL
    C. 10-20 mcg/mL
    D. 10-40 mcg/mL
    E. No therapeutic range is defined. Clinical outcome does not correlate to levels.

Case 42

7. What if SB's mother had presented with complaints of him staring into space for short periods of time where he was not responsive? What type of seizure is this characteristic of?

    A. Complex partial seizures
    B. Simple partial seizures
    C. Myoclonic seizures
    D. Absence seizures
    E. Atonic seizures

8. Four months later, SB returns to the neurologist. SB has had 3 seizures on carbamazepine monotherapy. The neurologist is debating whether to change monotherapy drugs or add an adjunct agent. Given SB's allergy history, which of the following anticonvulsants should NOT be considered when adjusting SB's current therapy?

    A. Lamotrigine
    B. Topiramate
    C. Phenytoin
    D. Valproic acid
    E. Zonisamide

9. Which of the following supplement should SB take while on anticonvulsant therapy?

    A. Vitamin C
    B. Vitamin D
    C. Vitamin B_{12}
    D. Vitamin B_3
    E. Vitamin E

10. SB's mom asks if he will ever come off anticonvulsant therapy completely and if so, when? You reply that SB may be given a trial off his medication when all of the following are met EXCEPT:

    A. SB must be seizure free for at least 2 years.
    B. SB must have an EEG that normalized with treatment.
    C. SB has only one seizure type.
    D. SB has remained on the same dose of medication for the last 6 months.
    E. SB has a normal IQ.

Neoplastic Disorders

Section Editor: Joseph Bubalo

Patient Name: Peter Lemon
Address: 123 Fletch Street
Age: 60   **Height:** 6' 0"
Weight: 178 lb   **Sex:** Male
Race: Caucasian
Allergies: NKDA

Chief Complaint

Stage IIIA IgA multiple myeloma. Admitted to hospital for high-dose melphalan on days -3 and -2 and autologous peripheral blood stem cell rescue on day 0.

History of Present Illness

Approximately 1 year previous, PL was found to have a pathologic fracture of left humerus, which was subsequently surgically repaired. Further workup revealed hypercalcemia (serum calcium: 11 mg/dL, serum albumin 4.1 g/dL) and serum IgA value of 1489 mg/dL. Bone marrow biopsy revealed 50% plasma cells. Skeletal bone survey demonstrated multiple lytic lesions in skull and thoracic vertebrae. The patient then received four cycles of lenalidomide plus low-dose dexamethasone. All four cycles were tolerated without serious adverse events. Posttreatment serum IgA level was 200 mg/dL with repeat bone marrow biopsy result showing 6% plasma cells, thus demonstrating a very good partial response to initial chemotherapy.

Social History

Retired New York City police officer. Fifteen pack-year tobacco history, quit 10 years ago. Alcohol only socially. No history of illicit substances. Married with four adult children, all healthy.

Family History

1) Father died from non-small cell lung cancer at age 64.

2) Mother died from acute myocardial infarction at age 68.

3) Brother died from non-small cell lung cancer at age 63.

All were heavy smokers up until time of death.

Review of Systems

Except as listed elsewhere in the history, all systems are negative

Physical Exam

GEN: Well-developed male in no apparent distress. Height is 72 in and weight is 178 lb. Tmax: 37.2°C, BP 128/83 mmHg, pulse 88 bpm, RR 18 rpm, pain score is 1/10.

HEENT: Grossly normal. PERRLA, EOMI. No sinus tenderness, normal funduscopic exam. Mucus membranes moist. No oral lesions.

NECK: Supple with normal ROM, no JVD, no carotid bruits, no thyromegaly.

CHEST: Clear to auscultation and percussion bilaterally. No rhonchi or rales appreciated. Triple-lumen central venous catheter present on right side of chest.

HEART: Regular rate and rhythm; no S_3 or S_4; no murmur, gallops, or rubs.

ABD: Soft, nontender. No palpable hepatosplenomegaly. Bowel sounds present and active in all 4 quadrants.

GU: Deferred

SKIN: No rash

NEURO: Grossly intact. Cranial nerves II thru XII intact. DTR present and symmetric in all extremities.

Laboratory Tests

Sodium 144 mEq/L	Chloride 106 mEq/L
BUN 9 mg/dL	Potassium 4.3 mEq/L
CO_2 29 mEq/L	Creatinine 0.9 mg/dL
Glucose 95 mg/dL	Albumin 3.6 g/dL
Calcium 8.6 mg/dL	Magnesium 1.7 mEq/L
Phosphate 2.2 mg/dL	WBC 4.37 x 10^3 cells/mm³
Hgb 12.9 g/dL	Hct 35.9%
Platelet count 238,000/µL	INR 1.0
Prothrombin time 11.2 sec	Protein 6.6 g/dL
Bilirubin total 0.7 mg/dL	AST 24 U/L
ALT 14 U/L	LDH 531 U/L
TSH 1.3 µU/mL	

24-hour measured creatinine clearance 115 mL/min

Diagnosis

Primary:

1) Stage IIIA IgA multiple myeloma

Secondary:

1) Major depression   2) Osteoarthritis

3) Benign prostatic hyperplasia   4) Hypothyroidism

Medical Note :

Chemotherapy regimen:

Melphalan 100 mg/m^2 IV on days -3 and -2

Ondansetron 24 mg po daily on days -3, -2, and -1

Dexamethasone 18 mg po daily on days -3, -2, and -1

Lorazepam 1 mg po/IV q 6 h PRN nausea/vomiting

Haloperidol 1 mg po/IV q 6 h PRN nausea/vomiting

Medications started on day -1:

Levofloxacin 500 mg 1 po daily

Fluconazole 200 mg 1 po daily

Acyclovir 800 mg 1 po BID

Normal saline rinses 15-mL swish and expectorate TID

 ## Pharmacist Note

10/10: All home medications verified with patient and mail order pharmacy where patient obtains medications. Patient orders prescriptions "like clockwork" from pharmacy.

10/10: Chemotherapy regimen checked and approved by clinical and compounding pharmacist.

 ## Medication Record

Date	Rx No	Physician	Drug/Strength	Quantity	Sig	Refills
7/10	27861	Babar	Sertraline 100 mg		1 po daily in the morning	
4/10	27710	Babar	Terazosin 10 mg		1 po daily at bedtime	
6/09	27368	Rosenrosen	Acetaminophen 1000 mg		1 po q 12 h	
6/09	27369	Rosenrosen	Levothyroxine 0.1 mg		1 po daily in the morning	
7/09	27869	Babar	Zolpidem 10 mg		1 po q hs prn insomnia	

Questions

1. Which of the following agents may decrease time to recovery of neutrophil count following high-dose chemotherapy?

    A. Filgrastim

    B. Darbopoietin

    C. Oprelvekin

    D. Rituximab

    E. Vancomycin

2. On day +7 (i.e., 7 days after stem cells were infused), PL has a temperature of 38.4°C with an increase in HR to 101 bpm. His blood pressure remains stable. Labs are as follows:

WBC: 0.01 k/μL, Plt: 18 k/μL, Na: 132, K: 3, BUN: 21, SCr: 1.2, T. bili: 0.6, AST: 23, ALT: 28.
What is most likely occurring in this patient?

    A. Neutropenic fever

    B. Delayed reaction from melphalan

    C. Febrile seizures

    D. Effects of bone marrow engraftment

    E. Adverse reaction from acyclovir

3. The chemotherapy order for PL states:
"Melphalan 200 mg/m$_2$ IV divided over 2 doses given daily."
What is the correct dose for PL?

Case 43

A. 400 mg IV q12 hr on day -3 at 0800 and 2000
B. 400 mg IV once daily on day -3 and day -2
C. 200 mg IV once daily on day -3 and day -2
D. 220 mg IV once daily on day -3 and day -2
E. 440 mg IV q12 hr on day -3 at 0800 and 2000

4. Which of the following medications would be best to give before melphalan to decrease incidence of nausea and vomiting?

A. Prochlorperazine 10 mg and haloperidol 1 mg
B. Metoclopramide 10 mg, diphenhydramine 50 mg, and ranitidine 150 mg
C. Granisetron 1 mg and prednisone 20 mg
D. Lorazepam 1mg, promethazine 25 mg, and dexamethasone 10 mg
E. Ondansetron 16mg, dexamethasone 20 mg, and lorazepam 1 mg

5. If neutropenic fever is suspected, which antibacterial(s) would be best choice?

A. Change levofloxacin to IV and add ceftriaxone IV
B. Add dicloxacillin po and gentamicin IV
C. Add cefazolin IV and ceftazidime IV
D. Add voriconazole IV
E. Discontinue levofloxacin; add vancomycin IV and cefepime IV

6. Which drug, when reconstituted, has short stability (less than 1 hour)?

A. Levofloxacin
B. Melphalan
C. Vancomycin
D. Dexamethasone
E. Lorazepam

7. Which of the following medications may reduce the incidence and duration of chemotherapy-induced oral mucositis when started prior to chemotherapy?

A. Viscous lidocaine
B. Becaplermin
C. Mesna
D. Palifermin
E. Dexamethasone

8. When counseling the patient regarding upcoming chemotherapy, which of the following would likely be a side effect of high-dose melphalan?

A. Skin rash
B. Hemorrhagic cystitis
C. Mucositis
D. Constipation
E. Tinnitus

9. When counseling the patient regarding side effects of filgrastim, what would you recommend to the patient to relieve bone pain?

A. Elevate legs
B. Apply cold compresses
C. Apply lidocaine patch to painful area
D. Administer diphenhydramine as it may be allergic reaction
E. Administer oxycodone

10. Which medication that PL was taking prior to admission should he stop taking and why?

A. Sertraline: transplant can cure him of cancer and, therefore, his depression
B. Acetaminophen: may mask some signs of fever
C. Zolpidem: may decrease effect of antinausea medications due to competitive inhibition
D. Acetaminophen: transplantation will decrease immune-mediated damage to joints
E. Terazosin: may interact with melphalan to decrease effect

Patient Name: Agnes Hall
Address: 124 South Street
Age: 65   **Sex:** Female
Height: 5' 5"   **Weight:** 176 lb
Race: Caucasian
Allergies: Penicillin (rash), Keflex (hives), iodine (unknown)

Chief Complaint

AH is a 65-yo white female who presents to the oncology clinic after falling and fracturing her hip while gardening.

History of Present Illness

AH presents to the oncology clinic after fracturing her hip. She had been gardening outside when she fell. She originally had the hip examined by her local family physician. An x-ray was performed that showed several osteolytic bone lesions present in her hip, femur, and spine. It was recommended she follow-up with her local oncologist due to suspicion of metastatic breast cancer. The oncology clinic performed a nuclear bone scan, chest x-ray, MRI of the abdomen, and blood work. The bone scan showed increased uptake in the L4 and L5 spine as well as the femur and right ileum. MRI of the abdomen reported a lesion in the liver suspicious for metastatic disease. All other workup was negative.

Past Medical History

AH was diagnosed with breast cancer 4 years ago. Her original tumor was a 2.3-cm adenocarcinoma (Stage IIa, T^2, No, Mo) with no metastasis noted at the time of resection. Hormonal receptors were estrogen receptor-85% (+), progesterone receptor-10% (+), and Her2/neu (IHC 2+, FISH+). She received adjuvant chemotherapy consisting of AC (Adriamycin and Cytoxan) x 6 cycles. She then took Tamoxifen for 3 years before stopping on her own. AH was also diagnosed with heart failure 2 years ago. She suffers from severe migraine headaches and occasional GERD. AH experienced menarche at age 12 and is Gravida$_2$, Para$_2$, Ab$_0$. She was 24 years old at the time of her first child's birth. She stopped menstruating at age 53 and took 5 years of hormonal replacement therapy. She has no history of oral contraceptive usage.

Social History

AH has been married for 46 years and works as a financial consultant at a local bank. She drinks an occasional glass of red wine and was a 15 pack/year smoker, quitting 26 years ago.

Family History

Mother diagnosed with breast cancer at age 70, died age 75.

Father died of a CVA at age 62.

Review of Systems

AH complains of increasing fatigue, which she attributes to not sleeping at night due to increasing pain in her lumbar spine. Her pain at night can increase up to a 7 or 8 out of 10, while during the day the pain decreases to the severity of 4 out of 10. AH continues to have migraine headaches that are becoming more frequent and severe. They are associated with nausea. She has occasional GERD symptoms when she eats fried or spicy food and is currently asymptomatic from her heart failure.

Physical Examination

General: Well-developed, well-nourished female in no apparent distress.

Vital Signs: BP 122/80, HR 72 bpm, RR 15 rpm, T 36.6°C, Ht 165.1 cm, Wt 82.3 kg. Oxygen saturation of 99% on room air, pain currently is 4/10.

HEENT: Normal, no palpable lymph nodes, fundi benign, throat is clear

Chest: Regular rate and rhythm; no rubs, murmurs, or gallops

Breasts: Without masses and symmetrical

Abdomen: Soft and without direct or rebound tenderness

Extremities: Normal with no edema

Neuro: Normal II through XII intact, normal cerebellar function

Laboratory and Diagnostic Tests

Sodium 143 mEq/L	Potassium 4.5 mEq/L
Chloride 108 mEq/L	CO_2 24 mEq/L
Magnesium 2.3 mg/dL	Calcium 9 mg/dL
BUN 9 mg/dL	Serum creatinine 0.7 mg/dL
Glucose 111 mg/dL	Phosphorous 3.1 mg/dL
Albumin 4.1 g/dL	CEA 54 ng/mL
T. bili 0.7 mg/dL	AlkPhos 170 U/mL
LDH 570 U/mL	SGPT 21 U/mL

WBC 5100 cells/mm³ with 73% PMN, 20% lymphocytes,

Case 44

6% monocytes, 2% eosinophils, 1% basophils

Hemoglobin 12.7 g/dL   Hematocrit 36.6%

Platelets 241,000 cells/mm³

MUGA: Ejection fraction was 44%

MRI Abdomen: Hypodensity located in the posterior portion of the right lobe of the liver worrisome for malignancy

Nuclear bone scan: Lesions in L4 and L5 vertebral bodies most likely representing metastatic disease

 ## Diagnosis

Metastatic breast cancer

 ## Pharmacist Notes and Other Patient Information

None available.

 ## Medication Record

Date	Rx No	Physician	Drug/Strength	Sig	Quantity	Refills
3/19	2925668	Fisher	Furosemide 20 mg	1 PO daily	30	6
3/19	2925667	Fisher	Lisinopril 10 mg	1 PO daily	30	6
5/13	2915620	Fisher	Hydrocodone/APAP 5/500 mg	1 PO Q4-6h PRN back pain	60	1
3/19	2925669	Fisher	Potassium chloride 10 mEq	1 PO daily	30	6
5/13	2901274	Johns	Sumatriptan 50 mg	1 PO at onset of headache. May repeat x 1	9	2
3/19	2925666	Fisher	Omeprazole 20 mg	1 PO daily	30	6

Questions

1. Which hormonal therapy option would be the most appropriate for AH?

   A. Tamoxifen 20 mg PO daily
   B. Faslodex (fulvestrant) 250 mg IM Q month
   C. Zoladex (goserelin) 3.6 mg SQ Q month
   D. Arimidex (anastrozole) 1 mg PO daily
   E. Megestrol acetate 40 mg PO QID

2. Which bisphosphonate(s) would be appropriate for treating her bone metastases?

   I. Zometa 4 mg IVPB over 15 minutes Q 3-4 weeks
   II. Aredia 90 mg IVPB over 2 hours Q 3-4 weeks
   III. Fosamax 70 mg PO Q week

   A. I only
   B. III only
   C. I and II only
   D. II and III only
   E. I, II, and III

3. Which adverse effect is not associated with Zometa therapy?

   A. Leg edema
   B. Renal toxicity
   C. Osteonecrosis of the jaw
   D. Hypomagnesemia and hypophosphatemia
   E. Ototoxicity

4. Which additional OTC product should AH ensure she is taking when initiating bisphosphonate therapy?

   A. Centrum Silver 1 tablet PO daily
   B. Vitamin D 400 IU PO daily
   C. Elemental calcium 500 mg PO daily + vitamin D 400 IU PO daily
   D. Aspirin 81 mg PO daily
   E. Elemental calcium 500 mg PO daily

5. Calculate an appropriate trastuzumab (Herceptin) dosage?

A. Herceptin 640 mg IVPB in 250 mL NS over 90 minutes Q 3 weeks

B. Herceptin 640 mg IVPB in 250 mL NS over 90 minutes loading dose on week 1, followed by 480 mg IVPB in 250 mL NS over 30 minutes Q week starting on week 2

C. Herceptin 320 mg IVPB in 250 mL NS over 90 minutes loading dose on week 1, followed by 160 mg IVPB in 250 mL NS over 30 minutes Q week starting on week 2

D. Herceptin 320 mg IVPB in 250 mL NS over 90 minutes loading dose on week 1, followed by 160 mg IVPB in 250 mL NS over 30 minutes Q 3 weeks starting on week 4

E. Herceptin 320 mg IVPB in 250 mL NS over 90 minutes Q week

6. Patients with which of the following WOULD NOT be good candidates for Herceptin (trastuzumab) therapy?

A. Her2/neu positivity
B. Metastatic breast cancer
C. Class III heart failure
D. Node positive breast cancer needing adjuvant treatment
E. Renal failure

7. AH's progressive disease is making her symptomatic. Initiation of chemotherapy is recommended. AH is concerned about developing an infection due to low blood counts. What advice would be inappropriate to give AH about neutropenia?

A. Wait 48 hours prior to calling the clinic if you're having diarrhea, nausea, or vomiting.
B. If you develop a fever of 100.4°F, call the clinic immediately.
C. Avoid large crowds and sick people, especially children.
D. Avoid eating undercooked fish, chicken, and meat.
E. Diligently take prophylactic medications for prevention of viral, fungal, and bacterial infections if prescribed.

8. What analgesic would be effective in managing AH's cancer-related bone pain?

I. Neurontin 600 mg PO TID
II. Dexamethasone 4 mg PO Q 12h
III. Naproxen 500 mg PO Q 12h

A. I only
B. III only
C. I and II only
D. II and III only
E. I, II, and III

9. Which statement is inappropriate information to tell AH about starting an opioid regimen?

A. Constipation can be a problematic side effect and is often managed with a stool softener/stimulant laxative, such as Senokot-S.
B. Urinary retention is a rare side effect. If it does occur, all opioid medications must be stopped.
C. Pruritus is a common side effect and can be managed with Benadryl PO since it is histamine related.
D. Opioids can make you drowsy. Do not operate machinery or drive after taking medication.
E. Nausea and vomiting may occur. Be sure to take your medication with food or milk.

10. If the patient were to become refractory to her hormonal therapy or symptomatic from her cancer, it would be appropriate to add chemotherapy. Which agent is NOT FDA-approved for treatment of breast cancer?

A. Taxol (paclitaxel) 80 mg/m^2 IVPB over 1 hour Q week
B. Gemzar (gemcitabine) 1000 mg/m^2 IVPB over 30 min, days 1 and 8
C. Cytosar-U (cytarabine) 3000 mg/m^2 IVPB over 1 hour Q 12h x 6 doses
D. Taxotere (docetaxel) 75 mg/m^2 IVPB over 1 hour Q 3 weeks
E. Xeloda (capecitabine) 1250 mg/m^2 PO BID 14 days on, 7 days off as a 21-day cycle

Patient Name: Edward Anderson
Address: 25 Park Street
Age: 68   **Sex:** Male
Height: 5' 10"   **Weight:** 71.8 kg
Race: African American
Allergies: Penicillin (rash)

 ## Chief Complaint

EA is a 68-yo male who returns to the clinic 3 weeks after completing his first course of cisplatin and etoposide for small-cell lung cancer (SCLC). He states that he was extremely nauseated the first few days after receiving his chemotherapy.

 ## History of Present Illness

This patient was seen in the ED approximately 1 month ago after being involved in a motor vehicle accident (MVA). After complaining of right-sided rib pain, a chest x-ray was obtained and the patient was found to have a right anterior rib fracture as well as an incidental finding of a left hilar mass and postobstructive pneumonia. He was sent to his PCP and worked up for possible lung cancer. Bronchoscopy with biopsy and the CT of the chest confirmed the diagnosis of limited disease SCLC. Over the years, he has had several episodes of pneumonia; all were treated successfully with antibiotics. For the past 10 months he has had a nonproductive cough. Every once in awhile he does cough up some white-colored sputum that sometimes has a tinge of reddish-brown in it. Five years ago, he noticed he was more short of breath and his physician diagnosed him with mild CHF. The shortness of breath has worsened recently in the last few months and he has noticed problems with climbing more than two flights of stairs. His wife states that his appetite is not what it used to be, and that he has lost approximately 15 lb over the past 3 or 4 months.

 ## Past Medical History

EA was diagnosed with CHF 5 years ago after complaining of mild shortness of breath and retention of fluid. This has been well controlled with medication. The remainder of his history is unremarkable other than constipation and hemorrhoids. Today, he is scheduled to receive his second course of chemotherapy.

 ## Social History

Tobacco use: 55 pack-year history; quit following the diagnosis of lung cancer

Alcohol use: 1-2 servings of beer a week

Illicit drug use: none

 ## Family History

Sister died of colon cancer at age 54. The other sister is alive with breast cancer. Father died of MI at age 61.

 ## Review of Systems

Complains of occasional pain from rib fracture and nonproductive cough. Denies headache, diplopia, or blurred vision.

 ## Physical Examination

GEN: Pale, cachectic male in NAD

VS: BP 148/85 mmHg, HR 92 bpm, RR 27 rpm, T 37.9°C, Wt 71.8 kg, Ht 177.8 cm, BSA 1.88 mm²

HEENT: Head atraumatic and normocephalic, PERRLA, oropharynx nonerythematous and without mucositis

LUNGS: Decreased breath sounds and wheezes bilaterally

CV: RRR, no murmurs

EXT: No signs of clubbing, cyanosis, or edema

NEURO: A&O x3

LYMPHS: Negative

 ## Laboratory and Diagnostic Tests

Sodium 139 mEq/L	Potassium 3.9 mEq/L
Chloride 111 mEq/L	CO_2 content 29 mEq/L
BUN 15 mg/dL	Serum creatinine 1.2 mg/dL
Glucose 89 mg/dL	T. bili 1.0 mg/dL
LDH 386 u/L	Alk phos 86 u/L
SGPT 48 u/L	Calcium 8.2 mg/dL
Inorganic phos 3.5 mg/dL	Albumin 2.5 g/dL

WBC 4500 cells/mm³ with 72% neutrophils, 23% lymphocytes, 5% monocytes

Hgb 10.2 g/dL	Hct 35.8 %

Platelets 204,000 cells/mm³

CXR: Postobstructive pneumonia, left hilar mass, and right anterior rib fracture

CT chest: 6 x 3 x 2 cm mediastinal mass with postobstructive pneumonia

CT abdomen: Negative for metastasis

CT brain: Negative for metastasis

Bone scan: Only significant for rib fracture from MVA

Bronchoscopy: Microbiology significant for *Klebsiella* pneumonia. Pathology significant for small-cell lung cancer

 ## Diagnosis

Small cell Lung Cancer

 ## Medication Record

Colace 100 mg, 1 po bid prn constipation (physician orders)

Cisplatin 75 mg/m^2 IV on day 1, q 21 days (for 4 cycles)

Etoposide 100 mg/m^2 IV qd on day 1-3, q 21 days (for 4 cycles)

Ondansetron 8 mg IV premedication for cisplatin, 8 mg po premedication for each dose of etoposide

Dexamethasone 12 mg IV premedication for cisplatin, then 8 mg PO daily days 2-4

Aprepitant 125 mg PO before cisplatin, 80 mg PO prior to etoposide on days 2 & 3

Date	Rx No	Physician	Drug/Strength	Quantity	Sig	Refills
4/29	32048	Smith	Tylenol 3	60	1 PO every 4 h PRN pain	1
5/2	33892	Gasper	Promethazine 25 mg	30	1 PO every 4 h PRN N/V	3
3/13	20986	Smith	Furosemide 40 mg	30	1 PO every AM	6
4/29	32047	Smith	Robitussin AC	240	5-10 mL PO every 4 h PRN cough	1
2/7	34556	Smith	Anusol HC	20	Apply to affected area PRN hemorrhoids	2

 ## Pharmacist Notes and Other Patient Information

None available.

Questions

1. The dose of cisplatin to be administered to EA is:
   A. 4.14 g.
   B. 1.41 g.
   C. 141 mg.
   D. 1.41 mg.
   E. 14 g.

2. In what volume of normal saline will etoposide need to be diluted in order to be stable for up to 48 hours (maximum concentration not to exceed 0.4 mg/mL)?
   A. 30 mL
   B. 313 mL
   C. 470 mL
   D. 940 mL
   E. 1148 mL

3. What would be the advantage if carboplatin were substituted for cisplatin in this patient?
   A. Increased survival
   B. Reduced nausea/vomiting, especially delayed emesis
   C. Less cycles of treatment
   D. Reduced myelosuppression
   E. Single agent therapy

4. Etoposide must be administered as an IV infusion over 30 minutes or longer to avoid which of the following from occurring?

Case 45

A. Sudden onset of abdominal cramps
B. Cardiotoxicity
C. Hypotension
D. Palmar-plantar erythrodysesthesia
E. Hemorrhagic cystitis

5. The prescription for prochlorperazine can be appropriately filled with:

   A. Kytril.
   B. Zofran.
   C. Compazine.
   D. Phenergan.
   E. Ativan.

6. Which of the following nonpharmacologic items could be offered to EA in an attempt to reduce emetogenicity?

   A. Psychotherapy for obsessive compulsive disorder
   B. Avoid sucking on cold items such as ice or frozen fruit
   C. Physiotherapy: change diet to large, frequent, spicy meals
   D. Cognitive distraction or counseling
   E. Increased physical activity prior to therapy

7. Which of the following statement(s) are TRUE regarding the pharmacokinetics of etoposide?

   I. Disposition is triphasic
   II. Cleared by both renal and nonrenal processes
   III. Highly protein bound

   A. I only
   B. III only
   C. I and II only
   D. II and III only
   E. I, II, and III

8. Ondansetron acts by:

   A. competing for the binding sites of dopamine receptors.
   B. competing for the binding sites of serotonin receptors.
   C. blocking histamine H_1 receptors.
   D. facilitating the neurotransmitter gamma-aminobutyric acid.
   E. blocking alpha$_2$ receptors.

9. As part of the health care team, you are asked by the lead oncologist to provide him with information on the best way to prevent cisplatin-induced nephrotoxicity. Which of the following would you recommend?

   A. Sodium thiosulfate
   B. Leucovorin
   C. Hydration
   D. Vitamin B$_{12}$
   E. Pegfilgrastim

10. What has been the single greatest health care change that has lead to declining lung cancer mortality among men and woman?

    A. Utilization of three drug regimens
    B. Use of radiographic imaging as a screening tool
    C. Decreased cigarette smoking rates
    D. Surgical intervention
    E. Addition of radiation in conjunction with chemotherapy agents

Infectious Diseases

Section Editors: John L. Woon and Catherine M. Oliphant

Patient Name: Monica Clarins
Address: CVICU Bed 4
Age: 67
Sex: Female
Height: 5' 4''
Weight: 161 lb
Race: African American
Allergies: NKDA

Chief Complaint

MC is a 67-yo female hospitalized 1 week ago for coronary bypass surgery after suffering an acute myocardial infarction. She had an uneventful postoperative period and is currently in the step-down unit, where you are the clinical pharmacist.

History of Present Illness

This morning MC spiked a temperature of 102°F. The nurse also noticed an area of erythema and swelling around her central line during a routine dressing change. The central line was replaced, and two sets of blood cultures were drawn. One specimen of each set was obtained via the central line, and one specimen was taken from a peripheral venipuncture. These specimens were sent for gram stain, culture, and sensitivity.

Past Medical History

MC has a 20-year history of HTN that has been moderately controlled with a various number of agents. In the last 6 months, MC had been complaining of increased shortness of breath and mild angina. She had a cholecystectomy in 1973 and had two children via normal vaginal delivery in 1955 and 1957.

Social History

Tobacco use: Quit 25 years ago

Alcohol use: None

Marital status: Married

Family History

Father died of heart disease at age 63. Mother died of breast cancer at age 69.

Review of Systems

A 67-yo African American female postoperative for triple-vessel bypass presents this morning with fever and erythema, swelling, and tenderness at the site of a central line.

Physical Examination

VS: (This morning) BP 144/88 mmHg, HR 80 bpm, RR 25 rpm, T 102.6°F, Wt 73 kg

Area around central venous IV site is erythematous and indurated

Laboratory and Diagnostic Tests

Sodium 142 mEq/L	Potassium 4.2 mEq/L
Chloride 110 mEq/L	CO_2 content 30 mEq/L
BUN 15 mg/dL	Serum creatinine 1.2 mg/dL
Glucose 141 mg/dL	Hemoglobin 12.1 g/dL
Hematocrit 35%	Platelets 250,000 cells/mm³

WBC 21,000 cells/mm³ with 60% PMN, 6% bands

ECG: NSR

CXR: Patchy infiltrates consistent with CHF

MICRO: Gram stain: gram-positive cocci in clusters, in 2 of 4 culture specimens

Final C&S: MRSA

Diagnosis

Postop Day 7: suspected central line infection

Medication Record

Cefazolin 1 gm IVPB preop x1

Cefazolin 1 gm IVPB q 8 h (D/C'd)

Vancomycin 1 gm IV q12 h

Metoprolol 100 mg 1 tab PO bid

Losartan 50 mg 1 tab PO daily

Atorvastatin 10 mg 1 tab PO daily

Meperidine 50 mg IM q 4 h prn severe pain

APAP 325/oxycodone 5 mg 1 tab PO q 4 h prn pain

Pharmacist Notes and Other Patient Information

Home medication list

Metoprolol 100 mg 1 tab PO bid

Losartan 50 mg 1 tab PO daily

Atorvastatin 10 mg 1 tab PO daily

MVI 1 tab po daily

Vitamin E 400 IU 1 cap PO daily

Questions

1. The most likely cause of MC's bacteremia is:

   A. Bacteroides fragilis
   B. Escherichia coli
   C. Pseudomonas aeruginosa
   D. *Staphylococcus* species
   E. *Streptococcus* species

2. MC's estimated creatinine clearance, based on her IBW and using the Cockcroft-Gault equation, is:

   A. 39 mL/min.
   B. 46 mL/min.
   C. 52 mL/min.
   D. 62 mL/min.
   E. 75 mL/min.

3. An M4 medical student asks you about guidelines for preventing central catheter-related infections. Which of the following would be an appropriate recommendation?

   A. Designate one port of a multi-lumen catheter exclusively for TPN.
   B. Change tunneled catheter site dressings every 2 days until the site has healed.
   C. Give a dose of prophylactic antibiotics 1 hour before catheter insertion.
   D. Replace the CVC catheter every 2 weeks.
   E. Use a vancomycin antibiotic lock solution for all idle central catheter ports.

4. When monitoring vancomycin serum concentrations, the recommended trough level range for the treatment of bacteremia is:

   A. <5 mg/L.
   B. 5-15 mg/L.
   C. 15-20 mg/L.
   D. 20-25 mg/L.
   E. 30-40 mg/L.

5. The Centers for Disease Control (CDC) has developed guidelines for the appropriate use of vancomycin in an attempt to control the emergence of bacterial resistance. Which of the following is NOT a recommendation from the CDC as far as appropriate use of vancomycin?

   A. Treatment of serious infections caused by beta-lactam resistant gram-positive microorganisms
   B. Treatment of infections caused by gram-positive microorganisms in patients who have a serious (type I) allergy to beta-lactam antimicrobials
   C. As first-line empiric therapy for the treatment of antibiotic-associated enterocolitis

   D. As prophylaxis for major surgical procedures involving implantation of prosthetic materials or devices (i.e., cardiac and vascular procedures and total hip replacement) when methicillin-resistant *Staphylococcus aureus* (MRSA) or methicillin-resistant *Staphylococcus epidermidis* (MRSE) infections are prevalent
   E. Prophylaxis, as recommended by the American Heart Association, for endocarditis following certain procedures in patients at high risk for endocarditis

6. Which of the following steps do you take before dispensing parenteral vancomycin to the unit?

   I. Wrap the bag in aluminum foil to protect from light.
   II. Inspect the bag for particulate matter and discoloration.
   III. Place a label on the bag with instructions to infuse over 60 minutes.

   A. I only
   B. III only
   C. I and II only
   D. II and III only
   E. I, II, and III

7. You receive a call from MC's nurse stating that MC became slightly hypotensive (110/60 mmHg) and developed a rash on her trunk and arms when receiving her first dose of vancomycin. You recommend to:

   A. discontinue the vancomycin immediately as MC appears to be allergic to the drug.
   B. administer diphenhydramine or hydrocortisone before administering subsequent doses.
   C. continue the vancomycin but infuse it over 90-120 minutes.
   D. change the dose of vancomycin to 375 mg IVPB every 18 hours.
   E. begin a desensitization protocol to be able to continue therapy.

8. Vancomycin belongs to which class of antibiotics?

   A. Beta-lactam
   B. Monobactam
   C. Macrolide
   D. Glycopeptide
   E. Aminoglycoside

9. By day 7 of therapy with vancomycin, MC is clinically stable, but a recent chemistry panel shows an increase in her serum creatinine to 1.9 mg/dL. Aside from making an adjustment to her vancomycin regimen, which of her other medications do you need to adjust for renal function?

Case 46

A. Losartan
B. Metoprolol
C. APAP + oxycodone
D. Meperidine
E. Atorvastatin

10. After 10 days on intravenous vancomycin, the fellow wants to convert this patient to oral vancomycin. The fellow wants to know whether an oral formulation of vancomycin is available and the most appropriate dose for the oral formulation of vancomycin for this patient. You respond:

    A. an oral formulation is available and should be dosed 500 mg PO every 6 hours.

    B. an oral formulation is available and should be dosed 750 mg PO every 12 hours.

    C. an oral dosage form is available and due to its poor absorption, the oral dose is double the IV dose.

    D. there used to be an oral formulation, but it was removed from the market due to poor absorption and bioavailability.

    E. an oral formulation is available but it is very poorly absorbed and should not be used to treat any infection outside the alimentary canal.

Case 47

Patient Name: Jack Dillon
Address: 101 Hoosiers Avenue
Age: 40   **Sex:** Male
Height: 6'2"   **Weight:** 92 kg
Race: White
Allergies: NKDA

 ## Chief Complaint

JD is a 40-year-old white male who presents to the hospital complaining of pain, worsening redness, and cloudy drainage from a surgical wound on his left lower extremity.

 ## History of Present Illness

Two weeks prior to admission, JD was involved in a farming accident, resulting in a deep laceration on his left calf and shin that was heavily contaminated with soil. The patient underwent surgery to repair the laceration and wash out the contaminated area. The patient was sent home with a closed wound and a prescription for cephalexin 500 mg four times daily for 7 days. Three days after the antibiotics were discontinued, the patient began noticing increased pain, erythema, and purulent discharge from the surgical wound site. The patient presented to the emergency room this morning when he developed a fever, and he was subsequently admitted to the hospital for both infectious disease and surgical consults.

 ## Past Medical History

No prior history of serious diseases or infections.

 ## Social History

Tobacco use: 1 pack per day; 20 pack-year history

Alcohol use: Six-pack of beer daily

 ## Family History

Mother with diabetes. Father's history is unremarkable.

 ## Review of Systems

Primary symptoms include pain, erythema, and purulent discharge from surgical wound site.

 ## Medication Record

Date	Rx No	Physician	Drug/Strength	Quantity	Sig	Refills
7/31	55412	Smith	Cephalexin 500 mg	28	1 po QID	0

 ## Physical Examination

GEN: Alert, well-developed male complaining of left leg pain and malaise

VS: BP 140/85 mmHg, HR 82 bpm, RR 16 rpm, T 101.5°F, Wt 92 kg

HEENT: PERRLA

EXT: Left inguinal lymphadenopathy

5-cm margin of erythema surrounding the 10-cm scar from the previous surgery. Area is warm and painful to the touch. The distal 2 cm of the surgical scar are now open, with purulent discharge.

 ## Laboratory and Diagnostic Tests

Sodium 141 mEq/L	Potassium 4.1 mEq/L
Chloride 104 mEq/L	CO_2 26 mEq/L
BUN 16 mg/dL	Serum creatinine 1.0 mg/dL
Glucose 94 mg/dL	ESR 95 mm/hr
CRP 15 mg/dL	Hemoglobin 16 g/dL
Hematocrit 45%	Platelets 195,000/mL

WBC 17,000/mm^3 with 81% PMNs, 8% bands, 9% lymphocytes, 2% monocytes

Miscellaneous results:

Left extremity radiograph: Periosteal elevation and bony destruction of the left distal tibia consistent with osteomyelitis

Culture results of wound drainage: Heavy growth of Pseudomonas aeruginosa

 ## Diagnosis

Acute osteomyelitis

 ## Pharmacist Notes and Other Patient Information

7/31 Instructed patient on the appropriate use of cephalexin: Take the full prescription (7 days).

Case 47

Questions

1. Which of the following patient data is NOT consistent with a diagnosis of osteomyelitis?

   A. Decreased platelet count
   B. Elevated CRP
   C. Local tenderness and swelling
   D. Fever
   E. Elevated WBC count

2. What is the primary selection criteria for choosing an antibiotic for the treatment of osteomyelitis?

   A. Cost
   B. Adequate bone penetration
   C. Convenience
   D. Safety
   E. Adverse effect profile

3. Which of the following factors contributed to the development of osteomyelitis in this patient?

   I. Deep, open wound
   II. Contamination of wound
   III. Patient's age

   A. I only
   B. III only
   C. I and II only
   D. II and III only
   E. I, II, and III

4. Which of the following statements explains the main reason why oral cephalexin therapy was ineffective in this patient?

   A. Cephalexin does not have activity against Pseudomonas aeruginosa.
   B. Cephalexin was dosed incorrectly for the treatment of osteomyelitis.
   C. Cephalexin was not taken on an empty stomach.
   D. The patient was not compliant with his cephalexin therapy.
   E. Cephalexin was not initially administered intravenously.

5. While waiting for the drug susceptibilities to return, the physician empirically starts JD on IV antibiotic therapy. Which of the following regimens would NOT be appropriate for initial treatment of osteomyelitis caused by Pseudomonas aeruginosa?

   A. Ceftazidime plus gentamicin
   B. Piperacillin/tazobactam plus ciprofloxacin
   C. Cefazolin plus clindamycin
   D. Cefepime plus tobramycin
   E. Piperacillin/tazobactam plus tobramycin

6. What is the appropriate length of therapy for the treatment of acute osteomyelitis?

   A. 3-5 days
   B. 7-14 days
   C. 2-3 weeks
   D. 4-6 weeks
   E. 3-4 months

7. The physician decides to start JD on an empiric antibiotic regimen containing IV piperacillin/tazobactam. However, due to a national shortage of this medication, only the pharmacy bulk packages are being supplied rather than the individual vial strengths. When reconstituted, these large bulk vials provide a solution containing 200 mg/mL of piperacillin and 25 mg/mL of tazobactam. How much of this reconstituted solution should be added to a compatible IV piggyback solution when compounding 4 g of piperacillin and 0.5 g of tazobactam?

   A. 10 mL
   B. 20 mL
   C. 30 mL
   D. 40 mL
   E. 50 mL

8. The following day, susceptibilities return on the wound drainage culture growing Pseudomonas aeruginosa and indicate that the organism is susceptible to various antibiotics, including ciprofloxacin, ceftazidime, and the aminoglycosides, but is only intermediate to piperacillin. JD's initial empiric regimen includes only IV piperacillin/tazobactam. The physician asks you if JD's antibiotic regimen should be altered. You instruct him to:

   A. Discontinue all antibiotics since this is a very resistant strain of Pseudomonas.
   B. Continue the IV piperacillin/tazobactam but add oral rifampin for synergy and better activity against the Pseudomonas.
   C. Switch to oral moxifloxacin as the sole agent for the duration of treatment.
   D. Call the lab and have them rerun the sensitivities because Pseudomonas is always sensitive to piperacillin.
   E. Change to the combination of IV ceftazidime plus IV tobramycin.

9. JD responds well to the new IV antibiotic regimen and receives treatment as an outpatient. However, just before his final week of therapy, he loses IV access. Since JD is clinically improving, the physician wants to change him to an oral antibiotic to complete treatment. Which of the following antibiotics is available in an oral formulation?

A. Ceftazidime
B. Cefepime
C. Ciprofloxacin
D. Tobramycin
E. Meropenem

10. When JD comes to your pharmacy to pick up his new oral antibiotic prescription, he asks you if there is anything that he can do to improve his treatment outcomes. You notice that he has a six-pack of beer in his left hand. You offer the following suggestions:

I. Reduce alcohol intake because excessive consumption may alter immune function and reduce the body's ability to fight off infection.
II. Compliance with oral antibiotics is essential if treatment is to be successful.
III. Add the dietary supplement saw palmetto to his antibiotic regimen to stimulate the immune system and promote wound healing.

A. I only
B. III only
C. I and II only
D. II and III only
E. I, II, and III

Case 48

Patient Name: Lori Daniels
Address: 78 Marigold
Age: 27 **Sex:** Female
Height: 5′ 4″ **Weight:** 135 lb
Race: White
Allergies: Fluoroquinolones (hives)

Chief Complaint

LD complains of a thick, white vaginal discharge. She states that she has intense itching and burning in the vaginal area.

History of Present Illness

LD's current symptoms began 5 days ago. Patient had sinusitis and finished up a course of Augmentin 4 days ago.

Past Medical History

Gravida 1, Para 1

LMP was 16 days ago

Occasional heartburn

Social History

Alcohol: Rare

Tobacco: None

Occupation: Elementary school teacher

Married; 1 child, 3 years old

Family History

Both mother and father alive and well

Review of Systems

Negative except for above

Physical Examination

GEN: Pleasant female in NAD

VS: BP 130/70 mmHg, HR 68 bpm, T 37.1°C

PELVIC: White, malodorous vaginal discharge

Laboratory and Diagnostic Tests

Wet mount (KOH) reveals yeast

Diagnosis

Vaginitis, unspecified cause

Medication Record

7/17, Macquire, Ortho-Novum 1/35

Pharmacist Notes and Other Patient Information

None available.

Questions

1. What is the most common cause of vulvovaginal candidiasis?

    A. *Gardnerella vaginalis*
    B. *Candida albicans*
    C. *Candida tropicalis*
    D. *Trichomonas vaginalis*
    E. *Candida glabrata*

2. Risk factors for vaginal candidiasis include all of the following EXCEPT:

    A. pregnancy.
    B. broad-spectrum antibiotic use.
    C. high estrogen-containing oral contraceptives.
    D. diabetes mellitus.
    E. condom use.

3. Over-the-counter (OTC) vaginal candidiasis products are appropriate for:

    I. patients with similar symptoms who have had a previously diagnosed vaginal yeast infection.
    II. pregnant women.
    III. recurrent (more than four episodes per year) vaginal candidiasis.

    A. I only
    B. III only
    C. I and II only
    D. II and III only
    E. I, II, and III

4. Appropriate therapy for vulvovaginal candidiasis includes all of the following EXCEPT:

    A. metronidazole.

    B. butoconazole.

    C. fluconazole.

    D terconazole.

    E. clotrimazole.

5. LD presents with a prescription for Terazol 3. What is the active ingredient in Terazol 3?

    A. Clotrimazole

    B. Nystatin

    C. Miconazole

    D. Terconazole

    E. Butoconazole

6. Which of the following statements regarding fluconazole in the treatment of vaginal candidiasis is FALSE?

    A Approved as a single 150-mg oral dose

    B. Improves patient compliance

    C. Reduces the time to relief of symptoms

    D. More costly

    E. Available by prescription only

7. Systemic azole antifungal agents (ketoconazole, itraconazole, and fluconazole) have many drug interactions. All of the following drugs interact with the azoles EXCEPT:

    A. atorvastatin.

    B. hydrochlorothiazide.

    C. phenytoin.

    D. warfarin.

    E. cyclosporine.

8. You are asked to counsel a patient receiving itraconazole capsules. Which of the following statements is appropriate?

    I. Take with a meal

    II. Avoid H_2 blockers, proton pump inhibitors, and antacids

    III. Take on an empty stomach

    A. I only

    B. III only

    C. I and II only

    D. II and III only

    E. I, II, and III

9. All of the following statements are appropriate counseling points for LD EXCEPT:

    A. signs and symptoms should improve in 48-72 hours.

    B. common adverse effects associated with intravaginal antifungal products include vulvovaginal irritation, burning, and pruritus.

    C. complete the full course of therapy.

    D. stop using the medication if menstruation begins.

    E. certain products are oil-based and may weaken a latex condom or diaphragm.

10. Common signs and symptoms of vaginal candidiasis include all of the following EXCEPT:

    A. foul-smelling (fishy odor) vaginal discharge.

    B. thick, white vaginal discharge.

    C. vulvar/vaginal pruritus.

    D. vulvar burning.

    E. dyspareunia.

Patient Name: Marko Ramius
Address: 1140 Red Oak Drive
Age: 30　　**Gender:** Male
Height: 5' 10"　　**Weight:** 102 kg
Race: Caucasian
Allergies: NKDA

Chief Complaint

MR was found to be diaphoretic and slightly confused by the evening staff nurse at Shadyside Rehabilitation Hospital.

History of Present Illness

The onset of symptoms was within the previous 8 hours; however, MR reported feeling "under the weather" for the past few days.

Past Medical History

C-6 spinal fracture secondary to motor vehicle accident: 2 years ago

Partial colectomy: 2 years ago

Hospitalized for community-acquired pneumonia: 2 weeks ago

Hospitalized for urinary tract infection: 4 weeks ago

Social History

Not married; no children

Family History

Mother, father, and 2 older siblings alive and well

Review of Systems

Fever present; (+) anxiety; bilateral lower extremity paralysis

Physical Examination

GEN: Well-nourished, ill-appearing adult male

VS: BP 90/60 mmHg, HR 110 bpm, RR 16 rpm, T 38.5°C, Wt 102 kg, Ht 5' 10"

SKIN: Subclavian catheter site is erythematous and warm to touch. Multiple scars on abdomen and neck from injuries and surgery.

CHEST: CTA bilaterally with no wheezes or crackles

CV: Tachycardic with no m/r/g appreciated

ABD: Soft, NT/ND, normo-active bowel sounds

MS/EXT: Motor and sensory activity is absent in the lower extremities and diminished in upper extremities

NEURO: A&O x 3

Laboratory and Diagnostic Tests

Na 142 mEq/L	K 4.1 mEq/L
Cl 109 mEq/L	CO_2 21 mEq/L
BUN 5 mg/dL	Scr 0.3 mg/dL
Gluc 90 mg/dL	

Blood cultures in the ER:

Gram stain: Gram-positive cocci in clusters

Blood cultures: Positive 2 out of 2 for *Staphylococcus aureus*; susceptibilities pending

Diagnosis

Catheter-related bloodstream infection

Medication Record

Piperacillin/tazobactam 4.5 g IV every 6 hours

Vancomycin 1 g IV every 12 hours

Pantoprazole 40 mg IV every 24 hours

Heparin 5,000 units SQ every 12 hours

Baclofen 10 mg PO three times a day

Docusate sodium 100 mg PO twice a day

Morphine 2 mg IV every 2 hours as needed for pain

Senna 8.6 mg 1 tab PO every evening as needed for constipation

Bisacodyl suppository 10 mg PR every evening as needed for constipation

Pharmacist Notes and Other Patient Information

None available.

Questions

1. The tazobactam component of piperacillin/tazobactam will:

    A. prevent degradation of piperacillin by renal dehydropeptidase.

    B. inhibit extended-spectrum beta-lactamase production by the organism in blood cultures.

    C. broaden coverage of piperacillin to include methicillin-resistant *S. aureus*.

    D. ensure activity against methicillin-susceptible *Staphylococcus aureus*.

    E. expand coverage of piperacillin to include vancomycin-resistant *Enterococcus*.

2. What if the organism isolated in MR's blood cultures was susceptible to oxacillin, but resistant to penicillin G. What would be the most likely mechanism of resistance?

    A. Production of penicillinase

    B. Production of a penicillin efflux pump

    C. Alteration of penicillin-binding protein 2a

    D. Alteration of DNA gyrase

    E. Loss of a porin channel in the outer membrane

3. Suppose the organism isolated in MR's blood cultures returned as MRSA. What would be the most likely mechanism of methicillin resistance?

    A. Change from D-ala-D-ala to D-ala-D-lactate

    B. Alteration of penicillin-binding protein 2a

    C. Production of an extended-spectrum β-lactamase

    D. Efflux of β-lactam antibiotics

    E. Alteration of the 50S ribosomal subunit

4. The microbiology lab performed a D-test on the organism isolated in MR's blood cultures and a D-zone was observed, suggesting that inducible MLS resistance was present. Which antibiotic(s) would be considered resistant to this isolate?

    I. Erythromycin

    II. Clindamycin

    III. Quinupristin-dalfopristin

    A. I only

    B. III only

    C. I and II only

    D. II and III only

    E. I, II and III

5. If the organism isolated in MR's blood cultures returned with a susceptibility profile suggesting a community-associated MRSA strain, which antibiotic would be most appropriate for MR?

    A. Vancomycin

    B. Piperacillin-tazobactam

    C. Ciprofloxacin

    D. Clindamycin

    E. Erythromycin

6. Which empiric vancomycin regimen would be most appropriate for MR?

    A. Vancomycin 750 mg IV every 12 hours

    B. Vancomycin 1000 mg IV every 12 hours

    C. Vancomycin 2000 mg given as a 24 hour continuous IV infusion

    D. Vancomycin 2500 mg IV x 1, then 1000 mg IV every 12 hours

    E. Vancomycin 2500 mg IV x 1, then 1500 mg IV every 12 hours

7. The recommended vancomycin infusion period is e"30 minutes for every 500 mg administered. If the final concentration of vancomycin is 5 mg/mL, the rate should not exceed:

    A. 3 mL/min.

    B. 5 mL/min.

    C. 16 mL/min.

    D. 33 mL/min.

    E. 100 mL/min.

8. In order to ensure that the final concentration of vancomycin is 5 mg/mL or less, MR's current dose of vancomycin should be diluted in a total volume of:

    A. 5 mL.

    B. 50 mL.

    C. 100 mL.

    D. 150 mL.

    E. 250 mL.

9. Given MR's nasal swab results, he should be:

    A. placed on droplet precautions.

    B. placed on airborne precautions.

    C. placed on contact precautions.

    D. treated for MRSA sinusitis.

    E. given intranasal Bactroban.

10. Which of the following strategies would be most effective for preventing future catheter-related bloodstream infections in MR?

A. Changing the catheter site to the internal jugular vein

B. Administering IV vancomycin for prophylaxis

C. Flushing the catheter daily with heparin

D. Using an inline filter when infusing drugs

E. Using aseptic technique when inserting a new catheter

Patient Name: Joanna Johnson
Address: 346 N.E. 4th Street
Age: 62   **Sex:** Female
Height: 5′ 5″   **Weight:** 175 lb
Race: White
Allergies: NKDA

Chief Complaint

JJ presents to the emergency department (ED) complaining of pain, burning in her chest, and difficulty breathing.

History of Present Illness

JJ states that she has felt ill for the last 8 to 9 days. She presented to the ED 2 days ago and was given a prescription for a pain medication, a sedative, and an antibiotic. She has not been able to keep the oral medications down. She presents to the ED today with fever, chills, and sweats. A blood gas performed in ED reports a pO$_2$ of 77 mmHg on room air. She has no previous history of pulmonary disease.

Past Medical History

Past medical history is only significant for hypertension, which was diagnosed last year. According to the patient's daughter, she does have frequent headaches for which she takes 250 Excedrin every month.

Social History

She drinks a glass of wine occasionally and denies smoking.

Family History

Noncontributory

Review of Systems

Patient has no previous history of heart disease, lung disease, kidney disease, or diabetes. Other than her recent respiratory tract disorder her only complaint is diarrhea, which has persisted over the last couple of days.

Physical Examination

GEN: The patient is alert and oriented yet appears tired and is quite dyspneic. Her extremities are pale and mottled.

VS: Temp 96.6°F, HR 115 bpm, RR 40 rpm, BP 80/50 mmHg, O$_2$ saturation 88%

LUNGS: Bilateral rhonchi with decreased breath sounds in the right quadrant

CV: Tachycardia with a regular rhythm

Urine output: 25 mL/h over the last 2 hours

Laboratory and Diagnostic Tests

Sodium 134 mEq/L	Potassium 5.5 mEq/L
Chloride 105 mEq/L	CO$_2$ content 13 mEq/L
BUN 52 mg/dL	Creatinine 4.1 mg/dL
Glucose 215 mg/dL	Hemoglobin 13.8 g/dL
Hematocrit 41%	Platelets 188,000 cells/mm^3
WBC 4400 cells/mm^3	PMNs 7%, bands 73%

Arterial blood gases (prior to intubation): pH 7.19, paO$_2$ 80 mmHg, pCO$_2$ 46 mmHg, O$_2$ saturation 88.9%, bicarbonate 17 mEq/L, FiO$_2$ 15 L/min, base excess -9.8

Chest x-ray: Bilateral effusions with bibasilar consolidation

Cardiac enzymes: CK 217 IU/L (elevated), CKMB 5.8 IU/L (elevated), troponin 2.6 ng/mL (elevated)

EKG: ST segment elevation

Diagnosis

1) Community-acquired pneumonia
2) Severe sepsis secondary to pneumonia
3) Acute renal failure secondary to sepsis or excessive Excedrin ingestion
4) Myocardial infarction possibly due to hypotension secondary to sepsis

Medication Record

Medications prior to admission:

Atenolol 50 mg po qday

Conjugated estrogens (0.625 mg)/medroxyprogesterone (2.5 mg) one po qday

Levofloxacin 750 mg po qday

Zaleplon 10 mg po qhs

Hydrocodone (5 mg) and acetaminophen (500 mg) po 6 hr as needed for pain

Initial inpatient medication profile:

Ceftriaxone 2 g IVPB q 24 h

Azithromycin 500 mg IVPB q 24 h

Famotidine 20 mg IVP q 12 h

Case 50

Sodium bicarbonate 50 mEq IVP x 2

Morphine 1-4 mg IVP q 2 h prn

Lactated Ringer's continuous infusion at 150 mL/h

Midazolam 1 mg IVP x 1

Dopamine continuous infusion at 10 mcg/kg/min

Normal saline infusion wide open

D_5 NS infusion at 200 mL/h

Drotrecogin alfa infusion per pharmacy

Discontinue ceftriaxone

Penicillin 2 million units IVPB q 6 h

Clindamycin 900 mg IVPB q 8 h

 Pharmacist Notes and Other Patient Information

None available.

Questions

1. According to the American College of Chest Physicians (ACCP)/Society of Critical Care Medicine (SCCM) 1991 consensus conference, sepsis is defined by an infectious process in the presence of the systemic inflammatory response syndrome (SIRS). SIRS includes the presence of two or more of the following criteria EXCEPT:

    A. temperature over 100.4°F or under 96.8°F.
    B. heart rate over 90 bpm.
    C. tachypnea, as manifested by a respiratory rate over 20 breaths per minute, or hyperventilation, as indicated by a $PaCO_2$ under 32 mmHg.
    D. alteration of white blood cell count over 12,000 cells/mm³ or under 4000 cells/mm³ with 10% or more bands (immature neutrophils)
    E. serum creatinine over 1.5 mg/dL.

2. The pathophysiology of severe sepsis includes which of the following?

    I. Increased inflammation as demonstrated by increases in inflammatory cytokines such as tumor necrosis factor-alpha (TNF-alpha) and interleukin 1 and 6
    II. Increased coagulation as demonstrated by increases in release of tissue factor, reduced levels of protein C and thrombomodulin, and increased production of thrombin

III. Increased fibrinolysis as demonstrated by reductions in plasminogen activator inhibitor-1 (PAI-I)

    A. I only
    B. III only
    C. I and II only
    D. II and III only
    E. I, II, and III

3. On rounds in the ICU, the medical team asks you for your recommendations on whether JJ should be placed on steroids for treating severe sepsis. Your response is:

    A. intravenous high dose steroids (e.g., methylprednisolone 2 g/day) are indicated as controlled clinical trials have shown that steroids in this dose are associated with a reduction in mortality.
    B. intravenous steroids in moderate doses (hydrocortisone 200 mg to 300 mg IVPB per day) for 7 days in 3 to 4 divided doses are recommended in patients who remain in septic shock after adequate fluid replacement and vasopressor support as they have been shown to reduce mortality.
    C. steroids have not been shown to improve outcomes in patients with severe sepsis and should not be used in JJ.
    D. oral steroids in physiologic doses have been shown to improve outcomes in patients with severe sepsis and are indicated in JJ.
    E. while studies have shown some benefit to the use of steroids in severe sepsis, their potential side effects negate any positive effects on outcomes and therefore are not indicated in JJ.

4. On the basis of JJ's blood gas results and impending respiratory failure, the decision is made to intubate her. A bronchoscopy is performed, and a bronch wash is sent for culture. Over the next 3 hours, her blood pressure continues to fall in spite of aggressive volume resuscitation. Her blood pressure is now 70/40 with a mean arterial pressure (MAP) of 50. The decision is made to start dopamine at 10 mcg/kg/min. During rounds, a discussion occurs as to whether or not JJ is a candidate for drotrecogin alfa (recombinant human activated protein C). On the basis of your assessment of the literature, which of the following are true?

    I. Drotrecogin alfa was associated with a statistically significant absolute 6% reduction in the risk of death in the Recombinant Human Activated Protein C Worldwide Evaluation of Severe Sepsis (PROWESS) trial in patients with severe sepsis.
    II. In the PROWESS trial, the reduction in the risk of death was significant only in those patients that were the sickest as defined by the Acute Physiology and Chronic Health Evaluation II (APACHE II) scores that were greater than 25.

III. A more recent trial, the ADDRESS trial, examined the use of drotrecogin alfa in severe sepsis patients who are at a lower risk of death as defined by APACHE II scores of less than 25 and single organ dysfunction. This study showed no reduction in mortality from the use of drotrecogin alfa in these patients.

A. I only
B. III only
C. I and II only
D. II and III only
E. I, II, and III

5. Drotrecogin alfa's proposed mechanism in reducing mortality in severe sepsis includes all of the following EXCEPT:

A. reduction in the release of inflammatory cytokines.
B. reduction in the production of thrombin.
C. improvement in the endogenous fibrinolysis system.
D. inhibition of leukocyte adhesion.
E. decrease in bleeding time.

6. JJ showed moderate hyperglycemia, blood glucose of 215 mg/dL. What is the most appropriate response?

A. Manage her hyperglycemia by changing all IV solutions to normal saline
B. Initiate a sliding scale insulin dose, monitoring blood glucose via finger sticks every 6 hours
C. Discontinue all steroids as these could be contributing to her hyperglycemia
D. Initiate glyburide 5 mg po daily to control her hyperglycemia
E. Initiate a titrated insulin infusion with initial glucose monitoring every 30-60 minutes, then every 4 hours once the glucose is stabilized between 140 and 180 mg/dL

7. It is postulated that JJ's myocardial infarction may have been a result of sepsis-induced hypotension. How is the treatment of her myocardial infarction impacted by her severe sepsis?

A. The treatment of her myocardial infarction is not impacted by the fact that she has severe sepsis.
B. The septic shock and drotrecogin alfa treatment prevent her from being a candidate for using fibrinolytics.
C. Despite septic shock and drotrecogin alfa treatment, she is able to receive fibrinolytics.
D. Despite septic shock and drotrecogin alfa treatment, she is able to receive beta blockers and ACE inhibitors as part of normal medical therapy for myocardial infarction.

E. The septic shock and drotrecogin alfa treatment prevent her from receiving aspirin as part of the normal medical therapy for myocardial infarction.

8. JJ's culture result from the bronch wash comes back reporting 4+ group A *Streptococcus*. Her antibiotics are changed from ceftriaxone to penicillin G 2 million units IVPB every 6 hours and clindamycin 900 mg IVPB every 8 hours. Which of the following are true regarding the use of clindamycin in this situation?

A. The combination of clindamycin and penicillin is not rational due to a significant drug interaction, i.e., clindamycin is bacteriostatic and reduces the effectiveness of cell-wall acting antibiotics, such as penicillin.
B. There is some evidence to suggest that clindamycin may suppress the production of bacterial toxin production, making it a rational choice in treating aggressive group A streptococcal infections.
C. The dose of clindamycin is too high for JJ's current renal function and should be reduced.
D. Clindamycin is ineffective in treating streptococcal infections.
E. Clindamycin has a high potential of causing *Clostridium difficile* infections and should be avoided.

9. You are need to make a drotrecogin alfa drip for this patient. Which of the following trade names applies to drotrecogin alfa?

A. Zosyn
B. Cleocin
C. Keppra
D. Xigris
E. Doribax

10. In evaluating the results of the PROWESS trial, you find that the number needed to treat (NNT) to prevent one death in the patients that received drotrecogin alfa versus placebo is 16. Which of the following are correct statements regarding the NNT?

A. The NNT can be calculated by dividing the absolute difference between the study groups into 1 (i.e., 1/absolute difference).
B. The NNT is simply another way of displaying the relative risk difference between groups.
C. The NNT is identical to the relative risk reduction.
D. The NNT can be calculated by dividing the relative difference between the study groups into 1 (i.e., 1/relative difference).
E. The NNT can be calculated by multiplying the absolute difference between the study groups by 10 (i.e., 10*absolute difference).

Patient Name: George Jones
Address: 4775 Cheshire Court #108
Age: 50   **Sex:** Male
Height: 6′ 4″   **Weight:** 233 lb
Race: White
Allergies: Penicillin (anaphylaxis)

Chief Complaint

GJ is a 50-yo white male who is admitted to the hospital for treatment of asymptomatic neurosyphilis. GJ is without complaints and reports no manifestations of infection. Presence of infection was identified when a routine screening test, conducted in conjunction with application for a marriage license, was positive for syphilis reagin antibody. Follow-up specific treponemal tests of serum and CSF confirmed the presence of infection.

History of Present Illness

GJ reports no complaints at present. He notes that he received treatment with unknown antibiotics 7 years ago for an STD that he acquired during "a period of sexual indiscretion" following his divorce. At that time, he presented with dysuria and a purulent urethral discharge and was informed that he had gonorrhea. He noted at that time that the infection was most likely acquired from one of several one-night encounters with women he had met in a bar. He was unable to identify the index source, so follow-up and treatment of the reference case did not occur. Following treatment, he reports rapid resolution of symptoms and no subsequent sequela. He denies observing the occurrence of any manifestations or symptoms suggestive of syphilis following this course of treatment.

Past Medical History

GJ has a history of HTN that is currently controlled and a history of STD exposure as noted above. He also reports a history of a severe allergic reaction to penicillin. He notes that 23 years ago, he received a prescription for penicillin for treatment of a sore throat. Immediately after taking the first dose, he noted shortness of breath accompanied by swelling of his face, neck, and tongue. He was rushed to the ED, where he received a "shot of adrenaline" and was observed until symptoms abated. He was informed at that time that he should avoid penicillin or all penicillin-like antibiotics in the future. The remainder of his history is unremarkable and is noncontributory.

Social History

GJ has been divorced from his first wife for 8 years and has been involved in a monogamous relationship with his current partner, to whom he is engaged, for the last 2 years. He reports that he used condoms with all his sexual contacts following diagnosis and treatment of the STD 7 years ago up to his current partner. He reports that he and his fiancé quit using condoms about 3 months into their relationship.

Tobacco use: chewing tobacco, 2 cans per week

Alcohol use: 3-4 beers or glasses of wine per week

Caffeine use: 3-4 cups of decaffeinated coffee per day

Family History

Father died in an MVA at age 58. Mother alive at age 72. Two brothers, ages 58 and 52, and one sister, age 44. Three children, ages 26, 24, and 19.

Review of Systems

Normal

Physical Examination

GEN: Well-nourished, white male in NAD

VS: BP 134/82 mmHg, HR 72 bpm, RR 20 rpm, T 37.5°C, Ht 6′ 4″, Wt 106 kg

HEENT: Normal, no adenopathy palpable

LUNGS: Clear breath sounds

CV: RRR with normal S_1/S_2 & no audible murmur

SKIN: No erythema or petechiae

GU: Normal

NEURO: Alert and oriented; normal reflexes elicited and normal gait observed

Laboratory and Diagnostic Tests

Sodium 144 mEq/L	Potassium 4.5 mEq/L
Chloride 103 mEq/L	CO_2 content 22 mEq/L
BUN 25 mg/dL	Serum creatinine 1.2 mg/dL
Glucose 110 mg/dL	Hemoglobin 12.4 g/dL
Hematocrit 37%	Platelets 385,000 cells/mm³

WBC 5600 cells/mm³ with 75% PMN, 20% lymphocytes, 4% monocytes, 1% eosinophils

Serum: RPR-1:256, FTA-ABS-Reactive

CSF: VDRL-1:32

Medication Record

Date	Rx No	Physician	Drug	Strength	Quantity	Sig	Refills
10/30	12345	Jones	Amlodipine	5 mg	100	1 po daily	3

Diagnosis

Neurosyphilis

Pharmacist Notes and Other Patient Information

None available.

Questions

1. The drug and route of choice for treating neurosyphilis is:

    A. penicillin IV.
    B. penicillin IM.
    C. ceftriaxone IV.
    D. doxycycline po.
    E. chloramphenicol IV.

2. What is the best option for the treatment of primary syphilis in a penicillin-allergic patient?

    A. Doxycycline 100 mg po bid x 7 days
    B. Tetracycline 500 mg po bid x 14 days
    C. Azithromycin 1 g po x 1
    D. Doxycycline 100 mg po bid x 14 days
    E. Minocycline 100 mg po bid x 7 days

3. A patient being treated for primary syphilis with penicillin benzathine may appropriately receive:

    I. bicillin L-A.
    II. bicillin C-R.
    III. bicillin G.

    A. I only
    B. III only
    C. I and II only
    D. II and III only
    E. I, II, and III

4. What is a finding characteristic of secondary syphilis?

    A. Rash on palms of hands and soles of feet
    B. Mucopurulent discharge
    C. Gummas
    D. Meningitis
    E. Penile chancre

5. A patient calls the clinic at 8 a.m. complaining of fever, headache, and sore muscles. The previous afternoon at his clinic appointment, the patient received an IM injection of penicillin benzathine. On questioning, the patient reports that he has received amoxicillin/clavulanate for a sinus infection in the past, which he tolerated well. What do you recommend to the patient?

    A. Ibuprofen
    B. Acetaminophen
    C. Epinephrine
    D. Hydroxyzine
    E. Diphenhydramine

6. What is the drug of choice for the treatment of syphilis in a pregnant patient with a penicillin allergy?

    A. Doxycycline
    B. Ciprofloxacin
    C. Penicillin
    D. Cefixime
    E. Azithromycin

7. A single, painless genital ulcer is most characteristic of what sexually transmitted infection?

    A. Herpes simplex virus
    B. Syphilis
    C. Gonorrhea
    D. Chlamydia
    E. Pelvic inflammatory disease

8. In monitoring a patient for the treatment of syphilis, what lab change would indicate efficacy of treatment?

    A. Four-fold decrease in RPR
    B. Four-fold decrease in FTA-ABS
    C. Two-fold decrease in RPR
    D. Two-fold increase in RPR
    E. Two-fold increase in FTA-ABS

9. What combination of labs and clinical disease meets the definition of latent syphilis?

    A. (+) RPR, (-) FTA-ABS, (-) clinical disease
    B. (+) RPR, (+) FTA-ABS, (+) clinical disease
    C. (+) RPR, (+) FTA-ABS, (-) clinical disease
    D. (-) RPR, (+) FTA-ABS, (+) clinical disease
    E. (+) RPR, (-) FTA-ABS, (+) clinical disease

Case 51

10. In general, sexually transmitted diseases in a female patient may result in which of the following?

    I. Transmission to the fetus or baby
    II. Pregnancy complications
    III. Damage to reproductive organs

    A. I only
    B. III only
    C. I and II only
    D. II and III only
    E. I, II, and III

Patient Name: Darius Jones
Address: 1387 Summerset Drive
Age: 4   **Sex:** Male
Height: 3′ 0″   **Weight:** 20 kg
Race: Caucasian
Allergies: Penicillin (rash)

Chief Complaint

DJ is a 4-yo male who presents to his pediatrician with complaints of crusted lesions around the nose that itch.

History of Present Illness

DJ was in his usual state of health until 3 days ago when his mother noticed the opening to his right nostril was red, sore, and inflamed, and that he seemed to be scratching and picking at it almost constantly. The next morning, the rash spread around his mouth and chin and had changed in appearance to flat, reddened areas with fluid-filled pustules. His mother applied some topical hydrocortisone and Neosporin cream to the area with no improvement overnight. Today, the affected area has crusted over and several other small patches of vesicles and pustules are noticed on his face, which he continuously picks at. He had prolonged sun exposure with a localized sun-burn on his nose 1 week prior to presentation.

Past Medical History

Acute otitis media x 2 (last episode 2 years ago)

Social History

Lives with his parents and has two younger siblings, ages 3 and 11 months. Attends daycare 4 days per week.

Family History

Grandfather died at age 76 of cancer

Review of Systems

Unremarkable except for acute presentation

Physical Examination

GEN: Sitting in NAD, growth parameters normal for age

VS: T 99.1°F, BP 120/70, P 89 bpm, RR 20

HEENT: EOMI, PERRLA, no regional lymphadenopathy, mucus membranes moist, no oral lesions noted

LUNGS: No wheezes or crackles

CV: Regular rhythm and rate, normal S_1 and S_2

ABD: Normal BS, soft and nontender

NEURO: CN II-XII grossly intact

GENITOURINARY: Unremarkable

EXT: Normal ROM

SKIN: Thick, honey-colored crusted lesions around right nare, with satellite lesions on his cheek and chin that are crusted over. Several clear vesicles present as well. No vesicles or bullae on the buttocks, trunk, or extremities. Small amount of yellow discharge from most lesions noted. Lesions are nontender.

Laboratory and Diagnostic Tests

WBC: 10.9 K/uL

RBC: 4.9 m/uL

Hgb: 15.3 g/dL

Hct: 46.0%

Plt: 235 K/uL, with Neut%: 70.0, Lymph%: 13.0, Mono%: 9.0, Eos%: 2.0, Baso%: 1.0, and Bands%: 5.0

Diagnosis

Impetigo

Medication Record

No current medications

Pharmacist Notes and Other Patient Information

None available.

Questions

1. What is the most likely causative organism(s) implicated in impetigo?

    I.   Group A *Streptococci*

   II.   *Staphylococcus aureus*

  III.   *Propionibacterium acnes*

    A.   I only

    B.   III only

    C.   I and II only

D. II and III only

E. I, II, and III

2. Which antibiotic is NOT considered appropriate for outpatient treatment of impetigo?

   A. Cephalexin
   B. Mupirocin
   C. Dicloxacillin
   D. Levofloxacin
   E. Erythromycin

3. Which of the following antibiotics is NOT an acceptable treatment for DJ's impetigo?

   A. Mupirocin
   B. Clindamycin
   C. Dicloxacillin
   D. Cephalexin
   E. Cefuroxime

4. Which of the following is TRUE regarding the treatment of impetigo with topical mupirocin?

   I. Drug of choice for cases involving lesions that are small or few in number in the absence of lymphadenopathy
   II. Associated with fewer adverse effects than other therapies
   III. Lesions usually resolve completely in 2-3 days with treatment

   A. I only
   B. III only
   C. I and II only
   D. II and III only
   E. I, II, and III

5. Non-bullous impetigo can resemble what other dermatological condition?

   A. Acne
   B. Herpes simplex infection
   C. Shingles infection
   D. Atopic dermatitis
   E. Erysipelas

6. Which of the following are TRUE regarding topical therapy for impetigo?

   A. Topical therapy is the preferred first-line therapy for patients with limited disease.
   B. Topical therapy is not as effective against MRSA as oral therapy.
   C. Topical therapy has a similar side effect profile to oral therapy.

D. Bacitracin or bacitracin/neomycin is as effective as other topical therapies.

E. Topical therapy is more effective than systemic therapy.

7. Which of the following side effect is commonly associated with Neosporin?

   A. Dermatomycosis
   B. Stevens-Johnson syndrome
   C. Contact dermatitis
   D. Diarrhea
   E. Ototoxicity

8. Which of the following are common complications can occur up to several weeks after initiating treatment for impetigo?

   A. Pain and scarring at the initial site of impetigo
   B. New patches of impetigo in new anatomical locations
   C. Rheumatic fever
   D. Post-streptococcal glomerular nephritis
   E. Systemic bacterial infection such as sepsis

9. To prevent the spread of impetigo to others, DJ's parents should do all of the following EXCEPT:

   A. keep DJ home from daycare for 24 hours.
   B. wash the affected areas with warm soap and water several times a day and then cover lightly with gauze.
   C. use separate bed linens and towels for DJ and wash daily.
   D. quarantine DJ from any physical contact with siblings for the duration of treatment for impetigo.
   E. all of the above are true.

10. Which of the following topical antibiotics does not possess activity against *Staphylococcus* and *Streptococcus* species?

    A. Mupirocin
    B. Bacitracin
    C. Polymyxin
    D. Retapamulin
    E. Chlorhexidine

Patient Name: Melvin Rogers
Address: 510 North 24th Avenue, Apt. 5A
Age: 43   **Sex:** Male
Height: 5′ 10″   **Weight:** 174 lb
Race: African American
Allergies: Bee stings

Chief Complaint

MR is a 43-yo male who recently returned to the United States after working as a bellman for the past year at a resort in Mexico City. MR presents to the ER complaining of cough, low-grade fever, and night sweats. He states that he has lost approximately 15 lb over the past month since his return to the United States.

History of Present Illness

He states that he started coughing while in Mexico, but he thought it was just his lung disease from smoking. Since his return to the states, however, he has noticed that his coughing is worse, and at times he notices blood in the sputum. He states that he remembers his neighbor in Mexico being treated for "consumption" and that he was taking several medications, but he does not know what they were.

Past Medical History

History of COPD with multiple episodes of acute bacterial exacerbations of chronic bronchitis. He has never been tested for HIV.

Social History

Smokes approximately 2 ppd and drinks approximately 2-4 beers per day. He regularly uses marijuana and methamphetamines and continues to have unprotected sex with multiple partners.

Family History

Noncontributory

Review of Systems

Negative except as noted previously

Physical Examination

GEN: Black male who appears stated age and is noticeably short of breath when talking

VS: T 100.8°F, HR 84 bpm, RR 26 rpm, BP 146/90 mmHg

LUNGS: Wheezing, rhonchi, and rales on inspiration

NEURO: A&O x3

CV: Distant heart sounds; no murmur or gallop appreciated

ABD: Soft, nontender

EXT: No clubbing, cyanosis, or edema

Laboratory and Diagnostic Tests

Sodium 133 mEq/L

Potassium 4.5 mEq/L

Serum creatinine 1.0 mg/dL

WBC 7200 cells/mm^3

Hemoglobin 17 g/dL

Hematocrit 45%

ALT 44 IU/L

AST 40 IU/L

Chest x-ray: Bilateral flat diaphragms. Right upper lobe atelectasis. Cavitary disease (R>L).

Sputum: Kinyoun stain +; culture pending

HIV antibody: POSITIVE

Diagnosis

New diagnosis of HIV r/o tuberculosis

Medication Record

None available.

Pharmacist Notes and Other Patient Information

None available.

Questions

1. What is an acceptable initial recommendation for therapy of MR's TB infection pending susceptibility test results?

Case 53

A. Isoniazid plus rifampin plus pyrazinamide plus ethambutol

B. Isoniazid plus rifampin plus pyrazinamide

C. Isoniazid plus rifampin plus streptomycin

D. Isoniazid plus pyrazinamide plus streptomycin plus pyridoxine

E. Isoniazid plus rifampin plus pyridoxine

2. MR's organism susceptibility tests demonstrate resistance to rifampin. At this time, no other susceptibility test results are available. Which of the following represents a correct adjustment in MR's current drug regimen (isoniazid, rifampin, pyrazinamide, and ethambutol)?

A. Discontinue the rifampin.

B. Discontinue the rifampin. Add moxifloxacin to the INH, pyrazinamide, and ethambutol.

C. Discontinue the rifampin. Add amikacin and streptomycin to INH, pyrazinamide, and ethambutol.

D. Continue INH, rifampin, pyrazinamide, and ethambutol until all final susceptibility results are available, then make changes in regimen.

E. Discontinue the rifampin. Add rifapentine to the INH, pyrazinamide, and ethambutol.

3. Which of the following is an appropriate length of therapy for MR's drug-resistant TB?

A. 2-4 months after culture conversion

B. 6 months total

C. 9 months total

D. 12-18 months total

E. Lifetime therapy

4. You are called by MR's physician and asked for the recommended oral dose of ciprofloxacin to treat MR's TB. What is your response?

A. Ciprofloxacin 250 mg bid

B. Ciprofloxacin 500 mg daily

C. Ciprofloxacin 750 mg bid

D. Ciprofloxacin 250 mg daily

E. Ciprofloxacin 500 mg every other day

5. Which of the following antitubercular agents can cause optic neuritis and, thus, requires monitoring for vision changes and color blindness during therapy?

A. Ethambutol

B. Pyrazinamide

C. Isoniazid

D. Streptomycin

E. Rifampin

6. Which of the following drugs requires dosage adjustment in patients with renal insufficiency?

A. Ethambutol

B. Isoniazid

C. Rifampin

D. Moxifloxacin

E. Pyridoxine

7. You are asked to provide an inservice on drug-resistant TB to a local group of nurses. As you prepare for this presentation, you learn that the term "multidrug-resistant TB" actually specifically refers to TB that is resistant to which of the following agents?

I. Rifampin

II. Isoniazid

III. Streptomycin

A. I only

B. III only

C. I and II only

D. II and III only

E. I, II, and III

8. As you are dispensing MR's new medications to him (moxifloxacin, ethambutol, pyrazinamide, and INH), you should counsel him on which of the following points?

I. He should refrain from drinking alcoholic beverages during his therapy since it will increase the hepatotoxicity of some of the drugs he is taking.

II. He should take the medications exactly as instructed.

III. He should inform his doctor if he notices any dizziness, vertigo, insomnia, or nightmares.

A. I only

B. III only

C. I and II only

D. II and III only

E. I, II, and III

9. Because MR appears to have a problem understanding the treatment regimen and adherence is in question, which of the following is an appropriate suggestion to increase medication adherence?

A. Discontinue two of the TB drugs after 6 months of directly observed therapy (DOT)

B. Give the total daily dose of each drug in the morning

C. DOT for the entire treatment course

D. Give all of the drugs twice weekly instead of daily for the planned treatment duration

E. Discontinue two of the drugs after sputum conversion is reported as negative

10. Because TB is a concern to public safety, which of the following agencies should be notified of MR's diagnosis?

    A. Centers for Disease Control and Prevention (CDC)
    B. Local police department
    C. Local office of the state health department
    D. Local chapter of the American Lung Association
    E. His employer

Patient Name: Sarah Nelson
Address: 1015 Cynthia Street
Age: 27   **Sex:** Female
Height: 5′ 6″   **Weight:** 136 lb
Race: White
Allergies: Sulfa (rash)

Chief Complaint

SN is a 27-yo white female who presents to the clinic complaining of a greenish nasal discharge, facial pain, tooth pain, fever, chills, and a cough.

History of Present Illness

SN had a cold that began approximately 10 days ago. She had been feeling better for 3 days but then developed a fever to 101.8°F, chills, facial pain, dental pain, worsening cough, and greenish nasal discharge.

Past Medical History

Migraines

Endometriosis diagnosed 7 years ago

Social History

Tobacco use: 1/2 ppd; 2 pack-year history

Alcohol use: social drinking on weekends

Caffeine use: 4 diet sodas/day

Family History

Both parents alive. Mother with COPD. Father's history is unremarkable. Four siblings in good health, except for one sister with mitral valve prolapse.

Review of Systems

Primary symptoms include cough, nasal discharge, fever, chills, facial pain, and dental pain. Patient also complains of a headache that worsens when she bends over.

Medication Record

Date	Rx No	Physician	Drug/Strength	Quantity	Sig	Refills
2/7	15289	Craig	Ortho Tri-Cyclen	28	1 po daily	11
2/10	15998	Craig	Rizatriptan 10 mg	6	1 po prn	9

Physical Examination

GEN: Well-developed female complaining of nasal discharge, facial pain, tooth pain, and fever

VS: On presentation to the clinic: BP 120/78 mmHg, HR 75 bpm, RR 14 rpm, T 38°C, Wt 62 kg

HEENT: PERRLA, yellow-green nasal discharge, nasal membranes mild erythema

CHEST: CTA

NEURO: Alert and oriented x3

Laboratory and Diagnostic Tests

Sodium 143 mEq/L	Potassium 4.8 mEq/L
Chloride 112 mEq/L	CO_2 content 28 mEq/L
BUN 14 mg/dL	Serum creatinine 0.8 mg/dL
Glucose 84 mg/dL	Hemoglobin 14 g/dL
Hematocrit 40%	Platelets 150,000 cells/mm³

WBC 14,000 cells/mm³ with 75% PMNs, 6% bands, 11% lymphocytes, 8% monocytes

Sinus radiograph: Bilateral opaque maxillary sinuses

Diagnosis

Acute sinusitis

Pharmacist Notes and Other Patient Information

None available.

Questions

1. Which one of the following signs and symptoms is not consistent with acute sinusitis?

A. Facial and tooth pain

B. Fever

C. Nasal discharge

D. Symptoms persisting for less than 5 days

E. Headache

2. What pathogen is most likely causing sinusitis in SN?

A. Rhinovirus

B. *Bacteroides* species

C. *Staphylococcus aureus*

D. *Streptococcus pneumoniae*

E. *Pseudomonas aeruginosa*

3. Appropriate supportive therapy for SN's sinusitis may include which of the following?

A. Saline nasal sprays

B. Decongestants

C. Topical nasal steroids

D. Antihistamines

E. Systemic corticosteroids

4. What antimicrobial regimen is most appropriate for SN?

A. Amoxicillin

B. Levofloxacin

C. Trimethoprim/sulfamethoxazole

D. Linezolid

E. Amoxicillin/clavulanate

5. SN's physician prescribes amoxicillin/clavulanate. What agent would be dispensed for this prescription?

A. Levaquin

B. Ketek

C. Ceftin

D. Zithromax

E. Augmentin

6. How long should SN be treated for acute sinusitis?

A. 3 days

B. 5 days

C. 7 days

D. 14 days

E. 21 days

7. What is the purpose of the clavulanate in the antibiotic combination?

A. To increase the absorption of the amoxicillin

B. To inhibit the bacterial enzyme that inactivates the amoxicillin

C. To prevent alteration of the penicillin-binding protein on the bacteria

D. To reduce the adverse effects of the amoxicillin

E. It is another antibiotic

8. SN's physician also recommends that she use a topical nasal decongestant such as Afrin (oxymetazoline) and an analgesic such as ibuprofen. How would you counsel SN regarding these products?

I. Decongestants are safe to use in any patient.

II. Take the ibuprofen with food.

III. Do not use the Afrin for >3 days or more frequently than directed as more frequent or prolonged use may lead to rebound congestion.

A. I only

B. III only

C. I and II only

D. II and III only

E. I, II, and III

9. SN is still experiencing signs and symptoms 96 hours after initiation of therapy. Her physician changes her antibiotic to levofloxacin. How would you counsel SN about her new antibiotic prescription?

I. If taking antacids, vitamins, or products containing iron, zinc, or calcium, separate these products and the levofloxacin by at least 2 hours.

II. You may experience headache or dizziness.

III. Discontinue the antibiotic when your signs and symptoms resolve.

A. I only

B. III only

C. I and II only

D. II and III only

E. I, II, and III

10. What is the mechanism of penicillin resistance for *Streptococcus pneumoniae*?

A. Alteration of the penicillin-binding protein

B. Beta-lactamase production

C. Efflux pump

D. Poor penetration

E. Porins that do not allow passage of the penicillin

Patient Name: John Sampson
Address: 4 West 305th Street
Age: 78 **Sex:** Male
Height: 5′ 10″ **Weight:** 145 lb
Race: White
Allergies: Penicillin (rash)

Chief Complaint

JS is a 78-yo male who was admitted to the hospital from an area nursing home with fever, chills, vomiting, and flank pain.

History of Present Illness

He was seen by the nursing home physician last evening and treated with a single IM dose of ceftriaxone 1 gram. He was transferred to the hospital this morning due to continued fever, chills, vomiting, and flank pain.

Past Medical History

JS had a stroke 3 years ago and has been in a wheelchair since that time due to residual hemiparesis. In addition, he often requires catheterization to facilitate urination. He also has prostatic hypertrophy, HTN, mild CHF, and glaucoma, which are all controlled with medication.

Social History

Noncontributory

Family History

Noncontributory

Review of Systems

Fever, chills, vomiting, and flank pain

Physical Examination

GEN: Pale, ill-looking, thin white male with poor skin turgor

VS: BP 92/65 mmHg, HR 100 bpm, RR 22 rpm, T 39.5°C, Wt 66 kg

HEENT: PERRLA, oral cavity is dry

CHEST: Equal shallow breath sounds, tachypnic, tachycardic

NEURO: Not easily arousable, disoriented to place and time

BACK/ABD: Costovertebral angle tenderness, suprapubic tenderness

Laboratory and Diagnostic Tests

Sodium 146 mEq/L	Potassium 4.4 mEq/L
Chloride 105 mEq/L	CO_2 25 mEq/L
BUN 35 mg/dL	Serum creatinine 1.5 mg/dL
Glucose 66 mg/dL	Hemoglobin 13 g/dL
Hematocrit 39%	Platelets 225,000 cells/mm³

WBC 18,000 cells/mm³ with 80% neutrophils, 8% bands, 10% lymphocytes, and 2% monocytes

Urinalysis (from Foley catheter): Appearance amber-colored, specific gravity 1.030, pH 6.5, WBC 20-25 cells/hpf RBC 2-5 rbc/hpf, protein negative, glucose negative, ketones trace, nitrite negative, leukocyte esterase positive, bacteria many

Urine culture 100,000 cfu/mL gram-negative rods, identification pending

Blood culture gram-negative rods, identification pending

Diagnosis

Complicated urinary tract infection

Pharmacist Notes and Other Patient Information

None available.

Medication Record

Date	Rx No	Physician	Drug/Strength	Quantity	Sig	Refills
5/3		Sarloff	Accupril 10 mg	180	bid	3
5/3		Sarloff	Doxazosin 1 mg	90	qd	3
5/3		Sarloff	Furosemide 40 mg	90	qd	3
5/22		Sarloff	Ceftriaxone 1 gram IM	1	Stat	0
5/3		Sarloff	Timolol 0.5%	15 mL	1 gtt OU bid	6
5/3		Sarloff	MVI	100	qd	

Questions

1. Which of the following factors or characteristics did NOT contribute to the development of a complicated urinary tract infection in JS?

    A. Catheterization of the urinary tract
    B. Incomplete bladder emptying
    C. Prostatic hypertrophy
    D. Previous stroke with residual hemiparesis
    E. Use of immunosuppressive medications

2. Which of the following should NOT be considered as a potential pathogen causing urosepsis in JS?

    A. *Escherichia coli*
    B. *Proteus mirabilis*
    C. *Streptococcus pneumoniae*
    D. *Klebsiella pneumoniae*
    E. *Pseudomonas aeruginosa*

3. In order to determine an appropriate antibiotic dose to treat this patient's infection, what is the patient's estimated creatinine clearance using the Cockcroft-Gault equation?

    A. 28 mL/min
    B. 38 mL/min
    C. 56 mL/min
    D. 74 mL/min
    E. 100 mL/min

4. Which of the following signs/symptoms, physical examination findings, and laboratory findings are NOT suggestive of a complicated urinary tract infection (urosepsis or pyelonephritis) in this patient?

    A. Costovertebral angle tenderness
    B. Fever
    C. Low serum glucose
    D. Altered mental status
    E. Pyuria with positive urine and blood cultures

5. Based on the initial gram stain results from the urine and blood cultures, which of the following antibiotic regimens is most appropriate for the empiric treatment of JS' complicated urinary tract infection?

    A. Cefepime 1 g IVPB every 12 hours
    B. Ertapenem 1g IVPB every 24 hours
    C. TMP/SMX DS 1 tablet PO every 12 hours
    D. Ampicillin 2 grams IVPB every 6 hours
    E. Doxycycline 100mg PO every 12 hours

6. The results of the urine and blood culture and susceptibility results yield *Escherichia coli* susceptible to TMP/SMX, ampicillin/sulbactam, piperacillin/tazobactam, cefazolin, ceftriaxone, cefepime, imipenem, meropenem, levofloxacin, and gentamicin. Which of the following antibiotic regimens should be used for the continued treatment of JS's infection (as directed therapy)?

    A. Cefepime 1 g IVPB every 12 hours
    B. Meropenem 500 mg IVPB every 12 hours
    C. Cefazolin 1g IVPB every 8 hours
    D. Gentamicin 80 mg IVPB every 8 hours
    E. Aztreonam 1 gram IVPB every 8 hours

7. Which of the following antibiotics should be used with caution in a patient with congestive heart failure or hypertension due to the high content of sodium in parenteral formulations?

    A. Cefepime
    B. Ticarcillin/clavulanate
    C. Levofloxacin
    D. Meropenem
    E. Aztreonam

8. What is the recommended duration of antibiotic therapy for a patient with a complicated urinary tract infection such as urosepsis and pyelonephritis?

    A. Single-dose therapy
    B. 3 days
    C. 7 days
    D. 14 days
    E. 28 days

9. Which of the following statements regarding urinary catheter use is NOT true with regard to the development of urinary tract infections?

    A. Urinary catheters do not increase the risk of developing urinary tract infections.
    B. Bacteria may be introduced directly into the bladder during catheterization of the urinary tract.
    C. The longer the patient has a urinary catheter, the greater the chances of developing a urinary tract infection.
    D. In patients with long-term urinary catheters who develop symptomatic urinary tract infections, replacement of the urinary catheter may decrease the incidence of reinfection.
    E. Antibiotic prophylaxis is not recommended in patients with long-term indwelling catheters to prevent the development of urinary tract infections because it may lead to the emergence of resistant bacteria.

Case 55

10. If it is determined that JS also has chronic prostatitis, which of the following treatment regimens would be most appropriate for his treatment?

    A. Ampicillin 500 mg PO every 6 hours for 28 days
    B. TMP/SMX DS one tablet PO BID for 42 days
    C. Levofloxacin 500 mg PO QD for 14 days
    D. Azithromycin 1 g PO as a single dose
    E. Ceftriaxone 1 g IVPB QD for 28 days

OB/GYN Disorders and Women's Health

Section Editor: C. Brock Woodis

Patient Name: Emma Johnson
Address: 1612 East College Street, Apt. 5-A
Age: 20   **Sex:** Female
Height: 5′ 4″   **Weight:** 112 lb (50.9 kg)
Race: Caucasian
Allergies: Codeine (nausea)

Chief Complaint

EJ is a 20yo female who presents today to her university's student health center. She is currently in a monogamous relationship of 6 months and is interested in starting hormonal contraception. Up until this time, she has only used barrier methods (e.g., male condoms) as her means of contraception.

History of Present Illness

EJ reports 8 sexual partners over the last 3 years. She denies any symptoms of sexually transmitted diseases (STDs) and has never been diagnosed with a STD. She has never been pregnant. Her last menstrual period began 8 days ago. She has mild cramping with menses that last approximately 4 days.

Past Medical History

EJ was diagnosed with seizure disorder following a motor vehicle accident 2 years ago. EJ had her first gynecological examination 1 year ago. EJ reports that her Papanicolaou (Pap) smear was negative. She has twice self-treated in the past with an OTC antifungal vaginal product for vaginal itching and discharge.

Social History

Tobacco use: none

Alcohol use: 4–5 drinks per day on the weekends

Occupation: Student at a local university

Family History

Mother has no significant medical history

Father has HTN

Medication Record

Date	Rx No	Physician	Drug/Strength	Quantity	Sig	Refills
5/7	172645	Ramirez	Phenytoin kapseals 100 mg	90	3 caps po qhs	5
10/12	168577	Ramirez	Naproxen 500 mg	24	1 tab po q 12 hr prn cramping	0

Review of Systems

Negative except as noted previously

Physical Examination

GEN: Well-nourished, well-developed, healthy appearing female in NAD

VS: BP 118/68 mmHg, HR 68 bpm

Laboratory and Diagnostic Tests

Serum phenytoin 11.2 µg/mL (approximately 3 months ago)

Diagnosis

Primary:
Contraception

Secondary:
History of seizures secondary to MVA

Pharmacist Notes and Other Patient Information

Student health plan (covers most generic medications)

Questions

1. If the patient desires an OTC contraceptive, all the following would be a choice **EXCEPT**:

    A. male condom.

    B. female condom.

    C. diaphragm and gel.

    D. spermicidal jelly.

    E. nonoxynol9 vaginal suppositories.

2. All of the following are important counseling points for combined oral contraceptives **EXCEPT**:

   A. oral contraceptives provide protection from sexually transmitted diseases.

   B. it is important to take the oral contraceptive at the same time each day.

   C. there is a risk of venous thromboembolism associated with combined oral contraceptive use.

   D. in addition to preventing pregnancy, some combined oral contraceptives may treat acne and help improve mood.

   E. there is a decreased risk of ovarian cancer with long-term use.

3. All of the following are contraindications to using oral contraceptives **EXCEPT**:

   A. breast cancer.

   B. deep venous thrombosis 3 years ago.

   C. HIV-positive status.

   D. hepatic adenoma.

   E. two-vessel coronary artery bypass graft.

4. Which of the following progestins is **LEAST** androgenic?

   A. Norethindrone

   B. Norgestrel

   C. Levonorgestrel

   D. Ethynodiol acetate

   E. Desogestrel

5. Because EJ has never taken combined oral contraceptives, she asks about possible side effects. All of the following have been seen in clinical trials or clinical use **EXCEPT**:

   A. weight gain.

   B. elevation in blood pressure.

   C. elevation in serum glucose.

   D. breakthrough bleeding.

   E. development of pancreatic tumors.

6. EJ returns to student health 3 months after starting a combined oral contraceptive (COC). She complains of frequent episodes of nausea and severe breast tenderness. Which of the following would be the **MOST** appropriate intervention?

   A. Recommend to EJ's prescribing physician that her current COC contains too little estrogen and that EJ should be switched to a product containing more estrogen.

   B. Recommend to EJ's prescribing physician that her current COC contains too much estrogen and that EJ should be switched to a product containing less estrogen.

   C. Recommend to EJ's prescribing physician that her current COC contains too little progestin and that EJ should be switched to a product containing more progestin.

   D. Recommend to EJ's prescribing physician that her current COC contains too much progestin that that EJ should be switched to a product containing less progestin.

   E. Recommend to EJ's prescribing physician that EJ discontinue the COC and only use barrier methods of contraception.

7. Three months later, EJ returns to student health and asks the physician for a different type of birth control because she is having a difficult time remembering to take her oral contraceptive each day. All of the following contraceptive options were discussed. The following pairings list a correct counseling point for the contraceptive method **EXCEPT**:

   A. depot medroxyprogesterone acetate: irregular menstrual bleeding.

   B. copper intrauterine device: increased dysmenorrhea.

   C. diaphragm and contraceptive gel: vaginal itching.

   D. depot medroxyprogesterone acetate: high failure rate.

   E. levonorgestrel intrauterine system: irregular bleeding initially.

8. EJ calls the student health center one afternoon with questions regarding emergency contraception (EC). All of the following statements regarding EC are correct **EXCEPT**:

   A. Both women and men aged 17 years and older who provide appropriate age verification may purchase Plan B One-Step or Next Choice over the counter (OTC).

   B. Many oral contraceptives have been declared safe and effective for EC by the United States Food and Drug Administration.

   C. Antiemetics such as meclizine or promethazine should be taken 30–60 minutes before progestin-only EC due to the high likelihood of vomiting.

   D. Levonorgestrel-only EC does not interfere with pregnancy once implantation has occurred.

   E. There appear to be no long-term complications associated with levonorgestrel-only EC.

9. Oral contraceptives are commonly used for other gynecological or hormonally related problems. All of the following are such uses **EXCEPT**:

Case 56

    A.   acne.

    B.   recurrent yeast vaginitis.

    C.   premenstrual symptoms.

    D.   dysmenorrhea symptoms.

    E.   irregular menstrual bleeding.

10. EJ confirms that she has been adherent with her phenytoin. Which of the following is **TRUE** regarding phenytoin and oral contraceptives?

    A.   Phenytoin slows the intestinal absorption of estrogens.

    B.   Phenytoin increases the hepatic metabolism of estrogens.

    C.   Estrogens decrease the seizure threshold.

    D.   Phenytoin does not interact with oral contraceptives.

    E.   Estrogens decrease the renal elimination of phenytoin.

Patient Name: Christina Lopez
Address: 1848 Magnolia Place
Age: 39   **Sex:** Female
Height: 5′ 3″   **Weight:** 142 lb (64.5 kg)
Race: Hispanic
Allergies: TMP-SMX (causes hives)

Chief Complaint

CL is a married 39-yo female presently 41/3 weeks pregnant by transvaginal ultrasound. She is gravida 3, para 2. She was admitted to the Women's and Children's hospital this morning for a scheduled labor induction.

History of Present Illness

The estimation of gestational age based on CL's last menstrual period (LMP) correlated with transvaginal ultrasounddating performed at 18 weeks. The only complication she has experienced during this pregnancy is her asthma for which she has had two exacerbations requiring prednisone.

Past Medical History

Moderate persistent asthma

Genital herpes simplex virus

Vaginal delivery of an infant boy at 39 weeks gestational age without complications (at age 31)

Vaginal delivery of an infant female at 40 weeks gestational age without complications (at age 34)

Social History

Married, husband is an police officer

Alcohol use: none

Tobacco use: 10 pack-year history, but quit smoking during her first pregnancy

Occupation: high-school teacher

Family History

Nothing significant

Review of Systems

Negative except as noted previously

Physical Examination

GEN: Pregnant, appears to be at term, NAD

VS: BP 138/88 mmHg, HR 86 bpm, RR 18 rpm

CHEST: Lungs clear

PELVIC: Bishop score of 3 (cervix unfavorable for delivery)

EXT: 2+ pedal edema

Laboratory and Diagnostic Tests

All prenatal tests were normal during pregnancy

1 hr 50 g oral glucose tolerance test (at 26 weeks) 128 mg/dL

Urine culture was negative at both 8 weeks (first prenatal visit) and at 38 weeks

Diagnosis

Primary:
Labor induction

Medication Record

Symbicort (budesonide/formoterol 80 mcg/4.5 mcg) 2 puffs INH bid

Albuterol MDI 2 puffs INH prn

Prenatal vitamin 1 tablet po qday

Medication Orders on Admission to Labor and Delivery

1) Lactated ringer's IV 100 mL/hour

2) Oxytocin 20 units/1000 mL Lactated ringer's; begin infusion at 2 mU/min; increase by 2 mU/min every 30 minutes up to maximum of 20 mU/min. If contractions become every 2-3 minutes or last longer than 45-60 seconds, decrease dose by 1 mU/min and contact prescriber.

3) Advair (fluticasone/salmeterol 250 mcg/50 mcg) 1 puff INH bid (formulary substitution for Symbicort)

4) Albuterol MDI 2 puffs INH q 4h prn

Pharmacist Notes and Other Patient Information

None available.

Case 57

Questions

1. The standard drug for labor induction is oxytocin. The half-life in late pregnancy is approximately eight minutes. Which of the following is/are correct regarding the dosing and pharmacokinetics of this agent?

   I. The dose should not be increased more rapidly than once per hour.
   II. A bolus dose should be given before the constant infusion is started.
   III. After a dosage change, steady state should occur within 40 minutes.

   A. I only
   B. III only
   C. I and II only
   D. II and III only
   E. I, II, and III

2. Since oxytocin has the potential to cause water intoxication, symptomatic hyponatremia could result if high concentrations of oxytocin are given in hypotonic fluids for an extended amount of time. Oxytocin is both functionally and structurally similar to which pituitary hormone that causes this effect?

   A. Growth hormone
   B. Vasopressin
   C. Corticotropin
   D. Thyrotropin
   E. Prolactin

3. CL was concerned about how her medications could affect her pregnancy. When assessing the placental transfer of medications from mother to fetus, basic characteristics of drugs and the developing fetus are considered. Which of the following characteristics is MOST likely to cause significant morphological effects in the developing fetus through placental transfer?

   A. A drug the mother took during the thirty-second week after conception
   B. A highly ionized drug
   C. A drug with a small molecular weight
   D. A weakly basic drug
   E. A drug administered as a single dose only

4. CL has concerns regarding taking prednisone during her pregnancy. All of the following are concerns regarding the child or mother EXCEPT:

   A. adrenal suppression of the fetus.
   B. growth restriction.
   C. neonatal sepsis.
   D. neonatal cataracts.
   E. gestational diabetes.

5. CL delivers a 7-pound, 8-ounce infant girl and begins breastfeeding. When evaluating drug transfer into breast milk, all of the following drug characteristics generally promote transfer into milk EXCEPT:

   A. low molecular weight.
   B. weakly basic pKa.
   C. highly protein bound.
   D. low ionization.
   E. high lipid solubility.

6. Since CL experienced four herpes outbreaks in the last year, she and her physician decide to start suppressive therapy. In trying to determine the safety of using this drug in lactation, what is/are the most appropriate reference(s) to find information based on available studies and databases?

   I. Package inserts
   II. Publication on drugs in lactation by the American Academy of Pediatrics
   III. Drugs in Pregnancy and Lactation: A Reference Guide to Fetal and Neonatal Risk

   A. I only
   B. III only
   C. I and II only
   D. II and III only
   E. I, II, and III

7. The pharmacy student that is interning with you is unsure of the pregnancy designations she has seen in patient charts. CL is G$_3$ P$_2$. Which of the following is true regarding what this information tells you?

   A. She has been pregnant twice.
   B. She appears to be in her third pregnancy.
   C. She has delivered twins.
   D. She has one living child.
   E. She delivered the child(ren) by vaginal delivery.

8. CL comes to your pharmacy to pick up a refill on her doxycycline that was originally filled eleven months ago. You know that CL is breastfeeding and you inquire whether she was instructed to refill this prescription by her obstetrician. She states that she decided that she needed the refill. When she comes to the prescription counter, she is planning on purchasing two cans of infant formula and three baby bottles. You ask her several questions. CL responds that her left breast feels warm, has a reddish discoloration, and hurts when her baby is nursing. Based on your knowledge and her response, which of these is most likely?

A. CL has another upper respiratory infection and is trying to self-treat. She does not have the energy to breas-feed and is going to start her infant on formula.

B. CL's husband is ill with a fever and cough and she is going to give him her prescription medication. Also she thinks her milk supply is waning so she wants to supplement with formula.

C. CL likes to keep an antibiotic on hand at home and is buying the formula for later use because it is on sale.

D. CL takes doxycycline at least once per year and wants to get the prescription filled prior to its expiration. She is also planning to go back to work half-time and wants to get formula for the babysitter.

E. CL has developed mastitis and is trying to self-treat. Breastfeeding is too painful at this time and she is going to switch her infant to formula.

9. CL is appropriately started on clindamycin 300 mg po q 6 hours for mastitis. What is the most common infecting organism in mastitis?

A. Peptostreptococcus

B. Group B streptococcus

C. *Staphylococcus aureus*

D. *Staphylococcus epidermidis*

E. Group A streptococcus

10. CL plans to discontinue breastfeeding and start formula milk. All of the following are true regarding formula EXCEPT:

A. formula milk is considered to be inferior nutrition to breast milk.

B. soy protein is usually reserved for infants intolerant of animal fats and vegetable oil for their protein source.

C. breast milk promotes the development of obesity in later life.

D. low-iron formulas should not be used unless recommended by a physician.

E. powders and concentrated liquids should not be diluted greater than recommended on packaging.

Patient Name: Beverly Dupuis
Address: 132 Lake Ridge Drive
Age: 50   **Sex:** Female
Height: 5′ 5″   **Weight:** 132 lb (60 kg)
Race: Caucasian
Allergies: Amoxicillin causes rash

Chief Complaint

BD is a 50-yo female who presents to her gynecologist with complaints of hot flashes, irritability, and frequent awakenings at night. She states this has been occurring intermittently for approximately 6 months but has become more severe in the last 8 weeks. She also mentions that her interest in sexual intercourse has drastically decreased over the past 6 months.

History of Present Illness

BD states her periods have become lighter and are occurring more erratically-. Her last three menstrual periods were October 15, January 4,, and May 20. She wakes up -approximately 2 times a week and has to change her nightgown due to sweating. BD states that she sleeps better with the air conditioner turned to a cooler temperature but her husband has difficulty with the low temperature. She also notes she becomes tearful over "little things" that did not affect her in the past. Her decreased interest in sex started approximately 6 months ago. This is a change for her and she feels that it is negatively affecting her relationship with her husband.

Past Medical History

Gravida 3, para 3 (BD has had three pregnancies and has three living children)

HTN

Hyperlipidemia, presently controlled by diet

Frequent UTIs; takes prophylactic antibiotics

Social History

Alcohol use: 5–6 drinks/week

Tobacco use: none

Illicit drug use: none

Occupation: business consultant

Has one daughter and two sons all in their twenties. Remarried 3 years ago.

Family History

Mother suffered a nontraumatic fracture in her sixties

Father has hyperlipidemia and suffered an MI (nonfatal) at age 56.

Negative for DM, cancer, HTN

Review of Systems

Otherwise negative except for occasional tension headaches relieved by acetaminophen. Patient denies any recent changes in weight, appetite, or bowel habits.

Physical Examination

VS: BP 146/86 mmHg (sitting), HR 78 bpm, Temperature 97.9°F

GEN: thin female in NAD

PELVIC: no adnexal tenderness or masses

RECTAL: hemoccult negative

Laboratory and Diagnostic Tests

Total cholesterol 208 mg/dL	Triglycerides 166 mg/dL
LDL 126 mg/dL	HDL 52 mg/dL
TSH 2.7 mU/L	FSH 85 mIU/mL

Diagnosis

Primary:
1. Perimenopause
2. Decreased libido

Pharmacist Notes and Other Patient Information

Use of nitrofurantoin has slowly dropped based on refill history; assess compliance issues versus improvement in disease state.

Medication Record

Date	Rx No	Physician	Drug/Strength	Quantity	Sig	Refills
2/22 3/14	97102	Walsh	Nitrofurantoin 100 mg Acetaminophen 500 mg	60	1 po qd UTI prn pain, HA	3
12/16	87933	Taylor	Lisinopril 20 mg 30 1 tab po qd	11		

Questions

1. BD's obstetrician assesses her and decides to treat her menopausal symptoms. All of the following are appropriate estrogen replacement products on the market EXCEPT:

   A. ogen.
   B. evista.
   C. climara.
   D. menest.
   E. premarin.

2. Which of the following is the primary reason a progestin is added to an estrogen?

   A. Increase bone mineral density over estrogen alone
   B. Offset the negative lipoprotein effects of estrogens
   C. Protect the endometrium from estrogen-induced proliferation
   D. Improve the acceptability to women
   E. Provide protection against development of breast cancer

3. Although BD is given a prescription, she inquires about the different types of estrogens. She wonders if she is "getting a strong one." As part of your explanation, you list the most important biological estrogens. Which of the following series contains the biological estrogens in the correct order from most potent to least potent?

   A. 17-estradiol; ethinyl estradiol; estrone
   B. Ethinyl estradiol; estrone sulfate; estriol
   C. 17-estradiol; estrone; estriol
   D. Equilin sulfate; estrone; estriol
   E. Estriol; estrone; 17-estradiol

4. BD wants to think about starting estrogen supplementation, but in the meantime she wants to know what she can do for painful intercourse. The physician asks that you recommend therapy for vaginal dryness. Which of the following is an estrogen with only local effects (as BD wants time to consider systemic therapy)?

   A. Maxilube vaginal lubricant
   B. Femring (estradiol acetate)
   C. Depo-Estradiol (estradiol cypionate in oil)
   D. Estring (estradiol)
   E. Estrasorb topical emulsion (estradiol hemihydrate)

5. Findings from the Women's Health Initiative (WHI) study have greatly influenced current prescribing of hormone replacement therapy. All of the following are pertinent study design issues/findings EXCEPT:

   A. approximately 65% of the women enrolled in the study were age 60 or over.
   B. contrary to previous studies, both the estrogen and estrogen plus progestin arms showed increased fracture risk compared to placebo.
   C. the study discouraged women who were having significant vasomotor symptoms from enrolling in WHI.
   D. the attributable risk due to hormone replacement therapy was actually low; treatment of 10,000 women for 1 year would result in 7 additional cardiovascular disease events, 8 strokes, and 8 cases of invasive breast cancer.
   E. the combination therapy (PremPro) arm was stopped early due to crossing a predetermined boundary of invasive breast cancer cases while the estrogen-only (Premarin) arm was allowed to continue at that time

6. BD says that her friend Maureen told her that some medications that are used to treat menopausal hot flashes do not contain any estrogen. Which of the following nonhormonal options for menopausal hot flashes is incorrectly paired with a possible adverse event?

   A. Gabapentin; somnolence
   B. Clonidine; postural hypotension
   C. Ginseng; warfarin potentiation
   D. Black cohosh; hepatotoxicity
   E. Duloxetine; urinary incontinence

7. BD takes an estrogen and progestin for 3 years before she self-discontinues it after her mother develops breast cancer. Which of the following agents stimulates breast tissue?

   A. Estropipate
   B. Raloxifene
   C. Alendronate
   D. Tamoxifen
   E. Toremifene

8. BD has noted some return in hot flashes and wants to restart estrogen but at a lower dose. Of note, her cholesterol and triglycerides have worsened. You as the pharmacist recommend transdermal estrogen that is changed once weekly. Which of the following estrogen preparations fits both of these criteria?

   A. Vivelle-Dot
   B. EstroGel
   C. CombiPatch
   D. Alora
   E. Climara

Case 58

9. BD inquires about therapy for her loss of libido. Which of the following products has been used in clinical practice (although not necessarily FDA-approved for this indication)?

   A. Estratest
   B. Methyltestosterone tablets
   C. AndroGel 1%
   D. Fluoxymesterone
   E. Estradiol valerate in oil

10. BD reports she has one other problem that has worsened recently: urinary incontinence. A description of her symptoms includes a loss of urine if she cannot reach a restroom quickly once the urge to urinate occurs. She is diagnosed with urge incontinence. She is considering drug therapy. Which of the following is/are differences between oxybutynin and tolterodine?

   I. Tolterodine is available in immediate-release, extended release, and transdermal products while oxybutynin is only available in immediate-release and extended release products.
   II. Tolterodine is a competitive antagonist at muscarinic receptors while oxybutynin has both anticholinergic activity and smooth muscle relaxant properties.
   III. Tolterodine is primarily metabolized by the CYP2D6 isoenzyme with accompanying drug interactions. Oxybutynin does not have this type of drug interaction.

   A. I only
   B. III only
   C. I and II only
   D. II and III only
   E. I, II, and III

Pediatric Therapy

Patient Name: Baby girl Hill
Address: 524 Juniper Street
Age: 0 days   **Sex:** Female
Height: 43.2 cm **Weight:** 3 lb 14 oz
Race: Caucasian
Allergies: NKDA

Chief Complaint

Baby Hill is a 31-week old premature infant admitted to the neonatal intensive care unit immediately after birth to rule out the possibility of sepsis.

History of Present Illness

Baby Hill was born by vaginal delivery at 31 weeks gestation to a 29yo mother (gravida 4, para 3, spontaneous Ab 1) at 12:45 p.m. today. APGAR's were 6 and 8 at 1 and 5 minutes, respectively. Cord pH was 7.32.

Past Medical History

Maternal history positive for rupture of membranes x 20 hours, pregnancy-induced hypertension (beginning 3 weeks ago), and Group B *Streptococcus* (GBS) positive. Medication use during pregnancy included prenatal vitamins, Zantac, and Tylenol.

Maternal Screen

GBS: pos (no treatment)

RPR: neg

HIV: neg

Hep B: neg

HSV: neg

Chlamydia: neg

Rubella immune

Social History

None

Family History

Will live with Mom, Dad, two sisters (8 and 4 yo) and one brother (2 yo) at home.

Maternal grandmother: HTN

Sister (8 yo): Asthma

Review of Systems

Negative except as previously noted

Physical Examination

GEN: Mottled color, active

VS: T 98.4°F, HR 137 bpm, RR 42 bpm, BP 43/32 rpm, O_2 sat 97% RA, Ht: 43.2 cm, head circumference 30 cm

HEENT: Anterior fontanelle present, no cleft palate or lip

CHEST: Bilateral breath sounds

CV: RRR, no murmur

ABD: Soft, NTND, positive BS

GU: Normal female genitalia, patent anus

NEURO: Good tone

EXT: 20 Digits, cap refill 4 sec

Laboratory and Diagnostic Tests

Sodium 139 mEq/L	Potassium 5.2 mEq/L
Chloride 108 mEq/L	CO_2 content 25 mEq/L
BUN 14 mg/dL	Creatine 0.8 mg/dL
Glucose 60 mg/dL	Calcium 7.2 mg/dL
Protein 4.2 g/dL	Albumin 2.6 g/dL
Total bili. 4.0 mg/dL	ALP 118 U/L
AST 50 U/L	ALT 13 U/L

WBC 9800/mm³ with 52 segs, 5 bands, 38 lymphs, and 5 monos

Hgb 15.7 g/dL, Hct 46.3 %, platelets 319,000/mm³

Blood cx: Pending

CSF cx: Pending

Diagnosis

Primary:
1) Suspected sepsis; GBS infection
2) Prematurity

Medication Record

Ampicillin 176 mg IV q 12 h

Gentamicin 7 mg IV q 24 h

D_{10} W at 6 mL/h

Pharmacist Notes and Other Patient Information

Obtain gentamicin levels with the 4th dose

Questions

1. The age of a neonate is defined as:
   A. Birth to 1 week of life
   B. Birth to 1 month of life
   C. Birth to 2 months of life
   D. Birth to 6 months of life
   E. Birth to 1 year of life

2. On initial assessment, Baby Hill has:
   I. normal hepatic enzymes
   II. hyperkalemia
   III. hyperchloremia

   A. I only
   B. III only
   C. I and II only
   D. II and III only
   E. I, II, and III

3. Which of the following bacteria is a gram negative rod organism that causes early-onset sepsis in the neonate?
   A. Group B *Streptococcus*
   B. *Listeria monocytogenes*
   C. *Escherichia coli*
   D. *Staphylococcus epidermidis*
   E. *Bacteroides*

4. BG Hill is currently being administered _____ mg/kg/d of ampicillin.
   A. 0.1
   B. 0.2
   C. 20
   D. 100
   E. 200

5. Gentamicin levels return for BG Hill. The trough is 0.9 μg/mL and the peak is 7.8 μg/mL. How would you adjust her current dose of 7 mg IV q 24 hours?
   A. Increase the dose
   B. Decrease the dose
   C. No change
   D. Increase the interval
   E. Decrease the interval

6. Ampicillin injection is available in the following dosage form(s):
   A. sodium only.
   B. sulfate only.
   C. sodium and trihydrate.
   D. trihydrate and sulfate.
   E. sodium, trihydrate, and sulfate.

7. BG Hill is receiving maintenance fluids of $D_{10}W$ at 6 mL/hr. How many kcal/kg/day is the baby receiving?
   A. 82
   B. 49
   C. 28
   D. 144
   E. 64

8. Which of the following is TRUE regarding the risk of RSV and subsequent need for prophylaxis with palivizumab for BG Hill?
   A. She should receive prophylaxis if she is d" 6 months at the beginning of RSV season.
   B. She is at risk only if she has chronic lung disease.
   C. All neonates born during RSV season should receive prophylaxis.
   D. She should receive prophylaxis only if she has additional risk factors such as day care attendance, siblings, or smoking in the home.
   E. She should not receive prophylaxis.

9. Which of the following describes best the mechanism of action(s) of gentamicin?
   I. Binds to the 30S ribosomal subunit and causes an inhibition of protein synthesis
   II. Binds to the 50S ribosomal subunit and causes an inhibition of protein synthesis
   III. Binds to binding proteins and causes cell wall death

   A. I only
   B. III only
   C. I and II only
   D. II and III only
   E. I, II, and III

10. An investigator wants to establish a causal relationship between the use of sulfonamides in neonates and the incidence of kernicterus. Which of the following study designs should be used?
    A. Case series
    B. Randomized controlled
    C. Retrospective cohort
    D. Crossover study
    E. None of the above

Patient Name: Katie Taylor
Address: 425 Bristol Way
Age: 1   **Sex:** Female
Height: 2' 4"   **Weight:** 8.8 kg
Race: White
Allergies: NKDA

Chief Complaint

KT is a 1–yo infant brought to her pediatrician's office with complaints of a fever, irritability, and decreased oral intake.

History of Present Illness

Two days ago KT became irritable and her mother noticed she felt warm. KT's temperature was 102.3°F (max) over the last 2 days. Yesterday she did not eat as much as she usually does and only had 1 cup of milk.

Past Medical History

Acute otitis media (right) 4 months ago (first episode)

Immunizations up-to-date

Social History

KT lives at home with her parents and older sister (3 yo). KT attends day care Mon-Fri for 4 hours a day. Father smokes. No animals in the home or outside.

Family History

Hypertension: maternal grandmother

Diabetes: paternal father

Review of Systems

Negative except as noted previously

Physical Examination

GEN: WD/WN white female, irritable

VS: BP 92/56 mmHg, HR 124 bpm, RR 24 rpm, T 101.8°F, Wt 8.8 kg, Ht 72 cm

HEENT: Rt. tympanic membrane (TM) red and bulging, immobile

CHEST: Unremarkable

CV: RRR

ABD: Palpable, nontender

EXT: WNL

NEURO: WNL

Laboratory and Diagnostic Tests

WNL

Diagnosis

Right acute otitis media

Medication Record

Prescriptions written:

Motrin (100 mg/5mL) 4 mL po q 8 hours PRN pain/irritability

Amoxicillin (400 mg/5 mL) 1 tsp po bid x 10 days

Pharmacist Notes and Other Patient Information

None available.

Questions

1. Listed are the common symptoms of acute otitis media EXCEPT:

    A. otalgia.
    B. otorrhea.
    C. partial deafness.
    D. dizziness.
    E. fever.

2. A resident asks you about the use of TMP/SMX in acute otitis media. The following statements regarding the role of TMP/SMX are true EXCEPT:

    A. in the past it was useful as a first-line agent in treating otitis media.
    B. incidence of pneumococcal resistance is higher than that of penicillins.
    C. numerous skin reactions may occur during therapy.
    D. approximately 10% of *Haemophilus influenzae* isolates are resistant.
    E. cross-resistance to beta-lactams is nonexistent.

3. The most common bacteria causing acute otitis media is:

    A. *Staphylococcus aureus.*
    B. *Streptococcus pyogenes.*
    C. *Streptococcus pneumoniae.*
    D. *Haemophilus influenzae.*
    E. *Moraxella catarrhalis.*

4. Nonpenicillin-susceptible *Streptococcus pneumoniae* may be resistant to all of the following antibiotics EXCEPT:

    A. vancomycin.
    B. TMP/SMX.
    C. azithromycin.
    D. cefprozil.
    E. cefuroxime axetil.

5. Which of the following mechanisms describes how *Streptococcus pneu*moniae develops antimicrobial resistance to beta-lactam agents?

    A. Beta-lactamase production
    B. Efflux pump
    C. Alteration in the PCN-binding proteins
    D. Alteration in the ribosomal binding site
    E. Alteration of the mec A binding site

6. Which of the following does NOT lead to a higher incidence of or increase the risk of developing acute otitis media?

    A. Eustachian tube dysfunction
    B. Breastfeeding
    C. Patient age
    D. Allergies
    E. Secondhand smoke

7. Developmental differences of the Eustachian tube between young children and adults have been postulated to increase the incidence of acute otitis media in children. These differences include all the following EXCEPT:

    A. the tensor veli palatini muscle is less efficient at opening the Eustachian tube in children.
    B. the Eustachian tube in children is shorter than in adults.
    C. the angle of the tube is 45 degrees in adults and only 10 degrees in children.
    D. there are no differences that increase the risk of acute otitis media.
    E. the clearing function of the cilia in the Eustachian tube improves with age.

8. How many mg/kg/day of amoxicillin is KT prescribed?

    A. 20 mg/kg/day
    B. 45 mg/kg/day
    C. 90 mg/kg/day
    D. 100 mg/kg/day
    E. 180 mg/kg/day

9. KT returns to her pediatrician 5 days after the initial visit. She is still having fever and is irritable. The physician feels she failed amoxicillin therapy due to a resistant organism and asks you what antibiotic KT should be prescribed. What antibiotic do you recommend?

    A. Amoxicillin/clavulanic acid
    B. TMP/SMX
    C. Cefdinir
    D. Ceftriaxone
    E. Azithromycin

10. Which of the following vaccinations would you administer if you needed to provide the pneumococcal vaccine to KT?

    A. Menactra
    B. Fluvirin
    C. Varivax
    D. Prevnar 13
    E. Adacel

Patient Name: Brian Thornton
Address: 1210 Mesa Drive
Age: 15
Sex: Male
Height: 5' 6"
Weight: 50 kg
Race: Caucasian
Allergies: NDKA; allergic to ragweed

Chief Complaint

"I had bloody diarrhea, and I fainted for about 5 minutes."

History of Present Illness

BT experienced three bloody bowel movements (BMs) (midnight, 2 a.m., and 5 a.m.) on the day of admission. He reported that the toilet was filled with red blood. He began to feel faint after his last BM and passed out for about 5 minutes. He denies any seizures. This is the first time he has ever fainted in association with bloody diarrhea. He denies any nausea, vomiting, fever, abdominal pain, palpitations, changes in vision, headache, or dysuria. He has had no recent changes to his diet.

A decision to start antibiotics and bowel rest was determined.

Past Medical History

Crohn's disease (CD) (diagnosed 6 years ago): Last CD admission 7/21 for exacerbation of CD symptoms

Allergic rhinitis (receives allergy shots once monthly)

Exercise-induced asthma

No history of surgeries (just endoscopy/proctoscopy for dx of CD)

Social History

Residence: Home with parents
Occupation: Student
Smoking: Denies
EtOH: Denies
Illicit drugs: Denies (other than prescribed for CD)
Diet: Typical adolescent diet (fatty foods)
Education: 9th grade, poor student
Family/social environment: Intact, stable

Family History

No family history of CD
Father: 40 yo; no complaints

Mother: 38 yo; healthy, no complaints

Siblings: 12-yo brother, no complaints

14-yo sister, + ADHD

Children: N/A

Other: Paternal GF, + DM

Maternal GM, + pancreatic CA (deceased)

Review of Systems

Well-nourished, young man in no apparent distress

Physical Examination

GEN: Fairly well-nourished young man in no apparent distress

VS: BP 100/60 mmHg, P 90 bpm, RR 20 rpm, T 37°C, weight 50 kg (24%), and height 5' 6", 167.6 cm (37%)

HEENT: Moist mucous membranes

LUNGS: Clear to auscultation, no wheezes, no shortness of breath

CV: No chest pain or palpitations WNL

GI: Soft, nontender, nondistended, + bowel sounds (hyperactive)

GU: WNL

EXT/SKIN: No joint pain; WNL

CNS: WNL

MS: WNL

GI: Per HPI

GU: No complaints

HEME: No abnormal clotting, bruising, or infections

Laboratory and Diagnostic Tests

Results from 8/13:

Sodium 140 mEq/L	Potassium 4.1 mEq/L
Chloride 110 mEq/L	CO2 24 mEq/L
BUN 8 mg/dL	Creatine 0.5 mg/dL
Glucose 90 mg/dL	Calcium 8.7 mg/dL
Protein 5.7 g/dL	Albumin 3.1 g/dL
Total bili 0.2 mg/dL	ALP 375 U/L

AST 12 U/L

ALT 30 U/L

Amylase 62 U/L

Lipase 58 U/L

WBC 4.4 x 103/mm³

RBC 2.93/mm³

Hgb 8.2 g/dL

Hct 25.9%

Platelets 488,000/mm³

Retic count 2.5%

ANC 2700

ESR 34 mm/hour

Transferrin 125 mg/dL

Ferritin 10 ng/mL

Results from 8/16:

Sodium 140 mEq/L

Potassium 4.3 mEq/L

Chloride 105 mEq/L

CO2 26 mEq/L

BUN 9 mg/dL

Creatine 0.6 mg/dL

Glucose 95 mg/dL

Calcium 8.9 mg/dL

Protein 5.7 g/dL

Albumin 3.1 g/dL

Total bili 0.2 mg/dL

ALP 390 U/L

AST 14 U/L

ALT 29 U/L WBC 7.4 x 103/mm³

RBC 2.95/mm³

Hgb 8.4 g/dL

Hct 26.5%

Platelets 439,000/mm³

ANC 4600

ESR 20 mm/hour

Clostridium difficile Toxin A - negative

Stool culture

Normal flora, negative for *Salmonella, Shigella, Campylobacter, Yersinia,* or *Aeromonas*

Ova and parasite: Negative

Diagnosis

Crohn's Disease Flare

Medication Record

Albuterol 2 puffs INH prn prior to exercise (last used 1 week ago)

Sulfasalazine 1 g PO bid

6-Mercaptopurine 50 mg PO q day

Metronidazole 500 mg IV q 8 h

TPN w/ famotidine150 mg/day (to start today)

Methylprednisolone 15 mg IV q 8 h

Infliximab 225 mg/250 mL NS x1

Pharmacist Notes and Other Patient Information

None available.

Questions

1. Which multivitamin in the parenteral nutrition would be the best choice for this patient?

   I.   Pediatric multivitamins
   II. No multivitamins are required
   III. Adult multivitamins with vitamin K

   A. I only
   B. III only
   C. I and II only
   D. II and III only
   E. I, II, and III

2. Calculate BT's maintenance fluids for 24 hours.

   A. 1248 mL/day
   B. 1512 mL/day
   C. 2304 mL/day
   D. 2406 mL/day
   E. 4992 mL/day

3. The best technique to avoid calcium phosphorus precipitation in parenteral nutrition is to:

   A. use amino acid solutions with a high pH.
   B. use the proper order of mixing.
   C. protect the solutions from light and cold temperatures.
   D. use calcium chloride salts in solution.
   E. add additional magnesium salts to the solution.

4. Which PN solution would you recommend for BT's first day of therapy? A percutaneous catheter (PICC) was placed by the radiologist upon admission.

   A. AA 1% - D_5W solution at 160 mL/h with fat emulsion 20% 500 mL
   B. AA 2.5% - $D_{10}W$ solution at 85 mL/h with fat emulsion 20% 250 mL
   C. AA 3% - $D_{25}W$ solution at 20 mL/h with fat emulsion 20% 100 mL
   D. AA 4% - D_5W solution at 125 mL/h with fat emulsion 20% 1000 mL
   E. AA 5% - $D_{15}W$ solution at 45 mL/h with fat emulsion 20% 50 mL

Case 61

5. BT's PICC line was accidentally removed. Which is NOT a consideration in administering PN by peripheral access?

   A. PN solution osmolarity of 900 mOsm/L
   B. Calcium concentration of 5 mEq/L
   C. Dextrose concentration of 10%
   D. Lipid concentration of 20%
   E. All should be assessed when peripheral parenteral nutrition is used

6. It is found that BT has an enterocutaneous fistula (ileum). He will require at least 2 weeks of parenteral nutrition and bowel rest. His albumin level has continued to decrease and he has had a weight loss of 2 kg since being admitted. What would you recommend as a protein goal in the PN solution?

   A. 0.5 g/kg
   B. 1 g/kg
   C. 1.5 g/kg
   D. 3 g/kg
   E. 3.5 g/kg

7. Since BT has an enterocutaneous fistula, he may be at risk for wasting certain nutrients. What trace element might you suggest increasing in his PN solution?

   A. Aluminum
   B. Copper
   C. Manganese
   D. Iodine
   E. Zinc

8. BT's physician is concerned that he is losing too much fluid from his fistula. What solution would you recommend using to replace his losses?

   A. 0.45% sodium chloride with potassium chloride 10 mEq/L
   B. 0.45% sodium chloride with sodium bicarbonate 30 mEq/L
   C. D_5W
   D. 0.9% sodium chloride with potassium chloride 40 mEq/L
   E. D5 0.225% sodium chloride with sodium bicarbonate 5 mEq/L

9. Since BT is 15 yo, which protein solution would you recommend for compounding his PN solution?

   A. FreeAmine (adult formulation)
   B. Premasol (pediatric specialty formulation)
   C. Trophamine (pediatric specialty formulation)
   D. Aminosyn-HF (hepatic failure formulation)
   E. RenAmin (renal failure formulation)

10. BT was found to have megaloblastic anemia in addition to his anemia contributed from his acute gastrointestinal bleeding. Which of BT's medications could be responsible for this?

    A. Infliximab
    B. Mercaptopurine
    C. Metronidazole
    D. Famotidine
    E. Sulfasalazine

Patient Name: Bridget Anderson
Address: 110 Washington Street
Age: 11 months **Sex:** Female
Height: 31 in **Weight:** 10 kg
Race: Caucasian
Allergies: NKDA

Chief Complaint

BA is an 11-month old female who presents with a 6-day history of fever, URI symptoms, and respiratory distress.

History of Present Illness

BA is an 11-month old female who has just been transported from a referring hospital for further management of respiratory distress. The patient was in good health until 6 days prior to admission when she developed fever (T_{max} 101°F) and nasal congestion. She did well until 2 days prior to admission, when she was seen by her PMD for URI symptoms and sent home with Tylenol prn. One day prior to admission, she had increased congestion and fever to 103°F. She was seen in an outside hospital's ER, where chest x-ray showed suspicion of pneumonia with bronchiolitis. The patient was given one dose of ceftriaxone, an albuterol nebulizer treatment, and a dose of Orapred and discharged home on Zithromax, albuterol syrup, and Orapred. That evening, the patient experienced increased work of breathing, retractions, grunting, and tachypnea and was taken back to the outside hospital, where she was admitted and started on oxygen, albuterol continuous nebulizer, and IV antibiotics and steroids. She was then transferred to the PICU of another hospital for further management. In that PICU, the patient decompensated and had to be intubated. Chest x-ray in that PICU showed right pleural effusion and left pneumothorax. Despite high settings with a conventional ventilator, the patient's O_2 saturations remained in the 60s. Due to an inability to maintain adequate oxygen saturations, the patient was transported to this PICU for further management with a high frequency oscillating ventilator (HFOV) and possible extracorporeal membrane oxygenation (ECMO).

Past Medical History

The patient has no significant past medical history. Immunizations are up to date.

Social History

Patient lives with both parents. She has no siblings. Her development is normal.

Family History

Unremarkable

Review of Systems

Patient is sedated and intubated

Physical Examination

Vital signs: Temp 35°C, Pulse 167, RR 48, BP 67/28

Head: AFOSF, NCAT

Skin: Pink, capillary refill less than 2 seconds

Eyes: Pinpoint secondary to sedation

Ears: TMs red

Nose: Clear

Mouth and throat: Intubated

Neck: Supple, slightly enlarged posterior cervical nodes B/L

Lungs: Significantly decreased breath sounds bilaterally (right more than left); crackles bilaterally

Heart: RRR, normal S_1/S_2, no murmur

Abdomen: Soft, nontender, nondistended, + bowel sounds, no hepatosplenomegaly

Genitalia: Normal female genitalia, anus patent

Neuro: Sedated

Laboratory and Diagnostic Tests

Sodium 152 mEq/L	Potassium 2.9 mEq/L
Chloride 116 mEq/L	CO_2 19 mEq/L
BUN 16 mg/dL	Creatinine 0.7 mg/dL
Glucose 193 mg/dL	Calcium 6.7 mg/dL
AST 65 units/L	ALT 27 units/L
Alk phos 68 units/L	T bili 0.3 mg/dL
Albumin 2.8 g/dL	WBC 1000 per mm³
Hemoglobin 8.8 g/dL	Hematocrit 26.0%
Platelets 107,000 per mm³	Segs 12%
Lymphocytes 61%	pH 7.15
pCO_2 42 mmHg	pO_2 27 mmHg
CO_2 15 mmol/L	O_2 saturation 42%

Case 62

Base deficit 14 mmol/L   RSV negative

PTT 102   PT 17.4

INR 1.7   CRP 9.0 mg/L

Chest x-ray: Diffuse infiltrates throughout both lung fields, right-sided pleural effusion, left-sided pneumothorax

 Diagnosis

Severe pneumonia, ARDS, shock, HFOV, and possible ECMO

 Medication Record

D_5W/0.2% NaCl with potassium chloride 20 mEq/L to run at 40 mL/hour (1 x M)

Albumin 5% 10 g/200 mL IV x 2

Dobutamine 15 μg/kg/min

Dopamine 15 μg/kg/min

Norepinephrine 0.02 μg/kg/min

Fentanyl 1 μg/kg/hour

Midazolam 0.1 mg/kg/hour

Insulin sliding scale q 4h

Ceftriaxone 500 mg IV q 12h (50 mg/kg/dose)

Tobramycin 25 mg IV q 8h (2.5 mg/kg/dose)

Vancomycin 200 mg IV q 8h (20 mg/kg/dose)

TPN and lipids

 Pharmacist Notes and Other Patient Information

Chest tubes placed bilaterally, O_2 sats on HFOV 80s, decision to put patient on ECMO

Questions

1. During a pediatric emergency, each of the following routes would be acceptable for administration of drugs, fluids, or blood products EXCEPT:
   A. intraosseus.
   B. peripheral venous access.
   C. umbilical artery access.
   D. central venous access.
   E. intrathecal.

2. How would you classify the type of shock present in BA on admission to the PICU?
   A. Hypovolemic shock
   B. Cardiogenic shock
   C. Septic shock
   D. Neurogenic shock
   E. Hypervolemic shock

3. BA's admission ABG indicates:
   A. no acid-base derangement.
   B. metabolic acidosis.
   C. metabolic alkalosis.
   D. respiratory acidosis.
   E. respiratory alkalosis.

4. Initial resuscitation of pediatric septic shock centers on the early and frequent administration of fluid infusions with either crystalloid or colloid solutions. Which of the following solutions is NOT a crystalloid?
   A. Lactated Ringer's solution
   B. 0.9% normal saline
   C. Dextran-40
   D. 5% dextrose
   E. 0.45% sodium chloride

5. BA's norepinephrine drip is initiated at 0.02 μg/kg/min. Given a standard concentration of 8 mg in 250 mL, what will be the rate of the drip?
   A. 3.75 mL/hr
   B. 375 mL/hr
   C. 6.3 mL/hr
   D. 0.38 mL/hr
   E. 0.006 mL/hr

6. After receiving repeated fluid boluses of 20 mL/kg in the first hour of treatment, BA's blood pressure remains 78/34 mmHg. The patient does not exhibit any signs or symptoms of fluid overload. The resident physician asks you to recommend alternative therapy for this patient's emergency resuscitation. Which of the following would you suggest?
   A. Fentanyl infusion
   B. Cisatracurium infusion
   C. Phenylephrine infusion
   D. Dopamine infusion
   E. Ketamine infusion

7. At a dose of 15 μg/kg/min, the effect of dopamine may best be defined as:
   A. dopaminergic.
   B. beta-1 adrenergic.

C. alpha-adrenergic.

D. beta-2 adrenergic.

E. omega-adrenergic.

8. Tobramycin levels have returned for this patient. The peak is 5.3 μg/mL and the trough is 1.0 μg/mL. The resident asks you if any change to the tobramycin order should be made. Before you make any recommendation for change, you should evaluate each of the following EXCEPT:

A. time of tobramycin administration.

B. time of trough sampling.

C. liver function tests.

D. at which dose the levels were drawn.

E. time of peak sampling.

9. After evaluating all information associated with the tobramycin levels, you determine that the measured levels are accurate. In order to adequately treat BA's pneumonia, which of the following changes would you recommend to the tobramycin regimen?

A. Increase the dose

B. Extend the interval

C. No changes are needed

D. Shorten the interval

E. Increase the dose and extend the interval

10. BA is started on a vecuronium drip at 0.1 mg/kg/hour. As the team pharmacist, which of the following interventions would you recommend for a patient on a neuromuscular blocker continuous infusion?

A. Medical restraints

B. Artificial tears

C. Saline nasal spray

D. Incentive spirometry

E. Physical therapy

Diseases of the Eye and Ear

Section Editor: Celtina K. Reinert

Patient Name: Darlene Miller
Address: 7201 Rose Street
Age: 23   **Sex:** Female
Height: 5'4"   **Weight:** 128 lb
Race: White
Allergies: NKDA

Chief Complaint

DM is a 23-yo female who presents to her primary care doctor complaining of red and itchy eyes for 2 days. She is a kindergarten teacher and several of her students have had pink eye recently.

History of Present Illness

DM has seasonal allergies but usually doesn't get red eyes with it. Several of her students have been sent home in the last week for possible pink eye, and DM's eyes started itching 2 days ago. This morning she woke up with matted eyes and wants to know if she needs to be treated.

Past Medical History

DM uses an oral contraceptive to manage irregular menstrual cycles and uses an OTC antihistamine to treat seasonal allergies. She is generally healthy, except for an occasional cold.

Social History

DM lives with her fiancé. She works full-time as a kindergarten teacher and has an active social life. Tobacco use: none. Alcohol use: occasional. Illicit drug use: none.

Family History

Parents are alive and well. Father, age 56, has hypertension and mother, age 53, has anxiety; both treated with lifestyle modifications and medications. Sibling has no known medical conditions

Review of Symptoms

Denies any pain or vision changes. Denies symptoms of allergies (runny nose, sneezing, post nasal drainage). Patient complains of itchy eyes with increased discharge and noticed matting upon waking this morning.

Physical Examination

GEN: WDWNWF, slightly anxious, but in NAD

VS: BP 112/76 mmHg, HR 72 bpm, RR 18 rpm, Temperature 98.4°F

HEENT: Conjunctiva reddened bilaterally, PERRLA.

Laboratory and Diagnostic Test

Deferred at this time.

Diagnosis

Primary:

1) Bacterial conjunctivitis

Secondary:

1) Menstrual regulation

2) Seasonal allergies

Pharmacist Notes and Other Patient Information

4/13 Aided patient selection of antihistamine, patient given information on seasonal allergies.

9/3 Patient instructed on proper oral contraceptive use.

10/14 Reviewed use of eye drops with patients.

Medication Record

Date	Rx No	Physician	Drug/Strength	Quantity	Sig	Refills
4/14			Loratadine 10 mg	90	1 po qd prn	
9/3	85743	Smith	Loestrin 24	1 pack	1 po qd	11
10/14	86901	Smith	Sulfacetamide 10% drops	15 mL	1 gtt ou qid x 7-10 days	

Case 63

Questions

1. Which of the following ophthalmic medications would duplicate the action of loratadine?

   A. Xibrom
   B. Crolom
   C. Patanol
   D. Azopt
   E. Vigamox

2. If DM had a sulfonamide allergy, which of the following would be appropriate to treat her current symptoms?

   A. Blephamide
   B. Tobramycin
   C. Trifluridine
   D. Ketotifen
   E. Olopatadine

3. Which of the following is more likely to occur in allergic conjunctivitis rather than bacterial conjunctivitis?

   A. Itching rather than irritation
   B. Acute rather than chronic symptoms
   C. Purulent discharge
   D. Rash
   E. Headaches

4. Which of the following would NOT help to prevent the spread of pink eye?

   A. Proper handwashing techniques
   B. Avoidance of those with diagnosed pink eye
   C. Sanitizing contaminated surfaces
   D. Touching or rubbing the eye
   E. Using a clean washcloth daily

5. If DM wants to try something over the counter for her symptoms, what would be most appropriate to tell her?

   A. Any eye drops will treat with pink eye.
   B. Artificial tears will help the itchiness of pink eye.
   C. An antibiotic eye drop is needed for pink eye.
   D. Visine will relieve the redness caused by pink eye.
   E. Allergy eye drops are used for pink eye.

6. If DM had allergic conjunctivitis instead of bacterial conjunctivitis, which of the following would be most appropriate for treatment?

   A. Tobramycin ophthalmic drops
   B. Sulfamethoxazole/trimethoprim oral tablets
   C. Ketotifen ophthalmic drops
   D. Brimodine ophthalmic drops
   E. Prednisolone oral suspension

7. Conjunctivitis can be caused by which of the following:

   I. Allergens
   II. Bacteria
   III. Viruses

   A. I only
   B. III only
   C. I and II only
   D. II and III only
   E. All of the above

8. Which of the following is NOT a symptom of conjunctivitis:

   A. Redness in the eye(s)
   B. Itchy eye(s)
   C. Gritty feeling in the eye(s)
   D. Color change in the iris(es)
   E. Discharge that forms a crust on the eye(s)

9. Pink eye is also known as:

   A. Blepharitis
   B. Bacterial conjunctivitis
   C. Glaucoma
   D. Stye
   E. Acanthamoeba keratitis

10. Which of the following is recommended to install eye drops in children:

    A. Self-installation
    B. Place drops in the outside corner of the eye
    C. Place drops in the conjunctival sac created by pulling down on the lower lid
    D. Place drops on closed lashes and have child blink several times quickly
    E. Place drops on inner corner of closed eye and slowly open eyes

Patient Name: Lisa Rossi
Address: 14624 Brentwood Drive
Age: 18   **Sex:** Female
Height: 5′ 4″   **Weight:** 54 kg
Race: White
Allergies: Grass and tree pollen

Chief Complaint

LR is an 18-yo female who presents to her PCP with redness and tenderness of her left ear.

History Of Present Illness

LR states that she has noticed that her left ear has been tender for approximately 1 week. Over the past few days, her ear has become increasingly tender and somewhat red ("raw" as she describes it) to the point where she cannot lie on her left side or put in her earrings. She states that her ear "feels full" but denies any loss of hearing.

Past Medical History

Febrile seizures as an infant

Occasional reactive airway disease, for which she uses an inhaler on a prn basis

Menarche at age 13

Mild facial acne

Social History

LR lives with her parents and a pet cat. She is a swimmer in high school and spends extended periods of time in the pool. She is sexually active with a single, male partner.

Tobacco use: has tried in the past but denies regular use

Alcohol use: none

Illicit drug use: admits to trying marijuana but denies regular use

Medication Record

Family History

Parents are alive and well. Mother has hypothyroidism; father has HTN.

Review of Systems

Ear as described above. Denies any headache, blurred vision, photophobia, fever, facial or neck stiffness or tenderness, or jaw/tooth pain.

Physical Examination

GEN: Healthy-looking female in mild distress due to otalgia

VS: BP 100/70 mmHg, HR 82 bpm, RR 20 rpm, T 37.0°C (oral), Wt 54 kg

HEENT: NC/AT, PERRLA. Examination of the left external ear (AS) reveals a tender, erythematous, macerated ear canal. No obvious pus, TM is intact. No apparent involvement of surrounding tissues. Right ear is normal.

NECK: No stiffness; mild cervical lymphadenopathy

LUNGS: CTA

NEURO: CN II-XII intact

The remainder of her physical exam is normal.

Laboratory and Diagnostic Tests

Gram's stain and microscopic examination of a swab of the external ear canal revealed Gram positive cocci in clusters. No hyphae or WBCs were seen.

Diagnosis

Primary:
1) Acute otitis externa (AS), bacterial

Secondary:
1) Acne
2) Reactive airway disease
3) Contraception

Date	Rx No	Physician	Drug/Strength	Quantity	Sig	Refills
4/1	34564	Watkins	Ventolin HFA	1	2 puffs prn	6
4/1			Claritin 10 mg	60	1 tab qd	
5/20	36008	Watkins	Ortho-Novum 1/28	1 pkg	1 tab qd	12
8/4			Benzoyl peroxide 10%		apply to face	
9/1			Naproxen 220 mg		prn menstrual cramps	

Case 64

Pharmacist Notes and Other Patient Information

4/1 Instructed patient on use of inhaler and peak flow meter.

4/1 Advised patient on allergy treatment options.

5/20 Provided patient with information regarding STD prevention.

8/1 Advised patient on facial skin care products.

Questions

1. A common synonym for otitis externa is:

    A. pinkeye.
    B. trench mouth.
    C. ringworm.
    D. earache.
    E. swimmer's ear.

2. Which of the following patient groups are affected by otitis externa?

    I. Children
    II. Adolescent/adults
    III. Elderly

    A. I only
    B. III only
    C. I and II only
    D. II and III only
    E. I, II, and III

3. The only otic product that may be used when the tympanic membrane (eardrum) is perforated is:

    A. ofloxacin otic solution.
    B. antipyrine-benzocaine otic solution.
    C. ciprofloxacin-hydrocortisone otic solution.
    D. neomycin-hydrocortisone-polymyxin B otic solution.
    E. acetic acid otic solution.

4. A common adverse effect of antibiotics found in topical otic preparations is:

    A. diarrhea.
    B. contact dermatitis.
    C. anaphylaxis.
    D. drug fever.
    E. photosensitivity.

5. Patients should be instructed to enhance the contact of an otic solution with the affected area by using which of the following techniques?

    I. Slightly warming the solution prior to instillation
    II. Placing a cotton wick in the ear following instillation
    III. Manipulating the tragus to effect adequate distribution in the canal

    A. I only
    B. III only
    C. I and II only
    D. II and III only
    E. I, II, and III

6. The antimicrobial properties of acetic acid, which is a component of some otic preparations, are attributable to its:

    A. drying properties.
    B. hypertonicity.
    C. viscosity.
    D. acidity.
    E. detergent properties.

7. Which of the following is a risk factor for acute otitis externa?

    A. Short ear canal.
    B. Co-morbid diabetes mellitus.
    C. Injury to ear canal by excessive cleaning.
    D. Family history of otitis externa.
    E. History of perforated tympanic membrane.

8. What information should be provided to the patient to prevent otitis externa from recurring?

    A. Meticulous aural hygiene
    B. Prophylactic systemic antimicrobial agents
    C. Prophylactic topical antimicrobial agents
    D. Daily use of otic drops containing a corticosteroid
    E. Ear plugs

9. An uncommon complication of otitis externa in which the surrounding bone and soft tissues are affected is known as:

    A. invasive external otitis.
    B. suppurative external otitis.
    C. malignant external otitis.
    D. regional external otitis.
    E. temporal external otitis.

10. Auralgan otic contains antipyrine for its property as an:

    A. analgesic.
    B. anesthetic.
    C. antiseptic.
    D. anti-inflammatory agent.
    E. antimicrobial agent.

Skin Disorders

Case 65

Patient Name: Antoine D'Angelo
Address: 716 Milton Street
Age: 15 **Sex:** Male
Height: 5' 9" **Weight:** 146 lb
Race: African American
Allergies: NKDA

Chief Complaint

"I finally got serious about my acne and got prescriptions from the doctor."

History of Present Illness

AD's acne began 2 years ago, but he says it "wasn't that bad" until 4 months ago. At that point he began washing his face every night with a salicylic acid-containing cleanser marketed for acne-prone skin and applying an over-the-counter benzoyl peroxide product to any pimples, but these measures didn't seem to be helping much. Increasingly frustrated, he was spurred to seek medical treatment and get prescription therapy when he realized his family's trip to Europe was only several weeks away. He knows he will be in many photos, and would like to meet European girls, so he hopes there is time to check the acne's progression before then. Today he presents new prescriptions for erythromycin 250 mg, 60 count, 1 po bid, and Differin 0.1% gel, 45 g, apply to affected area q hs.

Past Medical History

AD was relatively healthy until 3 years ago, when he had his first seizure since having two febrile seizures at ages 3 and 4. He was hospitalized for the recent seizure, his EEG was abnormal, and he was placed on medication. The medicine (Depakote) made him too sleepy and caused him to gain weight, so he was switched to Tegretol about 1.5 years ago. Last year, he fractured his left wrist while rollerblading.

Social History

The patient lives with his parents and two older brothers. He denies being sexually active or drinking alcohol. He also denies using illicit drugs or tobacco. He enjoys athletics and plays basketball and baseball. He has been working at McDonald's for about 6 months, which has increased his fast food intake considerably.

Medication Record

Date	Rx No	Physician	Drug/Strength	Quantity	Sig	Refills
8/2010	2297	Kato	Tegretol XR 200 mg	90	1 po q am 2 po q hs	4

Family History

The patient's father is healthy except for multiple dental problems. His mother has hypertension and cholecystitis.

Review of Systems

Positive for 3-4 days of mild scratchy throat and runny nose (clear, watery drainage). The patient denies any seizures in the last 8 months, as well as any dizziness, nausea or vomiting, fever, rash, or abdominal pain.

Physical Examination

VS: BP 126/72 mmHg, HR 64 bpm, RR 14 rpm, T 98.0°F

GEN: Well-developed, well-nourished young African American male in no acute distress

HEENT: Without trauma; pupils equal; no nystagmus; oropharynx slightly red without exudate; nasal mucous membranes with clear discharge; no sinus tenderness; no lymphadenopathy

SKIN: Face with about 10 pustules and many open and closed comedones on nose, cheeks, chin, and forehead; also has about 10 pustules and several closed comedones on his back and shoulders; no nodules or cysts

CV: Regular rate and rhythm; no murmurs, rubs, or gallops

CHEST: Clear to auscultation and percussion bilaterally

ABD: Thin, soft, nontender, normal active bowel sounds; no organomegaly

Laboratory and Diagnostic Tests

(1 month ago)

AST 22 IU/L   ALT 46 IU/L

T. bili 0.4 mg/dL

WBC 4.1 K/mm³, normal differential

H/H 14.0 g/dL/42.2%   Platelets 267 K/mm³

Serum carbamazepine 8.4 mg/dL

Diagnosis

Acne vulgaris

Case 65

 Pharmacist Notes and Other Patient Information

None available.

Questions

1. Before filling AD's erythromycin prescription, the pharmacist decides to call the physician regarding the potential for Tegretol toxicity. What is the mechanism of the drug interaction that could cause such toxicity?

   A. Tegretol may induce erythromycin metabolism.
   B. Tegretol may inhibit erythromycin metabolism.
   C. Erythromycin may induce Tegretol metabolism.
   D. Erythromycin may inhibit Tegretol metabolism.
   E. Erythromycin may enhance Tegretol absorption.

2. What is an open comedo?

   A. A whitehead
   B. A blackhead
   C. A ruptured papule
   D. A nodule
   E. A pustule

3. The most common adverse effect of benzoyl peroxide is:

   A. skin irritation.
   B. hepatotoxicity.
   C. drug allergy.
   D. skin cancer.
   E. skin discoloration.

4. Which topical therapies have synergistic effects on acne when used together?

   A. Adapalene plus tretinoin
   B. Azelaic acid plus salicylic acid
   C. Benzoyl peroxide plus salicylic acid
   D. Clindamycin plus erythromycin
   E. Clindamycin plus benzoyl peroxide

5. AD was prescribed Differin. Pharmacologically, this agent is most like:

   A. benzoyl peroxide.
   B. clindamycin.
   C. erythromycin.
   D. tretinoin.
   E. tetracycline.

6. Which of the following are acne risk factors or aggravating factors for AD?

   A. Family history
   B. High intake of fast food
   C. African American race
   D. Exposure to volatilized grease at his job
   E. Obesity

7. Patients should be counseled to keep which of the following products refrigerated?

   A. Ziana gel 60 g
   B. Azelex cream 50 g
   C. Benzamycin gel 46 g
   D. Aczone gel 30 g
   E. Epiduo gel 45 g

8. Which of the following is the most likely reason that AD has not noticed any improvement from his use of benzoyl peroxide and anti-acne cleanser?

   A. He has not given the regimen enough time to work.
   B. Over-the-counter treatments are not strong enough to affect acne as severe as AD's.
   C. He is only using the cleanser once a day.
   D. He is applying benzoyl peroxide only to existing pimples, not to the entire area affected by acne.
   E. He is applying benzoyl peroxide after using the cleanser containing salicylic acid.

9. Which topical agent is best tolerated?

   A. Benzoyl peroxide
   B. Azelex
   C. Clindamycin
   D. Retin-A Micro
   E. Tazorac

10. "Pledget" describes what kind of product?

    A. A wipe
    B. A foam
    C. A vanishing cream
    D. A rinse
    E. A liquid polymer

Patient Name: Natalie Christensen
Address: 1956 Orange Street, Apartment C
Age: 49   **Sex:** Female
Height: 5′ 4″   **Weight:** 162 lb
Race: Caucasian
Allergies: TMP/SMX (rash); codeine (pruritus)

Chief Complaint

"My face is so red and broken out."

History of Present Illness

In her early 40s, NC began to be bothered by persistent redness in her cheeks and nose. "It was like I was always blushing, or had just come in from out in the cold." The problem has gotten steadily worse, and now she also complains of "bumps" in these areas. Sometimes her face stings and burns. She tried using an over-the-counter benzoyl peroxide gel, but it dried and irritated her skin, making the redness worse. She remembers her father had ruddy cheeks and a red, swollen, disfigured nose when he was older, and was teased that he drank excessively. She is embarrassed by her appearance and worries that people will think she is an alcoholic.

Past Medical History

Generalized anxiety disorder, currently controlled; history of major depressive disorder

Social History

NC, single, is a university administrator. She does not drink alcohol or use tobacco or illicit drugs. She drinks 3-5 cans of diet cola per day. She eats a healthy diet with lots of whole grains, fruits, and vegetables, but rarely finds time to exercise and leads a sedentary lifestyle.

Family History

Noncontributory, except for her father's rosacea as noted above

Medication Record

Date	Rx No	Physician	Drug/Strength	Quantity	Sig	Refills
8/2010	5693	Patel	Sertraline 100 mg	30	1 po qd	4
			Acetaminophen 325 mg	100	1-2 po q6h prn HA	
			One-A-Day Women's Tablets	60	1 po qd	

Review of Systems

Remarkable only for irregular menstrual periods and occasional headaches associated with job stress. She denies anxiety, depressed mood, and anhedonia, although she does note that she is often fatigued and sleepy due to overwork. She does not complain of any dryness or irritation in her eyes.

Physical Examination

VS: BP 134/88 mmHg, HR 80 bpm, RR 18 rpm, T 97.9°F

GEN: Overweight white woman in no acute distress

SKIN: Intense erythema and slight dryness give cheeks a chapped appearance. Nose is also red. Eight papules are scattered on and near the nose. Mild telangiectasia.

CV: Regular rate and rhythm; no murmurs, rubs or gallops

CHEST: Clear to auscultation and percussion bilaterally

EXT: 2+ dorsal pedal pulses bilaterally; no edema

Laboratory and Diagnostic Tests

None available.

Diagnosis

Rosacea

Pharmacist Notes and Other Patient Information

None available.

Case 66

Questions

1. Which of the following measures will help NC control her rosacea?

   A. Use an astringent or toner several times a week
   B. Lose weight
   C. Clear pores with warm compresses or steamy showers several times a week
   D. Protect her face from cold, heat, and wind
   E. Avoid high glycemic load foods

2. Which of the following actions could <u>worsen</u> NC's rosacea?

   A. Using sunscreen daily
   B. Washing the face daily with a mild cleanser
   C. Using moisturizer when skin feels tight
   D. Exfoliating weekly with a facial scrub
   E. Increasing her dose of sertraline

3. The changes in NC's father's nose are the hallmark of which presentation of rosacea?

   A. Papulopustular
   B. Atypical
   C. Phymatous
   D. Erythematotelangiectatic
   E. Glandular

4. Telangiectasia is best described as:

   A. slowed capillary refill.
   B. dilation of superficial skin capillaries.
   C. increased skin thickness.
   D. unusual skin firmness.
   E. failure of red skin to turn white when pressure is applied.

5. Oracea, a formulation of doxycycline, is approved by the FDA to treat rosacea at doses of 40 mg po daily. Why is it believed that the effective dose for rosacea is so much lower than usual doses of doxycycline?

   A. Doxycycline achieves high concentrations in sebum relative to serum.
   B. The *Demodex folliculorum* mites responsible for rosacea have high susceptibility to doxycycline.
   C. Oracea is approved for use only when used concomitantly with benzoyl peroxide.
   D. Therapy only needs to curb *Demodex* overgrowth, not eradicate the organism, to achieve clinical effectiveness.
   E. Doxycycline has anti-inflammatory effects independent of its antibiotic effects.

6. Patients with rosacea have sensitive skin, as NC learned when she tried to use benzoyl peroxide gel. Which drug and formulation would be least irritating for NC to use on her face?

   A. Clindamycin solution
   B. Azelaic acid gel
   C. Metronidazole cream
   D. Adapalene gel
   E. Benzoyl peroxide cream

7. Which of the following is NOT a risk factor for rosacea?

   A. Middle age
   B. Male gender
   C. Fair hair and skin, light eyes
   D. Tendency to blush easily
   E. Alcohol consumption

8. Which statement regarding rosacea and acne is true?

   A. Patients who develop rosacea are likelier to have had acne earlier in life than patients who do not.
   B. Acne has a protective effect against developing rosacea.
   C. Unlike acne patients, who generally must use maintenance therapies, rosacea patients do not usually experience relapse or recurrence after a successful course of drug treatment.
   D. Rosacea and acne are both marked by persistent erythema and telangiectasia.
   E. Rosacea can be distinguished from acne by the absence of comedones.

9. Which of the following topical agents is FDA-approved for the treatment of rosacea?

   A. Tazorac
   B. Cleocin T
   C. Protopic
   D. Finacea
   E. DUAC

10. If NC starts topical pharmacotherapy for her rosacea, what therapeutic outcome can she reasonably expect?

    A. The papules will resolve within a few days, and the erythema within a week. The telangiectasia will resolve slowly over weeks. Once her face is clear, she can discontinue therapy.
    B. The erythema will resolve within a few days, but the papules and telangiectasia will slowly resolve over weeks. Once her face is clear, she can discontinue therapy.

C. The papules will resolve over weeks, but the erythema and telangiectasia will probably not resolve completely. She will likely need to continue therapy to maintain benefit.

D. The erythema will resolve over weeks, but the papules and telangiectasia will probably not resolve completely. She will likely need to continue therapy to maintain benefit.

E. Although the erythema may resolve somewhat, therapy will mainly prevent progression of rosacea rather than resolve existing lesions. She will likely need to continue therapy to maintain benefit.

Patient Name: Charles Reynolds
Address: 1618 Chelan Avenue
Age: 65   Sex: Male
Height: 6' 2''   Weight: 211 lb
Race: African American
Allergies: NKDA

Chief Complaint

During a routine follow-up visit, CR, a 65-yo male, complains that a rash he has had "off and on" for years is bothering him again, this time on his elbows and on the right forearm around an old scar from a motorcycle accident.

History of Present Illness

CR says this rash, which consists of dry, itchy, raised, scaly patches, probably began when he was in his 30s; he isn't sure when because he thought the flares were isolated incidents at first. About 20 years ago he first sought medical attention, eventually being diagnosed with psoriasis by a dermatologist. Plaques usually appear on his elbows, knees, and scalp. He has never had arthritis symptoms or issues with his nails. He has used courses of various topical corticosteroids over the years. He notes the problem seems worse in spring and fall. The last couple years the psoriasis has been present more often than not, and the pruritus is becoming increasingly annoying. He is also self-conscious about the lesions and feels like he has to wear long sleeves, adding, "My wife thinks it is disgusting."

Past Medical History

Diabetes mellitus type 2 x 20 years

Hypertension x 20 years

Parkinson's x 3 years

Social History

CR is a retired aeronautical engineer. He lives with his wife and has 3 adult children and 4 grandchildren. He is monogamous and denies using illegal drugs. He quit smoking about 10 years ago. He drinks a beer about every other day. He has a fairly sedentary lifestyle.

Family History

Patient's father, who also had psoriasis, died at age 76 from a heart attack. His mother died at age 81 from pneumonia after extended hospitalization for a hip fracture. His children are healthy.

Review of Systems

Positive for occasional nocturia. He denies chest pain, shortness of breath, palpitations, hypoglycemic episodes, dizziness, nausea or vomiting, fever, or abdominal pain. He has no joint pain. Although he is satisfied with his Parkinson's treatment overall, he still notices it can be hard to "get going" when initiating movement.

Physical Examination

VS: Ht 6' 2", Wt 211 lb, BP 132/74 mmHg, HR 80 bpm and regular, RR 18 rpm, T 98.5°F

GEN: Overweight African American male in no acute distress

HEENT: Normocephalic, atraumatic. Pupils equal, round, and reactive to light. Oropharynx normal; no lymphadenopathy.

SKIN: 3 x 5 cm erythematous, scaly, lichenified plaque on extensor surface of left elbow. Right arm has similar 4 x 6 cm plaque on the elbow and two 2 x 2 cm plaques on the extensor surface of the forearm. There is mild excoriation but no significant swelling, tenderness, heat, pus, or streaking. Nails appear normal.

CV: Regular rate and rhythm; no murmurs, rubs, or gallops

CHEST: Clear to auscultation and percussion bilaterally

ABD: Soft, nontender, + bowel sounds in all four quadrants. No organomegaly.

EXT: 2+ dorsal pedal pulses. Slightly decreased vibratory sensation in feet but no loss of sensation by monofilament test.

Laboratory and Diagnostic Tests

(Fasting, 2 days ago)

Na 142 mEq/L	K 4.8 mEq/L
Cl 101 mEq/L	CO_2 26 mEq/L
BUN 20 mg/dL	SCr 1.2 mg/dL
Glucose 121 mg/dL	

(1 month ago)

AST 19 IU/L	ALP 69 IU/L
T. bili 1.1 mg/dL	

(6 months ago)

Hgb_{A1c} 7.1 %

WBC 8.3 K/mm³, normal differential

H/H 15.0 g/dL/45.2%   Platelets 302 K/mm³

Urinary albumin: Creatinine ratio 133 g/mg

Diagnosis

Psoriasis vulgaris

 Pharmacist Notes and Other Patient Information

7/2004 Patient replaced BG monitor; reviewed self-monitoring of blood glucose.

 Medication Record

Date	Rx No	Physician	Drug/Strength	Quantity	Sig	Refills
8/2010			Aspirin 81 mg	100	1 po q am	
8/2010			Centrum Silver	100	1 po q am	
8/2010	1134	Lin	Metformin 1000 mg	60	1 po bid	1
1/2010			Psorent 15% coal tar solution	100 mL	Apply q hs	
8/2010	1132	Lin	Carbidopa/levodopa CR 50/200	60	1 po bid	0
8/2010	1131	Lin	Lisinopril/HCTZ 20/25 mg	30	1 po q am	1
8/2010	1130	Lin	Glyburide 10 mg	60	1 po bid	1
8/2010	1129	Lin	Metoprolol succinate 50 mg	60	1 po q am	1
11/2009			Eucerin cream	480 g	Apply bid prn	

Questions

1. Which is the best choice of initial agent to treat the acute flare-up of psoriasis in this patient?

   A. Anthralin 1% cream
   B. Dovonex 0.005% ointment
   C. Elidel 1% cream
   D. Hydrocortisone 1% cream
   E. Lidex 0.05% ointment

2. Which adverse effect may occur during continuous long-term therapy with topical corticosteroids, particularly of higher potency?

   A. Skin striation
   B. Paradoxical exacerbation
   C. Skin sensitization
   D. Hyperpigmentation
   E. Hypoesthesia

3. Which of the following aspects of CR's presentation is a hallmark of psoriasis vulgaris, distinguishing it from other disorders such as atopic dermatitis or seborrheic dermatitis?

   A. Scale
   B. Need for emollient adjunct therapy
   C. Erythema and pruritus
   D. Involvement of scalp
   E. Location at site of former trauma

4. A systemic drug used in combination with ultraviolet light to treat psoriasis is:

   A. methoxsalen.
   B. coal tar.
   C. calcipotriene.
   D. adalimumab.
   E. methotrexate.

5. Which of the following of CR's medications is likeliest to be associated with psoriasis flares?

   A. Metformin
   B. Hydrochlorothiazide
   C. Metoprolol succinate
   D. Carbidopa/levodopa
   E. Glyburide

6. Which of the following lifestyle factors has no known effect on psoriasis, positive or negative?

   A. Sun exposure
   B. Stress level
   C. Intake of acidic foods
   D. Product fragrances
   E. Cold weather

7. Which of the following nonprescription products contains a keratinolytic agent?

   A. Campho-Phenique
   B. Caladryl

Case 67

C. Eucerin

D. AmLactin

E. Cortaid

8. After a few weeks of appropriate therapy, when CR's psoriasis flare is under reasonable control, his therapy is changed to calcipotriene for maintenance. This drug is best described as a(n):

A. synthetic retinoid.

B. vitamin D analog.

C. antimitotic agent.

D. calcineurin inhibitor.

E. keratinolytic.

9. Which counseling point applies to patients receiving PUVA therapy?

A. Effective courses of therapy require at least 200 treatments.

B. To maintain therapeutic benefit, continue treatments at least 3 times per week.

C. Therapy is at adequate intensity if treatment generates mild-to-moderate erythema.

D. Allow at least 48 hours between treatments.

E. Discontinue therapy if there is no response after 10 treatments.

10. Which product is likeliest to benefit patients with psoriasis?

A. Oral zinc

B. Topical colloidal silver

C. Oral pregnenolone

D. Topical aloe

E. Oral gotu kola

Organ Transplantation

Section Editors: Pamela R. Maxwell and Rebecca Brady

Name: Juan Garcia
Address: 10 SW Merlin Court
Age: 60   **Sex:** Male
Height: 170 cm   **Weight:** 80 kg
Race: Hispanic
Allergies: NKDA

Chief Complaint

Presented for bilateral lung transplant

History of Present Illness

Patient JG is a 60-yo Hispanic male who was called in from home for a bilateral lung transplant. He is currently post-op day 5.

Past Medical History

Bronchiectasis and idiopathic pulmonary fibrosis

Osteoarthritis

GERD

Social History

Married

Worked in construction; exposed to concrete and crushed limestone

Quit smoking > 1 yr ago; previously smoked 0.5 pack per day for 20 years

Negative for IVDA

Family History

Father with Parkinson's disease, mother and siblings alive and well

Review of Systems

Today patient is complaining of hand tremors in the late morning and evening. All other systems negative.

Physical Examination

GENERAL: No apparent distress; afebrile; alert & oriented x 3

NEURO: Cranial nerves II-XII intact; able to follow commands and verbalize properly with good speech volume; good eye contact

CARDIO: RRR; no M/R/G; S_1, S_2 present; no aggregates

PULMONARY: Nasal canula 4L; O_2 sats 94%

ABDOMEN: Soft; mildly tender to palpation; BS +

EXTREMITIES: Motor strength 5/5; sensitivity conserved and intact; peripheral pulses + 2; no peripheral edema

Laboratory and Diagnostic Tests

Sodium: 143 mEq/L	Potassium: 4.1 mEq/L
Chloride: 106 mEq/L	HCO_3: 28 mEq/L
Fasting blood glucose: 129 mg/dL	
BUN: 19 mg/dL	SCr: 1.0 mg/dL
Ca: 8.4 mg/dL	Mg: 2.3 mg/dL
Phos: 1.6 mg/dL	WBC: 5,100/mm^3
Hemoglobin: 12.1 g/dL	Hematocrit: 34.6%
Platelets: 93,000 cells/mm^3	

CMV Status: Donor IgG positive/Recipient IgG negative

Diagnosis

Bilateral lung transplant, post-operative day 5

Medications Record

Tacrolimus 1 mg PO twice daily

Mycophenolate mofetil 1000 mg PO twice daily

Prednisone 50 mg PO once daily

Trimethoprim-sulfamethoxazole 80-400 mg PO once daily

Itraconazole oral solution 200 mg PO once daily before breakfast

Amphotericin B 10 mg INH per nebulizer q12h

Valganciclovir 900 mg PO once daily

Cytomegalovirus IVIG 12.5 g IV infusion every 2 weeks for 3 times

Acetaminophen-hydrocodone 325 mg-10mg PO q6h PRN pain

Pantoprazole 40 mg PO once daily

Bisacodyl suppository 10 mg PR once daily PRN constipation

Piperacillin-tazobactam 4.5 g IVPB q8h

Vancomycin 1 g IVPB q8h

Questions

1. Which of the following statements is FALSE regarding exposure to second-hand smoke?

   A. Second-hand smoke increases the risk for heart disease.
   B. Second-hand smoke increases the risk lung cancer.
   C. Second-hand smoke increases the risk diabetes.
   D. Second-hand smoke increases the risk for sudden-infant death syndrome.
   E. Brief exposure to second-hand smoke increases the risk for exposure-related diseases.

2. All of the following strategies/medications can be used for smoking cessation EXCEPT:

   A. amitriptyline.
   B. bupropion.
   C. varenicline.
   D. individual or group counseling.
   E. behavioral cessation therapies.

3. What is the smoking pack-year history for this patient?

   A. Half-a-pack
   B. 5 years
   C. 10 years
   D. 15 years
   E. 20 years

4. Which of the following medications can increase the risk for gastrointestinal ulcers?

   A. Corticosteroids
   B. Tacrolimus
   C. Mycophenolate mofetil
   D. Cyclosporine
   E. Valganciclovir

5. Which of the following anti-fungal agents has no activity for *Aspergillus* species?

   A. Micafungin
   B. Itraconazole
   C. Posaconazole
   D. Fluconazole
   E. Voriconazole

6. Which of the following medications is most likely contributing to the patient's hand tremors?

   A. Valganciclovir
   B. Itraconazole
   C. Tacrolimus
   D. Mycophenolate mofetil
   E. Pantoprazole

7. The patient was taking indomethacin at home for his osteoarthritis. Which of the following medications has a possible interaction with indomethacin?

   A. Valganciclovir
   B. Itraconazole
   C. Tacrolimus
   D. Mycophenolate mofetil
   E. Pantoprazole

8. Which of the following medications can increase the risk for post-transplant diabetes mellitus?

   A. Tacrolimus and mycophenolate mofetil
   B. Tacrolimus and corticosteroids
   C. Corticosteroids and mycophenolate mofetil
   D. Valganciclovir and corticosteroids
   E. Valganciclovir and itraconazole

9. What is the patient's ideal body weight?

   A. 59 kg
   B. 66 kg
   C. 73 kg
   D. 78 kg
   E. 85 kg

10. What dose of valganciclovir would you recommend based on the patient's creatinine clearance (Cockcroft and Gault method: use actual body weight when weight no more than 30% greater than ideal body weight)?

   A. CrCl is 90 mL/min; regular dose 900 mg PO daily
   B. CrCl is 90 mL/min; renally adjust dose to 450 mg PO daily
   C. CrCl is 70 mL/min; regular dose of 900 mg PO daily
   D. CrCl is 50 mL/min; renally adjust dose to 450 mg PO daily
   E. CrCl is 50 mL/min; renally adjust dose to 450 mg PO every 48 hours

Patient Name: Stephen Caldwell
Address: 428 Evansville Road
Age: 52 **Sex:** Male
Height: 5' 9" **Weight:** 184 lb
Race: Caucasian
Allergies: NKDA

Chief Complaint

SC is post-renal transplant presenting to clinic for follow-up.

History of Present Illness

SC is a 52–yo Caucasian male who received a living donor renal transplant 4 months ago from his sister. He is presenting to clinic for a routine follow-up appointment.

Past Medical History

Renal transplant 4 months ago

DM 2

ESRD secondary to DM 2

Social History

No alcohol, tobacco, or IVDA

Family History

Mother with diabetes

Review of Systems

Normal

Physical Examination

GEN: WD male with no apparent signs of distress

Vitals

VS: BP 136/82 mmHg, HR 74 bpm, RR 16 rpm, T afebrile

Laboratory and Diagnostic Tests

Sodium 140 mEq/L   Potassium 4.2 mEq/L

Chloride 110 mEq/L CO_2 25 mEq/L

BUN 17 mg/dL

Serum creatinine 1.3 mg/dL (nadir 1.3)

Glucose 110 mg/dL   Total cholesterol: 270 mg/dL

Triglycerides: 460 mg/dL   Sirolimus: 5 ng/mL

Tacrolimus: 3 ng/mL

Medication Record

Acetaminophen 500 mg PO q4h PRN pain

Insulin glargine 20 units subcutaneously at bedtime

Mycophenolate mofetil 500 mg PO twice daily

Prednisone 15 mg PO once daily

Ranitidine 150 mg PO once daily

Sirolimus 2 mg PO once daily

Sulfamethoxazole/trimethoprim SS PO daily

Tacrolimus 1 mg PO twice daily

Valganciclovir 900 mg PO once daily

Questions

1. Which of the following medications is MOST likely the cause for the patient's elevated cholesterol and triglycerides?

   A. Mycophenolate
   B. Ranitidine
   C. Sirolimus
   D. Tacrolimus
   E. Valganciclovir

2. All of the following over-the-counter products/items could interact with the patient's tacrolimus EXCEPT:

   A. cimetidine.
   B. St. John's wort.
   C. grapefruit juice.
   D. apple juice.
   E. ibuprofen.

3. Which of the following medications is most likely to cause mouth ulcers?

   A. Valganciclovir
   B. Sirolimus
   C. Mycophenolate
   D. Tacrolimus
   E. Prednisone

4. What is the most likely reason for dosing sirolimus once daily in this patient?

    A. Avoid impaired wound healing after surgery
    B. Target a specific blood concentration
    C. Prevent peripheral edema
    D. Dosed according to the half-life
    E. Dosed daily for better compliance

5. Which of the following parameters would LEAST likely be used to monitor renal function?

    A. Serum creatinine
    B. Blood urea nitrogen
    C. Alanine aminotransferase
    D. Urine chemical analysis
    E. Creatinine clearance

6. In a landmark trial reported by Paya and colleagues in 2004, valganciclovir (the experimental agent) was compared to ganciclovir (the control agent) for prevention of cytomegalovirus (CMV) disease in high-risk solid organ transplant recipients. The incidence of CMV disease in kidney recipients was 6% for those receiving valganciclovir and 23% for those receiving ganciclovir. What is the absolute risk reduction in CMV disease for kidney transplant recipients receiving valganciclovir versus ganciclovir?

    A. 6%
    B. 17%
    C. 23%
    D. 29%
    E. 71%

7. In a landmark trial reported by Paya and colleagues in 2004, valganciclovir (the experimental agent) was compared to ganciclovir (the control agent) for prevention of cytomegalovirus (CMV) disease in high-risk solid organ transplant recipients. The incidence of CMV disease in kidney recipients was 6% for those receiving valganciclovir and 23% for those receiving ganciclovir. What is the number-needed-to-treat with valganciclovir to prevent CMV disease in one kidney transplant recipient?

    A. 0.06
    B. 0.2
    C. 2
    D. 3
    E. 5

8. In a landmark trial reported by Paya and colleagues in 2004, valganciclovir (the experimental agent) was compared to ganciclovir (the control agent) for prevention of cytomegalovirus (CMV) disease in high-risk solid organ transplant recipients. The incidence of CMV disease in kidney recipients was 6% for those receiving valganciclovir and 23% for those receiving ganciclovir. What is the relative risk reduction in CMV disease for kidney transplant recipients receiving valganciclovir versus ganciclovir?

    A. 4%
    B. 17%
    C. 23%
    D. 29%
    E. 74%

9. Which of the following infections is the patient LEAST likely to develop being 4 months post-transplantation?

    A. Wound infection
    B. Opportunistic infections
    C. Polyomavirus
    D. Reactivation of latent infection from the donor
    E. Reactivation of latent infection from the recipient

10. Sirolimus belongs to which of the following drug classes?

    A. Calcineurin inhibitor
    B. Anti-microbial agent
    C. Purine synthesis inhibitor
    D. Mammalian target of rapamycin (mTOR) inhibitor
    E. Interleukin-2 (IL-2) receptor antagonist

Geriatric Disorders

Case 70

Patient Name: Chris Craxton
Address: 7605 Best Park Road
Age: 77   **Sex:** Male
Height: 72 in   **Weight:** 75 kg
Race: Caucasian
Allergies: NKDA

Chief Complaint

CC is a 77-year-old Caucasian male with increased problems of memory loss, disorientation, and irritability. He has an 8-year history of confusion that has slowly progressed.

History of Present Illness

More recently, the patient has experienced disorientation, anxiety, confusion, and appears to have a tremor. Approximately 2 years ago, CC's family physician started him on Aricept 5 mg at bedtime. It is difficult to determine if the donepezil helped the patient's condition. His family wants to start alternative therapies after reading about their benefit in health magazines.

Past Medical History

Hypertension x 10 years (well controlled)

Hyperlipidemia x 15 years

Dementia x 8 years

Social History

CC lives with his daughter, son-in-law, and their two children. Since his retirement from an accounting firm, he took an active role in the care of his grandchildren until the onset of his dementia 8 years ago. He denies tobacco and alcohol. CC tries to stay active but cannot leave the house by himself anymore, so he is generally sedentary.

Family History

CC's father passed away from a stroke at the age of 70. His mother died from unknown causes at age 57. She had dementia as did CC's maternal grandmother and maternal uncle. His sister is alive, 62 years old, and has hypertension.

Review of Systems

Unremarkable

Physical Examination

GEN: The patient is alert, not oriented to time or place. Looks his stated age and in no apparent distress.

VS: BP 128/80 mmHg, HR 72 bpm, RR 18 rpm, T 98.9°F, Wt 75 kg, Ht 72 inches

HEENT: PERRLA. EOMI. Funduscopic exam reveals no AV nicking, hemorrhages or exudates. Dentures present. Oropharynx clear. TMs intact.

NECK: Supple; no JVD or thyromegaly

CHEST: Lungs CTA

CARDIOVASCULAR: Normal S_1, S_2; no m/r/g

ABD: NT/ND, (+) BS

NEURO: CN II-XII intact; DTRs 2+

EXT: No edema; pulses 2+ throughout

Laboratory and Diagnostic Tests

Na 141 mEq/L	K 4 mEq/L
Cl 105 mEq/L	BUN 10 mg/dL
Scr 1.2 mg/dL	Glu 80 mg/dL
Total cholesterol 190 mg/dL	LDL 80 mg/dL
HDL 35 mg/dL	Triglycerides 108 mg/dL
Vit B12 WNL	RBC folate WNL
TSH 3.79 IU/mL	RPR NR
Urinalysis pending	MMSE 20/30

Diagnosis

Primary:
1) Progressive dementia

Secondary:
1) Hypertension
2) Hyperlipidemia

Medication Record

1) Aricept 5 mg po at bedtime
2) ASA 81 mg po daily
3) Lipitor 20 mg po daily
4) Vitamin E 1000 IU po daily
5) Temazepam 15 mg po at bedtime
6) Metamucil 1 tablespoonful with water at bedtime

Case 70

Pharmacist Notes and Other Patient Information

None available.

Questions

1. Which symptom is characteristic of Alzheimer's type dementia?

   A. Memory loss
   B. Tremor
   C. Hallucinations
   D. Shuffling gait
   E. Acute onset

2. In order to determine the true cause of CC's symptoms, other diagnoses must first be considered and ruled out. Which of the following conditions can cause symptoms of dementia in the elderly?

   I. Urinary tract infection
   II. Pain
   III. Ischemic stroke

   A. I only
   B. III only
   C. I and II only
   D. II and III only
   E. I, II, and III

3. CC is taking Aricept for dementia. What is the most likely mechanism of action?

   A. Increases acetylcholine activity through reversible inhibition of acetylcholinesterase
   B. Decreases acetylcholine activity through stimulation of choline acetyltransferase
   C. Increases serotonin activity through stimulation of serotonin 5-HT1 receptors
   D. Increases norepinephrine activity through blockade of reuptake at nerve endings
   E. Decreases monoamine oxidase type B activity through blockade of intracellular metabolism of biogenic amines

4. Which of CC's medications may be contributing to his disorientation?

   I. Aricept
   II. Vitamin E
   III. Temazepam

   A. I only
   B. III only
   C. I and II only
   D. II and III only
   E. I, II, and III

5. CC's physician discusses initiating Risperdal therapy with you. What is your most appropriate response?

   A. Risperdal is an antipsychotic and should be used in this patient.
   B. CC's symptoms of disorientation and confusion are likely to improve with Risperdal therapy.
   C. CC's symptoms of memory loss and tremor are unlikely to improve with Risperdal therapy.
   D. Risperdal has been found to be safe in the elderly population.
   E. A baseline ECG is required before initiation of Risperdal.

6. Which of the following examinations or imaging studies are used to evaluate the presence of cognitive impairment?

   A. Mini-Mental Status Exam (MMSE)
   B. Hamilton Depression Rating Scale (HamD)
   C. Electrocardiogram (ECG)
   D. Computerized tomography (CT) of head
   E. Glasgow Coma Scale (GCS)

7. Several theories exist regarding the cause of dementia and Alzheimer's disease. Which of the following is the most likely contributor to CC's dementia?

   A. Family history
   B. Hyperlipidemia
   C. Hyperkalemia
   D. Social history
   E. Ischemic stroke

8. Which of the following would least benefit CC's caregiver to minimize frustration in dealing with CC's disease state?

   A. Locating a support group for caregivers of Alzheimer's disease patients
   B. Hiring an outside caregiver to take care of CC at least 2-4 hours weekly
   C. Seeking counseling with a licensed provider at least monthly
   D. Communicating minimally about family milestones and holidays
   E. Exercising daily to maintain cardiovascular health and well being

9. Which of the following side effects may occur in CC with the use of a cholinesterase inhibitor?

    A. Dry mouth
    B. Cough
    C. Diarrhea
    D. Thrombocytopenia
    E. Hypokalemia

10. CC's family wants to start the following alternative therapies after reading about their benefit in health magazines. Which has been reported to lead to additive adverse effects when used with CC's medications?

    A. Gingko biloba
    B. Glucosamine
    C. Selenium
    D. Saw palmetto
    E. Green tea

Urological Disorders

Patient Name: Gary Smith
Address: 9876 Republic Avenue
Age: 66   **Sex:** Male
Height: 5′ 11″   **Weight:** 85 kg
Race: Caucasian
Allergies: NKDA

Chief Complaint

GS is a 66-yo white male who came to the Primary Care Clinic after a blood pressure screening at a local independent pharmacy. He was told by the pharmacist that his blood pressure was high and he should go see a physician. He does not remember the blood pressure numbers.

History of Present Illness

GS has a history of hypertension and admits to being non-compliant with the medication that was prescribed for his condition. He admits to having seen a physician a few years ago, but stopped taking his blood pressure medication shortly after that time. He has not been receiving regular medical care for at least 2 years. He states his health is generally good.

He states that he is very happy, and has no real complaints other than he doesn't move as quickly as he used to. He has a few aches and pains which he attributes to work during the weekend. However, he states that he has been having some problems urinating lately, and he sometimes has to get out of bed two or three times a night to urinate. He also states that he must make an effort to "get things moving."

The only medications he takes are occasional ibuprofen (Advil) for his aches, a daily multivitamin, and a Ginseng tablet for energy.

Past Medical History

Appendectomy 1952

Hypertension for last 2 years

Social History

Semi-retired teacher. Denies drug or tobacco use. Social drinker, has wine with meals and an occasional Scotch. Lives with wife of 40 years. Has a ranch outside the city. Active in raising horses and maintaining the horse ranch. Has three grown children who are alive and in good health.

Family History

His mother died in her eighties of a heart attack. His father is still alive in his eighties with multiple health problems, including Parkinson's disease. The father resides in a nursing home. GS has two siblings, both younger, and still alive and in good health.

Review of Systems

Fairly unremarkable. He denies any symptoms of chest pain, shortness of breath, headache, serious vision changes, light headedness, or episodes of limb or facial paralysis. He does mention occasional difficulty in urination, and waking up at night frequently to urinate.

Physical Examination

VS: Temp. 97.8º F, BP 165/90 mmHg, HR 75, RR 12

GENERAL: Appears to be an elderly male in no acute distress.

HEENT: WNL

CARDIOVASCULAR: Regular rate and rhythm, no murmurs, rubs, or gallops. No JVD. 2+ pulses bilaterally—dorsalis pedis and radial.

LUNGS: Clear to auscultation.

ABD: No tenderness, no distension. Normoactive bowel sounds

RECTAL: The prostate is enlarged and rubbery without nodules or undue hardness.

NEURO: Alert and oriented to person, place, and time. Cranial nerves II-XII in tact. Deep tendon reflexes normal and unremarkable. Motor strength and coordination within normal limits.

Laboratory and Diagnostic Tests

Sodium: 143 mEq/L	Potassium: 4 mEq/L
Chloride: 105 mEq/L	HCO3: 26 mEq/L
BUN: 20 mg/dL	Serum creatinine: 1.3 mg/dL
Glucose: 88 mg/dL	Total protein: 6 g/dL
Albumin: 3.5 g/dL	PSA: 9 ng/mL

Dipstick urinary analysis was unremarkable

Diagnosis

Benign prostatic hyperplasia (BPH)

Case 71

Medication Record

No current prescribed medications

OTC: Ibuprofen (Advil) 200 mg 1 or 2 tabs occasionally; multivitamin 1 tab daily; Ginseng 1 tab daily

Pharmacist Notes and Other Patient Information

Patient is known to be noncompliant with previous hypertension medication.

Questions

1. Which of the following symptoms found in GS does NOT support the diagnosis of benign prostatic hyperplasia (BPH)?

   A. Hypertension
   B. Nocturia
   C. Enlarged prostate
   D. Urinary hesitancy
   E. Urinary frequency

2. Which of the following is NOT an appropriate nonpharmacological means of treating BPH?

   A. Transurethral needle ablation (TUNA)
   B. Watchful waiting
   C. Salt restriction
   D. Decreasing fluid intake around bedtime
   E. Decreasing alcohol/coffee intake generally

3. In the case of severe BPH, including urinary retention and hydronephrosis, which of the following is the gold standard of treatment?

   A. Leuprolide
   B. Nafarelin
   C. Transurethral resection of the prostate (TURP)
   D. Megestrol acetate
   E. Thermal-based therapies

4. Mild cases of BPH are treated with alpha-1-adrenoceptor antagonists. This class of drug works in BPH by which of the following mechanism(s)?

A. Promote contraction of prostatic smooth muscle
B. Relieve bladder outlet obstruction and decrease urinary outflow resistance
C. Inhibit parasympathetic tone in the prostate
D. Promote parasympathetic tone in the prostate
E. Increase urinary outflow resistance

5. Which lifestyle changes are recommended for BPH patients?

A. Decreasing fluid intake throughout the day
B. Increasing fluid intake throughout the day to avoid fluid intake at bedtime
C. Replacing coffee intake with soda to prevent nocturia
D. Avoiding smoked meats and aged cheese
E. Avoiding alcohol and coffee after dinner

6. Which of the following agents would you recommend in GS's case for treatment of BPH?

A. Silodosin
B. Tamsulosin
C. Dutasteride
D. Doxazosin
E. Prazosin

7. If GS failed alpha-1-adrenoceptor antagonist therapy for his BPH, what would be your next recommended course of action?

A. Watchful waiting
B. Transurethral needle ablation (TUNA)
C. Transurethral Resection of the prostate (TURP)
D. Lifestyle changes
E. An alpha-2-adrenoceptor antagonist

8. When initiating alpha-1-adrenoceptor antagonist therapy on GS, what would be the major adverse effect you would counsel him about?

A. Constipation
B. Hypotension
C. Nausea and vomiting
D. Diarrhea
E. Insomnia

9. What are possible post-procedure complications for patients who have undergone a TURP?

A. TURP syndrome
B. Pneumonia
C. Hypotension
D. Hyperkalemia
E. Headache

10. Silodosin is a new oral alpha-1a-adrenoceptor antagonist, effective for the treatment of BPH. Silodosin is similar to tamsulosin and is as effective as tamsulosin for improving lower urinary tract symptoms associated with BPH. Which of the following is TRUE for the correct dosing of this medication?

    A. Adjustment required for renal impairment
    B. Adjustment required for the mild and moderate hepatic impairment
    C. Adjustment required for the elderly
    D. No adjustment required for renal impairment
    E. Adjustment is required for patients taking dutasteride

Patient Name: Rose Jackson
Address: 1165 Chase Drive
Age: 62   **Sex:** Female
Height: 5' 6"   **Weight:** 190 lb
Race: African American
Allergies: PCN (rash)

Chief Compliant

RJ is a 62–yo African American female who is admitted to an inpatient rehabilitation facility. She is admitted for management of spasticity and neurogenic bladder.

History of Present Illness

RJ has had an ischemic stroke that has left her with compromised motor function on her left side. Additionally, she now has increased bladder issues, including the inability to empty her bladder and frequent urinary tract infections.

She has been seen by urology, which diagnosed her with neurogenic bladder. The physician first prescribed bethanechol, which lead to some improvement in her symptoms, but she is still having problems voiding.

Past Medical History

CAD with history of PTCA 5 years ago

Hypothyroidism

Anxiety and depression

Social History

She used to smoke 1 pack every week. She has not had any alcohol for months because she has been hospitalized.

Family History

Positive for diabetes and CAD

Review of Systems

No fevers, no chills, no chest pain, no SOB, no headaches, no nausea, no vomiting, no abdominal pain, sensation of not being able to pass urine, urgency, occasional incontinence.

Physical Examination

GENERAL: She is in no acute distress, overall healthy appearing

VITAL SIGNS: Blood pressure 133/86, heart rate 81, temperature 98.8°F, sat 100% on room air and respiratory rate 14

NECK: No JVD

CHEST: Clear to auscultation bilaterally

CARDIOVASCULAR: S_1, S_2; no murmurs, gallops, or rubs

ABDOMEN: Soft, nontender, bowel sounds present

EXTREMITIES: No clubbing, cyanosis or edema

NEURO: CN 2-12 grossly intact, diminished strength in upper and lower extremities on the left side

Laboratory Data

Labs are within normal limits. Urinalysis: leukocyte esterase positive and nitrite negative, with 10 WBCs on micro, occasional bacteria.

Diagnosis

Neurogenic bladder

Medication Record

Lorazepam 2 mg p.o. at bedtime

Alprazolam 0.5 p.o. b.i.d. p.r.n. anxiety

Amitriptyline 50 mg p.o. at bedtime

Multivitamin 1 p.o. daily

Hydrocodone/APAP 10/325 1 p.o. every 4 hours p.r.n. pain

Morphine sulfate ER 30 mg p.o. q.12h.

Bethanechol 50 mg p.o. t.i.d

Calcium carbonate 500 mg chewable t.i.d

Escitalopram 20 mg p.o. daily

Heparin 5000 units subq every 8 hours

Levothyroxine 0.112 mg p.o. daily

Questions

1. Which of the following is an important counseling point about complications for patients with neurogenic bladder, especially in the case of RJ's symptoms?

    A. Advise to void bladder every 24 hours to avoid complications.

    B. Educate patient on signs and symptoms of urinary tract infections.

    C. Advise patient not to buy absorbent liners as they do not help at all.

    D. Educate patient on possible liver complications.

    E. Tell patient to avoid smoking since it is proven to make neurogenic bladder symptoms worse.

2. Which one of these is not a risk factors for developing neurogenic bladder?

    A. Brain injury

    B. Spinal cord injury

    C. Depression

    D. Multiple sclerosis

    E. Spina bifida

3. Which one of these is a nonpharmacologic treatment for patient with symptoms of urinary retention?

    A. Increase fluid intake over 3 liters a day

    B. Pelvic floor exercise (Kegel exercises)

    C. Intermittent catherizations every 4-6 hours

    D. For diabetics, keep blood glucose >250 most times of the day

    E. Avoid valsalva maneuver

4. What is a major side effect of bethanechol that you would council the patient about?

    A. Makes glaucoma worse

    B. May induce bronchospasms, especially in asthma patients

    C. Causes GI reflux

    D. Caution in patient with hypothyroidism

    E. Will increase blood pressure

5. What is the mechanism of action of bethanechol?

    A. Muscarinic receptor agonist, works on the bladder M_2 and M_3 receptors

    B. Works on the serotonergic receptors on the bladder

    C. Muscarinic receptor antagonists, works on the bladder M_3 receptors

    D. Alpha-receptor agonists on the bladder smooth muscle

    E. Alpha-receptor antagonist on the bladder smooth muscle

6. Which one of these is NOT used to treat various symptoms of neurogenic bladder?

    A. Oxybutynin

    B. Baclofen

    C. Doxazosin

    D. Solifenacin

    E. Sildenafil

7. Which drug is likely causing an interaction with bethanechol and making it hard to treat the RJ's urologic symptoms?

    A. Alprazolam

    B. Escitalopram

    C. Amitriptyline

    D. Lorazepam

    E. Levothyroxine

8. What disease state complicates and may contribute to RJ's worsening urologic symptoms?

    A. Diabetes

    B. Depression

    C. Anxiety

    D. Hypothyroidism

    E. CAD

9. Oxybutynin should NOT be added to this patient's medication regimen because it can cause:

    A. diarrhea.

    B. nausea.

    C. worsening of wide angle glaucoma.

    D. urinary retention.

    E. depression.

10. To help better control RJ's urologic symptoms, the following are options EXCEPT:

    A. stop amitriptyline.

    B. increase dose of bethanechol.

    C. stop bethanechol and start tolterodine.

    D. start intermittent catherizations.

    E. dose bethanechol 1 hour before meals.

Perioperative Care

Patient Name: Angie Perry
Address: 1640 Ridge Drive
Age: 38 **Sex:** Female
Height: 5′ 5″ **Weight:** 80 kg
Race: Caucasian
Allergies: NKDA

Chief Complaint

AP is a 38-year-old gravida 1, para 0, female at 35 4/7 weeks gestation undergoing an emergency cesarean section.

History of Present Illness

AP's pregnancy was relatively uneventful until 3 days ago when she presented to the triage center with dilated cardiomyopathy and worsening cardiac status. Her weight and blood pressure had been slightly increasing, with 2+ proteinuria at her previous two visits to her obstetrician. She has iron-deficiency anemia, which was treated with ferrous sulfate 300 mg TID (started 1 month ago).

Past Medical History

Polycystic kidney disease

Nephrolithiasis

Social History

Tobacco use: 1/2 pack of cigarettes/day for past 4 years, quit 1 month ago

Denies alcohol or drug use

Family History

Noncontributory

Review of Systems

AP has significantly increasing shortness of breath, cough, and edema in her extremities. She is in congestive heart failure, NYHA Class III-IV.

Physical Examination

VS: BP 110/55, HR 136 bpm, RR 32 rpm, Wt 80 kg (pre-pregnancy weight = 55 kg, IBW = 57 kg), T 97.7°F

LUNGS: Inspiratory rales and rhonchi bilaterally, 95% oxygen via face mask

CV: Soft heart murmur, tachycardia

NEURO: Unremarkable

GI: c/o moderate reflux esophagitis (heartburn), worse when supine

EXT: 2+ pitting edema of lower extremities

GU: Vaginal exam normal

Laboratory and Diagnostic Tests

Sodium 137 mEq/L Potassium 4.7 mEq/L

Chloride 106 mEq/L CO_2 27 mEq/L

BUN 16 mg/dL Serum creatinine 1 mg/dL

Glucose 85 mg/dL Calcium 9.1 mg/dL

Albumin 2.8 g/dL HCT 30.5%

Hgb 10.7 g/dL

Alkaline phosphatase 109 units/L

Ultrasound: Normal for gestational age

CXR: Pulmonary edema, cardiomegaly

Diagnosis

Labor, congestive heart failure

Medication Record

Medications prior to surgery:

Digoxin 0.25 mg q day

Isosorbide dinitrate 20 mg TID

Enoxaparin 40 mg SC daily

Calcium carbonate (Tums) 1000 mg po prn

Medications on call to OR (to be administered in preop holding area):

Famotidine 20 mg IV x1

Metoclopramide 10 mg IV x1

Sodium citrate/citric acid (Bicitra) 30 mL po x1

Pharmacist Notes and Other Patient Information

None available.

Case 73

Questions

1. Which of the following IV anesthetic agents should be used to induce general anesthesia (produce unconsciousness) in AP?

   A. Etomidate
   B. Thiopental
   C. Propofol
   D. Methohexital
   E. Ketamine

2. The first-year anesthesia resident assisting in the case is not familiar with etomidate and inquires as to its major adverse effects. What do you tell him?

   I. Myoclonus
   II. Nausea and vomiting on emergence from anesthesia
   III. Pain on injection

   A. I only
   B. III only
   C. I and II only
   D. II and III only
   E. I, II, and III

3. Premedication with which of the following agents can decrease the chances of myoclonus occurring in AP?

   A. Labetalol
   B. Fentanyl
   C. Esmolol
   D. Metoprolol
   E. Famotidine

4. Rapid sequence induction will be employed in AP. Which of the following medications is not a good choice for inducing general anesthesia using this technique?

   A. Etomidate
   B. Midazolam
   C. Propofol
   D. Ketamine
   E. Thiopental

5. The anesthesia resident asks you if etomidate has analgesic properties that would allow less opioid to be administered to AP during the procedure. You inform him that which of the following IV anesthetic agents produces analgesia?

   A. Ketamine
   B. Etomidate
   C. Thiopental
   D. Methohexital
   E. Propofol

6. Sevoflurane is selected by the anesthesiologist to maintain general anesthesia in AP. What type of drug is sevoflurane?

   A. Benzodiazepine
   B. Volatile inhalation agent
   C. Gas
   D. Opioid
   E. Barbiturate

7. AP's caesarean section lasted 90 minutes. Since etomidate has a half-life of 2.5 hours, why was sevoflurane needed to maintain general anesthesia?

   I. Etomidate is rapidly redistributed from the brain to other sites in the body.
   II. Etomidate is rapidly metabolized in the liver.
   III. Etomidate has a significant hangover effect.

   A. I only
   B. III only
   C. I and II only
   D. II and III only
   E. I, II, and III

8. Which of the following devices can be used to measure the degree of hypnosis in AP during general anesthesia?

   A. Precordial stethoscope
   B. Pulse oximeter
   C. Bispectral Index (BIS) monitor
   D. Pulmonary artery catheter
   E. Capnometer

9. Since AP has CHF, the anesthesia resident is concerned that blood flow to the liver is decreased. This may result in agents metabolized hepatically to have a decreased elimination and the potential for a prolonged effect. Since sevoflurane is going to be used to maintain general anesthesia in AP, he would like to know what percent of sevoflurane is metabolized in the liver. What do you tell him?

   A. 3%
   B. 0.2%
   C. 0.02%
   D. 15% to 45%
   E. 2%

10. Which of the following physiologic or pharmacologic factors present in AP may decrease the amount of sevoflurane required to maintain general anesthesia?

    A. Tachycardia
    B. Heparin administration
    C. Pregnancy
    D. Edema
    E. Digoxin administration

Patient Name: Michael Perez
Address: 155 Beechwood Lane
Age: 33 **Sex:** Male
Height: 5' 4" **Weight:** 75 kg
Race: Hispanic
Allergies: NKDA

Chief Complaint

MP presents to the emergency department with confusion and a complaint that "sometimes things looking small" in his left eye.

History of Present Illness

MP is a 33-yo Spanish-speaking gentleman who presents to the emergency department with altered mental status, cognitive deficits, and impaired balance. MP is admitted to the hospital and scheduled for a surgical procedure to relieve the excess buildup of cerebrospinal fluid that is causing his worsening mental status and balance. MP's surgery, a ventriculoperitoneal (VP) shunt placement, is expected to last approximately 1 hour.

Past Medical History

None

Social History

Tobacco use: denies

Alcohol use: denies

Substance abuse: denies

Illnesses: none

Injuries: remote history of being punched in left eye

Surgeries: none

Family History

No glaucoma or other eye disorders

Review of Systems

ENT: Negative

Eye: Pupils unequal in size with L>R, no pain

Cardiovascular: Negative

Gastrointestinal: Negative

Hematologic/lymphatic: Negative

Respiratory: Negative

Allergic/Immunological: Negative

Dermatologic: Negative

Musculoskeletal: Negative

Neurological: Patient feeling that he may be only slightly confused

Physical Examination

General Appearance: Well-nourished, lying in bed in NAD

VS: BP 112/68 mmHg, T 98.2°F, P 74 bpm, RR 18 bpm, SaO_2 97%

HEENT: Good range of motion, no masses, neck vein flat, no bruits, PERRLA, EOMI

Peripheral pulses: Normal

Abdomen: soft, nt, bs+

Lungs: Clear bilaterally

CV: RRR, no murmurs, normal S_1 & S_2, no gallop

Extremities: no lower extremity edema

Mental Status: Alert, awake, oriented to person, but does not know that he is in a hospital, the day of the week, and the current month. Moderate cognitive deficits are noted in areas of orientation, memory, judgment, and executive functions.

Cranial nerves: Intact bilaterally II-XII, except pupils unequal in size with L>R

Gait and Station: Slow gait, able to ambulate fairly steady with slight unsteadiness during turns, able to walk on toes and heels. MP is able to balance on one foot, but on the left foot he is more unsteady than the right foot. When he balances on both feet, MP is less balanced than would have been expected for his age.

Laboratory and Diagnostic Tests

Electrolytes

NA: 139 mEq/L

K: 4.6 mEq/L

CL: 104 mEq/L

CO2: 28 mEq/L

AGAP: 11

Case 74

CA: 9.5 mg/dL

Ionized CA: 4.7 mEq/L

MG: 2.1 mg/dL

PHOS: 5.3 mg/dL

Renal/Metabolic Tests

BUN: 10 mg/dL

CREAT: 0.7 mg/dL

GLUC: 96 mg/dL

Anticonvulsant Assays

Free phenytoin: 1.1 mcg/mL

Coagulation

PT: 13.3 seconds

INR: 0.960

PTT: 32.2 seconds

MRI: hydrocephalus and calcifications in right frontal lobe and 4th ventricle thought be consistent with neurocysticercosis

Head MRI: signs of elevated intracranial pressure and prominent superior ophthalmic veins

Medication Record

Docuaste 100 mg po BID

Famotidine 20 mg po Q12H

Heparin 5,000 units SC Q12H

Nafcillin 1 gram IV Q6H

Phenytoin ER 200 mg po Q12H

Acetaminophen 650 mg po Q6H PRN for pain or if temp above 101.0°F

Acetaminophen-hydrocodone 500 mg/5 mg 2 tabs po Q6H PRN for pain

Bisacodyl 10 mg suppository rectally daily PRN for constipation

Zolpidem 10 mg po QHS PRN for insomnia

Diagnosis

MP has been diagnosed with hydrocephalus (an abnormal accumulation of cerebrospinal fluid [CSF] in the ventricles, or cavities, of the brain). To relieve his symptoms, MP will undergo placement of a ventriculoperitoneal (VP) shunt.

Pharmacist Notes and Other Patient Information

None available.

Questions

1. Rocuronium exerts its therapeutic effect by:
    A. blocking the effect of acetylcholine at the nicotinic receptor.
    B. blocking the effect of acetylcholine at the muscarinic receptor.
    C. acting like acetylcholine at the nicotinic receptor.
    D. facilitating the action of GABA in the central nervous system.
    E. acting in the brainstem to reduce somatic motor activity.

2. Which test should be used in the operating room by the anesthesia care provider to assess the degree of neuromuscular blockade in MP?
    A. Train-of-Four (TOF)
    B. Electroencephalogram (EEG)
    C. Electrocardiogram (ECG, EKG)
    D. Nerve conduction study (NCS)
    E. Myelogram

3. When emergency control of the airway is required and there is no intravenous access, the most appropriate NMBA to administer is:
    A. cisatracurium (Nimbex).
    B. midazolam (Versed).
    C. propofol (Diprivan).
    D. succinylcholine (Quelicin).
    E. remifentanil (Ultiva).

4. At the end of surgery, MP is experiencing residual neuromuscular blockade from a non-depolarizing NMBA. It is deemed necessary to utilize reversal agents in order to extubate him. Which of the following would you recommend?
    A. Naloxone and flumazenil
    B. Epinephrine and vasopressin
    C. Diphenhydramine and famotidine
    D. Neostigmine and glycopyrrolate
    E. Midazolam and fentanyl

5. According to the Institute for Safe Medication Practices (ISMP), which of the following stickers are recommended to be affixed to each vial, syringe, bag, and storage box of NMBAs?

A. Do Not Refrigerate
B. Protect From Light
C. Warning: Paralyzing Agent-Causes Respiratory Arrest
D. Caution: May Cause Drowsiness
E. Must Be Diluted Before Use

6. What is the correct order, from shortest to longest onset of action, for these non-depolarizing NMBAs?

A. Rocuronium > vecuronium > pancuronium
B. Cisatracurium > vecuronium > rocuronium
C. Atracurium > rocuronium > pancuronium
D. Pancuronium > vecuronium > cisatracurium
E. Rocuronium > pancuronium > cisatracurium

7. All of the following are adverse affects of succinylcholine EXCEPT:

A. hyperkalemia.
B. malignant hyperthermia trigger.
C. increased intracranial pressure.
D. fasciculations.
E. metabolic acidosis.

8. NMBAs are utilized in the operating room and/or an intensive care setting to provide:

I. sedation.
II. analgesia.
III. muscle paralysis.

A. I only
B. III only
C. I and II only
D. II and III only
E. I, II, and III

9. A 77-yo man is rushed to the emergency department via ambulance following a motor vehicle accident. He is unresponsive, bleeding internally, and requires emergency surgery. Etomidate and succinylcholine are administered, he's intubated, and anesthesia is maintained with sevoflurane. About an hour into the surgery, his heart rate is 120 beats per minute and his end tidal carbon dioxide is 60 mmHg. His family arrived at the hospital and they explain that the man has a family history of malignant hyperthermia.

Appropriate management of this patient's malignant hyperthermia crisis includes all of the following EXCEPT:

A. stop the sevoflurane and switch to propofol to maintain anesthesia.
B. stop the sevoflurane and switch to desflurane to maintain anesthesia.
C. treat with dantrolene in an initial dose of 2.5 mg/kg IV.
D. cool the patient using iced normal saline.
E. call for help.

10. Which of the following provides the best patient and health care provider information about malignant hyperthermia?

I. Malignant Hyperthermia Association of the United States
II. Up to Date
III. Pharmacist's Letter

A. I only
B. III only
C. I and II only
D. II and III only
E. I, II, and III

Over-the-Counter Medication Cases

Section Editor: W. Reneé Acosta

Patient Name: Gerald Morgan
Address: 2955 Old Town Road
Age: 40   **Sex:** Male
Height: 5'11"   **Weight:** 160 lb
Race: White
Allergies: Penicillin (rash)

Chief Complaint

GM is a 40-yo male who presents to your ambulatory care clinic pharmacy on 12/28 with paroxysmal sneezing, rhinorrhea, watery eyes, and a hacking cough. He is complaining of constant sneezing and an irritating cough that is preventing him from sleeping at night. He states "I can't seem to get rid of this tickle in my throat, and it's making me cough" and has a "runny nose that won't quit." During an attempt to speak to the pharmacist, GM suffered a sneezing episode that lasted for approximately 90 seconds. Punctuating the conversation after the sneezing episode had passed was an occasional dry, hacking cough. GM states that he is "sick and tired of being sick," and he would like to be well to celebrate with his wife at a big New Year's Eve event to which they have been invited (in 3 days).

History of Present Illness

GM states that the sneezing and runny nose started approximately 3 days ago when, according to the allergy forecast on the local news, the mountain cedar blew in, a potent allergen in this part of the country and the cause of a 1.5- to 2-month long allergy season. However, several weeks ago GM had seen the doctor for a "pretty bad infection" that lasted for about 7 days. When asked to describe this infection, GM states that he had had a stuffy nose and head, a constant headache, a rattling cough, and a temperature of 102°F. He had seen a doctor in the clinic who had prescribed an antibiotic and something for the congestion. Following this illness, he had been symptom-free until he began sneezing 3 days ago. He does complain of some fatigue, which he attributes to working overtime to make some extra money for holiday gifts for his family.

Past Medical History

GM has been treated for precancerous spots on his face and arms due to occupational sun exposure (as a construction worker) and for a broken leg suffered in a construction accident about 2 years ago. He has been assigned to a supervisory position rather than actual labor since this accident. He has also been treated for periodic respiratory infections. The remainder of his history is unremarkable.

Social History

Tobacco use: 1 ppd

Alcohol use: 1-2 servings of beer most weeknights;

Caffeine use: drinks coffee all morning (pours 1 ten-cup pot into a thermos)

Family History

Both parents are still living. Father is overweight and smokes.

Review of Systems

Negative except as noted previously

Physical Examination

(Performed by clinic doctor 12/28)

GEN: Well-developed, fatigued-looking male with profuse rhinorrhea; paroxysmal sneezing; nasal congestion; dry, hacking cough; and red, watery eyes

VS: BP 140/90 mmHg, HR 95 bpm

Laboratory and Diagnostic Tests

None available.

Diagnosis

Primary:
Suspected seasonal allergic rhinitis

Medication Record

Date	Rx No	Physician	Drug/Strength	Quantity	Sig	Refills
9/10	87421	Smith	Fluorouracil Cr 1%	30	Apply bid	2
12/1		Smith	Pseudoephedrine 30 mg	24	1-2 q 4-6 h prn	
12/1	95002	Smith	Z-Pak	1	ud	
12/20		Jones	Ibuprofen 200 mg	24	1-2 q 6 h prn pain	
12/20		Jones	Diphenhydramine 25 mg	24	1-2 q 4-6 h	
12/20	89994	Jones	Medrol Dosepak	1	ud	

Case 75

Pharmacist Notes and Other Patient Information

12/1 Counseled patient on correct use of Z-Pak

12/20 Advised patient to return in 3-5 days if no apparent relief of symptoms

12/24 Patient complains of drowsiness

Questions

1. What additional questions should be asked of GM to supplement the information provided in the case description prior to making a therapeutic recommendation?
   I. Have you had any fever with this latest episode of sneezing and coughing?
   II. Are you currently taking anything for any of these symptoms?
   III. Are any of your family members experiencing the same symptoms?

   A. I only
   B. III only
   C. I and II only
   D. II and III only
   E. I, II, and III

2. This episode of sneezing and coughing, based on the case, is likely caused by:

   A. seasonal allergic rhinitis.
   B. a viral infection.
   C. an acute bacterial infection.
   D. his previous infection.
   E. perennial allergic rhinitis.

3. Assuming no nasal congestion is present, which of the following is the most appropriate recommendation(s)?

   A. Expectorant
   B. First-generation antihistamine
   C. Decongestant
   D. Cough suppressant
   E. Nonsedating antihistamine

4. Which of the following is the most sedating nonprescription antihistamine?

A. Chlorpheniramine maleate
B. Cetirizine
C. Diphenhydramine hydrochloride
D. Loratadine
E. Dexbrompheniramine

5. Which of the following is a nonprescription mast-cell stabilizer?

A. Afrin
B. Neo-Synephrine 0.5%
C. Nasalcrom
D. Flonase
E. Vanceril

6. The side effects of dry mouth and eyes and urinary retention that are caused by first-generation antihistamines are due to:

A. alpha-adrenergic agonistic effect.
B. beta-adrenergic agonistic effect.
C. muscarinic cholinergic receptor blockade.
D. alpha-adrenergic antagonistic effect
E. beta-adrenergic antagonistic effect

7. The most appropriate initial OTC eye drop recommendation for GM for short-term use would be:

A. Tobrex.
B. Vasocon-A.
C. Visine Original.
D. Refresh.
E. Collyrium.

8. GM is considering allergy shots as a preventive treatment for his seasonal allergic rhinitis. Which of the following would be considered a contraindication to therapy?

A. History of cancer or precancer
B. History of respiratory infections
C. Patient is HIV positive
D. Patient smokes
E. Patient consumes alcohol most days of the week

9. Steps that patients can take to avoid allergy triggers include:

   I. check your local allergy forecast to know when pollen counts are elevated.
   II. use a high-efficiency particulate air (HEPA) filter.
   III. dusting with a damp cloth.

   A. I only
   B. III only
   C. I and II only
   D. II and III only
   E. I, II, and III

10. Which of the following preparations is the most appropriate recommendation for GM's dry, hacking cough?

    A. Robitussin DM Max (dextromethorphan, guaifenesin)
    B. Triaminic Cough and Sore Throat (acetaminophen, dextromethorphan)
    C. Chlor-Trimeton (chlorpheniramine)
    D. Robitussin AC (guaifenesin, codeine)
    E. Delsym (dextromethorphan)

Patient Name: Steven Carmichael
Address: 2718 Barton Springs Court
Age: 45   **Sex:** Male
Height: 5′ 11″   **Weight:** 185 lb
Race: Caucasian
Allergies: Sulfonamides (rash)

Chief Complaint

SC is a 45-yo white male who seeks recommendation from his community pharmacist on Monday afternoon, September 2, for treatment of a dermatological condition. He complains of a red rash on both hands and arms characterized by intense itching and burning.

History of Present Illness

SC has returned the previous weekend from a 3-day camping trip on Friday through Sunday with the Boy Scout troop for which he serves as scoutmaster. The primitive campsite included no running water or bathroom facilities. On questioning, you learn that the camping trip included daily expeditions involving crawling on the hands and knees through low brushy undergrowth for exploration and retrieval of local flora and fossils. One such exploration on Saturday morning resulted in a small laceration (1/4-inch in length and shallow) to the patient's left palm caused by a sharp rock, which was subsequently cleaned with a nonprescription antiseptic cleanser from the first-aid kit and bandaged with a topical antiinfective agent. The itching and rash were first noticed on Sunday evening at home on return from the camping trip. The patient then showered with mild soap at home and has applied only a nonallergenic topical emollient lotion once following the shower in an attempt to relieve the itching. Patient denies use of any new or unusual chemical agents that may have caused irritant contact dermatitis. His clothing on the camping trip included long khaki pants, a short-sleeved scout uniform shirt, socks, and boots. No topical agents have been applied other than the nonallergenic emollient lotion and the topical antiinfective cream, which was used unilaterally.

Past Medical History

SC has a history of atopic dermatitis as a child. Patient was diagnosed with HTN approximately 6 years ago and has modified his diet and used the prescription drug telmisartan to maintain good control of HTN. He was diagnosed with hyperlipidemia 2 years ago; 12 months of dietary modification failed to decrease his cholesterol levels below borderline levels, so his PCP initiated treatment with lovastatin 11 months ago, with successful control of cholesterol levels resulting.

The patient also describes current nonprescription therapies including the following: an aerosol spray liquid for athlete's foot, a topical cream for jock itch, and the topical antibiotic cream and bandages for the recent palm injury.

Social History

Tobacco use: none

Alcohol use: 1-2 glasses of wine or beer 2-3 times/week

Caffeine use: 2 cups of coffee each morning and 1-2 caffeine-containing diet soft drinks daily

Family History

Father died of complications from hepatitis B at age 56. Mother survived MI at age 50 and is being treated for HTN. Negative for CVA, DM, and cancer.

Review of Systems

Incidence and appearance of dermatitis consistent with allergic contact dermatitis, possibly due to exposure to poison ivy, poison oak, or poison sumac during camping trip. Otherwise negative. Denies recent chemical contact or atopic dermatitis. Denies change in weight, appetite, or bowel habits.

Physical Examination

GEN: Healthy, well-developed male with bilateral linear red streaks on dorsal sides of hands and forearms; no large bullae present

VS: BP 144/89 mmHg, HR 135 bpm, T 38.4°C, Wt 84 kg

HEENT: PERRLA, TM normal, oral cavity without lesions

CHEST: Clear

NEURO: A&O x2

Laboratory and Diagnostic Tests

None available.

Diagnosis

Primary:
1) Mild-to-moderate rhus dermatitis secondary to poison ivy exposure
2) Minor laceration of palm of left hand

Secondary:
1) Hypertension
2) Hyperlipidemia
3) Tinea pedis
4) Tinea cruris

Medication Record

Date	Rx No	Physician	Drug/Strength	Quantity	Sig	Refills
8/12	4562609	Johansen	Telmisartan 80 mg	30	1 qd	6
8/12	4562610	Johansen	Lovastatin 20 mg	30	1 qd	6
8/27			Tolnaftate 1% spray liquid	1 oz	apply to feet bid	
8/27			Terbinafine 1% cream	30 g	apply to groin bid	
8/31			Neomycin sulfate cream	15 g	apply to palm qid	

Pharmacist Notes and Other Patient Information

8/27 OTC consult by RPh. Advised patient on selection and use of products for treatment of acute exacerbation of athlete's foot and jock itch.

Questions

1. Which of the following drug products is NOT available on an OTC basis for potential pharmacist recommendation in the treatment of rhus dermatitis?

    A. Burow's solution
    B. Betamethasone valerate cream 0.1%
    C. Aluminum acetate solution 1:40
    D. Hydrocortisone cream 1%
    E. Diphenhydramine 25-mg capsules

2. The pharmacist may choose to recommend an OTC product for symptomatic relief of rhus dermatitis with which of the following agents?

    I. Hydrocortisone 0.5% cream
    II. Colloidal oatmeal 100% powder as bath treatment
    III. Aluminum acetate solution 1:40 soaks

    A. I only
    B. III only
    C. I and II only
    D. II and III only
    E. I, II, and III

3. If the pharmacist chooses to recommend the use of topical diphenhydramine 2% cream for relief from itching caused by rhus dermatitis, which of the following warnings or precautions should be communicated to SC?

    A. SC should be warned of the high incidence of drowsiness and advised not to operate a vehicle or dangerous machinery while using the product.
    B. The product has a high incidence of anticholinergic side effects, including dry mouth and urinary retention.

    C. The use of topical antihistamines may occasionally result in sensitization and, thus, aggravation of contact dermatitis.
    D. SC should be warned that topical antihistamines should not be used since it can exacerbate his hypertension.
    E. SC should not use topical antihistamines because of the increased systemic absorption they have.

4. SC should be counseled on all of the following measures for prevention of future episodes of rhus dermatitis EXCEPT:

    A. recognition and avoidance of poison ivy, poison oak, and poison sumac.
    B. use of alkaline soap or organic solvents such as alcohol for thorough washing of the skin.
    C. when camping, be sure to wear lightweight clothing to stay cool and prevent exposure by wearing protective clothing, such as short-sleeve shirts, shorts, and sandals.
    D. wear protective clothing including long pants, long-sleeved shirts, socks, and shoes when exposure to the plants is possible.
    E. wash all objects, such as clothing, that may have come into contact with damaged plants.

5. Which of the following symptoms of rhus dermatitis is an indication for physician referral rather than initiation or continuation of self-treatment?

    A. Widespread reaction associated with major swelling or eye involvement
    B. Linear streaks of papules and vesicles
    C. Intense itching
    D. Presence of small fluid-filled bullae
    E. Presence of lesions on the hands

6. Treated or untreated rhus dermatitis will generally resolve in approximately 10-21 days. Which of the following would NOT be a goal or expected outcome of self-treatment of this condition?

    A. Relief of itching
    B. Prevention of secondary infection
    C. Prevention of complications arising from oozing, crusting, or scaling

D. Desensitization is effective either by chewing leafs or having commercially prepared extracts injected

E. Prevention of excessive scratching

7. Which of the following may be an adverse effect of topical neomycin use?

I. Allergic contact dermatitis
II. Secondary fungal infection
III. Hyperpigmentation of the skin

A. I only
B. III only
C. I and II only
D. II and III only
E. I, II, and III

8. The brand name for the OTC product (tolnaftate) that was recommended by the pharmacist for athlete's foot for SC is:

A. Betadine.
B. Micatin.
C. Lotrimin AF.
D. Lamisil AT.
E. Tinactin.

9. SC should be advised by the pharmacist to continue antifungal therapy with terbinafine 1% cream for what length of time for complete clearing of the tinea cruris infection?

A. 3-5 days
B. 7-10 days
C. 2-4 weeks
D. 6-8 weeks
E. 3-6 months

10. Additional drug or nondrug measures appropriate for use along with the antifungal agents used in this case for treatment of the two cutaneous fungal infections should include:

A. minimizing or avoiding the use of occlusive clothing or shoes.

B. daily cleansing of the affected areas with selenium sulfide lotion.

C. application of occlusive dressings on the affected areas following application of the antifungal.

D. liberal quantities of an emollient cream or ointment should be applied daily to prevent dryness and/or cracking.

E. occlusive clothing, shoes, or bandages should be used during treatment time to ensure area stays clean.

Patient Name: Nell Basinger
Address: 805 West 6th Street
Age: 47   **Sex:** Female
Height: 5′ 2″   **Weight:** 110 lb
Race: White
Allergies: NKDA

Chief Complaint

"I am experiencing vaginal dryness, and pain during intercourse because of it."

History of Present Illness

NB is a 47-yo female who presents to the pharmacy complaining of vaginal dryness for the past 4 months. Recently, she has begun experiencing pain during intercourse due to the dryness. Her last natural menstrual period was 2 weeks ago. She is generally in good health, and exercises three times weekly.

Past Medical History

Hyperlipidemia, presently controlled by diet

Social History

Alcohol use: 1-2 drinks/week

Tobacco use: none

Occupation: Attorney

Married, with 2 teenage children

Family History

Mother is currently being treated for asthma and osteoporosis.

Father has hyperlipidemia.

Medication Record

Date	Rx No	Physician	Drug/Strength	Quantity	Sig	Refills
4/1	44580	Watts	Benazepril 40 mg	30	1 po q am	prn
4/1	44582	Watts	Furosemide 20 mg	30	1 po q am	prn
4/1	44578	Watts	ASA EC 325 mg	30	1 po q am	prn
4/1	44579	Watts	Atorvastatin 40 mg	30	1 po qd	prn
4/1	44581	Watts	Digoxin 0.125 mg	30	1 po qd	prn
10/15			Calcium carb 500 mg		1 po qd	
10/15			Multivitamin		1 po qd	

Review of Systems

Otherwise negative except for occasional tension headaches due to job-related stress. Headaches are relieved by acetaminophen or ibuprofen. Patient denies any recent changes in bowel habits, weight, or appetite.

Physical Examination

VS: BP 120/60 mmHg, HR 65 bpm, Temperature 98.6°F

Pelvic: No tenderness or masses (self-reported by patient)

Laboratory and Diagnostic Tests

Total cholesterol 200 mg/dL

Diagnosis

Primary:

1. Atrophic vaginitis

Pharmacist Notes and Other Patient Information

None available.

Questions

1. Which of the following factors could be contributing to the patient's recent vaginal dryness?

    I.   The patient is perimenopausal.
    II. The patient is stressed and/or fatigued.
    III. The patient and her husband are using nonlubricated condoms for birth control.

Case 77

A. I only
B. III only
C. I and II only
D. II and III only
E. I, II, and III

2. Which of the following would NOT be an appropriate treatment option for vaginal dryness?

   A. Astroglide (glycerin, propylene glycol)
   B. Replens Gel (glycerin, mineral oil)
   C. Lubrin Suppositories (caprylic/capric triglyceride, glycerin)
   D. Massengill Disposable Douche (purified water, sodium citrate, citric acid, vinegar)
   E. H-R Lubricating Jelly (hydroxypropyl methylcellulose)

3. How often should a vaginal lubricant be used?

   A. As often as needed
   B. Prior to intercourse only
   C. Once daily at bedtime
   D. Once daily in the morning
   E. Twice daily in the morning and at bedtime

4. If the patient uses a vaginal lubricant and sees no improvement after 2 weeks, what would be the next appropriate step?

   A. Refer to a physician for an oral estrogen
   B. Refer to a physician for a vaginal estrogen product
   C. Switch lubrication products
   D. Switch birth control method to spermicide-lubricated condoms
   E. Switch birth control method to a spermicidal sponge

5. What other recommendation could you make to the patient to help improve vaginal lubrication?

   A. Try a petroleum-based lubricant such as petroleum jelly
   B. Regular sexual activity
   C. Baths instead of showers
   D. Regular exercise
   E. Sitz bath daily

6. NB has been using a nonlubricated latex condom for birth control. Which of the following would be an appropriate lubricant for use with the latex condom?

   A. Mineral oil
   B. Miconazole vaginal cream
   C. Petroleum jelly
   D. Glycerin
   E. Baby oil

7. NB is interested in other birth control options. Which of the following recommendations would you provide in private consultation with this patient?

   I. Female condom
   II. Sponge
   III. Lubricated latex condom

   A. I only
   B. III only
   C. I and II only
   D. II and III only
   E. I, II, and III

8. If NB chooses the sponge, what counseling information would NOT be appropriate regarding the proper use of a contraceptive sponge?

   A. The sponge must be left in place for at least 6 to 8 hours after intercourse.
   B. The sponge can be left in place for up to 24 hours.
   C. The sponge can be inserted up to 24 hours prior to intercourse.
   D. The sponge should be inserted at least 15 minutes prior to intercourse.
   E. The sponge can be removed by pulling on the loop attached to the sponge.

9. Which of the following vaginal lubricants does not contain a spermicide?

   A. Ortho Options Delfen Foam
   B. K-Y Plus Lubricating Gel
   C. Encare Vaginal Inserts
   D. VCF Vaginal Film
   E. Astroglide

10. NB tries the sponge and does not like it. She comes in requesting information on the female condom. Which of the following would be appropriate counseling points for the female condom?

    A. It can be reused, but should be inspected for tears each time before use.
    B. It can be combined with a male latex condom to ensure more effective birth control.
    C. Additional lubrication can be added during intercourse without removing the condom.
    D. It can be left in place for up to 24 hours before it must be removed.
    E. It is not effective for preventing sexually transmitted diseases.

Federal Law Review

Section Editor: Jesse Vivian

Background

A majority of states and jurisdictions assess the pharmacy law competencies of individuals applying for a pharmacist license through administration of the National Association of Boards of Pharmacy's (NABP) Multistate Pharmacy Jurisprudence Examination™ (MPJE™). The MPJE uses questions that are applicable to all jurisdictions through the federal laws, but also tailors questions to the individual states and territories. The states that do not administer the MPJE use examinations that are developed by each individual state. However, even these examinations almost always include questions dealing with federal laws, especially controlled substances. As such, no matter where the exam is taken, licensure applicants must be proficient in both state and federal laws pertaining to pharmacy. In any event, candidates must take a separate law exam for each state in which they are seeking licensure.

License applicants should consult the competency statements provided by NABP with the MPJE materials as a starting point for determining which subjects should be studied. This advice applies to candidates in non-MPJE states as well, because the subject matter of pharmacy law is similar in all jurisdictions. The MPJE competency statements and other study tools may be accessed at the NABP website: www.nabp.net. There is a wealth of information about the examination located there and applicants should take advantage of those materials.

The exam consists of 90 multiple choice questions; however, 30 of those questions will not be counted for the purpose of calculating your score. These "pre-test" questions are dispersed throughout the examination and there is no way that candidates can tell which questions are counted and which are not. Candidates will be given 2 hours to complete the exam. If a candidate answers fewer than 77 questions, the exam will not be scored. Candidates should try to answer all 90 questions because there is a penalty for not answering questions. No two exams are the same because there is a large block of test questions. The difficulty of subsequent questions depends on whether or not the prior question was answered correctly. Candidates will not know whether a question was answered correctly while taking the exam or afterwards because only scores are reported. The minimum passing score is 75.

Unlike the NAPLEX exam, scores for the MJPE are not transferable between the states or jurisdictions that use the MPJE because the MPJE is uniquely tailored for each state.

The law exam is administered as a "computer adaptive" format. This means that a candidate cannot go back and forth between questions and change an answer after the question is finished. This testing format is very different from traditional paper-and-pencil exams commonly used in academic settings. Please consult the NABP materials for further explanation of the test-taking procedures. It is also important to know the competencies the MJPE is attempting to assess. In its Registration Bulletin, the NABP states: "The MPJE Competency Statements serve as a blueprint of the topics covered on the examination. They offer important information about the knowledge, judgment, and skills you are expected to demonstrate while taking the MPJE. A strong understanding of the Competency Statements will aid you in your preparation to take the examination."

Definitions, Abbreviations, and Explanations

Think of studying pharmacy law as learning a new language. Understanding words and phrases in a foreign language requires knowledge of how those words and terms are defined. In studying pharmacy law, it is most helpful to start with common legal definitions. For example knowing the difference between a "drug," a "food," a "dietary supplement," and a "cosmetic" will determine which records, if any, a pharmacist must keep or what labels must be provided when "distributing" or "dispensing" these various "articles." It is also important to know what the terms "label" and "labeling" mean. Likewise, it is helpful to know which activities are encompassed in the legal notion of the "practice of pharmacy" to understand what is meant by a statute that contains a statement such as "no one is allowed to engage in the practice of pharmacy unless properly licensed." Equally important, it is necessary to understand what "delegation" means to determine what acts, tasks, or functions normally associated with the practice of pharmacy may be delegated by a pharmacist to nonpharmacist supportive personnel, including pharmacy interns and technicians. Some of these terms, such as "drug" and "food," are defined primarily by federal laws like the Food Drug and Cosmetic Act (FDCA). Others, such as the "practice of pharmacy," will be determined by state law. It is also important to understand that context might change the definitions of these words or phrases. For example, when one refers to a "label" the content included thereon will differ if the term is used in connection with a manufacturer's label, the pharmacy's dispensing label, or a patient-package label.

Another useful review activity is to consider common abbreviations associated with pharmacy laws. Knowing what NDA, ANDA, SNDA, DEA, DESI, FDA, USP/NF, and similar abbreviations stand for may make studying much easier. Recognize that the context in which these abbreviations are used may also change the meaning. For example, an NDA might refer to a "new drug application" or a "new drug approval" depending on the status a drug is in during an FDA review.

Obviously, a review of this size cannot list definitions and abbreviations for all key terms from all jurisdictions. Furthermore, it is important to note that several of these terms may have additional or different definitions under other federal or state laws. Some of the more important terms and abbreviations (in alphabetical order) associated with federal laws are listed below.

Adulterate

A drug is deemed to be adulterated when it is produced under conditions that are not sanitary. Any drug produced under conditions that violate the CGMPs (discussed below) will be deemed adulterated. Drugs that are listed in any of the official compendia (e.g., USP/NF, defined further below) but fail to meet the purity or strength standards established by the compendia will also be deemed adulterated. Students sometimes mix up the concepts of adulteration and misbranding (see below). Adulteration deals with the quality of the drug itself. Misbranding deals with the packaging and labeling of the drug. Note that drugs may be both adulterated and misbranded under certain conditions.

Adequate Directions for Use

This term is defined as directions under which the layman can use a drug safely and for the purposes for which it is intended. All OTC drugs must bear a label containing adequate directions for use. For Rx-only drugs, the manufacturer or distributors labeling must include adequate directions for use up and until drugs are dispensed pursuant to a prescription when the labeling requirements change. The directions must include a statement of all conditions, purposes, or uses for which such drug is intended, quantity of dose, frequency of administration, duration of use, time of administration (in relation to time of meals, time of onset of symptoms, or other time factors), route or method of administration, and preparation for use (shaking, dilution, adjustment of temperature, or other manipulation or process).

ANDA

Abbreviated New Drug Approval (or Application) is the process by which a generic manufacturer of a drug already on the market with an NDA obtained by the innovator company obtains pre-market approval from the FDA. In order to have an application for an ANDA approved, the applicant must prove that the generic active drug component is the exact same chemical entity as and is bioequivalent to the innovator product. The generic company is not required to submit safety and efficacy data because that evidence is already on file from the innovator company.

CGMP (or GMP)

Current Good Manufacturing Practices (or just Good Manufacturing Practices) are FDA regulations that dictate the conditions under which all drugs are produced in the United States. This includes drugs that are exempt from NDA requirements for safety and efficacy data under the grandfather clauses of the FDCA. See NDA (below) for a discussion of the grandfather clause. In other words, all drugs manufactured in the United States or for importation into the country must be manufactured under the CGMP standards irrespective of whether they are grandfathered or if they are OTC drugs or Rx-only drugs.

Cosmetic

This is defined as something that is intended to be rubbed, poured, sprinkled, sprayed on, introduced into, or applied to the human body for purposes of cleaning, beautifying, or promoting human attractiveness. Soap (see below) is *generally* excluded from the categories of articles that constitute cosmetics.

DEA

The Drug Enforcement Administration is a division of the Department of Justice. It is responsible for administering and enforcing the Controlled Substances Act.

DESI

In 1968, the FDA established the Drug Efficacy Study Implementation program to implement recommendations of the National Academy of Sciences investigation of effectiveness of new drugs that were marketed between 1938 and 1962. Drugs on the market before 1938 were exempted from having to prove their safety. Drugs put on the market after 1938 had to obtain the pre-market approval of the FDA through the NDA process. The efficacy requirement did not go into effect until 1962, after which manufacturers had to prove that new drugs were both safe and effective. For drugs put on the market between 1938 and 1962, manufacturers had to only prove the drug's safety. The DESI program was established to provide a mechanism for the federal government to establish evidence as to whether or not these groups of drugs were also efficacious for intended purposes.

Dietary Supplement

An item other than tobacco that is intended to supplement the diet and contains a vitamin, mineral, herb, or other botanical ingredient; or an amino acid; or is a dietary substance taken by humans to supplement total dietary intake. The definition also includes many other items that are not likely the topic of license exams.

Dispense

This term is defined as the act of a pharmacist preparing a medication for a patient pursuant to a prescription issued by a licensed practitioner and delivery of that medication to the patient or patient caregiver.

Distribute

In pharmacy, this term means the act of transferring a drug by means other than dispensing between individuals or persons who are licensed or registered to handle the drug. For example, a physician might wish to purchase an office supply of a prescription-only medication directly from a pharmacy. The act of taking the drug out of the pharmacy's inventory and selling it to a physician's office constitutes distribution, not dispensing.

Drug

This is defined as an item listed in the USP/NF (see below) or the Homeopathic Pharmacopeia of the United States; an item intended for use in the diagnosis, cure, mitigation, treatment, or prevention of disease in humans or other animals; or an item (other than food) intended to affect the structure or function of humans or other animals. This includes components of any of these listed items.

FDA

The Food and Drug Administration is a division of the Department of Health and Human Services responsible for administering and enforcing the FDCA (see below) and its amendments. Note that the FDA has jurisdiction over the distribution of food, drugs, and cosmetics in interstate commerce. It has limited authority over dietary supplements. More important, the FDA has authority to regulate the manufacture, research, labeling, and distribution of all drugs including those available over the counter (OTC) and by prescription only (federal legend drugs). It also has authority to regulate the marketing of prescription-only drugs. The FTC (see below) regulates most of the advertising claims for OTC drugs and several aspects of the advertising of dietary supplements.

FDCA (sometimes abbreviated in other texts as "FD&CA")

The Food Drugs and Cosmetic Act is a law, originally enacted in 1938, that has been amended several times over the years. References to the FDCA may be to the whole Act, as amended, or may be only to portions of the Act or specific Amendments. For example, as explained in more detail below, the PDMA amended the Act in 1987 and affected the distribution of prescription-only drugs and drug samples. The Food and Drug Administration Modernization Act (FDAMA) was adopted in 1997 as an amendment to the FDCA and affects many FDA activities. Readers should take care in understanding the context under which references are made to any of these acts and amendments so as to avoid confusion.

Food

This term is defined as an item that is used for food or drink in humans and other animals. Chewing gum is always a food. Note that gum may be used as a drug delivery device as with nicotine gum, but the gum itself is still a food.

FTC

The Federal Trade Commission is a federal agency that has authority to investigate and prevent unfair trade practices including false and misleading advertising of OTC drugs and dietary supplements. For all intents and purposes, the FTC does not regulate the advertising or promotion of prescription-only drugs; this function is performed by the FDA.

Grandfather

The term "grandfather," when it comes to use in context with the FDCA, is used to denote drugs that were on the market before 1938 when the NDA process was adopted to require manufacturers to get pre-market approval from the FDA (in the form of an NDA) by showing that the drug is safe for its intended purposes. The "grandfather" provision exempts pre-1938 drugs from the NDA requirement. Had this provision not been written into the law there would have been a great deal of protest from manufacturers who were allowed to market their pre-1938 drugs without very much government regulation. This probably would be found in violation of the U.S. Constitution's prohibition about enacting "ex post facto" laws. It is very unlikely that the MPJE would ever ask about anything so esoteric as ex post facto laws. Nevertheless, the FDA has embarked on a program that will require manufacturers of grandfathered drugs to submit data showing effectiveness and safety or risk having the drug removed from the market under other unique enforcement provisions that the FDA has interpreted to give it this authority. http://www.fda.gov/ICECI/ComplianceManuals/CompliancePolicyGuidanceManual/ucm074382.htm (accessed 2010 Dec 2).

GRAS

A term used by the FDA for a vast variety of things that it regulates when those things are Generally Recognized As Safe.

IND

This is an abbreviation of Investigational New Drug. Whenever the maker of a "new" drug wishes to begin human testing to assemble evidence that the drug is safe and effective, the company files an IND application with the FDA. The IND application must disclose safety and efficacy data collected in animals and describe how the drug will be tested using human volunteers. An IND application is required when the maker of a drug on the market with an NDA wishes to test the drug in humans for uses not contemplated in the original NDA application. In other words, established drugs with an NDA, will be treated as "new" drugs when administered by methods or used in a manner not contemplated in the original NDA. Usually the applicant is required to perform three categories of human clinical testing beginning with small-scale testing on a few individuals and concluding with full-scale clinical research with multiple subjects.

Label

This term is defined as written or printed material on the immediate container of an item such as a drug. In pharmacy practice, this usually means the written matter that appears on the outside of a commercial or pharmacy bottle containing drugs.

Labeling

This term includes labels and any other written material on or accompanying an item. In pharmacy, this means the manufacturer's package insert and anything else that might accompany a drug. It also includes patient package inserts for the few drugs (e.g., oral contraceptives and estrogen products) that require them. The FDA must approve the content and appearance of all labels and labeling.

Drugs that have improper labels or labeling are considered misbranded. All OTC drugs must be marketed with a Drug Facts Label that complies with FDA regulations. http://www.fda.gov/Drugs/ResourcesForYou/Consumers/ucm143551.htm (accessed 2010 Dec 2).

Misbrand

A drug is considered misbranded when the labeling is false or misleading or when a label that is required by law is not provided. Drugs that are packaged without conforming to the child-resistant safety restrictions established by the Poison Prevention Packaging Act (see below) are also considered misbranded.

NDA

This is an abbreviation for New Drug Approval or New Drug Application. A manufacturer or distributor that wishes to introduce a new drug must obtain approval of its application before the drug may be sold (i.e., pre-market approval) in this country. In order to obtain an NDA, the applicant must prove that the drug is both safe and effective for its intended purpose. Evidence is gathered from testing the drugs in humans. Before human testing may begin, the applicant must obtain an IND (see above). Note that there are a few drugs on the market today that do not have an NDA. These drugs were on the market before the FDCA became effective in 1938. These drugs were allowed to remain on the market under a grandfather clause in the Act that exempted them from the NDA process for pre-market approval. As such, there is no evidence on file at the FDA that these drugs are safe. Multiple years of experience with the use of these few drugs has demonstrated that they are, in fact, safe when used as intended.

New Drug

Any drug that has not previously been marketed in the United States and is not generally recognized as safe and effective by qualified experts under conditions for use specified in the labeling of the drug. A new drug may be created from an existing FDA-approved drug if there are any changes in the dosage form, labeling claims, indications, or other significant changes in the marketing of the drug.

SNDA

Supplemental New Drug Approval (or Application) is needed when the maker of a drug already on the market with an NDA wishes to make new claims for the drug. It must seek approval from the FDA to change the approved labeling. This is done through the SNDA process whereby the applicant provides evidence that the drug is safe and effective for the newly claimed uses.

Soap

Soap is a category that needs special explanation. That's because the regulatory definition of soap is different from the way in which people commonly use the word. Products that meet the definition of soap are exempt from the provisions of the FDCA because even though the Act includes "articles...for cleansing" in the definition of a cosmetic, another section §201(i)(2) excludes soap from the definition of a cosmetic. Thus, for practical purposes, soap is neither a drug, cosmetic, nor food in terms of classifications.

USP/NF

The *United States Pharmacopeia–National Formulary* is a book of pharmacopeial standards that contains standards for medicines, dosage forms, drug substances, excipients, medical devices, and dietary supplements. Drugs that do not conform to these compendial standards may be deemed adulterated, misbranded, or both.

There are only a few historical facts that pharmacists need to know about regulations of drugs at the federal level. While the MPJE does not ask questions about when an amendment to the FDCA was passed into law or what the popular name of an amendment is, it may be easier to understand current regulations if a few drug law developments are kept in mind. There is one exception: know that the FDCA became law in 1938. This date is critical to determine which laws apply to specific drugs. For example, not every drug on the market in the United States has been proven safe and effective for its intended use. This is because drugs that were on the market before the original FDCA was enacted in 1938 were grandfathered from the mandates of the then-new law. As noted in the grandfather definition above, there is a move on the part of the FDA to eliminate this distinction. Nevertheless, under current law, any drug placed on the market after 1938 must be proven to be safe when used according to the labeled directions. This law also instituted the NDA process mandating that a drug manufacturer obtain pre-market approval from the FDA before offering a drug for sale. As explained below, it was a later amendment to the FDCA that added the requirement that manufacturers also must prove that a drug is efficacious for its intended purpose.

The FDCA was amended in 1951 by the "Durham-Humphrey Act" to establish two classes of drugs. OTC drugs are those that are considered safe to use according to the labeled directions. OTC labeling must include adequate directions for use, rendering them safe to use without further medical directions. Drugs that are not safe for use without medical direction are limited to sale to a patient only pursuant to a prescription issued by someone who is allowed to prescribe under state law. (Note that federal law defers to the states for determining who is allowed to prescribe.) These items are known as "prescription only" or "federal legend" drugs.

The term "federal legend" requires some special attention because the phrase is still widely used in pharmacy practice today. For many years, the commercial container from the manufacturer or distributor of these drugs had to bear a label stating, "Caution: Federal law prohibits dispensing without a prescription." This phrase was called the federal legend. The Food and Drug Administration Modernization Act of 1997 (FDAMA) amended this mandate; now federal legend drugs must be labeled, at a minimum, with the designation "Rx Only." In effect, this amendment changed the content of the federal legend to Rx Only. Thus the terms, federal legend, prescription only, and Rx only should be understood to mean the same thing.

Federal legend drugs are exempt from the adequate directions for use labeling requirements because they are otherwise properly labeled when they are dispensed pursuant to a prescription. Under federal law, a pharmacy label of a dispensed prescription must contain the name of the prescriber, the serial number (more commonly known as the prescription number), the name and address of the dispensing pharmacy, and the date the prescription was originally written, dispensed, or most recently refilled. This amendment also provides that federal legend drugs may be refilled according to the prescriber's directions. In addition, the name of the patient and any directions for use, including precautions must also appear on the pharmacy label if this information appears on the prescription. In other words, the patient's name and directions for use are not always required on the pharmacy label of a prescribed drug under federal law. It is important to note that this provision applies only to federal legend noncontrolled substances. As discussed below, labeling requirements for prescription legend controlled drugs that are dispensed from a pharmacy do require this information. Be aware, however, that every state has additional labeling requirements for dispensed medications. In addition to the

patient's name and directions for use, the vast majority of states also require the drug name to appear unless there are special circumstances. If questions arise as to the labeling mandates for a dispensed drug, responses should include considerations for both state and federal law.

The "Kefauver-Harris Amendment of 1962" (also called the "Drug Efficacy Amendment") added a section to the FDCA to mandate that manufacturers of drugs submit proof that a new drug is effective in addition to being safe, as mandated in the original 1938 Act. After implementation of this Amendment, manufacturers had to prove that new drugs are both safe and effective. Drugs placed on the market between 1938 and 1962 must also be shown to be effective; however, for this category of drugs, the FDA established the DESI program. Most, if not all, drugs subject to the DESI program have been removed from the market where evidence is not available to substantiate that they are effective.

This amendment also established the CGMPs that specify the conditions under which all drugs made in the United States must be produced. Note that the CGMPs apply to all drugs, both OTC and prescription-only and irrespective of when introduced to the market in the United States. In other words, a grandfathered drug, not subject to the NDA pre-market approval and safety requirements, is nevertheless subject to the CGMPs. This Amendment also gave the FDA authority to regulate prescription drug advertising. Keep in mind that the FTC has authority to regulate the advertising of OTC drugs. Under this scheme, the FDA regulates the labeling of all drugs, but a jurisdictional division exists between these classes of drugs insofar as advertising is concerned.

The FDCA was amended again in 1984 by the "Drug Price Competition and Patent Term Restoration Act" (also known as the "Waxman-Hatch Amendment") to exempt generic drug manufacturers or distributors from having to submit original safety and efficacy evidence for drugs already subject to an NDA from the innovator manufacturer. The generic company must prove that the generic drug is bioequivalent to the innovator drug. Successful applicants are awarded approval of an ANDA from the FDA. This event gave rise to the FDA's practice of rating the equivalency of drugs that are listed in the so-called "Orange Book," which is formally known as the *Approved Drug Products with Therapeutic Equivalence Evaluations*. The online version is often referred to as the "Electronic Orange Book" (http://www.fda.gov/cder/ob/default.htm). For applicants living in jurisdictions that use the Orange Book as a guide for pharmacists in making generic substitution (also called drug product selection or DPS) decisions, it is important to recall that drugs in the listings with a designation in the first letter or the equivalency rating (the FDA assigns two alphabetical letters for each listed drug) as an "A" are deemed to be equivalent with the innovator companies product. If the first letter is a "B," the FDA considers the generic drug to NOT be equivalent with that of the innovator company.

It is important to know that not all generic and innovator drugs are listed in the Orange Book. Only those that have an existing NDA are listed. Drugs that were grandfathered from the safety evidence requirement of the 1938 Act are not included in the Orange Book even though there may be generic products available. Note also that some states use the Orange Book as a reference for drug product selection or generic substitution activities as well as for formulary development.

The Prescription Drug Marketing Act (PDMA) of 1987 amended the FDCA to implement controls on the distribution of prescription drugs, prescription drug samples, and prescription drug coupons. The PDMA prohibits drug manufacturers and their representatives from distributing drug samples to physicians unless the physician makes a request in writing. Under federal law, hospital pharmacies may receive and maintain drug samples for and on behalf of prescribers when the prescriber has made a proper request. Community pharmacies are not allowed to have any drug samples in stock or on hand. The PDMA also prohibits, with a few rare exceptions, manufacturers and distributors from importing drugs into the United States after drugs have been exported. The sale of coupons for federal legend drugs is also prohibited under this Act.

The Prescription Drug User Fee Act (PDUFA) was originally enacted in 1992 as an amendment to the FDCA. It contains something called a sunset provision meaning that it will expire after a certain time unless it is renewed by Congress. It was most recently renewed in 2007 (called PDFUA IV) and will expire, unless renewed, in 2012. This Act had a substantial change in how the work of the FDA is funded. Prior to its enactment, the FDA was primarily supported through tax revenues collected by the federal government and distributed to its various agencies. After its enactment, the FDA was authorized to collect fees from the manufacturers that wanted to obtain the various licenses and registrations the FDA has authority to grant. On the good side, this change in funding revenue has played an important role in expediting the drug approval process (http://www.fda.gov/ForIndustry/UserFees/PrescriptionDrugUserFee/default.htm (accessed 2010 Dec 2). On the other hand the FDA, which is supposed to be the watchdog for making sure the American public is only exposed to safe and effective drugs, is now funded primarily by the very drug manufacturers that pay for and are dependent on the FDA for getting new drugs to market. In other words, the FDA is no longer funded primarily through taxpayer dollars. This has lead to some questions about where the primary allegiance of the FDA lays: with the taxpayers it is sworn to protect or the manufacturers who pay for its annual operations. Again, this is an esoteric question likely never to appear on the MPJE. It is offered only to make the reader think about the role of the FDA in the functioning of the American society.

Another important amendment to the FDCA is the Dietary Supplement Health and Education Act of 1994. This act often referred to as the DSHEA law carves out a regulatory scheme for dietary supplements separate and apart from drug regulation. The act severely limits the FDA from having jurisdiction to regulate many aspects of the marketing of dietary supplements. Instead, the FTC monitors advertising for dietary supplements to ensure that no false or misleading claims are made by the manufacturers or distributors. Effects of the DSHEA law are discussed in more detail in the section dealing with distinguishing between food, dietary supplements, cosmetics, and drugs.

Another amendment to the FDCA is the Food and Drug Administration Modernization Act (FDAMA) of 1997. This Act has far-reaching effects on how the FDA conducts its mandates for overseeing the marketing and distribution of drugs. As mentioned above, this is the Act that changed the traditional federal legend that has to appear on the manufacturer or distributor labels of drugs that are restricted to distribution pursuant to a prescription; following implementation, the drugs must bear a label that, at a minimum, states "Rx Only." This Act also eliminated the need for a warning label on certain habit-forming drugs. It also specifies that drugs and drug products compounded by pharmacists are exempt from FDA regulation under specified circumstances. This provision was included because the FDA had, in a few instances, attempted to restrict pharmacist compounding on the notion that the compounded product was a new drug subject to NDA and CGMP requirements. The U.S. Supreme Court ruled in 2002 that the FDAMA statute that restricts compounding to pharmacies that do not solicit or advertise this service is unconstitutional. Further

discussion of the implications of this decision is addressed below in the section entitled "Compounding Prescription Drugs."

There have been numerous other amendments to the FDCA over the years. The above descriptions only highlight some of the more important provisions that pharmacist licensure candidates should be aware of.

Distinguishing Foods, Dietary Supplements, Cosmetics, and Drugs

In the language of the FDCA, the things we put on, into, or around us are "articles" that fall into four distinct classifications: food, dietary supplements, cosmetics, or drugs. The key to understanding whether an article falls into one or another of the named categories is to focus on the intent of the manufacturer or marketer of the item. Intent is most often determined by looking at claims that are made for the item. For example, if the manufacturer of a cereal that contains naturally occurring oat-bran advertises that this cereal builds strong bones, then the cereal would likely be classified as just a food. If that manufacturer advertises that this product helps control cholesterol, it might be viewed as either a food or a dietary supplement. But if that manufacturer advertises the cereal will prevent heart attacks by lowering cholesterol levels, the FDA may view this claim as one for prevention of a disease and, therefore, deem this to be a drug claim.

There are serious ramifications in classifying an item as a drug or one of the other categories. If an item is a drug, it is subject to the whole array of FDA regulations including the need for a pre-market NDA approval, proof that the drug is safe and effective, that is manufactured by an FDA-registered manufacturer in accordance with the CGMPs, and that its labeling is proper and approved by the FDA. If the drug may be sold without a prescription, it must be labeled with adequate directions for use and packaged in accordance with federal anti-tamper proof and child-resistant regulations. Additional storage and labeling mandates apply to prescription drugs dispensed by a pharmacist. If the drug is packaged with the labeling required by the FDA for Rx-only drugs, the pharmacy label will replace the adequate directions for use requirement. A pharmacist who sells any drug, OTC, or Rx-only that does not comply with all legal mandates is subject to severe disciplinary sanctions including criminal prosecution. Improperly labeled drugs will be deemed misbranded under the FDCA. Drugs produced in violation of the CGMPs are considered adulterated under the federal law.

In comparison to drugs, cosmetics are subject to very few regulations. Foods and food supplements are subject to some labeling and packaging requirements at both the state and federal levels. However, with rare exceptions, pharmacists need not be concerned with these regulations. Perhaps the more difficult distinction, in terms of regulations, involves dietary supplements and claims made for their usefulness. There is a fine, and often vague, line between a claim for a dietary supplement and a claim that would cause such an item to be classified as a drug. While readers should be aware of these issues, it is unlikely that detailed questions would appear on a licensure exam because so many questions are unsettled and controversial. Readers should, however, recognize that dietary supplements, a classification that includes vitamins, herbs, botanicals, and anything else intended to supplement the diet, are exempt from most FDA scrutiny, including the need for an NDA and compliance with the CGMPs. Regulations adopted by the FDA do attempt to define what kinds of labeling and other claims will render a dietary supplement to be considered a drug. The FTC does review claims made for dietary supplements to make sure the claims are truthful and not misleading.

The 1994 DSHEA law establishes dietary supplements as a category distinct and separate from foods or drugs. Unlike drugs that must be pre-approved for the United States market by the FDA, DSHEA shifts the burden of proof to the FDA to prove a dietary supplement put on the market in the United States by a manufacturer or distributor is not safe before the FDA can take the item off of the market.

The most controversial part of the DSHEA law is its permission for dietary supplement makers to make certain function-structure claims for their products. It is often difficult to tell whether a manufacturer or distributor of a product is making a claim that the product does something to cure, treat, or mitigate a disease (which would classify the product as a drug) or is merely making a claim that the product will enhance nutrition (which would result in a dietary supplement categorization for the product). When a dietary supplement manufacturer makes a function-structure claim on the labeling of the product, the label must also carry a disclaimer stating: "This statement has not been evaluated by the Food and Drug Administration. This product is not intended to diagnose, treat, cure or prevent disease." The manufacturer or distributor of a product must notify the FDA of its actions within 30 days of putting the product on the market in the United States. Presumably, the 30-day notification requirement would give the FDA time to amass evidence that the product is unsafe or not effective for the claimed purpose.

While it is not likely that the MPJE would ask questions of a pharmacist licensure applicant, there is a fifth category of articles regulated to some extent by the FDA. Veterinary pharmaceuticals are drugs intended for animals other than humans, which must also meet safety and efficacy standards.

Poison Prevention Packaging Act (PPPA)

The PPPA requires that all *oral* drugs intended for use in humans be placed in special packaging that is child-resistant, as described in regulations adopted by the Consumer Products Safety Commission (CPSC). The intent of these laws is to prevent the poisoning of young children from common household products, including most drugs. In community pharmacy practice, this means that oral dosage forms of dispensed drugs must be delivered to the patient (or caregiver) with child-resistant safety caps irrespective of whether the drug is intended for adult or pediatric patients and irrespective of whether or not there are children present in the patient's home. Note that these regulations are mandated separate and apart from FDA packaging and labeling requirements. However, the FDA does consider drugs sold in packaging that does not conform to PPPA requirements to be misbranded. The PPPA does not apply to drugs dispensed to institutional or hospital patients.

A prescriber or patient may request that child-resistant packaging not be used. It is important to note that while the request does not have to be in writing under the PPPA, pharmacists should always note the request for non-child-resistant packaging has been made on the prescription or in the patient profile record.

There are 17 drug and drug categories that are expressly exempted from the mandates of this law. Pharmacist licensure applicants should know the drugs and drug categories that are exempted from the child-resistant packaging regulations. Only the most common are listed here: sublingual dosage forms of nitroglycerin, sublingual and chewable forms of isosorbide dinitrate in 10-mg or less strengths, progesterone or estrogen oral contraceptives dispensed in packages for cyclical administration, sodium fluoride when sold in containers with 264 mg or less per package, pred-

nisone tablets in packages containing no more than 105 mg, conjugated estrogen tablets in packages of no more than 32 mg, and erythromycin ethylsuccinate tablets in packages containing 16 g or less of erythromycin. *Readers should consult pharmacy law texts for a listing of drugs exempt from this law.* Note that the exceptions are narrowly construed. For example, the exception applies to sublingual nitroglycerin tablets, not to any other forms. Note also that the Act applies only to *oral* dosage forms of drugs. Therefore, creams, pastes, injectables, and patches are not covered by this law.

The law also prohibits reusing child-resistant packaging; glass containers may be reused only if a new safety closure is provided at the time the glass container is reused. In practical terms, this means, for the most part, that pharmacists cannot reuse patient vials for oral prescription drugs that are refilled. Essentially, commercial containers of federal legend drugs distributed to a pharmacy do not have to contain child-resistant closures. Exceptions exist when the commercial container is intended to be relabeled by a pharmacy and sold or otherwise transferred directly to a patient; in these cases, the commercial container must include child-resistant packaging.

Note also that the Act applies to OTC drugs. Regulations allow manufacturers and distributors of OTC drugs to package one size of a product that does not conform to the child-resistant requirement as long as the label clearly states that the product is not in child-resistant packaging.

Anti-Tampering Act

Tamper-resistant packaging is required for many consumer products, including most OTC drugs, cosmetics, and medical devices. Contact lens solutions and lubricants are also subject to these restrictions. Dentifrices, dermatological products, lozenges, and insulin are exempted from the regulations. Prescription drugs dispensed from a pharmacy are also exempted.
Tampering is defined as an intentional act of altering a product to make objectionable and unauthorized changes. Anyone charged with tampering with a product is subject to criminal charges. Three federal agencies have jurisdiction to enforce anti-tampering regulations. The Federal Bureau of Investigation (FBI), the U.S. Department of Agriculture, and the FDA each have authority to regulate products that must be marketed with these preventative measures. The FDA regulation applicable to OTC drugs requires a statement on the label indicating that it is packaged with tamper-resistant materials.

Other Packaging Requirements

Commercial containers of drugs must meet federal standards for maintaining the integrity of the drugs during distribution throughout the marketing chain. For all federal legend drugs, manufacturers' labeling (package insert) must contain a statement indicating to a pharmacist what kind of container a particular drug should be dispensed in to maintain its identity, strength, and purity. For the most part, the FDA regulations defer to standards established by the USP/NF for determining adequate container standards. Drugs that are not packaged in accordance with these standards are considered misbranded

Drug Recalls

Although the FDA does not have inherent authority to order a drug manufacturer or distributor to remove an adulterated or misbranded drug from the market, the FDCA prescribes the procedures followed by the FDA to obtain court-ordered recalls or seizures. Of course, a company may voluntarily engage in a product recall if it believes that a product is adulterated or misbranded. The law establishes three categories of recalls designed to alert practitioners and the public as to the level of concern that ought to be raised about the recall. A Class I recall indicates that there is reason to believe use of the drug will cause serious adverse health consequences or even death. A Class II recall means that use of the drug may cause medically reversible consequences but the likelihood of serious adverse results is remote. A Class III recall means that use of a drug will not likely cause adverse health reactions. The manufacturer or distributor of a recalled drug is responsible for notifying the organizations that received the drug. The FDA is responsible for notifying the public about drug recalls.

Some students of pharmacy law confuse the class of drug recall with controlled substances schedules due to the similarities in the numbering system. A simple way to recall the order of severity of a drug recall is it follows the kind of categorization for controlled substances. A schedule I controlled substance has the highest level of concern because of the addiction potential of a drug in this class. A class I drug recall is the one where serious harm or death might result. As the numbers increase the level of severity in both groups goes down.

Withdrawal of NDA

Although not much attention of the MPJE in the past has not been devoted to the authority of the FDA to withdraw an NDA after post-marketing surveys suggest there is evidence that an approved drug may be more dangerous than beneficial, there has been more recent activity by the FDA to engage in this type of conduct. For example, propoxyphene (Darvon) products have been on the market with an NDA since 1957. Late in 2010, the FDA concluded that there was sufficient evidence to show that risks associated with the use of these products outweighed the potential benefits and began the process of withdrawing the manufacturer's NDA, thereby effectively removing propoxyphene products from the U.S. market. See www.fda.gov/Drugs/DrugSafety/ PostmarketDrugSafetyInformationforPatientsandProviders/ ucm233800.htm (accessed 2010 Dec 6). The point is that once an NDA has been approved, the FDA retains the right to revoke that NDA where the appropriate circumstances are available to demonstrate the risks of a drug outweigh its potential benefits.

Omnibus Reconciliation Act of 1990 (OBRA-90)

The federal laws discussed up to this point generally deal with the manufacturing, packaging, and labeling of drugs and do not directly impact the practice of pharmacy as such. This is partly because the federal government does not have direct authority to regulate pharmacy practice. This right is, at least theoretically, reserved to the states. The law, commonly known as OBRA-90, is somewhat of an exception to this notion because it does mandate certain actions by pharmacists when dispensing drugs to certain patients. This law has much more impact because the vast majority of states have enacted provisions to make the OBRA-90 requirements apply to all patients. Readers will have to take care to determine the specific laws in the states where licensure is sought. Although it is unlikely to be a question on the MJPE, be aware that OBRA-90 did not take effect until 1993.

OBRA-90, insofar as outpatient pharmacy practice is concerned, requires that pharmacies that participate in Medicaid reimbursement programs perform a drug utilization review before dispensing a drug to a Medicaid-eligible patient. This review

requires that a pharmacist make an attempt to obtain and maintain a medication history of the patient and determine that a prescribed drug is both necessary and appropriate for the patient before the drug is dispensed. The pharmacist must also be available to counsel a patient on the proper administration of the drug, its common adverse effects, how to monitor the drug's use and effectiveness, and on proper storage techniques. An offer to counsel may be made by someone other than a pharmacist but the counseling itself must be performed by a pharmacist if the offer is accepted.

As noted, OBRA-90 applies only to outpatient drugs dispensed to Medicaid-eligible recipients. Congress has authority to regulate pharmacy practice to this limited extent because the federal government pays a portion of the Medicaid drug benefit. Medicaid programs are administered by each state but the states are allowed to seek reimbursement from the federal government for approximately 50 percent of the costs of drugs paid to pharmacies by the state. At the federal level, Medicaid is administered by the Centers for Medicare & Medicaid Services (http://cms.hhs.gov) (formerly known as the Health Care Financing Administration [HCFA]), which is a division within Health and Human Services. OBRA-90 sets forth the conditions that must be met by the state to be eligible for this reimbursement. As a result, every state has enacted some type of law to implement OBRA-90 mandates. However, very few states restricted the OBRA-90 provisions to just Medicaid patients. Instead, nearly every state has, in one form or another, made the drug utilization review process applicable to all patients. In other words, the duty of a pharmacist to offer to counsel all patients on drug use is almost standard across the country. MPJE candidates should consult the laws in the state where pharmacist licensure is sought.

Compounding

The FDAMA amendments to the FDCA (discussed in the FDCA section, above) contain restrictions on when pharmacists are allowed to compound prescription drugs. Basically, the statute permits pharmacists to compound drugs pursuant to valid prescriptions so long as the pharmacy does not solicit compounded prescriptions or advertise to the health care community or the general public that it performs compounding services. While the history underlying this policy is interesting, it is not likely to be the subject of licensure examination questions. Nevertheless it is important for applicants to understand that the U.S. Supreme Court struck down the entire compounding statute as an unconstitutional restriction on freedom of speech. The decision in *Thompson vs. Western States Medical Center* was released in 2002. In a close 5-4 decision, the majority of the members on the Court ruled that the restriction on advertising violated the First Amendment because the government failed to articulate why a ban on advertising was necessary to prevent manufacturing under the guise of compounding and because the government went too far in its restriction of advertising of compounded products.

It should be understood that before the FDAMA amendments went into effect, pharmacists always enjoyed the right to compound drugs for individual patients. The Supreme Court decision, in essence, returns the pharmacy compounding rules to where they were before FDAMA went into law. The FDA, however, issued internal guidelines for FDA field offices to use in trying to determine whether a pharmacy has crossed the line between accepted compounding practices and entered into the drug manufacturing role.

Suffice it to say, for examination purposes, that pharmacists may legally compound drugs pursuant to a prescription for an individual patient. The resulting compounded drug product will not be characterized as an unapproved new drug by the FDA under normal circumstances.

Controlled Substances Laws

Introduction

Significant portions of the MPJE are devoted to assessing licensure candidates' knowledge of both federal and state controlled substances laws. This is because pharmacists spend significant time complying with the laws regulating the ordering, delivery, storage, recordkeeping, and dispensing of these drugs. It is important to note at the outset that the state and federal governments share concurrent jurisdiction over the regulation of controlled substances. This means that at least two sets of laws need to be considered with reference to controlled substances.

While controlled substances laws have been in place for several years, there are a number of changes that must be taken into account. The DEA publishes a revised version of *The Pharmacist's Manual* frequently. At the time of printing this text, the most current edition of the Manual is available online at www.deadiversion.usdoj.gov/pubs/manuals/pharm2/pharm_manual.htm#8 (accessed 2010 Dec 2). Do not use any printed or online versions of *The Pharmacist's Manual* prior to the revised 2010 edition as a study reference. If a newer edition of the *Manual* is published, use the then-current version in preparation for the MPJE.

It cannot be overemphasized that studying from *The Pharmacist's Manual* will greatly improve the chance of success in taking the MJPE. This document has been the source of many questions that appear on the examination. Pay attention to the details. For example, knowing which DEA form is used for what purpose will be worth points.

Many states have adopted modifications that take into account newer practice settings such as group homes and assisted living arrangements and newer technologies such as the Internet, online prescribing, and electronic signatures. Because of this, it is important for applicants to recognize that some laws may have changed since taking a pharmacy law course in school. One of the most common issues that students raise is whether they will be asked questions about which drugs are designated as controlled substances and which schedule a drug is placed in. The answer is that the states take a wide variety of approaches to assessing a candidate's knowledge about these topics. The best advice is that all candidates should know the controlled substance status of the most commonly prescribed and dispensed controlled substances and non-controlled drugs. There are several lists of commonly prescribed drugs online. Try to find a list tailored to the state in which licensure is being sought.

The other important piece of advice is to pay attention to drugs that may be placed in different schedules by the DEA as compared with the state agency that regulates these drugs. In some cases, a state will place a drug into a higher classification at the state level compared to the schedule it is assigned by the DEA. For example, pentazocine (Talwin) is a Schedule 4 controlled substance under DEA regulations. In Michigan, however, it is classified as a Schedule 3 controlled substance. Another point of departure between state and federal laws is that some states will designate a drug as a controlled substance when the DEA has not put the drug into any schedule. The last issue to consider is drugs designated as OTC Schedule 5 drugs under federal law. Some states have elected to make the medication available only by prescription.

Historical Background

While it is highly unlikely that questions would appear on the MJPE about the history of controlled substances regulation, preparation for the exam might be easier if just a few historical developments are kept in mind. Congress adopted the federal Controlled Substances Act (CSA) in 1970. The CSA repealed many of the earlier laws and adopted a comprehensive approach to preventing drug abuse. The CSA is sometimes referred to as The Comprehensive Drug Abuse Prevention and Control Act of 1970. The provisions of Title 2 of that Act directly affect pharmacy practice and contain the laws most familiar to pharmacists.

At the time that the CSA was enacted, the FDA was given authority to make the scientific and medical findings that determined whether a drug would be controlled and, if so, how it would be scheduled. That authority changed over time. In 1973, the Drug Enforcement Administration (DEA) was created in the Department of Justice (DOJ), and the Bureau of Narcotics and Dangerous Drugs (BNDD), the agency that had responsibility over these drugs, was abolished. While most current laws have eliminated reference to the BNDD, a few still exist. Where a reference in state or federal law is made to the BNDD, it should be understood to mean the DEA as the successor federal agency. By 1986, the FDA's role in scheduling drugs was eliminated for the most part and the DEA assumed this authority. The DEA is now the organization that has primary responsibility for promulgating the regulations that implement, interpret, and enforce the CSA. As the head of the Department of Justice, the U.S. Attorney General is responsible for the DEA operations. The DEA Director reports to the Attorney General.

Goals and Objectives of the CSA

Prevention of drug abuse is one of the CSA's main goals. It attempts to accomplish this objective in several ways. Record-keeping mandates for manufacturers, distributors, prescribers, and dispensers of controlled substances are designed to reduce the diversion of drugs from the legitimate course of commerce into illegal markets. One of the major impacts of the CSA is the establishment of a closed system of distribution that regulates controlled substances from the moment of initial manufacture or harvest until they reach the hands of the ultimate user. An ultimate user is a person who lawfully obtains and possesses a controlled substance for his or her own use or use by a member (including an animal) of his or her household. No one is permitted to obtain or possess a controlled substance unless authorized under the provisions of the CSA. Another method of limiting drug diversion is through the requirement of federal registration of persons who handle controlled substances. As used in this law, the term "person" means both individuals and any legally recognized entity including corporations, partnerships, etc. The registration mandate is discussed in detail below.

Concurrent Jurisdiction

Controlled substances are regulated by both federal and state law. Many state laws require additional or different steps than those demanded by federal laws. For example, federal law mandates that a pharmacy maintain controlled substances records, including prescriptions, for a minimum of 2 years. Many states require a pharmacy to maintain all prescription records for a minimum of 5 years from the date the prescription was filled or last refilled. Using the rule that the stricter law controls, in this instance the pharmacy would have to keep the prescriptions on file for the longer period.

Regulatory Authority

From a constitutional standpoint, the federal government exerts jurisdiction over controlled substances under the interstate commerce clause on the presumed notion that these products will cross between state lines at some point in time. The Attorney General has the primary authority to enforce the CSA. As head of the DOJ, the Attorney General determines which substances will be controlled and which schedule the substance will be placed in. The

Attorney General also determines whether violations of the CSA and DEA regulations may have occurred and whether to seek penalties through the federal court system.

The CSA has been amended many times and the DEA has been given expanded authority. For example, in 1990, the DEA was given authority to regulate anabolic steroids. The agency also regulates precursor chemicals that may be used in producing controlled substances, machinery used in controlled substances manufacturing, and controlled substance analogues.

Schedules

The CSA regulates drugs and other substances by placing affected chemical entities into a hierarchy of five schedules that vary depending on the abuse and dependence-producing potential of an individual substance. It is significant that not all of the substances regulated under the CSA are drugs. By definition, Schedule 1 controlled substances do not have any accepted medical use in the United States and should not properly be referred to as drugs. Nevertheless, it is common to refer to all controlled substances as drugs, and that convention is followed here.

The listing of the various controlled substances in each of the five schedules was initially established by the CSA. The Attorney General, not the DEA director, is given authority to modify the substances in each schedule by adding, deleting, or rescheduling the substances. The schedules are updated and republished on an annual basis. The lists of which drugs are controlled and which schedule each controlled drug is placed in are available from a variety of sources. License applicants are presumed to know the schedule that the common controlled drugs are placed in. States may also place drugs into schedules established by the individual states. For the most part, the state schedules will track the federal schedule. However, there may be some differences making it worthwhile for license applicants to check the law of the state where a license is sought. It should also be useful to review the criteria for placing a substance into a particular schedule.

Schedule 1

(C-I): The drugs and other substances in this schedule are those that have (a) a high potential for abuse; (b) no current accepted medical use in the United States; or (c) there is a lack of accepted safety for use under medical supervision.

Pharmacies, other than those in facilities that are registered for investigative or research uses, should not have any Schedule 1 controlled substances in inventory. Further, physicians are not authorized to prescribe Schedule 1 controlled substances unless registered to perform investigations or do research under approved protocols. Most of the controlled substance analogues of drugs in other schedules, sometimes called "designer drugs," are classified as Schedule 1 controlled substances. Examples of substances classified in Schedule include heroin, LSD, marijuana, and MDMA (ecstasy).

Marijuana deserves some special attention. At the time of publication of this review, 14 states and the District of Columbia have approved the use of marijuana for medical purposes to one degree or another and another six states have pending legislation that would accomplish the same result (see http://medicalmarijuana.procon.org/view.resource.php?resource ID=000881 (accessed 2010 Dec 6). This website is updated frequently and should be checked to find the current status of marijuana in any given jurisdiction.

The fact that some states have recognized that marijuana does have recognized medical benefits for some people puts those states

in direct conflict with the DEA scheduling of marijuana as a Schedule I controlled substance, meaning the DEA considers that there is no currently accepted medical use for products containing marijuana in the United States. Under the Supremacy Clause of the U.S. Constitution, federal law preempts state law when there are direct conflicts such as this one. This situation could create a significant conflict for MPJE applicants in states where marijuana has been legalized for medical use. For this reason, it is likely the MPJE would avoid questions concerning the legal status of marijuana.

Schedule 2

(C-II): To be placed in this schedule, the drug or other substance must be determined to (a) have a high potential for abuse; (b) have a currently accepted medical use in treatment in the United States or a currently accepted use with severe restrictions; and (c) abuse may lead to severe psychological or physical dependence.

Schedule 1 and 2 drugs are subject to annual production quotas established by the DEA. The amount of any given drug subject to this regulation that may be manufactured and distributed is determined each year by medical usage in prior years as measured by studies conducted by the HHS. The quotas are revised once annually.

Some examples of Schedule 2 narcotics include morphine, codeine, hydrocodone, opium, hydromorphone (Dilaudid), methadone (Dolophine), meperidine (Demerol), oxycodone (Percodan), and fentanyl (Sublimaze). Some examples of Schedule 2 stimulants include amphetamine (Dexedrine), dextroamphetamine and amphetamine (Adderall), methamphetamine (Desoxyn), and methylphenidate (Ritalin). Other Schedule 2 substances include cocaine, amobarbital, glutethimide, pentobarbital, and secobarbital.

Schedule 3

(C-III): In order to be placed in this schedule, a drug or other substance must have (a) less potential for abuse than substances in Schedule 1 or 2; (b) a currently accepted medical use for treatment in the United States; and (c) a moderate or low physical or high psychological dependence potential when abused. Some examples of Schedule 3 narcotics include products containing less than 15 milligrams of hydrocodone per dosage unit (i.e., Vicodin, Lorcet, Tussionex, and products containing not more than 90 milligrams of codeine per dosage unit such as codeine with acetaminophen, aspirin or ibuprofen). Other Schedule 3 substances include anabolic steroids, benzphetamine (Didrex), phendimetrazine, buprenorphine (Buprenex), and any compound, mixture, preparation or suppository dosage form containing amobarbital, secobarbital, pentobarbital, dronabinol (Marinol), or ketamine.

Schedule 4

(C-IV): Drugs or other substances in this schedule have (a) a low potential for abuse relative to substances in Schedule 3; (b) a currently accepted use for treatment in the United States; and (c) a limited physical or psychological dependence potential when abused relative to substances in Schedule 3. Schedule 4 drugs include the benzodiazepines: alprazolam (Xanax), clonazepam (Klonopin), clorazepate (Tranxene), diazepam (Valium), flurazepam (Dalmane), halazepam (Paxipam), lorazepam (Ativan), midazolam (Versed), oxazepam (Serax), prazepam (Verstran), temazepam (Restoril), triazolam (Halcion), and quazepam (Doral). Other Schedule 4 substances include barbital, phenobarbital, chloral hydrate, ethchlorvynol (Placidyl), ethinamate, meprobamate, paraldehyde, methohexital, phentermine, diethylpropion, pemoline (Cyler), mazindol (Sanorex), and sibutramine (Meridia).

Schedule 5

(C-V): Drugs or other substances in this schedule must have been determined to (a) have a low, but still very real, potential for abuse relative to substances in Schedule 4; (b) have a currently accepted use for treatment in the United States; and (c) lead to a limited physical or psychological dependence potential when abused relative to the substances listed in Schedule 4. Some examples are cough preparations containing not more than 200 milligrams of codeine per 100 milliliters or per 100 grams (e.g., Robitussin AC, Phenergan with codeine).

OTC Schedule 5

It is noteworthy that there are some drugs on the market that are Schedule 5 controlled substances but do not require a prescription. Most of these are either codeine-based cough syrups or paregoric-based anti-diarrheals. This seemingly peculiar inconsistency exists because the FDA, which is part of the HHS, makes the determination as to whether a drug will be available on a prescription-only basis or available without a prescription as an OTC drug. The FDA uses scientific and medical data to make its decisions on the availability and access of drugs. Safety and efficacy are the primary concerns of the FDA. The DEA, which is a totally unrelated government agency, determines whether a substance or drug will be designated as a controlled substance. In addressing this decision, the DEA behaves more like a police agency that is concerned with crime prevention and prosecution of criminal activity. The DEA uses abuse potential and concerns over diversion as the primary factors in making decisions on the control and scheduling of drugs and other substances. In this respect, the jurisdiction of the agencies is separate and does not overlap. As far as Schedule 5 OTC drugs are concerned, the FDA has determined that they are safe and effective for use without the need of medical supervision, while the DEA has concluded that they have a potential, albeit small, for abuse.

Exempt Narcotics

Schedule 5 OTC drugs in the past were referred to as "exempt narcotics." This archaic but still common term dates back to an exemption from taxation for Class X drugs under the 1914 Harrison Narcotic Act. Take care to note how the state where the applicant is seeking licensure regulates nonprescription Schedule 5 drugs. Usually, these preparations are available only in a state-licensed, DEA-registered pharmacy and the pharmacist who sells these medications must keep a record of sales by filling out information about the purchaser and the date of the sale.

Sale of Controlled Substances Without a Prescription

DEA regulations permit a retail-based pharmacist to dispense certain controlled substances without a prescription if a particular drug has not been designated as a prescription-only substance by the FDA or under the applicable state law and the following procedures are followed.

1. The sale is made by a pharmacist (or pharmacist intern acting under the direct supervision of a licensed pharmacist), not by other nonpharmacist employees, even if under the direct supervision of a pharmacist. However, after the pharmacist has fulfilled professional and legal responsibilities, the actual cash, credit transaction, or delivery may be completed by a nonpharmacist.

2. The pharmacist must use professional judgment to ensure the medical necessity of the need for the product.

3. Not more than 240 mL or not more than 48 solid dosage units

of any substance containing opium, not more than 120 mL (4 fluid ounces), or not more than 24 solid dosage units of any other controlled substance may be distributed at retail to the same purchaser in any given 48-hour period without a valid prescription.

4. The purchaser is at least 18 years of age.

5. The pharmacist must obtain suitable identification, including proof of age, where appropriate if the pharmacist is not familiar with the purchaser.

6. A bound record book must be maintained containing the name and address of the purchaser, name and quantity of controlled substance purchased, date of each sale, and initials of the dispensing pharmacist. This record book must be maintained for a period of 2 years from the date of the last transaction and it must be made available for inspection and copying.

Chemical Control Requirements

In recent years, the DEA has recognized that some OTC drug products contain chemical precursors of controlled substances. For example, pseudoephedrine (Sudafed) can be converted to methamphetamine with rudimentary chemical procedures. Ephedrine and phenylpropanolamine are also commonly involved in the clandestine manufacture of controlled substances. These precursors have garnered the attention of regulators at both the state and federal levels. MPJE applicants should review the laws in the states where pharmacist licensure is sought to determine the current regulations for these products.

Persons who handle controlled chemicals need to register with the DEA. Community pharmacies that are registered to receive and dispense controlled substances do not have to register a second time to also carry the affected chemicals unless the pharmacy also engages in the wholesale distribution of the chemicals. DEA Form 510 is used to register as a chemical distributor.

Registration

Most persons (recall that this means both individuals and legal entities including corporations and partnerships) who handle controlled substances must be registered with the DEA unless specifically exempted from federal registration. Manufacturers and distributors of controlled substance drugs are usually required to register on an annual basis. Pharmacies and prescribers (both are often referred to as dispensers or practitioners in the regulations) usually are required to register once every 3 years.

Pharmacists (with the exception of sole proprietorships), pharmacy interns, technicians, and other agents or employees of a properly registered pharmacy do not have to register independently of the pharmacy. These individuals may handle controlled substances without registration so long as they do so while acting in the usual course of business and within the scope of their employment or agency relationship.

This same kind of exemption applies to most other DEA registrants. As such, the employees of manufacturers and distributors need not apply for registration and do not violate the law when possessing controlled substances in the course of their employment. Military officials, including Public Health Service employees, law enforcement agents, and civil defense workers are also exempted from registration so long as their employment situation requires them to handle controlled substances.

Medical students and residents associated with medical institutions including hospitals need not obtain a DEA registration as long as they are working under the supervision of a registered physician and the institution is registered. Physician's assistants and nurse practitioners (or nurse clinicians) must register as midlevel practitioners in almost all situations.

Separate registrations are required for each individual site where controlled substances are stored or dispensed. Each pharmacy must have its own separate registration and DEA number even if a single corporate entity operates several pharmacies. Thus, if a chain-store owns 100 pharmacies each operating at a separate street address, 100 separate registrations must be obtained. If a hospital or other health care facility operates more than one pharmacy at several satellites within the facility, only a single registration is necessary so long as the facility operates from a single street address. However, if that same facility operates hospital and several clinic pharmacies at different locations, multiple registrations will be required.

Separate registrations are also required for multiple activities even if they occur at the same location. For example, a large health care facility may manufacture, distribute, and dispense controlled substances. Each activity requires a separate registration. If research is also conducted at the facility, an additional registration is necessary.

A pharmacy applies for a DEA registration on DEA form 224, which is available online in the *Pharmacist's Manual*, and may be obtained from any DEA field office, or at the DEA Headquarters in Washington, D.C. Once the registration certificate is issued to the pharmacy, it must be kept on file in the pharmacy and made available for inspection upon request. The DEA should send the pharmacy an application for renewal 45 days before the end of the 3-year registration period. If the pharmacy does not receive the renewal registration by 30 days before its expiration date, the pharmacy will have to request a renewal form. Renewal requests are made on DEA Form 224a. Corporation or other forms of ownership that operate pharmacies at multiple locations use DEA Form 224.

The DEA requires a pharmacy engaged in co-op buying of controlled substances to also register as a distributor. As a distributor, a pharmacy must meet distributor (wholesaler) security and record-keeping requirements.

If a DEA-registered pharmacy moves locations or the postal address of the pharmacy changes, the pharmacy is responsible for submitting a written request for a new registration certificate from the DEA before the change occurs. The request should be made to the local DEA field office. Once the new location is noted by the DEA it will issue new DEA Form 222 (if the pharmacy is still using hard copy forms to order Schedule 2 controlled substances).

A DEA registration may be suspended or revoked, or an application for renewal or for a change in location may be denied if the DEA has reason to believe the registrant is involved in the diversion of controlled substances from legitimate channels into illegal markets. Decisions resulting in the suspension, revocation, or denial of renewals or change of locations are made by the U.S. Attorney General. The grounds for making these adverse decisions include false statements made by applicants; conviction of the applicant of a felony related to the use of controlled substances or controlled chemicals; revocation, suspension, or denial of a state-issued controlled substance or pharmacy license; exclusion from the Medicaid or Medicare programs; and performing an act that would render continuance of a DEA registration "inconsistent with the public interest."

The "inconsistent with the public interest" standard requires the U.S. Attorney General to take into account specific factors including:

1. The recommendation of the appropriate state licensing board or professional disciplinary authority;

2. The applicants experience in dispensing or conducting research with respect to controlled substances;

3. The applicant's conviction record under federal or state laws relating to the manufacture, distribution, or dispensing of controlled substances;

4. Compliance with applicable state, federal, or local laws relating to controlled substances; and

5. Such other conduct that may threaten the public health and safety.

If a DEA-registered pharmacy discontinues doing business or transfers ownership to another legal entity, the pharmacy is obligated to notify the nearest DEA field office in writing in advance of the termination or transfer. The pharmacy is required to return any unused DEA Form 222s with the word "VOID" written on each one. The notification must indicate where the controlled substances inventory and records will be located after the termination or transfer and how they were transferred or destroyed. Even though the pharmacy may be closing, the pharmacist-in-charge must make arrangements to have the records kept available for inspection up until 2 years after the final controlled substance transaction occurred.

If the pharmacy is being transferred to a different owner, the registered pharmacy is obligated to inform the nearest DEA field office of the change at least 14 days prior to the change. The notice must include:

1. The name, address, registration number of the registrant discontinuing business;

2. The name, address, registration number of the registrant acquiring the pharmacy;

3. Whether the business activities will be continued at the location registered by the current business owner or moved to another location (if the latter, give the address of the new location);

4. The date on which the controlled substances will be transferred to the person acquiring the pharmacy.

A complete and final controlled substances inventory must be conducted on the day the pharmacy is terminated or ownership is transferred and, if a transfer is involved, both the seller and the buyer should each keep a copy of the inventory for at least 2 years from the date the inventory was performed.

Electronic Prescribing and Communications

There are several methods by which an authorized prescriber may legitimately communicate a controlled substance prescription to a pharmacy. The traditional pen (or indelible pencil) and paper (hard copy) method is still available and widely used. A prescriber may delegate an agent to communicate a Schedule III-V prescription to a pharmacy by telephone. Note that while the prescriber may delegate *communication* of the prescription to an agent, such as a nurse or office receptionist, the prescriber cannot delegate *prescribing* authority. Fax machines may also be used to communicate Schedule III-V prescriptions to a pharmacy. Schedule II controlled substances prescriptions cannot be called into a community pharmacy unless there are specific emergency circumstances that warrant deviation from the normal rule.

In June 2010, the DEA revised its regulations, entitled "Electronic Prescriptions for Controlled Substances" to permit the electronic prescribing of Schedule II through V prescriptions to a pharmacy, providing that strict security credentialing procedures are followed by both the prescriber and the pharmacy (www.deadiversion.usdoj.gov/ecomm/e_rx/index.html [accessed 2010 Dec 3]). The security provisions are fairly technical and apply primarily to the software and hardware vendors that supply the equipment necessary for pharmacies and prescribers to utilize this technology. Both the prescriber and the pharmacy equipment, software, policies, and procedures for electronic prescribing must be certified by an organization recognized by the DEA as having the knowledge and capacity to identify compliant systems. Even so, the licensed and/or registered practitioners are fully responsible and accountable for compliance with the compliance requirements. Note that the regulations permit the pharmacy to receive, dispense, and archive electronic prescriptions.

Pharmacists should also be cognizant that while the DEA permits electronic prescribing of controlled substances prescriptions, there is no obligation on the part of a pharmacy or pharmacist to accept prescriptions transmitted in this format. In other words, electronic prescribing and dispensing is a voluntary option available to practitioners. Part of the impetuous for the change in regulations encouraging electronic prescribing is reduction of dispensing errors associated with handwritten or hard copy prescriptions as well as the notion that the electronic prescribing may be effective in reducing fraudulent, altered, or forged prescriptions.

Insofar as the pharmacy is concerned, the prescriber must use a two-factor authentication procedure to verify the prescriber's identity and verification that the prescriptions originated from the authorized prescriber. There are three factors available to prescribers that will satisfy the authentication credentials: something the prescriber knows, a "hard token" stored separately from the computer used to send the prescription, or biometric information. Any two of these three options are sufficient. The hard token, if used, must be a cryptographic device or a one-time password that meets federal standards. Use of this two-factor authentication process will constitute an "electronic signature." Some states may have differing definitions of what constitutes an electronic signature for a controlled substances prescription. The trick will be finding the method of combining federal and state laws to comply with both jurisdictional requirements.

If a pharmacy receives a controlled substances prescription electronically and uses that prescription as authority to dispense the medication, the DEA has created special record-keeping procedures. As stated in *The Pharmacist's Manual*:

1. If a prescription is created, signed, transmitted, and received electronically, all records related to that prescription must be retained electronically.

2. Electronic records must be maintained electronically for 2 years from the date of their creation or receipt. However, this record retention requirement shall not pre-empt any longer period of retention, which may be required now or in the future, by any other federal or state law or regulation, applicable to pharmacists or pharmacies.

3. Records regarding controlled substances must be readily retrievable from all other records. Electronic records must be easily readable or easily rendered into a format that a person can read.

As noted previously, readers should consult the online version of *The Pharmacist's Manual* for any additional or updated changes to the electronic prescribing requirements (www.deadiversion.usdoj.gov/pubs/manuals/pharm2/pharm_manual.htm#8. Section VI- Recordkeeping Requirements [accessed 2010 Dec 3]).

Classifications of Pharmacies and Special Provisions for Unique Practices

Traditionally, the DEA only recognized two kinds of pharmacies: the typical community "retail" pharmacy and the "institutional" or hospital-based pharmacy. Over time, the DEA started to accept that there are different sets of considerations that need to be made for long-term nursing homes. In DEA language, these institutions are known as "Long Term Care Facilities" (LTCFs). The DEA has not yet recognized pharmacy services to senior citizen independent living situations or assisted living institutions as anything other than community-based pharmacy. In one of the more recent developments, the DEA has developed rules for "central fill pharmacies" as described below. There are also some regulations pharmacists should know about using controlled substances in drug addiction and rehabilitation clinics.

LTCFs

Nursing homes, retirement care, mental health care, or other facilities or institutions that provide extended health care to resident patients are deemed to be LTCFs by the DEA. Despite the fact that these institutions are not routinely registered with the DEA, they do maintain inventories of controlled substances, usually in the form of medications dispensed by an outside pharmacy directly to the patients but held at nursing stations for administration by LTCF personnel. When patients of these institutions are discharged or expire, or there is a change in the medications of patients, the LTCF may need to dispose of controlled substances it was holding for the patients. The DEA advises operators of these facilities and pharmacists who dispense medications to patients to follow state laws with respect to handling controlled substances no longer needed for a patient or to contact the nearest DEA field office for instructions on how to proceed.

In October 2010, the DEA issued a statement of policy concerning the procedure by which a registrant-prescriber may use an agent, including a nurse in a LTCF, to communicate controlled substances prescriptions to a pharmacy. In summary, the policy states:

1. An agent may "prepare a written prescription for the signature of the practitioner," provided the practitioner has "in the usual course of professional practice" made the necessary determinations regarding the legitimate medical need and has specified the "required elements" of the prescription to the agent.

2. An agent may telephone a pharmacy concerning a prescription for a controlled substance in Schedules III through V and convey the practitioner's otherwise valid oral prescription provided the prescriber has specified all required prescription information.

3. Where otherwise permissible to fax a controlled substance prescription to a pharmacy, the agent may do the actual faxing.

The notice further states that due to the legal responsibilities of practitioners and pharmacists under the CSA and the potential harm to the public from inappropriate and unlawful prescribing and dispensing of controlled substances, the DEA advises practitioners and their agents to commit their agency authorization to writing (http://edocket.access.gpo.gov/2010/pdf/2010-25136.pdf [accessed 2010 December 4]).

Internet Pharmacies

Internet commerce has presented a number of challenges to the DEA because the majority of its experience and requirements deal with traditional community- and hospital-based pharmacy practices. The potential for drug diversion and need for new, innovative solutions takes on global proportions. In what will likely be the first of many attempts by the DEA to regulate controlled substance dispensing and distribution with this newer technology, the DEA issued some regulations addressed to pharmacies that pursue Internet opportunities.

As with all pharmacies, those that wish to use the Internet must be registered with the DEA at the pharmacy's physical location where controlled substances will be held in inventory if it plans on doing any controlled substances dispensing or distributing. There is no need to register the Internet homepage or Internet ownership information. The pharmacy must also be licensed by the state in which the pharmacy is physically located and, if required, in those states where it does business. In most cases, this means that if the pharmacy located in state X sends prescriptions ordered on the Internet to state Y, it would have to have the appropriate licenses from both state X and state Y, in addition to being registered with the DEA. All of the other DEA regulations apply to the Internet pharmacy as would apply to any retail pharmacy.

Note that the regulations for delivering drugs, including controlled substances by the U.S. Postal Services, are discussed below (see Mailing Prescription Drugs).

Narcotic Treatment Programs

Congress adopted laws specifically geared for the use of controlled substances in the treatment of addicted patients seeking rehabilitation. The laws deal with two different treatment programs. One is for maintenance treatments, usually in methadone clinics, and the other is for detoxification. Operators of either type of program must register with the DEA using DEA Form 363. The registrant will only be approved to use the narcotics listed on the form in treatment programs. Controlled substances cannot be used for any purpose other than maintenance or detoxification unless the practitioner who operates the program is also registered for normal practices associated with the controlled substances.

While the DEA has adopted regulations governing these programs, there is also a widely divergent set of regulations adopted by state agencies having jurisdiction over these treatment modalities. Regardless of these differences, narcotic treatment programs must use DEA Form 222 for all transactions involving Schedule II drugs. The electronic CSOS system replaces the need for use of the hard copy forms (www.deaecom.gov/csosmain.html).

Methadone

In addition to the use of methadone in narcotic maintenance programs, methadone is used as an analgesic to treat severe forms of pain. This raises concerns when methadone is used to treat pain in an individual who is also a narcotic addict. With one exception, the DEA has taken the position that practitioners who are not registered as operating a narcotic maintenance program cannot prescribe methadone to an addicted patient under the guise of treating pain. The exception occurs when a practitioner who is not part of a narcotic treatment facility prescribes methadone to a narcotic addict experiencing withdrawal while waiting to get into a treatment program. The methadone used in this manner is limited to a maximum 3-day supply under DEA regulations. There are some states that do not permit this practice.

Narcotics for Patients With Terminal Illnesses or Intractable Pain

The DEA recognizes that the use of narcotics for treatment of patients with intractable pain or pain associated with a terminal illness is effective, appropriate, and legitimate. The regulations require that prescriptions for controlled substances be issued for legitimate medical purposes by a practitioner (i.e., an individual authorized under state law to issue a controlled substances prescription) who is acting in the course of medical practice. The DEA has stated that pharmacists should not be concerned when dispensing controlled substances so long as they act with "good faith" when evaluating the legitimacy or appropriateness of a controlled substance prescription. While inappropriate use of narcotics is not acceptable, the DEA does acknowledge that appropriate narcotic drug use will often be accompanied by drug tolerance and physical dependence in individuals who have the need for high doses or prolonged treatment. The DEA has specifically stated that pharmacists receiving prescriptions for high strengths or large quantities of controlled substances for an individual patient should not fear DEA sanctions because "the quantity of drugs prescribed and frequency of prescriptions filled alone are not indicators of fraud or improper prescribing."

Medical Missions and Humanitarian Charitable Solicitations

In order for practitioners to hand carry controlled substances overseas while providing charitable medical, dental, or veterinary treatment in foreign countries, they must obtain approval from the DEA and the appropriate authority in the foreign country. In these situations, practitioners should allow at least 30 days to obtain the necessary approvals from a local DEA field office. If a pharmacy is asked to donate controlled substances, the pharmacist should contact the state agency that regulates controlled substances and the DEA field office for information on how to proceed.

Central Fill Pharmacies

In recent years the DEA has acknowledged that new technologies and differing market needs have developed so that there are more ways of delivering pharmacy services than the traditional retail and hospital settings. One of these developments has given rise to the concept of a "central fill pharmacy." The DEA describes a central fill pharmacy as one that "fills prescriptions for controlled substances on behalf of retail pharmacies with which central fill pharmacies have a contractual agreement to provide such services or with which the pharmacies share a common owner." In this scenario a retail pharmacy receives a prescription from a patient and transmits it to second pharmacy where the prescription medicine is prepared and delivered to the first retail pharmacy for dispensing to the patient.

In this kind of arrangement, records must be maintained by both the central fill pharmacy and the retail pharmacy that completely reflect the disposition of all controlled substance prescriptions dispensed. Central fill pharmacies, in essence, must comply with the same security requirements applicable to retail pharmacies. Note that retail pharmacies that also perform central fill activities may do so without a separate DEA registration, separate inventories, or separate records.

Central fill pharmacies are permitted to prepare both initial and refill prescriptions, subject to all applicable state and federal regulations. Both the central fill pharmacy and the retail pharmacy share responsibility for determining the validity of a controlled substance prescription. The procedures developed by the DEA for central fill pharmacies apply to all controlled substances prescriptions in Schedules II-V.

The DEA does not permit a central fill pharmacy to accept prescriptions from or deliver medications directly to patients by use of the mail. This seems odd given that patients may obtain controlled substance medication from a regular mail order pharmacy. The distinction between a mail order pharmacy and a central fill pharmacy may not make much logical sense but this is the way the DEA has indicated it will treat central fill pharmacies.

There are two ways for a retail pharmacy to submit prescriptions to a central fill pharmacy. The first is to permit faxed prescriptions between the entities. In this situation, the retail pharmacy keeps the original prescription and the central fill pharmacy uses the faxed prescription as its record of dispensing. All records must be retained in a readily retrievable manner. Interestingly, the DEA does allow the prescription information to be transmitted electronically through the Internet.

MPJE candidates should check the state laws in the state where licensure is sought to determine if state law permits central fill pharmacies. Many states have been adopting standards that follow the model described by the DEA. Other states have not done so or have unique variations.

Destruction or Transfer of Controlled Substances

When a pharmacy goes out of business, it may transfer its inventory of controlled substances to another pharmacy as described above. It may also transfer the drugs to a DEA-registered distributor or back to a DEA-registered manufacturer that is also registered by the DEA to destroy controlled substances. This process is known in DEA terms as "reverse distribution." Records detailing the transfer or destruction must be kept by the pharmacy owner for 2 years after the transfer or destruction, or longer if required by the laws of an individual state.

To transfer Schedule II substances, the receiving registrant must issue a DEA Form 222, to the registrant transferring the drugs or comply with the paperless controlled substances ordering system (CSOS) procedures.

When Schedule II-V controlled substances are transferred, the transaction must be recorded in writing to show the drug name, dosage form, strength, quantity, and date transferred. The document must include the names, addresses, and DEA registration numbers of the parties involved in the transfer of the controlled substances.

If the pharmacy going out of business is transferring its controlled substances back to a distributor or manufacturer, the pharmacy must maintain a written record showing:

1. The date of the transaction;
2. The name, strength, form, and quantity of the controlled substance;
3. The supplier's or manufacturer's name, address, and, if known, registration number; and
4. DEA Form 222 will be the official record for the transfer of Schedule II substances.

If the transfer is to a reverse distributor registered to dispose of controlled substances, the pharmacy is permitted to forward its controlled substances to DEA-registered reverse distributors who handle the disposal of drugs.

Destruction of Controlled Substances

The DEA asks that any pharmacy having controlled substances it needs to destroy because they are expired, become adulterated, or are misbranded to notify the local DEA field office for disposal instructions. There is no provision in the law for transferring drugs that should be destroyed between a pharmacy and the DEA. Once each calendar year, a pharmacy may request permission from the DEA to destroy controlled substances using DEA Form 41. All drugs proposed to be destroyed must be listed on the form together with the proposed date and method of destruction. Written notice to the DEA must also contain the names of at least two witnesses who will observe the destruction. Appropriate witnesses include a licensed physician, pharmacist, midlevel practitioner, nurse, or a state or local law enforcement officer.

Both the DEA form and the written notice must be received by the nearest DEA diversion field office at least 14 days prior to the proposed destruction date. After reviewing all available information, the DEA field office should notify the pharmacy in writing of its decision. Once the controlled substances have been destroyed, signed copies of the DEA Form 41 must be forwarded to DEA. It should be noted that this prior notification procedure need not be followed if an authorized member of a state law enforcement authority or regulatory agency witnesses the destruction. However, DEA Form 41 must still be filled out be the pharmacy and sent to the local DEA field office. Although not necessarily covered in the DEA regulations, the DEA suggests that pharmacists contact local environmental authorities prior to implementing the proposed method of destruction to ascertain that hazards are not associated with the destruction.

It should be noted that there is a procedure whereby the DEA will provide a blanket authorization for destruction of controlled substances on a very limited basis to registrants who are associated with hospitals, clinics, or other registrants having to dispose of used needles, syringes, or other injectable objects only. The DEA states that "this limited exception is granted because of the probability that those objects have been contaminated by hazardous bodily fluids." A pharmacist practicing in these kinds of environments should contact their local DEA field office for information about how to request such an authorization. DEA will evaluate requests for a blanket authorization.

If a pharmacy removes controlled substances from the regular inventory because the drugs are damaged, defective, adulterated, or misbranded, the drugs must be inventoried and the records maintained with the other controlled substances records. The document must include the following:

1. The inventory date,
2. The drug name,
3. The drug strength,
4. The drug form (e.g., tablet, capsule, etc.),
5. The total quantity or total number of units/volume,
6. The reason why the substance is being maintained, and
7. Whether substance is capable of being used in the manufacture of any controlled substance in finished form.

Labeling

Commercial containers (from a manufacturer or distributor) of controlled drugs must bear a label containing a specific symbol indicating the schedule that the drug has been placed in (e.g., C-II or CII). The symbol must be prominent and easily identifiable.

There are some exceptions, such as the circumstance that the container is too small to display the symbol or that the container is being used in the course of blinded drug research protocols.

For controlled substances that are dispensed pursuant to a prescription, the prescription label must contain (a) the name and address of the pharmacy (or dispenser), (b) the patient's name, (c) a prescription serial number, (d) the date that the medication is dispensed, (e) the prescriber's name, (f) directions for use, and (g) cautionary statements, if any are required by the prescription or other laws. Schedule II, III, and IV prescription labels must also contain the federal transfer warning statement. This statement must include these specific words: "Federal law prohibits the transfer of this drug to any person other that the patient for whom it was prescribed." Take specific notice that this transfer warning is not required on a Schedule V prescription label. These labeling requirements do not apply to drugs that are dispensed for or to patients who are admitted to a health care facility such as a hospital or nursing home if the drugs are to be administered on site. The DEA regulations do not recognize group homes for the physically or mentally disabled or assisted living homes. In these situations a pharmacist would label prescription drugs dispensed to residents of these facilities as for any other community-based patient.

There are almost as many variations in prescription drug labeling laws for controlled substances at the state level as there are states and territories. Reference must be made to individual state laws to determine what information must appear on the pharmacy label.

Security

Most practitioners are required to store all controlled substances in a "securely locked, substantially constructed cabinet." The DEA, however, allows some flexibility in how controlled substances are stored in a pharmacy and registered institutions. In these facilities, scheduled drugs may either be stored in an appropriate locked cabinet or be dispersed throughout the stock of noncontrolled drugs in a manner calculated to obstruct theft or diversion or a combination of both options may be used. For example, many pharmacies will lock Schedule II drugs in a cabinet or drawer and disperse Schedule III-V drugs throughout the pharmacy inventory. Although not required by the CSA statutes of DEA regulations, the DEA does recommend that pharmacies use a security alarm to deter thefts.

In recognition of the fact that DEA-registered pharmacies and other registrants can be the target of thefts, armed robberies, violence, and even death, Congress passed the Controlled Substance Registrant Protection Act of 1984 (CSRP). A federal investigation of thefts and robberies is mandated when controlled substances valued at $500.00 or more are lost, a registrant or other person is killed or suffers significant bodily injury during a robbery or theft of controlled substances, or a crime occurs or is planned involving the interstate transport of controlled substances. Breach of this law could result in federal criminal charges and punishment includes fines, imprisonment in a federal penitentiary, and the death penalty if a murder occurs during a controlled substances robbery.

Prescriptions

Introduction

Under the CSA, a prescription is just one of the means of moving a controlled substance drug from the inventory of a practitioner (i.e., a physician or a pharmacy) into the hands of a patient. This is the primary method of authorizing an ultimate user to obtain controlled substances in the community setting. Patients may also receive controlled substances without prescriptions when a drug is administered directly to a patient, when it is dispensed to a nursing unit for administration to a patient in a hospital, or when it is transferred directly from a physician to a patient for later use outside the physician's presence.

Pharmacists are considered "gatekeepers" when it comes to determining the validity of prescriptions. By authorizing pharmacists to dispense controlled substances only pursuant to legitimate prescriptions, the DEA attempts to minimize the diversion of controlled substances from legal markets into the hands of illegitimate users, sellers, and abusers. Understanding the regulations and duties imposed on pharmacists should help control drug diversion while insuring that legitimate and needy patients have access to necessary and appropriate drug treatments.

Purpose

A prescription for a controlled substance must be issued by a qualified prescriber and for a "legitimate medical purpose." Under the DEA regulations, an order (also referred to as a purported prescription) for a controlled substance may not necessarily be a prescription, even if that order is issued by an authorized prescriber. This means that a pharmacist must make a determination as to whether a controlled substance prescription is issued for a valid purpose before medication is dispensed. The appearance of an order, while an important factor, is not determinative of whether or not the order is truly a prescription. An order might appear to be proper in that it contains all the information necessary to constitute a prescription. It may be issued by an authorized prescriber (see Scope of Practice, below). It may even contain a valid DEA number. But the order is still not valid unless it is issued for a recognized medical use. While the prescriber may have responsibility for prescribing controlled substances for proper purposes, pharmacists also have a corresponding responsibility to determine the legitimacy of an order before controlled substances are dispensed.

Validity

There is no single acid test or bright-line determinant for assessing the validity of any one prescription. Instead, a list of factors must be considered in making a professional judgment as to whether a controlled substance order should be filled. The DEA suggests that prescribers who write large numbers of controlled substance prescriptions or write large quantities relative to other prescribers in the area should be suspect. Issuance of prescriptions for antagonistic drugs (depressants and stimulants) at the same time may be another cause for concern. Patterns of patients who appear frequently in the pharmacy with new controlled substance prescriptions or return for refills too soon suggests a problem may be occurring. Patients who present prescriptions in the names of other people or from multiple physicians could be involved in drug diversion. A number of patients appearing in the pharmacy within a short period of time with similar prescriptions from the same prescriber also ought to send up a red flag. A large number of strangers, people who have never been patients in the pharmacy before, who show up at the same time with controlled substance prescriptions from the same prescriber may be another factor to consider. A dramatic increase in the controlled substances inventory could be another sign that the pharmacy is being targeted by drug abusers.

Scope of Practice

The only individuals who are authorized to issue controlled substances prescriptions are those who are licensed by a state to prescribe controlled substances and who are either registered with the DEA or exempted from registration. State laws vary considerably on which practitioners are allowed to prescribe controlled substances. Prescribing is also limited by the scope of a practitioner's license. For example, a state-licensed medical doctor may be able to prescribe just about any controlled substance to treat a human disease. A dentist, however, is limited to prescribing controlled substances for treatment of conditions relating to the oral cavity and its supporting structures. Veterinarians are allowed to prescribe controlled substances for animals in most states, but a controlled substance prescription from a veterinarian for a human would not be valid. Some states also allow midlevel practitioners to prescribe controlled substances.

Verification

When a pharmacist is presented with a controlled substance prescription or an order that purports to be a prescription, the validity of the prescription should be verified. Knowledge of the prescriber and his or her prescribing habits is perhaps the most efficient means of verification. Validation of the prescriber's DEA registration number is important. A mathematical check should be performed to determine if the number is valid.

A DEA registration is usually composed of two letters followed by seven digits, the last of which is a "check" number. If the DEA number on a prescription, for example, showed AB1234563, the prescriber's last name should begin with a "B." The formula for determining the validity of the check number is to add the first, third, and fifth digits and note the last number of that addition. Then add the second, fourth, and sixth numbers and multiply that sum by 2. Take the last number in that calculation and add it to the number saved in the first equation. The last number in the product of this equation should be the same as the seventh digit in the DEA registration number. Using the number in the example above the calculation would look like this:

1 + 3 + 5 = 9;
2 + 4 +6 = 12 x 2 = 24.
Then add 9 + 4 to equal 13.

The last digit, 3, should be the same as the last digit of the registration number. Candidates taking the MPJE are expected to know this equation. In practice, if the math is too cumbersome, there are online sites that will do the math and indicate whether the check digit number is valid(e.g., www.msspnexus.com/ msspn_dea.asp). There are some variations including how the number is expressed if the first character in a registrant' name is a number, such as 123 Pharmacy Corp. See the *Pharmacist's Manual* for determining the validity of a registration number in these situations.

Prescription Formats and Transmittals

The regulations permit the use of fax transmittals for drugs listed in Schedules III-V. As such, prescriptions for drugs listed in these schedules may now be written, orally transmitted, or sent to the pharmacy via a fax machine. Again, state laws should be consulted to determine if there are any restrictions or modifications regarding the transmittal of controlled substance prescriptions.

A controlled substance prescription, if written, must be signed on the date issued; predated and postdated prescriptions are not valid. For Schedule II drugs, the prescription must be written in ink, indelible pencil, or typewritten and manually signed by the prescriber. Prescriptions may be prepared by a secretary or agent of the prescriber but the prescriber remains responsible for compliance with the legal requirements for issuing the prescription. Pharmacists also have a corresponding responsibility to insure the prescription contains all necessary information and conforms to the legal mandates. Secretaries and agents of a prescriber are permitted to communicate controlled substance prescriptions and refills to a pharmacy but only the authorized prescriber is permitted to actually prescribe.

Refills and Prescription Transfers

Unlike Schedule II drugs, which cannot be refilled, Schedule III-V drugs may be refilled if authorized by the prescriber. Schedule III and IV drugs may be refilled up to a maximum of five times within 6 months from the date of issuance. Schedule V prescriptions may be refilled as authorized up to the amount allowed under state law (frequently up to 1 year measured from the date the prescription was issued, not from the date the prescription was first filled). Schedule II drugs may be partially filled, giving the effective appearance of a refill, under limited circumstances such as in a long-term care facility or hospice services.

Where refills are permitted, transfers of controlled substance prescriptions between different pharmacies are allowed one time only. However, additional transfers between pharmacies that share an electronic real-time database of prescription information are permitted. In other words, there is a distinction between transfers between individually owned pharmacies and those that may share a common ownership such as a chain store. In this later situation, transfers are allowed up to the maximum number of refills authorized by the prescriber. The information that must be captured in making a transfer of this type is specific and detailed. License applicants and pharmacists should review state law and employer policies before attempting to transfer controlled substance prescriptions.

When a prescription for any controlled substance in Schedules III-V is refilled, the dispensing pharmacist's initials, the date the prescription was refilled, and the amount of drug dispensed on the refill must be recorded on the back of the prescription or, if the pharmacy uses computerized records, in accordance with the rules for using computerized records (see Record-Keeping, below). If the pharmacist only initials and dates the back of the prescription, it will be assumed that the full amount of the drug called for on the front of the prescription was dispensed on a refill.

Distributions of Controlled Substances

A clear distinction should be made between dispensing activities and controlled substances distributions because the record-keeping requirements are very different. Dispensing is the act of delivering a controlled substance to an ultimate user based on a legitimate prescription order. Distribution, on the other hand, is the delivery of a controlled substance to a person by means other than dispensing or administering. Distribution is the transactional method by which a pharmacy transmits or delivers controlled substances to another pharmacy, a wholesale distributor, or a prescriber or another entity that is registered with the DEA and has the right to possess controlled substances. The DEA has a regulation that permits a pharmacy to distribute up to 5% of its annual dispensed controlled substances before a distributor license will be required.

A prescription cannot be used by prescribers to obtain office supplies of controlled substances for the purpose of dispensing drugs directly to patients. DEA Order Form 222 or its electronic equivalent must be used to distribute Schedule II drugs from a pharmacy to a practitioner. An invoice should be used to distribute Schedule III-V drugs from a pharmacy to a practitioner.

Only Schedule I and II controlled substances are ordered with an official order form, DEA Form 222, or the electronic equivalent. A DEA Form 222 is required for each distribution, purchase, or transfer of a Schedule II controlled substance (www.deaecom.gov/ csosmain.html and www.deadiversion.usdoj.gov/pubs/manuals/ pharm2/pharm_manual.htm#8, Section VIII-Ordering Controlled Substances, *The Pharmacist's Manual* [accessed Dec 4]).

Record-Keeping

Under the CSA, one of the major responsibilities of pharmacies is to keep accurate and detailed records of activities relating to controlled substances. As with dispensing activities, there is a wide variation between the states in record-keeping mandates that must be followed in addition to the federal requirements.

The DEA requires that all controlled substances records be maintained in the registered pharmacy for a minimum period of 2 years dating from the last transaction pertinent to a particular record. For example, if a Schedule IV controlled substance prescription is authorized for up to five refills and the patient orders the last refill before the end of the 6 months since the prescription was issued, the pharmacy would have to maintain the prescription for at least 2 years after the date of the last refill.

All records dealing with controlled substances must be maintained in "readily retrievable" manner in the pharmacy. This term means controlled substances records kept in some form of computer database storage must be retrievable separate from all other records.

In terms of specific records, the DEA mandates pharmacies maintain the following documents in a readily retrievable fashion:

1. Official Order Forms (DEA Form 222);

2. Power of attorney authorization to sign Order Forms;

3. Receipts and invoices for Schedule III-V controlled substances as well as registered chemicals, if any;

4. All inventory records of controlled substances, including the initial and biennial inventories;

5. Records of controlled substances distributed or dispensed (i.e., prescriptions) and threshold amounts of List I chemicals distributed;

6. Report of Theft or Loss (DEA Form 106);

7. Inventory of Drugs Surrendered for Disposal (DEA Form 41);

8. Records of transfers of controlled substances between pharmacies; and

9. DEA registration certificate.

For entities that own two or more DEA-registered pharmacies, there is a provision for central record-keeping. Shipping and financial records may be stored at a headquarters or offices of the organization if it notifies the nearest DEA field office of the intent to do so. Once 14 days have passed after issuing this notice, the organization may start keeping these records at the intended location unless the DEA informs the organization that permission to store required records at the intended place is denied.

Inventories

Pharmacies are required to maintain a current and complete record of controlled substances inventories and perform an audit of these drugs every 2 years. The required date that the inventory is performed was altered somewhat under the 1997 amendments to the DEA regulations. Now the biennial inventory may be taken anytime within 2 years of the prior inventory. Inventory records for Schedule II drugs (and Schedule I drugs in the rare event that a pharmacy has any) must be maintained separate and apart from all other records. Schedule III-V inventory records must also be maintained separate and apart from all other records or maintained in a format that they will be readily retrievable from the ordinary records of the pharmacy. No special form is required for inventory records. However, all records must be written, typewritten, or printed. The name of the drug, its dosage form (i.e., 10-mg capsule), the size of the commercial container (i.e.,

100 tablets), and the number of commercial units on hand must be recorded. For open stock containers of Schedule II drugs, an exact count of the drugs on hand is required. For open stock of Schedule III-V drugs, an estimate of the amount on hand is permitted unless the container holds more than 1000 units in which case an exact count is necessary. All inventories, records of purchases, executed order forms (DEA Order Form 222), prescriptions, and distribution records must be kept on file at the pharmacy for a minimum of 2 years.

Prescription Records

Schedule II prescriptions must be maintained in a separate file. Similarly, Schedule III-V prescription records must be maintained separate and apart from all other prescriptions or maintained in a manner that allows them to be readily retrieved from all other prescriptions. There are, however, options available for filing Schedule III-V prescriptions. If separate prescription files are not kept for prescriptions in these schedules, the prescriptions may be mixed in with the Schedule II prescriptions or mixed in with the noncontrolled prescriptions. In either of these options, the Schedule III-V prescriptions must be stamped with red ink on the face of the prescription in the lower right hand corner with the letter "C" no less than 1-inch high. Another option is available for pharmacies that utilize automatic data processing (ADP) systems or some other form of electronic record-keeping. As in the prior option, Schedule III-V prescriptions may be mixed in with either the Schedule II prescriptions or the noncontrolled prescriptions. The red "C" stamp requirement is waived as long as the ADP or other system permits identification of the prescriptions by serial number and retrieval by prescriber name, patient name, drug name, and date dispensed. In addition, records have to be kept of the number of units or volume of scheduled drugs that are dispensed, including the name and address of the person to whom it was dispensed, the date of dispensing, the number of units or volume dispensed, and the written or typewritten name or initials of the pharmacist who dispensed or administered the drug. State laws vary on these procedures and may require other alternatives.

Distribution Records

The kind of information that must be recorded by a pharmacy when it receives controlled substances is complex. For each controlled substance distributed to a pharmacy, a record must be kept of the name of the drug, its finished dosage form (e.g., 10-mg tablet or 10-mg concentration per fluid ounce or mL) and the number of units or volume of finished form in each commercial container (e.g., 100-tablet bottle or 3-mL vial), the number of commercial containers acquired from other persons, including the date of and number of units and/or commercial containers in each acquisition to inventory and the name, address, and registration number of the person from whom the units were acquired. If a pharmacy distributes (as opposed to dispenses) controlled substances to other registrants, the number of commercial containers distributed, including the date of and number of containers in each reduction from inventory, and the name, address, and registration number of the person to whom the containers were distributed must be recorded. The pharmacy must also record the number of units of finished forms and/or commercial containers distributed or disposed of in any other manner, such as destruction, including the date and manner of distribution or disposal; the name, address, and, if applicable, the registration number of the person to whom distributed; and the quantity in finished form distributed or disposed.

Location of Records

Prescriptions, completed inventories, and executed order forms (DEA Order Form 222), if used instead of the electronic format, must be kept in the pharmacy where the prescription was originally filled for at least 2 years from the date the drugs were last dispensed. All controlled substance prescriptions and records maintained in the pharmacy are subject to inspection by DEA officers. Pharmacies may keep financial and shipping records, such as invoices and packing slips, at a central location like a chain store headquarters. Special permission to store the other records at a central location may be available in limited circumstances.

Employment Disqualifications and Requests for Waivers

The DEA prohibits pharmacies with controlled substances available from employing anyone with access to those controlled substances who has been convicted of a felony relating to controlled substances, or who, at any time, has had an application for DEA registration denied, revoked, or surrendered "for cause." This term is defined to mean "surrendering a registration in lieu of, or as a consequence of, any federal or state administrative, civil, or criminal action resulting from an investigation of the individual's handling of controlled substances." While there is a procedure that permits pharmacies to apply for a waiver of this provision, permission is rarely granted.

Reporting Controlled Substance Theft or Loss

Upon discovery of a significant loss or theft of controlled substances, a DEA-registered pharmacy must immediately notify the local DEA field office and the local police authority by telephone, fax, or by a brief written message explaining the circumstances. There is no bright-line test of how "significant" the loss or theft must be. Pharmacists should judge the situation in the context of the amount of theft or loss as compared to the general controlled substances inventory. Missing six or seven phenobarbital pills is not significant. Loss of a whole unopened bottle of 500 Valium tablets is definitely significant. The DEA asks pharmacists to err on the side of caution and report losses when not sure of whether or not the loss should be considered significant. Some factors to consider suggested by the DEA for determining significant loss include:

1. The schedule of the missing items.

2. The abuse potential of the missing items.

3. The abuse potential in your area of the missing substance.

4. The quantity missing (one tablet vs. one bottle or container).

5. Is this the first time this loss has occurred? Has a similar loss occurred before?

6. Was this loss reported to local law enforcement authorities?

In addition to the immediate notification requirement, a pharmacy must also complete DEA Form 106 and send it to the local DEA field office. Most states also require pharmacies to send a copy of this form to the state Board of Pharmacy or the agency that oversees pharmacy licensure. In any event, the pharmacy must also keep a copy of the Form 106 with its own controlled substances records for use if a controlled substances audit is performed. The Form 106 must also be made available for inspection upon request. Information on this form is to include the circumstances of the loss and theft and the quantity and names of the controlled substances involved. At a minimum the DEA Form 106 must include:

1. Name and address of the pharmacy,

2. DEA registration number,

3. Date of theft (or date that the theft was discovered),

4. Name and telephone number of local police department notified,

5. Type of theft (night break in, armed robbery, etc.),

6. Listing of symbols or cost code used by pharmacy in marking containers (if any), and

7. Listing of controlled substances missing from theft or significant loss.

If a pharmacy reports a theft or loss of controlled substances to the DEA and later discovers after an investigation that no loss or theft actually occurred (e.g., the missing bottle of 500 Valium tablets was found to have been accidentally thrown out and recovered from the trash), the DEA does not require that the reporting form be filed. However, the DEA should be given written notice of the circumstances as to why the pharmacy is not completing Form 106. The state agency and local police should also be informed.

Penalties

Introduction

Penalties for violation of the CSA and DEA regulations may be very severe. Many provisions require intent to violate or knowledge of an infraction of the CSA. There are other provisions, however, including many of the record-keeping mandates applied to pharmacists that impose a strict liability type of penalty where knowledge or intent is not considered. Both civil fines and criminal sanctions are possible. In addition, states may also impose penalties for controlled substance violations. Revocation of the federal registration and suspension or revocation of any state issued controlled substance licenses or registrations may also be administratively imposed. Penalties are not exclusive to any one jurisdictional body. In other words, the same act of wrongdoing could result in federal civil and/or criminal penalties, state criminal and/or civil penalties, and administrative sanctions against federal and state registrations and licenses. The prohibitions against double jeopardy in the U.S. Constitution do not apply to health care licensees who violate the multiple requirements of controlled substances laws. This means that one offending activity may result in multiple penalties. Therefore, it is in the best interest of pharmacists to know and follow the controlled substances laws.

Intentional or Knowledgeable Penalties

Pharmacists who knowingly dispense controlled substances based on orders that are not valid are subject to significant penalties. Imprisonment of up to 4 years and fines as high as $30,000 may be imposed for each violation. The knowledge requirement may be implied by the circumstances. Deliberate ignorance of objectively determined facts that should indicate that a prescription has been forged, altered, or issued for a nonlegitimate medical purpose will expose the dispensing pharmacist to criminal penalties. In other words, the "ostrich defense" (i.e., figuratively sticking one's head in the sand to ignore objectively verifiable facts), does not work in the pharmacist's favor. Studied avoidance of realities and circumstances may be used as evidence to create an inference that the pharmacist knew or should have known that a purported prescription was not legitimate.

Record-Keeping Penalties

The penalties for failure to keep records as mandated by the CSA and DEA regulations include monetary fines, loss of registration, and criminal sanctions. A pharmacy that is charged with a record-keeping violation may be subject to a civil penalty of $25,000 for each violation. Imprisonment is also possible for intentional record-keeping violations. However, for civil charges to apply, no knowledge or intent is needed. In other words, pharmacists and pharmacies are strictly liable for record-keeping violations. Innocent errors, mistakes, and negligent inadvertence to details could still lead to significant penalties under the applicable laws.

Applicants should be aware of all state laws in their jurisdictions that may modify the rules discussed above (see State Pharmacy Practice Laws, below).

Computerized Records

A DEA-registered pharmacy may use either manual records on hard copy or computerized records for keeping track of refills for controlled substances prescriptions. It cannot use one method some of the time and the other on different occasions. It must choose one or the other. State law should also be consulted to determine if there are any other requirements for computerized pharmacy data.

Any computer system used must provide a mechanism for accessing the original prescription information. At a minimum the original prescription number; date the prescription was issued; the name and home address of the patient; the prescriber's name, address, and DEA registration number; the name, dosage form, quantity dispensed, and strength of the drug dispensed; and number of refills authorized, if any, must be available on the computer. The database must also have refill information available. Computerized records must provide for a backup method in case there is a problem with retaining original information in the system.

If the system used by the pharmacy permits printouts of the daily controlled substances dispensing activities, a pharmacist must verify the accuracy of the printout information by signing and dating the document. This printout must be available within 72 hours of the date any refills were recorded.

If the system does not permit printouts as described above, the pharmacy must keep a bound record book that a pharmacist must sign and date showing that the refill records were reviewed and are accurate. All systems are required to have the capacity to print refill data that includes the prescriber's name, amount dispensed on the refill, the refill dispensing date, identification of the pharmacist (name or initials), and the prescription number. If the entity that owns the pharmacy is permitted to maintain records at a central office such as a headquarters, the refill records must be made available in the pharmacy within 48 hours upon request.

Mailing Prescription Drugs

Pharmacists may send nearly all OTC and prescription-only drugs to patients using the U.S. Postal Service (USPS), an agency of the federal government. The postal regulations still prohibit the mailing of abortive drugs or devices and the unsolicited mailing of contraceptives. About the only other special alert pharmacists should be aware of is that postal service bans mailing of powders that might be able to escape from their containers; however, if the powder is packed in leak-proof receptacles or sealed in durable, leak-proof outer containers they can be mailed. There are also provisions for shipping chemicals but they do not apply to pharmaceutical products.

The *Pharmacist's Manual* contains pertinent information about the mailing of controlled substances. Basically, these are the same as those for noncontrolled substances. The USPS regulations permit mailing any controlled substances, provided that they are not "outwardly dangerous or of their own force could cause injury to a person's life or health." In addition, the pharmacy packaging of the controlled substance must be properly labeled with all of the information the DEA mandates for dispensed medications including the name and address of the pharmacy. The visible outer wrapper should be securely wrapped in plain paper and should not have any indication as to the contents of the package.

Pharmacists are prohibited from shipping or delivering controlled substances dispensed pursuant to a valid prescription to a different country without authorization. This activity is deemed by the FDA to be drug exporting and is not permitted unless the pharmacy has a DEA exporter registration.

Private carriers like United Parcel Service and DHL Worldwide Express have their own rules and regulations about the products they will accept for delivery. The policies of private carriers are beyond the scope of this review.

Privacy Considerations

Confidentiality of patient records and information is regulated at both the state and federal level. The traditional methods of protecting individual's privacy concerns are governed primarily by state laws. The approach of the states varies greatly from simple statements such as "prescription records are not public records" (perhaps the lowest form of protection) all the way up to "prescription information and the information learned by a pharmacist in the course of serving a patient are privileged." Because there is such a diverse set of state laws, MJPE applicants are directed to state laws in the state where pharmacist licensure is being sought. At the federal level, there is a fairly new set of laws affecting privacy rights. The Health Insurance Portability and Accountability Act of 1996 (HIPAA) required the HHS to adopt regulations affecting the confidentiality of patient information. Even though the law was adopted in 1996, its provisions were not fully enacted until 2004.

The essential point to remember is that providers, including pharmacists and pharmacies, must obtain their patients' consent for uses and disclosures of protected health information (PHI) about the patient to carry out treatment, payment, or health care operations (TPO). Use of PHI beyond basic TPO requires additional patient authorization. Health care providers must have a documented privacy procedure in place. Each health care organization must train employees so that they understand the privacy procedures and there must be at least one designated individual responsible for seeing that the privacy procedures are adopted and followed.

Providers must also detail security measures for patient records containing individually identifiable health information with a goal of preventing access by those who have no express need for access.

The privacy rules apply to all business associates of providers. For example, a third party hired by a pharmacy to administer prescription claims or process bills would also have to adhere to the same rigid standards applicable to the pharmacy personnel.

State Pharmacy Practice Laws

Every state has legislation that regulates the profession of pharmacy. Even so, there is a great deal of variation in state laws pertaining to pharmacy practice. The laws of each state for which licensure candidates will be taking the pharmacy law exam should be reviewed individually. There are some general issues addressed by nearly all states. The NABP Survey of Pharmacy Law provides lists of the common issues and how they are addressed in each state. Some of the items that should be reviewed are listed below.

1. The minimum education, training, and experiential qualifications that license applicants must satisfy at the time of examination or registration.

2. The authority, makeup, and duties of the agency, usually known as the State Board of Pharmacy, charged with enforcement and administration of the pharmacy laws.

3. How licenses or other permits to engage in the practice of pharmacy are granted and renewed and for what period of time.

4. The conditions under which licenses or registrations to engage in the practice of pharmacy may be restricted, canceled, or revoked.

5. The activities included in the scope of pharmacy practice and what duties might be delegated to nonpharmacists.

6. The individual who is responsible for compliance with state and federal pharmacy laws.

7. Whether continuing education is necessary for maintaining a pharmacist license and what those requirements include

8. What kinds of labels, labeling, and record-keeping are required for controlled and noncontrolled prescription drugs dispensed in a pharmacy.

9. Whether there are any special rules that distinguish how pharmacy is practiced in community (retail) settings versus an institutional (hospital) setting.

10. Whether the state participates in reciprocal registration with other states and, if so, what conditions have to be satisfied before reciprocating.

11. Who is qualified to prescribe drugs and the conditions that must be met before a prescription is dispensed.

12. Whether the state has any laws regarding drug product selection, generic substitution, therapeutic substitution, or formularies.

13. Whether licensure, registration, or certification is required for pharmacy technicians and/or educational requirements for personnel who assist a pharmacist.

There are, of course, numerous other issues such as nuclear pharmacy regulations, prescription drug compounding, and third-party benefits laws that are too long and complex for a law review of this type. The above list is only a suggestion to help license applicants get started on studying for a pharmacy law examination.

On a broad scale, one of the more common issues confronted under state laws deals with the scope of pharmacy practice. Activities that are normally associated with the practice of pharmacy include evaluating and interpreting a prescription, selecting a drug product to be dispensed pursuant to a prescription, preparing of the patient label, and performing a drug utilization review to determine that a prescription medication is necessary and appropriate for a patient. Patient counseling on the proper use and storage of medications is usually included in the scope of pharmacy. In contrast, pharmacists rarely are assigned duties to make physical assessments of patients while engaging in the practice of pharmacy. Most state laws also make provisions for assigning responsibility for compliance with state and federal pharmacy laws to a pharmacist-in-charge or a pharmacist on duty. In addition, a corporate officer or other designated corporate employee may be designated as one of the responsible parties when the pharmacy is owned and operated as a corporation.

Questions

1. Under which of the following circumstances may a drug manufacturer's representative legally distribute a federal legend drug sample?

A. When requested by a community pharmacist

B. When requested by a hospital pharmacist

C. When requested in writing by a prescriber

D. All the time

E. When requested by a community-based mental health pharmacist

2. A DEA registration is NOT required for an individual who is legally recognized as a prescriber and is a:

A. doctor of medicine practicing as a family physician.

B. physician's assistant working in a hospital.

C. medical resident employed by a teaching and research hospital.

D. doctor of osteopathic medicine and surgery specializing in psychiatry.

E. nurse clinician (nurse-practitioner).

3. The pharmacist who is charged with responsibility for compliance with state and federal pharmacy laws is most often designated as the:

A. chief operating officer.

B. pharmacist-in-charge.

C. pharmacy manager.

D. responsible pharmacist.

E. pharmacy district manager.

4. Which of the following activities is NOT usually associated with the practice of pharmacy?

A. Selecting a specific drug product to be dispensed pursuant to a prescription

B. Monitoring a patient's drug therapy and use

C. Making a physical assessment of the patient

D. Counseling a patient on the safe use and storage of prescription medications

E. Interpreting and evaluating a prescription

5. Which of the following institutions or individuals is NOT ordinarily required to obtain a registration from the DEA before handling controlled substances?

A. A hospital

B. A staff physician performing research with controlled substances at a medical teaching hospital

C. A community pharmacy owned by a chain store corporation

D. A pharmacist employed by a hospital or community pharmacy

E. A nursing home

6. Assume that a podiatrist asks a community pharmacist to sell a 1-month supply of a prescription-only oral contraceptive to his wife, who also happens to be his office manager, using the podiatrist's prescription. Which of the following responses by the pharmacist are lawful?

   A. Ask the podiatrist write a prescription and dispense it as ordered.

   B. Decline the request because it is beyond the scope of practice of the podiatrist to prescribe oral contraceptives.

   C. Sell the oral contraceptives to the podiatrist as an office supply, using a pharmacy invoice to record the transaction.

   D. Sell the podiatrist a 2- or 3-day supply as a professional courtesy and tell him that this is a one-time favor.

   E. Dispense the oral contraceptive as written and make a call to the state podiatry board.

7. Which of the following statements regarding patient counseling about drugs is TRUE?

   A. All state laws require a pharmacist to counsel patients on all prescription drugs including refills.

   B. Any individual designated to work in a pharmacy department may provide counseling about prescription drug use.

   C. A pharmacist may counsel any patient about the use of OTC and prescription-only drugs at any time the pharmacist believes counseling is necessary and appropriate.

   D. Licensed pharmacy interns may counsel patients about prescription drug use without the supervision or presence of a pharmacist.

   E. Pharmacies employing the U.S. Postal Service to provide prescription drugs are exempt from all counseling requirements as long as written information about the drug is provided.

8. Pharmacies are licensed or registered to engage in the practice of pharmacy by which one of the following administrative agencies?

   A. Centers for Medicare & Medicaid Services (CMS)

   B. Joint Commission on Accreditation of Healthcare Organizations (JCAHO)

   C. Department of Health and Human Services (DHHS)

   D. State board of pharmacy or its equivalent and the Drug Enforcement Administration (DEA)

   E. Food and Drug Administration (FDA)

9. If a drug is placed in a schedule that is regulated by the Drug Enforcement Administration, that drug is classified as a:

   A. controlled substance.

   B. federal legend.

   C. sample.

   D. generic.

   E. investigational new drug (IND).

10. On June 1, 2011, a medical doctor legitimately issues a prescription for #35 diazepam, a prescription-only C-IV controlled substance, to a patient with directions to take one (1) dose every 4-6 hours as needed for anxiety. The prescription indicates that it may be refilled six (6) times. The patient has the prescription filled at First Community Pharmacy on June 1, 2011. The patient returns to that pharmacy on July 1, 2011, and obtains a refill. On August 1, 2011, the patient goes to ABC Retail Pharmacy, an independent pharmacy not affiliated in any way with First Community Pharmacy, and asks that the prescription be transferred and refilled. The prescription is filled and dispensed at ABC Retail Pharmacy on August 1, 2011. The patient returns to ABC Pharmacy on September 1, 2011, again on October 1, 2011, and again on November 1, 2011, and obtains refills of the prescription on each day.

    Under federal law, how long must First Community Pharmacy maintain the prescription in its records?

    A. Until at least June 30, 2013

    B. Until at least June 30, 2012

    C. Until at least November 1, 2013

    D. Until at least November 1, 2014

    E. Until the pharmacy is either closed or transferred to a new owner

11. On June 1, 2011, a medical doctor legitimately issues a prescription for #35 diazepam, a prescription-only C-IV controlled substance, to a patient with directions to take one (1) dose every 4-6 hours as needed for anxiety. The prescription indicates that it may be refilled six (6) times. The patient has the prescription filled at First Community Pharmacy on June 1, 2011. The patient returns to that pharmacy on July 1, 2011, and obtains a refill. On August 1, 2011, the patient goes to ABC Retail Pharmacy, an independent pharmacy not affiliated in any way with First Community Pharmacy, and asks that the prescription be transferred and refilled. The prescription is filled and dispensed at ABC Retail Pharmacy on August 1, 2011. The patient returns to ABC Pharmacy on September 1, 2011, again on October 1, 2011, and again on November 1, 2011, and obtains refills of the prescription on each day.

    Under federal law, how long is ABC Retail Pharmacy required to maintain the prescription in its records?

    A. Until at least October 31, 2013

    B. Until at least May 31, 2014

    C. Until at least October 31, 2013

    D. Until at least December 31, 2014

    E. Until the pharmacy is either closed or transferred to a new owner

12. On June 1, 2011, a medical doctor legitimately issues a prescription for #35 diazepam, a prescription-only C-IV controlled substance, to a patient with directions to take one (1) dose every 4-6 hours as needed for anxiety. The prescription indicates that it may be refilled six (6) times. The patient has the prescription filled at First Community Pharmacy on June 1, 2011. The patient returns to that

pharmacy on July 1, 2011, and obtains a refill. On August 1, 2011, the patient goes to ABC Retail Pharmacy, an independent pharmacy not affiliated in any way with First Community Pharmacy, and asks that the prescription be transferred and refilled. The prescription is filled and dispensed at ABC Retail Pharmacy on August 1, 2011. The patient returns to ABC Pharmacy on September 1, 2011, again on October 1, 2011, and again on November 1, 2011, and obtains refills of the prescription on each day.

Then the patient returns to ABC Retail Pharmacy on December 2, 2011, and asks for another refill. What is the pharmacist legally required to do?

A. Dispense the refill because the prescription is still valid.

B. Refuse to dispense the refill because the legal limit on the number of refills allowed would be exceeded.

C. Transfer the prescription back to First Community Pharmacy so that the patient may obtain the remaining refill called for in the original prescription.

D. Inform the local DEA office that the patient is attempting to obtain controlled substances on an illegally issued prescription.

E. Give the prescription order to the patient and ask that additional refills be obtained from a different pharmacy.

13. A hospital-based pharmacy is legally permitted to provide a limited quantity of controlled substances medications that are not under the control of a pharmacist to:

A. an emergency room supply cabinet that is secured under a protocol approved by the pharmacy director.

B. an unsecured cabinet in a nursing station.

C. a stockroom in the hospital basement.

D. an automobile owned and operated by the hospital for transferring patients between the hospital and off-site clinics.

E. a supply cabinet located just outside the pharmacy.

14. In most states, the board of pharmacy or equivalent administrative agency issues controlled substances licenses to:

A. pharmacies.

B. pharmacists.

C. physicians.

D. authorized prescribers.

E. all of the above.

15. Which federal agency determines whether drugs are safe and effective for intended uses?

A. FDA

B. DEA

C. DHHS

D. CMS

E. BNDD

16. Which federal agency determines whether drugs should be designated as controlled substances?

A. FDA

B. DEA

C. DHHS

D. CMS

E. BNDD

17. Which governmental agencies have authority to regulate controlled substances?

A. The federal government exclusively

B. State governments exclusively

C. World Trade Federation

D. State and federal governments concurrently

E. Local municipalities only

18. Who determines which schedule a drug designated as a controlled substance will be placed in?

A. President of the United States

B. FDA Commissioner

C. U.S. Attorney General

D. Secretary of Health and Human Services

E. Speaker of the House of Representatives

19. Who is required to register with the DEA?

A. All pharmacies that dispense controlled substances

B. All pharmacists who dispense controlled substances

C. All licensed pharmacy interns while working in a pharmacy that dispenses controlled substances

D. All employees of drug manufacturers that produce controlled substances

E. All police officers who might encounter controlled substances while on duty

20. Which of the following categories of drugs must be labeled with the federal transfer warning when dispensed from a community pharmacy?

I. Schedule II controlled substances

II. Schedule III and IV controlled substances

III. Schedule V controlled substances

A. I only

B. III only

C. I and II only

D. II and III only

E. I, II, and III

21. How are controlled substances to be stocked in a pharmacy?

A. In a locked cabinet in the pharmacy

B. Dispersed throughout the inventory of noncontrolled drugs in the pharmacy

C. In a separate storage room away from the pharmacy

D. In a safe that is accessible only by the pharmacist-in-charge

E. Either choice A or B or a combination of both

22. What is a "purported prescription"?

    A. An order for a controlled substance that has not been issued for a legitimate medical purpose

    B. An order for a controlled substance from a prescriber that has not yet been verified by a pharmacist

    C. A legitimately prescribed controlled substance order that was communicated to a pharmacist by the prescriber's agent

    D. A legitimately prescribed controlled substance order issued by a midlevel practitioner

    E. An order for a controlled substance issued by a prescriber whose practice is located in a different state than the pharmacy

23. How many times may a Schedule V drug be refilled according to federal law?

    A. Five times in a 6-month period

    B. Twelve times in a 12-month period

    C. For a maximum of 2 years

    D. As authorized by the prescriber

    E. Schedule V drugs cannot be refilled

24. Under federal law, how many times may a prescription for a refillable controlled substance be transferred between different (unrelated) pharmacies?

    A. As often as the patient and the prescriber agree

    B. A maximum of 3 times

    C. A maximum of 2 times

    D. One time only

    E. Never

25. Under federal law, how many times may a prescription for a refillable controlled substance be transferred between commonly owned pharmacies that share an electronic real-time database of prescription files?

    A. As often as the patient and the prescriber agree

    B. A maximum of three times

    C. One time only

    D. As many times as the prescription is legally refillable

    E. Never

26. According to federal law how does a prescriber obtain a supply of Schedule II controlled substance drugs from a pharmacy for use in the prescriber's office?

    A. The supply is obtained by using one of the prescriber's prescriptions marked "For Office Use" in the space designated for a patient's name.

    B. The supply is obtained by using a DEA Form 222 or the electronic equivalent.

    C. The supply is obtained by using a DEA Form 106.

    D. The supply is obtained by having the pharmacist record the transaction on a pharmacy invoice that is kept with the other Schedule II controlled substances records.

    E. This practice is not permitted. The prescriber must obtain the drugs from a wholesale distributor of the manufacturer.

27. According to federal law, how does a prescriber obtain a supply of Schedule III or IV controlled substance drugs from a pharmacy for use in the prescriber's office?

    A. The supply is obtained by using one of the prescriber's prescriptions marked "For Office Use" in the space designated for a patient's name and the document is filed in the pharmacy with its Schedule III and IV controlled substances prescriptions.

    B. The supply is obtained by using a DEA Form 222 or online CSOS.

    C. The supply is obtained by using a DEA Form 106.

    D. The supply is obtained by having the pharmacist record the transaction on a pharmacy invoice that is kept with the other Schedule III and IV controlled substances records.

    E. This practice is not permitted. The prescriber must obtain the drugs from a wholesale distributor of the manufacturer.

28. How often does federal law require a pharmacy to perform a controlled substance inventory?

    A. Monthly

    B. Once every year

    C. Every 2 years

    D. Every 3 years

    E. Every 4 years

29. According to federal law, how long does a pharmacy have to keep prescriptions, invoices, and inventory records for Schedule II drugs?

    A. 1 year

    B. 2 years

    C. 3 years

    D. 5 years

    E. Until the pharmacy is closed or transferred to a new owner

30. If the DEA believes that a pharmacy has knowingly violated the controlled substances laws, it may proceed against the pharmacy by:

    A. seeking criminal penalties.

    B. seeking civil penalties.

    C. seeking to have the pharmacy's DEA registration revoked.

    D. seeking to have the pharmacy's DEA registration suspended.

    E. seeking any and all of the above sanctions.

Compounding and Calculations Review

Section Editors: Robert O. (Bill) Williams III and Jason M. Vaughn

Compounding and Calculations Review

Compounding

Pharmaceutical Solid Dosage Forms

Important Terms

Comminution—the term describing the reduction in particle size of a powder.

Deliquescent—liquefying upon contact with the air; capable of attracting moisture from the atmosphere and becoming liquid

Efflorescent—will give off moisture or attract moisture, depending on the vapor pressure difference between the atmosphere and the powder.

Eutectic—solid substances that when mixed together reduce the melting point of each solid and cause liquid formation.

Geometric dilution—a mixing technique used to incorporate potent drugs or small quantities of powders in which equal volumes of drug and diluent are blended so as to ensure homogeneous mixing.

Hygroscopic—readily absorbing moisture from the atmosphere

Levigating agent—a dispersing agent used to wet powders for their incorporation into semisolid or suspension dosage forms.

Levigation—the formation of a paste by wetting a powder with a levigating agent and reducing the particle size of the powder.

Trituration—the process of grinding a drug in a mortar and pestle to reduce the particle size.

Powders

Description of Delivery System

Powders are homogeneous mixtures of finely divided drug and excipient combinations. They can be manufactured for both oral and topical uses. They are typically dispensed in dry form, but they may require the addition of a liquid, such as water, or food. Powders can be compounded into bulk products or into divided powders for unit-dose dispensing. Dry powders are typically not preferred by patients because of confusion with the method of administration and bitter or unpleasant tasting drugs or excipients. Also, the difficulty associated with protecting some powders from degradation, such as hygroscopic or deliquescent powders can make it difficult for pharmacists to find a suitable package for dispensing. The powder components must be homogeneously mixed, meaning the pharmacist must use the technique of geometric dilution when compounding such prescriptions. Also, the components of the powder must be appropriately sized (e.g., micronized). The USP/NF defines particle sizes as very coarse, coarse, moderately coarse, fine, and very fine. This is determined by the proportion of powder that is able to pass through a sieve of a defined size. Methods used to decrease the particle size of different powders are collectively termed comminution. Pharmacists compounding a powder or other dosage forms that include powders may need to decrease the particle size in order to have a uniform distribution of smaller diameter particles. The particle size is important because it can prevent segregation and is also important in the dissolution of oral powders. Trituration can be accomplished with a mortar and pestle, typically of the porcelain type, which has a coarser contact surface suitable for comminution. Powders used in ointments or suspensions are typically wetted with a levigating agent, such as propylene glycol, in order to form a paste prior to spatulation with the ointment base or for diluting. When blending powders, geometric dilution should be employed and can be accomplished by spatulation or using a glass mortar and pestle.

Interpreting the Prescription Order

Prescriptions for powders should include the intended use and ingredients for compounding. The prescription will typically call for the blending of powders, usually a drug and diluent mixture. Latin terms are usually employed to instruct the pharmacist on manufacturing procedure and dispensing instructions.

Calculating the Prescription

For most powders, the ingredients will be listed as % w/w or total weight of each substance. When calculating the amount and proportion of each ingredient, it is important to remember the basics of pharmaceutical calculations in order to ensure proper compounding and dispensing. When powders are needed in amounts less than the smallest amount weighable, the aliquot method should be used to ensure accurate weighing (see the Calculations section for further assistance).

Compounding and Calculations Review

Compounding the Product

Powders can be compounded by two well-known techniques. First, the method of spatulation involves the use of a pill tile or ointment slab to mix the powders. The drug and other excipients are mixed geometrically with the diluent using a spatula. This method is tedious, time-consuming, and does not result in a high degree of homogeneity compared to other techniques. Second, the pharmacist uses the mortar and pestle method most often to mix powders. The drug is admixed with the excipients by geometric dilution in the mortar by stirring or grinding the powders together using the pestle. This method is less time-consuming and shows a higher degree of homogeneity compared to the spatulation method.

Capsules

Description of Delivery System

Capsules comprise enclosure of a substance, typically a powder, within a capsule shell. The outer shell is generally made from some type of gelatin, but for patients refusing gelatin capsules, there are other alternatives available (e.g., HPMC, starch). Gelatin capsules are composed of hard or soft gelatin but, for compounding purposes, hard gelatin capsules are typically used. Because most capsules are intended for oral use, the size of the capsule becomes important when compounding such prescriptions. Capsule sizes range from the largest (#000) to the smallest size (#5), which can hold 1000 or 100 mg of aspirin, respectively (Table 1).

Table 1. Approximate Capacity of Empty Gelatin Capsules in Grams

No.	000	00	0	1	2	3	4	5
Quinine sulfate	0.65	0.40	0.32	0.25	0.20	0.15	0.10	0.06
Aspirin	1.00	0.65	0.50	0.32	0.25	0.20	0.15	0.10
Na pentobarbital	1.10	0.80	0.57	0.42	0.32	0.24	0.17	0.11
Powdered lactose	1.20	0.85	0.60	0.45	0.35	0.27	0.19	0.12
Na bicarbonate	1.50	1.00	0.72	0.52	0.40	0.32	0.25	0.15

When compounding prescriptions for specific patients, age and ability to swallow certain size capsules become important factors, as well as the amount of powder needed for each capsule. The size of the capsule determines the total amount of powder (diluent and drug) that can be encapsulated and the drug concentration within the diluent must be calculated accordingly. Filling the capsule shells is performed by various techniques, including the punch method or commercially available machines for the manufacture of capsules on a small scale. Compounded capsules should be dispensed and stored in appropriate child-resistant, tight, light-resistant containers.

Interpreting the Prescription Order

A prescription order will contain the number of capsules and the amount of drug per capsule, and may or may not give the capsule size to use. The pharmacist should use his or her professional judgment to choose the capsule size based on the patient's age, health status, and ability to swallow solid objects. Generally, the smallest capsule that will hold the desired amount of drug is used. The directions will be in abbreviations, as are most prescription orders, and must be translated into directions appropriate for the patient. The amount of powder in each capsule and the relative concentrations of drug in each capsule must be calculated. The pharmacist must be aware of compatibility of the drug with the excipients when compounding tablets, and should use available resources, such as the United States Pharmacopoeia, journal literature, or the Merck Index, to confirm that the ingredients are compatible.

Calculating the Prescription

If the prescription order calls for eight capsules that contain 30 mg of pseudoephedrine HCl, the total amount of powder required to fill eight capsules should be calculated. When using the punch method, a two-capsule overage is recommended in order to ensure that sufficient powder is available to yield the correct number of capsules. So in this example, the calculation would be for 10 capsules. If a #2 capsule shell is used and the diluent is lactose, the total weight of powder per capsule is 350 mg (Table 1). So the total weight of powder required for 10 capsules is 3500 mg or 3.5 g. The amount of pseudoephedrine HCl is 10 x 30 mg = 300 mg. By subtracting the 300 mg from the total of 3500 of pseudoephedrine HCL the pharmacist calculates the quantity of lactose required for the prescription (3500 mg - 300 mg = 3200 mg lactose).

Compounding the Product

Compounding a capsule using the punch method is typically done for smaller quantities, due to the enormous amount of time required to precisely fill the proper weight into each capsule shell. Commercial equipment is available for compounding of capsules on a slightly larger scale, ranging from manual to fully automated. To compound the prescription order using the punch method, the pharmacist must first calculate and weigh out the appropriate amounts of drug and diluents to deliver the desired amount of drug in each capsule.

Compounding and Calculations Review

The drug should be mixed by geometric dilution with the diluent using spatulation or using a glass mortar and pestle. Once the powders are thoroughly mixed to make a homogeneous dispersion, the powder should be positioned in a cone shape in the center of a glass pill tile. Gloves should be worn in order to prevent finger printing onto the outer shell walls. Prior to compounding, the empty capsule is weighed and subtracted from the final weight when determining the amount of powder in each capsule or the scale should be zeroed with an empty capsule. The first capsule shell should be opened and the body, which is the narrow half that fits inside the cap, should be removed. Now, with the filling half (body) in hand, place a small amount of powder into the body by dragging it horizontally across the glass pill tile. Then, in a smooth motion, invert the capsule shell and punch it into the powder cone. This will cause the powder to pack tightly into the capsule body. Each capsule (body and cap rejoined) should be weighed after each fill and adjusted to the desired weight by the removal or addition of powder. This procedure should be followed for each capsule in the prescription order.

Tablets

Description of Delivery System

Tablets are solid dosage forms prepared by the compression of powders using a tablet press or small-scale press. The formulation is designed to fulfill certain characteristics that improve bioavailability and patient compliance. Tablet hardness, disintegration time, friability, taste, color, stability, and size are all attributes of a tablet that must be optimized during the formulation process. Most pharmacies do not manufacture tablets on such a small scale. However, some compounding pharmacies do have the capability to manufacture tablets and should have formulations available that are optimized based on tablet properties. The choice of tablets over capsules would be one of judgment based on the patient's use of this medication, such as effervescent or chewable tablets, or as will be discussed further, the manufacture of lozenges and troches using a tablet press.

Interpreting the Prescription Order

The prescription order for tablets presented by the patient includes the ingredients and the number of tablets to be dispensed. It is important when making tablets that the ingredients used be physically and chemically compatible. The pharmacist must be aware of compatibility of the drug with the excipients when compounding tablets, and should use available resources to confirm that the ingredients are compatible.

Calculating the Prescription

The process for calculating prescription orders for tablets is similar to that used for capsules. The number of tablets and the weight of each tablet should be multiplied to get the total quantity of powder needed. An over amount should be added to ensure that sufficient powder is available for the prescription order. The concentration of drug in each tablet must be equal and precise. Because the tablet dimensions, size, and fill amount will vary according to the tooling and equipment, the tablet weight must be calculated for the specific apparatus used.

Compounding the Product

The drug should be mixed by geometric dilution with the diluent and other ingredients such that it is homogenously mixed. Then powder is loaded into the tableting machine and compressed to form the tablets. The compression force used affects the hardness of the tablet, which in turn affects the disintegration and dissolution properties of the tablet. The pharmacist should be aware of this and should consult the available literature to ensure proper tableting technique.

Troches and Lozenges

Description of Delivery System

Lozenges, which are synonymous with troches, are tablet-shaped solid dosage forms that are held in the oral cavity and allowed to slowly dissolve. They can be used to deliver topical antifungals to the mouth, or as a method to deliver systemic medications, such as hormones. Lozenges can be made by direct compression on a tablet press or by melting the components and adding them to a mold. The latter method is most useful to a compounding pharmacist, due to the lack of equipment for manufacturing tablets in most pharmacies. When melting pharmaceuticals, the pharmacist should be aware of the effect elevated temperatures have on drug stability.

Interpreting the Prescription Order

Prescriptions for lozenges include the ingredients (drug and excipients) and the number of lozenges to be made. The actual carrier or dissolving ingredient (e.g., sorbitol) used may vary and the choice is usually made by the pharmacist. The decision for this should be made based on literature citations or on previous formulations. If the drug being compounded is known to be bitter, a taste modifier should be added to improve patient compliance.

Compounding and Calculations Review

Calculating the Prescription

The calculations involved are the same as discussed for capsules and tablets. However, rather than being based on the capsule or tablet, calculations are usually based on the size of the mold used for compounding.

Compounding the Product

Lozenges or troches can be manufactured by the tableting method or by melting the ingredients together and pouring them into a mold. The tableting method is advantageous for heat labile drugs and for large-scale production. For most pharmacies, the melting technique is more convenient. The diluent, which is the carrier in this case, is melted to a molten state at which time the drug and other excipients are added and mixed. The molten mixture of drug and excipients are then poured into lozenge molds, which are similar to suppository molds, and then allowed to cool to room temperature to form the hardened final molded product.

Pharmaceutical Liquids

Important Terms

Agglomeration—the clumping of particles in air or liquid medium as an attempt to increase particle size and decrease the surface free energy

Aseptic—free of pathogenic microorganisms

Solubility—the amount of substance that can be dissolved in a given amount of solvent

Solution—a liquid preparation containing one or more chemical substances molecularly dissolved in a suitable solvent or mixture of mutually miscible solvents

Suspension—a system consisting of a solid dispersed in a liquid, in which the particles are typically larger than 5 microns.

Solutions

Description of Delivery System

A solution is a liquid preparation containing one or more chemical substances dissolved in a suitable solvent or mixture of mutually miscible solvents. Solutions can be used for oral, topical, and parenteral administration. Depending on the composition, solutions may be classified as syrups, elixirs, aromatic waters, tinctures, or fluid extracts. A syrup typically contains sucrose as a sweetening agent, the most common being Syrup NF which is 85% (w/v) sucrose solution. Elixirs contain various amounts of ethanol as a cosolvent, whereas aromatic waters contain aromatic compounds with or without alcohol (also known as spirits). Solutions that are made from drugs extracted from plants or other substances are termed tinctures or fluid extracts. When a solid or liquid is dissolved into another liquid, the solubility of the substance must be considered. If the level of material added to the solution exceeds the solubility, the substance may precipitate to form a suspension or phase separate in the case of liquid-in-liquid solutions.

Specialty Excipients for Compounding

Liquid Vehicle	Composition	pH	Alcohol Content (%)
Aromatic Elixir NF	Essential oils, syrup, alcohol, purified water	5.5-6.0	21-23
Compound Benzaldehyde Elixir NF	Benzaldehyde, flavoring, alcohol, purified water	6.0	0
Peppermint Water NF	Peppermint oil, purified water	-	0
Sorbitol Solution USP	65% D-sorbitol, purified water	-	0
Suspension Structured Vehicle NF	Potassium sorbate, xanthan gum, anhydrous citric acid, sucrose, purified water	-	0
Sugar-Free Suspension Structured Vehicle NF	Xanthan gum, saccharin sodium, potassium sorbate, citric acid, sorbitol, manitol, glycerin, purified water	-	0
Syrup NF	85% sucrose, purified water	-	0
Xanthan Gum Solution NF	Xanthan gum, methylparaben, propylparaben, purified water	-	0

Compounding and Calculations Review

Liquid Vehicle	Composition	pH	Alcohol Content (%)
Acacia Syrup	Acacia, sodium benzoate, vanilla tincture, sucrose, purified water	5.0	0
Cherry Syrup	Cherry juice, sucrose, alcohol, purified water	3.5-4.0	1-2
Citric Acid Syrup	Citric acid, syrup, lemon tincture	-	<1
Cocoa Syrup	Cocoa, sucrose, liquid glucose, glycerin, sodium chloride, vanillin, sodium benzoate, purified water	-	0
Raspberry Syrup	Raspberry juice, sucrose, alcohol, purified water	3.0	1-2
Tolu Syrup	Tolu balsam tincture, magnesium carbonate, sucrose, purified water	5.5	2-4
Wild Cherry Syrup	Wild cherry powder, sucrose, glycerin, alcohol, purified water	4.5	1-2
Ora-Sweet Syrup Vehicle	Citrus-berry flavoring, glycerin, sorbitol, sucrose, sodium phosphate, citric acid, potassium sorbate, methylparaben, purified water	4.0-4.5	0
Ora-Sweet SF Syrup Vehicle	Citrus-berry flavoring, glycerin, sorbitol, sodium saccharin, Xanthan gum, glycerin, sodium phosphate, citric acid, potassium sorbate, methylparaben, purified water	4.0-4.4	0

Interpreting the Prescription Order

Determination of the type of liquid desired by the physician is the first step in interpreting prescription orders for liquids. The components of the solution should be listed as % w/v, % v/v or g/mL. Depending on the availability of solubility data for the ingredients, it should be determined whether the liquid that is made will be a solution or a suspension, each of which have different properties and dispensing instructions. As previously stated, if the concentration of an ingredient is above the solubility, it will precipitate to form a suspension.

Calculating the Prescription

The calculations used to compound solutions involve converting directions, given in parts or in percents, into the actual amount needed for the prescription. Compounding directions typically give the amounts needed for an arbitrary volume, which may be different from the actual amount directed to be dispensed. The pharmacist must convert (reduce or enlarge) the amount needed for the prescription from the amount specified in the directions. This can involve proportions or if the quantity is given in a percentage, it can be calculated directly. Any stock solutions used must be accounted for in the final volume calculations. For example, if the prescription called for 1 gram of lidocaine HCl and a stock solution containing lidocaine HCL 100 mg/mL was available, then the pharmacist would need to account for and remove the 10-mL volume containing the lidocaine HCl from the water used to fill to the final volume.

Compounding the Product

When compounding a solution, the drug particles must be dissolved in a suitable solvent for the application in which it will be used. Solutions containing high alcoholic components should not be used for oral administration. Also, the solubility of the ingredients should be taken into account when choosing the solvent. The components should be mixed with the solvent in a beaker or mortar, and, in some cases, filtered prior to dispensing in order to prevent particulate material from being incorporated into the final preparation.

Suspensions

Description of Delivery System

Suspensions are liquid dosage forms that contain solid materials dispersed in a liquid vehicle. Suspensions are useful for chemically unstable drugs. This type of delivery system allows for the administration of medicines that are unstable in solution, as well as to patients unable to take solid dosage forms. Also, the dose of drug can be precisely titrated to deliver the required amount. Pediatric patients as well as the elderly benefit from this type of delivery system. Poor tasting or bitter compounds are more difficult to formulate into a suspension, but the problem can be overcome by the addition of a taste modifier. The suspension should be

Compounding and Calculations Review

formulated to prevent agglomeration and caking (formation of a solid pellet at the base of the container) of the suspended drug particles.

Interpreting the Prescription Order

A prescription order for a suspension will contain the desired ingredients (drug, excipients, and taste modifier) that should be added to the suspension formulation. Typically, the pharmacist is required to formulate a commercially available solid dosage form (e.g., tablet or capsule) into a suspension. The pharmacist must exercise caution to choose ingredients that are known to be compatible with the drug substance. If unsure, the pharmacist must consult the literature or other sources for stability and compatibility information (e.g., USP, Merck Index, journal literature).

Calculating the Prescription

The prescription is calculated based on the total volume of the prescription. If commercially available tablets are used, the volume used should be proportional to the number of tablets used. For example, if tablets containing 5 mg of active drugs are available and the prescription asks for 1 mg/mL, the volume used should be in multiples of 5 mL, since it would take one whole tablet for every 5 mL. Partially divided tablets should not be used, since it is unknown what the actual quantity of drug is in each subdivided part of the tablet.

Compounding the Product

Following the selection of an appropriate suspension formulation and completion of the calculations, the pharmacist can begin to combine and mix the ingredients to make the suspension. This is typically done using a mortar and pestle to disperse and thoroughly mix the ingredients. First, the powder or tablets (pulverized first in a ceramic mortar) should be added to the mortar and pestle and wetted with a levigating agent, such as propylene glycol. The suspending agent along with the liquid vehicle (usually water or flavored syrup) is added and mixed with the solid ingredients. The suspension is poured into the dispensing container and the mortar and pestle is rinsed with a portion of the water in order to ensure complete mass transfer of the drug substance. The suspension is brought to volume with the liquid vehicle.

Sterile Solutions

Description of Delivery System

Sterile solutions are used for injectable, ophthalmic and nasal/pulmonary delivery of drug substances. Solutions for intravenous administration must be in solution, while intramuscular, subcutaneous, ophthalmic, and nasal/pulmonary preparations can be administered as either a suspension or solution. When compounding prescriptions, it is difficult to prepare sterile suspensions because of the sterile filtering step that is required to make the preparation sterile that will collect the suspension particles on the filter membrane. Suspensions are reserved for pre-manufactured products that are reconstituted by the pharmacist. Sterile compounding is performed using a laminar flow hood or other suitable equipment to ensure an aseptic environment. The tonicity of the preparation is important when manufacturing injectable, ophthalmic and nasal/pulmonary preparations. If the tonicity is different from physiologic osmolarity, the patient may experience tissue irritation and pain at the site of administration. Therefore, the pharmacist must calculate the tonicity of the preparation and compare it to physiological parameters. Preservatives are used to maintain sterility of the preparation over the expected shelf life. Single-dose preparations do not necessarily require preservatives, but multiple-dose preparations must contain a preservative system. To ensure sterility and to prevent particulate matter within the sterile preparation, the final solution should be filtered through a 0.22-μm sterilizing filter using aseptic processing techniques.

Interpreting the Prescription Order

The mode of administration will determine whether the preparation should be sterile. Like other solutions, the concentration of ingredients is listed as parts or percentages and must be converted to the actual amounts for the prescribed preparation volume.

Calculating the Prescription

The calculations involved for sterile solutions are similar to nonsterile solution calculations. However, injectable or ophthalmic preparations should be formulated at a pH and osmolarity similar to those of the biological fluids which they contact.

Compounding the Product

Sterile preparations should be compounded in an approved aseptic environment, preferably in a laminar flow hood. The pharmacist should be trained in aseptic techniques and should be aware of the potential for contamination. Compounding of sterile solutions is similar to nonsterile solutions.

Compounding and Calculations Review

Topical Pharmaceutical Delivery Systems

Ointments

Ointments are semisolid preparations consisting of an ointment base with or without the incorporation of a medication. Nonmedicated ointments are often used as protectants, emollients, or lubricants.

Specialty Excipients for Compounding

Hydrocarbon Bases

Hydrocarbon bases, also known as oleaginous bases, have an emollient effect when placed on the skin. They prevent the escape of moisture and because they are hydrophobic in nature, they are difficult to wash from the skin using water. Typically, mineral oil is used as levigating agent when powdered substances are incorporated into hydrocarbon bases. Petrolatum, USP, is a purified mixture of semisolid hydrocarbons. It may vary in color from yellowish to light amber and melts between 38°C and 60°C. This product is also known as yellow petrolatum or petroleum jelly. White petrolatum, USP, has the same composition as petrolatum, USP, but has been decolorized. It has the same chemical attributes and melts within the same range as petrolatum, USP.

White ointment, USP, is a combination of yellow wax and petrolatum, USP. To make 1000 g of this ointment, 50 g of yellow wax is melted and mixed with 950 g of petrolatum, USP to make a uniform mixture.

White ointment, USP, is similar to yellow ointment, USP, but is made from white wax (decolorized yellow wax) and white petrolatum, USP.

Absorption Bases

Absorption bases are water-in-oil emulsions that permit the incorporation of aqueous solutions into the base. They are not easily washed from the skin with water because the continuous or external phase is oleaginous and they possess less significant emollient characteristics than hydrocarbon bases. Absorption bases act as adjuncts for the incorporation of aqueous solutions into hydrocarbon bases, synonymous with a co-solvent system. Examples of absorption bases include hydrophilic petrolatum and lanolin, USP.

Water-Removable Bases

Water-removable bases are oil-in-water emulsions that are easily washed from the skin with water. Because of the higher water content, they are paste-like and able to carry higher amounts of aqueous solutions, compared to oleaginous bases. One example is hydrophilic ointment, USP.

Water-Soluble Bases

Unlike the previous types of ointment bases described, water soluble-bases do not contain oleaginous components. They are easily washed from the skin and are considered "greaseless" bases. Water-soluble bases are typically used for the incorporation of solid substances into a base. One example is polyethylene glycol ointment, NF.

Interpreting the Prescription Order

The Latin abbreviation "ung" denotes ointment prescriptions. The pharmacist must note the amount to be dispensed and the relative amounts of each ingredient, usually given on a w/w basis or in parts. The stability (physical and chemical) of the ingredients should be confirmed.

Calculating the Prescription

When calculating for ointment prescriptions or other topical solid/semi-solid dosage forms, the pharmacist typically converts from percent w/w to the actual amount of a substance in grams.

Compounding the Product

Two methods are available for manufacture of compounded ointments. For most pharmacies, the method of spatulation is the most useful method for dispersing solid materials and other ingredients into an ointment base. A pill tile or ointment slab is used to geometrically dilute and disperse the ingredients into the ointment base. The ingredients are placed in the center of the ointment slab and pre-weighed ointment base is slowly added and mixed with the ingredients, geometrically, until the entire ointment base is added to the mixture. The second method involves heating of the ointment base and addition of the other ingredients into the molten base. This method works well as long as the drug, base and other ingredients are not heat labile. If any of the ingredients are heat sensitive, the first method must be used to disperse the ingredients into the ointment base.

Compounding and Calculations Review

Pastes

Description of Delivery System

Pastes contain higher solids content than ointments but are made in a similar manner. They contain the same bases, only in smaller amounts, which make a stiff semisolid base for the delivery of pharmaceutical products. Examples of pastes include oral pastes and topical pastes for the delivery of drugs or other therapeutic agents.

Compounding the Product

Two methods are available for manufacture of compounded ointments. For most pharmacies, the method of spatulation is the most useful method for dispersing solid materials and other ingredients into an ointment base. A pill tile or ointment slab is used to geometrically dilute and disperse the ingredients into the ointment base. The ingredients are placed in the center of the ointment slab and pre-weighed ointment base is slowly added and mixed with the ingredients, geometrically, until the entire ointment base is added to the mixture. The second method involves heating of the ointment base and addition of the other ingredients into the molten base. This method works well as long as the drug, base and other ingredients are not heat labile. If any of the ingredients are heat sensitive, the first method must be used to disperse the ingredients into the ointment base.

Interpreting the Prescription Order

The Latin abbreviation "ung" denotes ointment prescriptions. The pharmacist must note the amount to be dispensed and the relative amounts of each ingredient, usually given on a w/w basis or in parts. The stability (physical and chemical) of the ingredients should be confirmed.

Creams

Creams are semisolid oil-in-water emulsions containing medicinal substances used for topical administration. They are easily applied and spread effectively over the affected area. Unlike ointments, they are readily washed from the skin with water. Creams may also be used for rectal or vaginal administration because of their high water content.

Lotions

Description of Delivery System

Lotions are emulsion systems designed to hydrate the skin, act as an emollient in order to protect the skin, and act as a carrier for drugs. Lotions spread well on the skin and are useful to cover large surface areas of the skin. Emulsions are composed of a water phase and an oil phase that are dispersed, one within the other, either as an oil-in-water or water-in-oil emulsion, where the first term refers to the internal phase and the second term refers to the external phase. The surfactants and the relative amounts of each component determine the type of emulsion formed. Surfactants with a low hydrophilic/lipophilic balance (HLB) will make water-in-oil emulsions whereas surfactants with high HLB values tend to make oil-in-water emulsions. The type of emulsion formed will determine the washability of the lotion from the skin. Oil-in-water emulsions tend to be washed from the skin more easily than water-in-oil emulsions. If a drug is incorporated into the lotion, it should be added to the phase in which it is most soluble, prior to emulsification of the two phases.

Interpreting the Prescription Order

A prescription for a lotion typically contains the oil and water phases that should be mixed and, if one is needed, the drug substance. The relative amounts of each component are included but must be calculated (reduced or enlarged) for the given amount to be dispensed. The pharmacist must be aware of the properties of emulsions in order to prevent "breaking" of the emulsion, which is an irreversible phase separation of the emulsion.

Compounding the Product

To make a lotion, the procedure involves heating the two phases separately to melt the components and mixing them to form the emulsion. The order of addition is important to ensure proper emulsion preparation. To make an emulsion, the oil-soluble components are added together and melted and, in a separate beaker, the water-soluble components are mixed and heated a few degrees above the temperature of the oil phase. The internal phase is added to the external phase with mixing. The mixture must be stirred vigorously until the mixture cools and the emulsion is formed and set. If the stirring is not sufficient, the emulsion may break.

Compounding and Calculations Review

Gels

Description of Delivery System

Gels are water-based semisolid materials that may contain medicinal substances for topical, vaginal, rectal, and ophthalmologic administration. With the addition of a gelling agent, the viscosity of the aqueous solution increases due to cross-linking of the polymeric molecules. Gels can contain cosolvents such as alcohol or propylene glycol. Because of the high water content, they require the addition of a preservative such as a paraben or chlorhexidine gluconate

Specialty Excipients for Compounding

Pluronic TM (poloxamer) makes a thermoplastic gel that when dissolved in water has a low viscosity at low temperatures (e.g., 5° C), but the viscosity increases with increasing temperature (e.g., 25° C). It can be purchased in various grades that differ in molecular weight and gelling properties. Carbopol TM (carbomer) is a solid polymer of acrylic acid that is a weak acid. When dispersed in a suitable solvent and neutralized with a base (e.g., sodium hydroxide or triethanolamine [TEA]), cross-linking between the polymeric chains causes gelation. Carbopol is available in various molecular weight distributions that have different properties.

Interpreting the Prescription Order

Prescriptions involving gels typically list the active ingredient and some type of gelling material. Because not all gels are the same, and because the intended use can affect the choice of gelling agent, the pharmacist must ensure that the proper gelling agent be used for the specific application. Occasionally the gelling agent is not listed and the pharmacist must decide on the appropriate type and level. The ingredients may be listed on a percentage w/w or parts basis that must be converted to the amount needed for the prescription.

Calculating the Prescription

The prescription order for gels is calculated similarly to ointments and creams, since the final product is a semi-solid. However, during the compounding, some of the components are liquid, so proper volumes (based on density) are used for the weights given.

Compounding the Product

Following the calculations, the appropriate weights and/or volumes of the ingredients should be mixed in order to ensure homogeneity. Depending on the gelling agent used, the mode of gelation will determine the final step. For Pluronic gels, the final solution need only be allowed to warm to room temperature to increase the viscosity of the gel. The pharmacist should ensure that the preparation has fully gelled prior to dispensing. Since other ingredients were added to the preparation, the dilution effect can prevent the gel from solidifying at room temperature and may require additional amounts of the gelling agent Pluronic. When Carbopol is used as the gelling agent, the final step involves neutralization with a base to cause the cross-linking and gelation. The pharmacist should use caution when adding the neutralizing agent such that the gel formed is homogenous in nature and lacks clumps from poor mixing. Adding an overage of neutralizing agent, effectively alkalinizing the mixture, will cause the gel to break, resulting in a watery mass. Therefore, the neutralizing agent should be added just to the point of gelation.

Aqueous Nasal Sprays

Description of Delivery System

Aqueous Nasal Sprays must follow specific guidelines as described by the Food and Drug Administration. Nasal Spray Solutions or suspension are used for administration of topical or systemic medications via the nasal route. Because of their route of administration, it is important that the drug be sterile and be applied in a suitable fashion by a calibrated nasal spray pump. For the most part, the guidelines regarding nasal sprays regulate the pump and will not be discussed here. The contents of the nasal spray are typically filtered through a sterilizing membrane prior to dispensing, to prevent microbial contamination. Preservatives can also be added for prevention of microbial growth.

Interpreting the Prescription Order

The prescription order lists the ingredients, the mode of administration, and the dose of each administration. The pump used will determine the exact volume expelled during each spray that will be used in the calculations. Similar to solutions, the relative amounts of each ingredient will typically be listed as parts of percentages.

Compounding and Calculations Review

Suppositories

Rectal Suppositories

Description of Delivery System

Rectal Suppositories are cylindrical or cone shaped solid dosage forms that are intended to be inserted into the rectum for topical or systemic delivery of medications. Patients who are vomiting or are unable to take oral medications may benefit from this type of delivery route. Rectal suppositories are designed to either melt or dissolve in the rectal vault and release the medication to either be absorbed across the rectal membrane or exhibit a local effect on the membrane. The suppository base used will determine the release mechanism.

Specialty Excipients for Compounding

The excipients used for the manufacture of suppositories are the suppository bases along with a lubricant for the suppository mold. The lubricant is typically of an opposite hydrophilicity as the suppository base. Some common bases and lubricants are listed below.

Oleaginous Bases

Cocoa butter, NF is a triglyceride that melts between 30°C and 36°C; therefore, it melts at body temperature but is a solid at room temperature. However, cocoa butter exhibits several polymorphs or different crystalline forms that will display different melting behavior and rate. If cocoa butter is quickly heated well above the minimum melting temperature, the resulting crystal will be the metastable crystal, also known as the a crystal, which has a lower melting point than the original crystal (ß form) and may not solidify at room temperature. Therefore, it is important to slowly melt the cocoa butter. Also, the addition of other substances, such as drugs, may cause a melting point depression of the base. This can be alleviated by the addition of substances like cetyl esters wax or beeswax to increase the temperature of solidification of the cocoa butter. Witepsol is an oleaginous suppository base consisting of triglyceride esters, saturated fatty acids and mono- and diglycerides that has a melting point in the range of 40°C -45°C. Witepsol will not melt as fast during the insertion of the suppository, which is beneficial to the patient.

Water-soluble bases

Polyethylene glycol is designed to dissolve in the fluids of the rectum or vagina rather than melt. Because of this, the melting point of the suppository is well above body temperature. Furthermore, the suppository does not melt during handling and insertion.

Lubricants

Propylene glycol is useful for the lubrication of molds when using oleaginous bases. Mineral oil is useful for the lubrication of suppository molds when using water-soluble bases.

Interpreting the Prescription Order

The prescription will call for a certain amount of drug to be contained in each suppository. The calculations must take into account the size of the suppository mold and the amount of drug contained in each suppository. The size of the mold or the amount of base needed for each suppository may vary between pharmacies and even within pharmacies that have several molds. The mold should be calibrated to ensure that the pharmacist knows the amount of material needed for each type of suppository base. When dispensing to a patient, the directions should include the method for insertion as well as a statement to unwrap the suppository or remove it from its primary packaging.

Calculating the Prescription

The number of suppositories multiplied by the amount needed for each suppository is calculated. An overage amount of two suppositories is recommended in case there is some waste and to ensure enough material during manufacture. A typical mold can make 10-12 suppositories, so if a prescription called for 8 suppositories containing 10 mg of sumatriptan, the total amount of drug needed is 100 mg (assuming an overage of 2 suppositories). If the suppository mold holds 2 g of cocoa butter per suppository, the total amount of cocoa butter would be 10 x 2 g = 20 g -100 mg (sumatriptan) = 19.9 g of cocoa butter.

Compounding the Product

Using the previous example, the cocoa butter and drug are weighed. The cocoa butter is slowly heated to near 40°C with stirring. Once the base is melted, the drug is added slowly with mixing to disperse. After the mold has been lubricated with propylene glycol, the cocoa butter/drug dispersion is slowly poured into the mold, making sure each mold is filled completely, and allowed to cool. Once cooled to room temperature, the excess cocoa butter is scraped from the mold and the mold taken apart to release the suppositories. The finished suppositories are wrapped in a suitable primary wrap (aluminum foil) and dispensed. Plastic molds are also available for preparation and dispensing. Patients must be advised to unwrap the suppositories prior to insertion.

Compounding and Calculations Review

Vaginal Suppositories

Description of Delivery System

Vaginal suppositories are similar to rectal suppositories in shape and function. However, they are typically designed to dissolve in the vagina where the drug is released to exhibit a local effect, rather than a systemic effect. They are made in a similar fashion to rectal suppositories but the suppository bases may differ because of the physiologic differences between the rectum and the vagina. Diseases, such as yeast infections, bacterial infections, and many others are commonly treated with vaginal suppositories. Also, contraceptive vaginal suppositories are used that contain spermicidal agents, such as nonoxynol-9.

Parenteral Delivery Systems

Important Terms

Aseptic—lacking organisms or biological materials which may cause local infection or sepsis when injected directly into the blood stream.

Aseptic technique—a technique utilized by pharmacists to compound sterile parenteral medications that minimizes the introduction of biological materials such as bacteria.

Intraarterial injections (IA)—administration directly into arterial blood vessels.

Intracardiac injections (IC)—administration directly into the heart.

Intramuscular injection (IM)—administration into the muscular tissue. Typically to the arm, thigh or buttocks.

Intrathecal injections (IT)—administration into the space surround the spinal cord. Intravenous injection (IV)—injection into venous blood vessels which is the most common form of parenteral administration.

Subcutaneous injection (SC)—administration below the skin in the subcutaneous region.

Solutions

Description of Delivery System

As mentioned previously, solutions are homogeneous mixtures of drug and diluent combinations. Solutions for injection are sterile and may be used for SC, IA, IT, IC or IV administration. They may be supplied in vials or sterile polyethylene terephthalate (PET) bags which allow for admixture to form the final solution for administration. The most common diluents for solutions and suspensions for injection include isotonic solutions of NaCl and dextrose which is a 5% w/v solution of dextrose in sterile water for injection or 0.9% w/v NaCl (normal saline) in sterile water for injection. Suspensions for injection contain suspended particles and therefore cannot be injected directly into the blood stream. Intramuscular injection is typically utilized for suspensions and the product relies on the fluids within the muscle to dissolve the drug and release it into the blood stream.

Interpreting the Prescription Order

Prescriptions for solutions or suspensions for injection should include the intended use and ingredients for compounding. Typically the prescription will call for the admixture of powders, usually a drug and diluent mixture. Latin terms are usually employed to instruct the pharmacist on manufacturing procedure and dispensing instructions. The pharmacist will be required to follow product labeling or calculate concentrations that differ from that labeling.

Calculating the Prescription Order

For most solutions or suspensions for injection, the ingredients will be listed as % w/w, mEq or total amount of each substance. Typical calculations which are utilized for the compounding of sterile solutions and suspensions for injection can be found in the Calculations section of this book.

Compounding and Calculations Review

Questions

Powders

1. Example prescription order:

   Tolnaftate 1% foot powder
   Tolnaftate 1% w/w
   Zinc oxide 5% w/w
   Talc 20% w/w
   Fragrance 3 gtt
   Corn starch qs
   Mft pulv DTD 20 g
   Sig: Apply pulv to feet AD bid for rash

   How often should this prescription be administered?

   A. Twice daily
   B. Three times daily
   C. Four times daily
   D. Every other day
   E. Every 2 hours

2. How many grams of corn starch are needed to complete the prescription?

   A. 20 grams
   B. 10 grams
   C. 14.8 grams
   D. 7.4 grams
   E. 1.48 grams

3. How many grams of corn starch are needed if the prescription called for 30 grams to be dispensed?

   A. 22.2 grams
   B. 2.22 grams
   C. 4.44 grams
   D. 30 grams
   E. 7.88 grams

4. How many grams of tolnaftate are needed if the prescription called for 30 grams to be dispensed?

   A. 3 grams
   B. 0.3 grams
   C. 0.03 grams
   D. 30 grams
   E. 20 grams

5. How many parts tolnaftate are there contained in the total mixture?

   A. 1 part tolnaftate per 200 parts mixture
   B. 1 part tolnaftate per 100 parts mixture
   C. 1 part tolnaftate per 300 parts mixture
   D. 1 part tolnaftate per 50 parts mixture
   E. 1 part tolnaftate per 99 parts mixture

6. Which of the following auxiliary labels should be included with the prescription?

   A. Shake well
   B. Not to be taken by mouth
   C. For the ear
   D. For rectal use only
   E. For the eye

7. Example prescription order:

   Atropine sulfate   1.4 mg
   Blue tracer dye   1.4 mg
   Sodium bicarbonate qs 10 g
   Mft: pulv   DTD 300 g
   Sig: 2 tsp po for procedure

   What quantity of atropine is required for this prescription?

   A. 1.4 mg
   B. 1400 mg
   C. 42 g
   D. 0.42 g
   E. 0.042 g

8. How many grams of atropine are administered with each dose?

   A. 1.4 g
   B. 0.0014 g
   C. 4.2×10^{-6} g
   D. 4.2 g
   E. 0.0042 g

9. What is the % w/w of atropine in the prescription?

   A. 1.4%
   B. 2.5%
   C. 3.6%
   D. 0.014%
   E. 0.0014%

10. What is the intended site of administration of this powder?

    A. The right eye
    B. The left eye
    C. Both ears
    D. The left ear
    E. The right ear

11. How often should the prescription be administered?

    A. Three times daily
    B. Twice daily
    C. Four times daily
    D. Every other day
    E. Every 3 hours

12. How many grams of miconazole are needed to prepare the prescription?

    A. 5 grams
    B. 4 grams
    C. 6 grams
    D. 3 grams
    E. 2 grams

13. How many grams of boric acid powder will be needed to prepare the prescription?

    A. 90 grams
    B. 95 grams
    C. 5 grams
    D. 98 grams
    E. 15 grams

14. Which of the following auxiliary labels should be included on the prescription label?

    A. For external use only
    B. Keep in refrigerator
    C. Shake well
    D. For the ear
    E. A and D only

15. How many milligrams of misoprostol are needed to complete this prescription?

    Misoprostol 0.0027% mucoadhesive powder
    misoprostol   400 µg
    Polyethylene oxide   200 mg
    HPMC   qs   15 g
    Mft: pulv   DTD 30 g
    Sig: as directed

    A. 800 mg
    B. 400 mg
    C. 1 mg
    D. 0.4 mg
    E. 0.8 mg

16. How many grams of misoprostol are required if the prescription calls for 60 g to be dispensed?

    A. 0.0016 g
    B. 0.016 g
    C. 0.08 g
    D. 0.8 g
    E. 8 g

17. How many grains are to be dispensed for this prescription?

    A. 4.6296 gr
    B. 46.296 gr
    C. 462.96 gr
    D. 4629.6 gr
    E. 231.48 gr

18. If the specific gravity of this powder was 1.3, how many milliliters would the final preparation occupy?

    A. 30 mL
    B. 40 mL
    C. 39 mL
    D. 23.1 mL
    E. 231 mL

19. What does the term "pulv" mean on the prescription order?

    A. Powder
    B. Ointment
    C. Tablet
    D. Capsule
    E. Gel

20. How many parts of misoprostol are there per part of polyethylene oxide?

    A. 1 part misoprostol per 250 parts polyethylene oxide
    B. 1 part misoprostol per 500 parts polyethylene oxide
    C. 1 part misoprostol per 100 parts polyethylene oxide
    D. 1 part misoprostol per 750 parts polyethylene oxide
    E. 1 part misoprostol per 375 parts polyethylene oxide

21. What is the weight percent of misoprostol in the preparation?

    A. 2.7%
    B. 0.27%
    C. 27%
    D. 0.0027%
    E. 0.027%

22. Example prescription order:

    Camphor   0.3% w/w
    Menthol   0.7% w/w
    Talc   30% w/w
    Corn Starch   qs
    Mft: pulv   DTD 30 g
    Sig: Apply pulv affected area bid prn rash

    How many grams of camphor are required to fill 2 orders of this prescription?

23. How many milligrams of menthol are required to fill 1 order of this prescription?

24. How much corn starch, in grams, is needed to fill 1 order of this prescription?

25. How many times per day will the patient apply this formulation?

26. If the patient uses 2 grams of the formulation during each application, how many grams of menthol will be used in 1 week?

27. How many parts talc are contained in the total mixture (assuming 30 parts of a mixture)?

Compounding and Calculations Review

Capsules

1. Example prescription order:

   Acetaminophen 160 mg
   Chlorpheniramine maleate 2 mg
   Pseudoephedrine HCl 10 mg
   Lactose qs
   Mft caps (#2) DTD: 6
   Sig: 1-2 caps po tid prn allergies

   If the smallest amount weighable for the balance used to measure the ingredients is 70 mg, which of the following ingredients require the use of an aliquot?

   A. Acetaminophen
   B. Chlorpheniramine maleate
   C. Pseudoephedrine HCl
   D. Lactose
   E. Pseudoephedrine HCl and chlorpheniramine maleate

2. What weight of acetaminophen is required to fill eight capsules, in grains?

   A. 1.98 gr
   B. 19.8 gr
   C. 198 gr
   D. 1980 gr
   E. 0.198 gr

3. What weight of pseudoephedrine HCL is required to fill 10 capsules, in grains?

   A. 1.54 gr
   B. 15.4 gr
   C. 0.154 gr
   D. 154 gr
   E. 1540 gr

4. How many ounces of powder are required for the final preparation, if #2 capsules hold 350 mg lactose?

   A. 0.07 ounces
   B. 0.7 ounces
   C. 7 ounces
   D. 70 ounces
   E. 700 ounces

5. If a #2 capsule holds 350 mg lactose, how many milligrams of lactose are needed for each capsule?

   A. 200 mg
   B. 350 mg
   C. 178 mg
   D. 250 mg
   E. 300 mg

6. What is the percentage w/w of acetaminophen in the preparation?

   A. 45.7%
   B. 22.85%
   C. 30%
   D. 60%
   E. 42.5%

7. How often should this preparation be administered?

   A. Twice daily as needed
   B. Once daily as needed
   C. Three times daily as needed
   D. Four times daily as needed
   E. Every 3 hours

8. Which of the following auxiliary labels should be included on the prescription?

   A. Shake well
   B. Not to be taken by mouth
   C. For external use only
   D. For the ear
   E. None of the above

9. How often should this preparation be administered?

   Dehydroepiandrosterone   50 mg
   Lactose   qs
   Mft: caps (size #2)   DTD: 10
   Sig: 1 capsule po qid

   A. Once daily
   B. Twice daily
   C. Four times daily
   D. Three times daily
   E. Every four hours

10. If a #2 size capsule holds 350 mg of lactose, what is the percentage w/w of dehydroepiandrosterone in each capsule (assuming no overage)?

    A. 28%
    B. 14.3%
    C. 24.6%
    D. 30%
    E. 22.5%

11. How many grams of lactose will be required to fill this prescription?

    A. 3 grams
    B. 6 grams
    C. 3.5 grams
    D. 7 grams
    E. 1.75 grams

12. How many grams of dehydroepiandrosterone are required to fill 12 capsules?

    A. 600 g
    B. 60 g
    C. 0.6 g
    D. 6 g
    E. 0.06 g

Compounding and Calculations Review

13. How many grains of lactose are required to complete the prescription, if a #2 capsule will hold 350 mg lactose?

   A. 5.4 gr
   B. 5.4×10^4 gr
   C. 46.296 gr
   D. 0.54 gr
   E. 0.054 gr

14. How many parts of dehydroepiandrosterone are there per part of lactose?

   A. 1 part dehydroepiandrosterone per 7 parts lactose
   B. 1 part dehydroepiandrosterone per 6 parts lactose
   C. 1 part dehydroepiandrosterone per 10 parts lactose
   D. 1 part dehydroepiandrosterone per 5 parts lactose
   E. 1 part dehydroepiandrosterone per 4 parts lactose

15. What quantity of lactose is required to complete this prescription?

   Estradiol   1 mg
   Estriol   8 mg
   Estrone   1 mg
   Progesterone   150 mg
   Lactose   qs   280 mg
   Mft: 100 capsules
   Note: 1 capsule shell will hold 280 mg of lactose
   Sig: 1 capsule po bid

   A. 1.2g
   B. 120mg
   C. 12g
   D. 0.012g
   E. 24g

16. What is the concentration (%w/w) of estriol in the capsule formulation?

   A. 5.67%
   B. 2.23%
   C. 2.86%
   D. 1.25%
   E. 0.029%

17. How many grams of progesterone will be dosed to the patient after 30 days?

   A. 8 g
   B. 0.9 g
   C. 9 g
   D. 0.8 g
   E. 2.5 g

18. Example prescription order:

   Estriol   200 mg
   Estrone sulfate   25 mg
   Estradiol   25 mg
   Methocel K3   10 g
   Lactose   23.75 g
   Mft caps (#2)

What combined weight of Estriol, Estrone and Estradiol is required in grains to prepare this formulation?

19. If each #2 capsule holds 350 mg of the final powder, how many full capsules can be manufactured?

20. If each #2 capsule holds 350 mg of the final powder, how many milligrams of Estriol will be present in each capsule (nearest whole milligram)?

21. What is the percentage w/w of lactose in the formulation?

22. If each #2 capsule holds 350 mg of the final powder, what is the percentage w/w of Methocel K3 in each capsule?

23. How many parts estriol are present per part estradiol

24. Example prescription order:

   Ibuprofen   150 mg
   Lactose qs
   Mft caps (#2)
   Sig: 1–2 capsules po qid

   How many times each day is this patient to take their capsule(s)?

25. If each #2 capsule holds 350 mg of the formulation, and you have 1 ounce (avoirdupois) of lactose, how many full capsules could be produced?

26. How many grains of ibuprofen are present in each capsule?

27. How many grams of ibuprofen are required to make 5 capsules?

28. Based on the prescription, what is the maximum possible amount of ibuprofen a patient may take each day in grams?

29. You do not have bulk ibuprofen in your pharmacy however you have ibuprofen tablets at a different strength which may be ground and used to prepare these capsules. If the tablets available to you contain 200 mg of ibuprofen in each tablet, how many tablets must be ground to obtain enough ibuprofen to compound 20 capsules?

Tablets

1. Example prescription order:

   Loratadine 10 mg
   Pseudoephedrine HCl 15 mg
   Lactose 100 mg
   Microcrystalline cellulose 24 mg
   Magnesium stearate 1 mg
   Mft: 150 mg tablets DTD: 200
   Sig: 1 tab po tid prn allergies/congestion

Compounding and Calculations Review

What is the total amount of powder needed, including a 10% overage of powder?

A. 33 grams
B. 30.3 grams
C. 15 grams
D. 60 grams
E. 45 grams

2. How often should the product be administered?

A. Once daily
B. Twice daily as needed
C. Three times daily as needed
D. Every other day as needed
E. Every 3 hours

3. What percentage strength (w/w) is the pseudoephedrine in each tablet?

A. 5%
B. 10%
C. 1%
D. 1.5%
E. 0.1%

4. What weight of pseudoephedrine HCl, in grains, is required to fill the prescription, including a 10% overage?

A. 46.75 gr
B. 4.675 gr
C. 467.5 gr
D. 46750 gr
E. 4675 gr

5. What weight of loratadine, in grams, is required to complete the prescription, including a 10% overage?

A. 2.02 g
B. 202 g
C. 2020 g
D. 0.202 g
E. 20.2 g

6. What is the ratio strength for loratadine?

A. 1:2
B. 1:1.5
C. 2:1.5
D. 1:5
E. 1:0.75

7. Example prescription order:

Calcium carbonate	500 mg
Maltodextrin	150 mg
Powdered cellulose	320 mg
Lactose	25 mg
Talc	2.5 mg
Cherry flavor powder	2.5 mg

Mft 1000 mg tablets DTD: 200

Sig: chew 2–4 tablets prn indigestion

What is the percent w/w powdered cellulose in this formulation?

8. How many milligrams of talc will be present in the dispensed amount?

9. A patient takes 4 tablets during a single dosing. How many grains of lactose have they consumed in this dose?

10. How many parts maltodextrin are present per part lactose?

11. You decide to compound a single practice tablet. In order to obtain the correct amount of cherry flavor you decide to prepare an aliquot in powdered cellulose. You blend 70 mg of cherry flavor powder with powdered cellulose. If you use 10 mg of this blend to obtain the correct amount of flavor how much powdered cellulose was used?

12. If density of powdered cellulose is 1.5 g/cm^3 and that of calcium carbonate is 2.7 g/cm^3, how many milliliters, combined, of these ingredients are needed to prepare 200 tablets (Rounded to nearest whole number)?

Troches and Lozenges

1. Example prescription order:

Sodium fluoride 50 mg
Sorbitol qs
Mft 10 lozenges (each lozenge mold will hold 2 grams of material) Sig: 1 loz bid

How often should the preparation be administered?

A. Once daily
B. Twice daily
C. Four times daily
D. Three times daily
E. Every 2 hours

2. How many grams of sodium fluoride are required to complete the preparation including a 20% overage?

A. 600 g
B. 0.60 g
C. 6.0 g
D. 60 g
E. 0.51 g

3. If the specific gravity of the molten material is 0.98, how many milliliters will each mold hold?

A. 2.04 mL
B. 20.4 mL
C. 1.96 mL
D. 19.6 mL
E. 0.98 mL

Compounding and Calculations Review

4. How many total grams of sorbitol are needed to complete the preparation?

   A. 20 grams
   B. 19.5 grams
   C. 30 grams
   D. 10 grams
   E. 15 grams

5. What is the amount of sodium fluoride in ___% w/w?

   A. 2.5%
   B. 5%
   C. 10%
   D. 0.25%
   E. 0.025%

6. Example prescription order:

Menthol	8 mg
Eucalyptus oil	0.5% w/w
Sorbitol	qs

   Mft 15 lozenges
   Sig: 1 loz q2-3h prn cough

   Each lozenge mold holds 2.5 grams of material. How many grams of material must be produced to fill 1 order of this prescription?

7. Each lozenge mold holds 2.5 grams of material. How many grams of eucalyptus oil are needed to fill one prescription order?

8. The density of eucalyptus oil is 0.909 g/mL. How many milliliters of eucalyptus oil will be needed for 2 orders of this prescription?

9. Each lozenge mold holds 2.5 grams of material. How many grams of sorbitol are needed to fill 1 prescription order?

10. Each lozenge mold holds 2.5 grams of material. You decide to manufacture 10,000 grains of material. How many full orders can you fill with this amount (whole number)?

11. What is the maximum number of lozenges a patient may take in a 10 hour time period based on the sig?

Solutions

1. Example prescription order:

   Phenobarbital 20 mg
   Syrup NF 10% v/v
   Glycerin 5% v/v
   Alcohol 5% v/v
   Methylparaben 0.1% w/v
   Propylparaben 0.01% w/v
   Flavor 0.5 gtt
   Water qs 5 mL
   Mft syrup DTD ii oz
   Sig: ii tsp po tid for seizures

   How many milliliters of the preparation will be dispensed?

   A. 30 mL
   B. 15 mL
   C. 60 mL
   D. 120 mL
   E. 45 mL

2. If phenobarbital is available in a 25-mg/mL stock solution, how many milliliters are required to complete the preparation?

   A. 96 mL
   B. 9.6 mL
   C. 0.96 mL
   D. 960 mL
   E. 0.096 mL

3. If the specific gravity of Syrup NF is 1.3, how many grams would be required to complete the preparation?

   A. 4.6 g
   B. 0.46 g
   C. 7.8 g
   D. 0.78 g
   E. 2.3 g

4. How many milliliters should be administered for each dose?

   A. 15 mL
   B. 30 mL
   C. 10 mL
   D. 5 mL
   E. 60 mL

5. How often should the preparation be administered?

   A. Once daily
   B. Twice daily
   C. Three times daily
   D. Four times daily
   E. Every 3 hours

6. How many milligrams of phenobarbital are required to complete the preparation?

   A. 120 mg
   B. 240 mg
   C. 20 mg
   D. 40 mg
   E. 60 mg

7. How many milliliters of Syrup NF are needed to complete the preparation?

   A. 6 mL
   B. 12 mL
   C. 24 mL
   D. 48 ml
   E. 10 mL

8. How many parts of methylparaben are there per part of phenobarbital?

Compounding and Calculations Review

A.   1 part methylparaben to 4 parts phenobarbital
B.   1 part methylparaben to 8 parts phenobarbital
C.   1 part methylparaben to 1 part phenobarbital
D.   1 part methylparaben to 16 parts phenobarbital
E.   1 part methylparaben to 10 parts phenobarbital

9.   Example prescription order for questions 8, 9, and 10:

Meperidine HCl 2.5 g
Phenol 200 mg
Sterile water for injection qs 100 mL
Mft nasal solution DTD 15 mL
Sig: 2 gtt each nostril qid prn

What is the percentage w/v of meperidine in the preparation?

A.   0.25%
B.   2.5%
C.   5%
D.   10%
E.   15%

10. If meperidine is available in a 10% stock solution, how many milliliters are required to complete the preparation?

A.   3.75 mL
B.   375 mL
C.   37.5 mL
D.   0.375 mL
E.   0.0376 mL

11. How many milligrams of phenol are needed to compound the preparation?

A.   15 mg
B.   200 mg
C.   100 mg
D.   30 mg
E.   5 mg

12. How often should the preparation be administered?

A.   Three times daily as needed
B.   Four times daily as needed
C.   Twice daily as needed
D.   Every other day as needed
E.   Every 4 hours

13. Which of the following auxiliary labels should be included on the label of the preparation?

A.   For the nose
B.   Not to be taken by mouth
C.   Shake well
D.   A and B only
E.   None of the above

14. Example prescription order:

Liquid phenol	1.2 g
Tannic acid	4.0 g
Benzocaine	2.4 g
Ethanol	77 mL

| Propylene glycol | 15 % v/v |
| Water | qs 4 oz. |

MFT soln dtd iii oz.
Sig: Swish and spit one tsp q 3 hr prn ulcer pain

How many milliliters of propylene glycol will be needed to prepare this formulation?

15. If the liquid phenol is a stock solution of 200 mg/ mL, how many liters of the stock solution are needed for the preparation?

16. A 200 mg/ mL liquid phenol stock solution is dispensed via a dropper. You have determined that 20 drops fills a 10 mL graduated cylinder to the 4 mL mark. How many drops will be needed to prepare this prescription?

17. Assuming the patient uses this prescription every 3 hours, how many pints will be used in an 18 hour period?

18. If the patient uses the prescription 5 times a day for 14 days, how many fills will he/she require?

19. How many kilo grams of benzocaine will be used to fill 4 orders of this prescription?

Suspensions

1.   Example prescription order:

Metronidazole 0.24 g
Xanthan gum 0.9% w/v
Water qs 250 mL
Mft susp DTD 100 mL
Sig: Give 0.5 mg/kg body weight bid for intestinal parasite
     (cat weighs 10.5 lb)

How many grams of xanthan gum are needed for this preparation?

A.   0.9 g
B.   9 g
C.   0.09 g
D.   18 g
E.   2.7 g

2.   What is the percentage strength of metronidazole in this preparation?

A.   0.096%
B.   9.6%
C.   4.3%
D.   0.043%
E.   0.43%

3.   How many grains of metronidazole are required if the prescription calls for 150 mL to be dispensed?

A.   2.2 gr
B.   0.22 gr
C.   0.0093 gr

Compounding and Calculations Review

D. 9.3 gr

E. 93 gr

4. How often should this preparation be administered?

   A. Once daily
   B. Twice daily
   C. Three times daily
   D. Every other day
   E. Four times daily

5. How many milligrams of metronidazole are needed for the preparation?

   A. 0.96 mg
   B. 0.0096 mg
   C. 96 mg
   D. 0.096 mg
   E. 240 mg

6. How many milliliters of the preparation should be administered per dose?

   A. 5.37 mL
   B. 2.48 mL
   C. 4.8 mL
   D. 6.2 mL
   E. 10 mL

7. Which of the following auxiliary labels should be included with this preparation?

   A. Shake well
   B. For external use only
   C. Not to be taken by mouth
   D. A and B only
   E. All of the above

8. Example prescription order:

   Sulfamerazine 10.0 g
   Carbopol 934P 0.5 g
   Sodium lauryl sulfate 0.02 g
   Sodium saccharin 0.125 g
   Methylparaben 0.2% w/v
   Propylparaben 0.02% w/v
   Citric acid 0.2 g
   2 N Sodium hydroxide solution 5.0 mL
   Flavor 5 gtt
   40% w/v sucrose qs 100 mL
   Mft susp DTD 2 oz
   Sig: 3/4 tsp po qd for infection prophylaxis for 1 month

   How many milliliters of the final suspension will be dispensed?

   A. 20 mL
   B. 30 mL
   C. 60 mL
   D. 120 mL
   E. 240 mL

9. If the specific gravity of 2 N sodium hydroxide is 1.2, how many grams of 2 N sodium hydroxide are required to complete the preparation?

   A. 3.6 g
   B. 36 g
   C. 2.5 g
   D. 25 g
   E. 0.25 g

10. If the only sucrose solution available is Syrup NF (85% sucrose), how many parts Syrup NF and water are required to make the 40% sucrose solution?

    A. 4 parts Syrup NF and 4.5 parts water
    B. 6 parts Syrup NF and 6.5 parts water
    C. 1 part Syrup NF and 5 parts water
    D. 3 parts Syrup NF and 2 parts water
    E. 5 parts Syrup NF and 1 part water

11. How many milliliters of drug product are given for each dose?

    A. 2.5 mL
    B. 3.75 mL
    C. 11.25 mL
    D. 15 mL
    E. 5 mL

12. How often is the sulfamerazine suspension intended to be administered?

    A. Once daily
    B. Twice daily
    C. Four times daily
    D. Every other day
    E. Information not given

13. How many milliliters of sodium hydroxide are needed to compound the preparation?

    A. 5 mL
    B. 3 mL
    C. 6 mL
    D. 1.5 mL
    E. 10 mL

14. If the sodium lauryl sulfate is available as a 1% stock solution, how many milliliters are needed to prepare the preparation?

    A. 1.2 mL
    B. 2.4 mL
    C. 4.8 mL
    D. 0.2 mL
    E. 5 mL

15. Example prescription order:

    Clonazepam   0.5 mg
    Suspension vehicle   qs 5 mL
    Mft: susp dtd 2 fl. oz.
    Sig: f iss at hs prn tremor

Compounding and Calculations Review

How much clonazepam, in milligrams, is needed to fill this prescription?"

16. How many fluid drams are to be given at each dosing?"

17. How many milliliters will be dispensed to the patient?"

18. When is the patient to take his medication?

19. Assuming the suspension vehicle is a 40% w/v aqueous sucrose solution, how many grams of sucrose are present in 2 dispensed orders of this prescription?

20. What is the strength of this formulation in mg/mL?

21. What is the strength of this formulation in mg/dL?

Sterile Solutions

1. Example prescription orders:

   Albuterol sulfate 1 mg/mL
   Benzalkonium chloride 0.01% w/v
   Normal saline qs 1.0 mL
   Mft nebulizer solution DTD 20 mL
   Sig: Use 2 milliliters in nebulizer tqid prn wheezing

   How many mg of albuterol sulfate is delivered in each dose?

   A.   1 mg
   B.   2 mg
   C.   4 mg
   D.   8 mg
   E.   15 mg

2. How often should this preparation be administered?

   A.   Once daily as needed
   B.   Three times daily as needed
   C.   Three to four times daily as needed
   D.   Four times daily as needed
   E.   Every 3-4 hours

3. How many milligrams of benzalkonium chloride are needed for the preparation?

   A.   2 mg
   B.   4 mg
   C.   20 mg
   D.   40 mg
   E.   200 mg

4. If benzalkonium chloride is available as a 0.1% stock solution, how many milliliters of the stock solution are needed to make the prescription?

   A.   5 mL
   B.   2 mL
   C.   4 mL
   D.   6 mL
   E.   10 mL

Ointments

1. Example prescription order:

   Hydrocortisone 0.5% w/w
   Methylparaben 0.1% w/w
   Propylparaben 0.01% w/w
   White petrolatum qs
   Mft ung DTD 10 g
   Sig: Apply to affected area qod for 1 month

   How many grams of hydrocortisone are required in the preparation?

   A.   0.05 g
   B.   0.5 g
   C.   5 g
   D.   15 g
   E.   25 g

2. If the specific gravity of the final ointment preparation is 1.1, how many milliliters would it occupy?

   A.   9.09 mL
   B.   90.9 mL
   C.   11 mL
   D.   1.1 mL
   E.   110 mL

3. How many grams of white petrolatum are required to dilute to the desired weight of 10 grams?

   A.   9.94 g
   B.   99.4 g
   C.   4.97 g
   D.   0.497 g
   E.   14.9 g

4. How many grams of methylparaben are specified in the prescription drug order?

   A.   0.1 g
   B.   0.01 g
   C.   0.2 g
   D.   0.25 g
   E.   0.5 g

5. How often must the preparation be administered?

   A.   Four times daily
   B.   Three times daily
   C.   Once daily
   D.   Every other day
   E.   Every 12 hours

6. What does the term "ung" mean in the prescription order?

   A.   Powder
   B.   Cream
   C.   Gel
   D.   Ointment
   E.   Capsule

Compounding and Calculations Review

7. Which of the following auxiliary labels should be included on the prescription label?

A. Shake well
B. For external use only
C. Not to be taken by mouth
D. All of the above
E. B and C only

8. Example prescription order:

Anhydrous lanolin 10% w/w
Cetyl esters wax 18% w/w
Yellow wax 30% w/w
Liquid petrolatum 42% w/w
Mft ung DTD 15 g
Sig: Apply to lips q 2-3 h prn chapping

How often should this preparation be administered?

A. Once daily
B. Four times daily as needed
C. Every 2 to 3 hours as needed
D. 2 to 3 times per day as needed
E. Every 8 hours

9. How many grams of anhydrous lanolin are needed for this preparation?

A. 3 g
B. 5 g
C. 1.5 g
D. 15 g
E. 30 g

10. How many grams of cetyl esters wax are needed for this preparation?

A. 27 g
B. 2.7 g
C. 18 g
D. 36 g
E. 0.27 g

11. How many grams of yellow wax are needed for this preparation?

A. 18g
B. 36g
C. 30g
D. 9g
E. 4.5g

12. How many grams of liquid petrolatum are needed for this preparation?

A. 25.2 g
B. 12.6 g
C. 6.3 g
D. 42 g
E. 21 g

13. If the specific gravity of liquid petrolatum is 0.89, how many milliliters are used in the preparation?

A. 14.2 mL
B. 7.08 mL
C. 21 mL
D. 12.6 mL
E. 0.07 mL

14. How many parts of cetyl esters wax are required in the preparation, compared to liquid petrolatum?

A. 1 part cetyl esters wax per 10 parts liquid petrolatum
B. 1 part cetyl esters wax per 4.66 parts liquid petrolatum
C. 1 part cetyl esters wax per 2.33 parts liquid petrolatum
D. 1 part cetyl esters wax per 5.6 parts liquid petrolatum
E. 1 part cetyl esters wax per 2.5 parts liquid petrolatum

15. Which of the following auxiliary labels should be included on the prescription label?

A. Shake well
B. For external use only
C. Not to be taken by mouth
D. All of the above
E. B and C only

Example prescription order:
White wax   3 g
Anhydrous lanolin   30 g
Sweet almond oil   27 g
Mft un g DTD 10 g
Sig: Apply to nails AD tid

1. You decide to compound twice the amount of ointment to be dispensed in order to account for overage. How much ointment will you be preparing in grams?

2. How many milligrams of white wax will be required to prepare twice the amount required for dispensing?

3. How many ounces (avoirdupois) of anhydrous lanolin will be required to prepare twice the amount required for dispensing?

4. The density of sweet almond oil is 0.9 g/mL. How many milliliters will be required to prepare twice the amount required for dispensing?

5. What is the percent w/w of the sweet almond oil in the dispensed amount?

6. What does the abbreviation AD stand for?

7. How many times per week may the patient use this preparation?

Compounding and Calculations Review

8. Example prescription order:

Anhydrous lanolin	10% w/w
Spermaceti	18% w/w
Yellow wax	30% w/w
Liquid petrolatum	42% w/w

Mft un g DTD 5 g

Sig: Apply to lips q 2-3 h prn chapping

How many grams of spermaceti will be present in the dispensed preparation?

9. If the density of liquid petrolatum is 0.8 g/mL, how many milliliters will be present in the dispensed preparation?

10. If the dispensed amount perfectly fills an 8 mL container, what is the density of the final preparation?

11. You receive 3 orders for this preparation and decide to prepare all of them at once as well as 3 grams extra to account for overage. How many kilo grams will you be preparing?

12. You receive 3 orders for this preparation and decide to prepare all of them at once as well as 3 grams extra to account for overage. How many milligrams of yellow wax will be needed to prepare this amount?

13. When following the sig, what is the shortest amount of time a patient may go between applications?

14. The patient uses the prescription 6 times per day and uses 1 grain of the formulation per application. How many full days will the dispensed amount last?

Pastes

1. Example prescription order:

Zinc oxide ointment 53 g
White petrolatum 17 g
Mineral oil 25 g
White Wax 5 g
Mft dtd 30 g
Sig: apply to affected area qid prn

What is the amount of zinc oxide ointment needed for the preparation?

A. 53 g
B. 15.9 g
C. 31.8 g
D. 60 g
E. 30 g

2. If zinc oxide ointment contains 20% zinc oxide and 15% mineral oil in white petrolatum, how many total grams of white petrolatum are contained in the preparation?

A. 15.44 g
B. 1.544 g

C. 154.4 g
D. 27.34 g
E. 2.734 g

3. What is the amount of white petrolatum needed for the preparation?

A. 10 g
B. 17 g
C. 34 g
D. 5.1 g
E. 10.2 g

4. If the specific gravity of mineral oil is 0.89, how many milliliters are needed for the preparation?

A. 10 mL
B. 25 mL
C. 8.4 mL
D. 28.1 mL
E. 15 mL

5. How many grams of white wax are needed for the preparation?

A. 3 g
B. 5 g
C. 1.5 g
D. 10 g
E. 15 g

6. How many parts white wax is there, compared to zinc oxide ointment?

A. 1 part white wax per 5 parts zinc oxide ointment
B. 1 part white wax per 10.6 parts zinc oxide ointment
C. 1 part white wax per 20.4 parts zinc oxide ointment
D. 1 part white wax per 15 parts zinc oxide ointment
E. 1 part white wax per 1 part zinc oxide ointment

Creams

1. Example prescription order:

Cetyl esters wax 125 g
Yellow wax 100 g
Mineral oil 560 g
Sodium borate 5 g
Water qs 1000 g
Mft: cream DTD 15 g
Sig: apply to hands q 2-3 h prn dryness

If the density of the cream is 1.1 g/mL, how many milliliters will be dispensed to the patient?

A. 0.22 mL
B. 909 mL
C. 13.6 mL
D. 20 mL
E. 30 mL

Compounding and Calculations Review

2. If a 5% sodium borate stock solution in water is available, how many milliliters are required?

   A. 2 mL
   B. 1.5 mL
   C. 3 mL
   D. 15 mL
   E. 2.5 mL

3. How often should this prescription be administered?

   A. Every 4 hours
   B. Twice daily as needed
   C. Five times daily as needed
   D. Two to three times daily as needed
   E. Every 2-3 hours as needed

4. How many grams of cetyl esters wax are required to make the product?

   A. 1.875 g
   B. 2 g
   C. 5 g
   D. 5.245 g
   E. 125 g

5. What is the amount of cetyl esters wax required, in % w/w?

   A. 5%
   B. 10%
   C. 12.5%
   D. 15%
   E. 20%

6. If the density of mineral oil is 0.89 g/mL, how many milliliters will be added to make this preparation?

   A. 8 mL
   B. 10 mL
   C. 9.4 mL
   D. 15 mL
   E. 630 mL

7. How many parts of cetyl esters wax are in the preparation?

   A. 1 part cetyl esters wax per 100 parts cream
   B. 1 part cetyl esters wax per 8 parts cream
   C. 1 part cetyl esters wax per 10 parts cream
   D. 1 part cetyl esters wax per 1 part cream
   E. 1 part cetyl esters wax per 20 parts cream

8. Example prescription order:

Shea butter	35% w/w
Mango butter	10% w/w
Yellow wax	10% w/w
Apricot oil	5% w/w
Vitamin E oil	5% w/w
Water	qs 250 g

   Mft cream DTD 30 g
   Sig: apply to hands q 2 – 4 h prn dryness

   What percent w/w of the formulation is water?

9. How many grams of shea butter will be dispensed to the patient?

10. The density of the final formulation is 0.8 g/mL. How many milliliters will be dispensed to the patient?

11. How many milliliters will the full formulation prepare if the density of the final formulation is 0.8 g/mL?

12. The density of Shea butter is 0.9 g/mL. What is the percent v/v of Shea butter in the formulation if the density of the final formulation is 0.8 g/mL?

13. Over time, a patient receives their initial prescription plus an additional 3 refills. How many grams of apricot oil have they received?

14. Over time, a patient receives her initial prescription plus an additional 3 refills. How many grains of vitamin E oil has the patient received?

Lotions

1. Example prescription order:

   Dimethicone 0.75 g
   Cetyl alcohol 1.00 g
   Petrolatum 3.00 g
   Stearic acid 4.50 g
   Mineral oil 6.00 g
   Propylparaben 0.05 g
   Glycerin 5.00 g
   TEA 1.25 g
   MgAL silicate 0.50 g
   Methylparaben 0.10 g
   Lactic acid 0.50 g
   Water qs 100 g
   Mft lotion DTD 15 g
   Sig: Apply to face bid ud. Discontinue if redness occurs.

   If the specific gravity of the final preparation is 1.2, how many milliliters will the lotion occupy?

   A. 12.5 mL
   B. 18 mL
   C. 1.25 mL
   D. 125 mL
   E . 180 mL

2. If lactic acid is available in a 25-mg/mL stock solution in water, how many milliliters of the stock solution are required?

   A. 3 mL
   B. 4 mL
   C. 3.5 mL
   D. 5 mL
   E. 10 mL

Compounding and Calculations Review

3. What percent lactic acid is included in this preparation, in w/w?

   A. 0.25%
   B. 0.5%
   C. 0.75%
   D. 1%
   E. 2%

4. How many parts of methylparaben are required compared to lactic acid?

   A. 1 part methylparaben per 2 parts lactic acid
   B. 1 part methylparaben per 4 parts lactic acid
   C. 1 part methylparaben per 10 parts lactic acid
   D. 1 part methylparaben per 5 parts lactic acid
   E. 1 part methylparaben per 20 parts lactic acid

5. If the specific gravity of mineral oil is 0.89, how many milliliters are needed for compounding this prescription drug order?

   A. 3 mL
   B. 5 mL
   C. 1.01 mL
   D. 2.37 mL
   E. 10 mL

6. Example prescription order:

Rose water	75% v/v	
Aloe vera juice	5% v/v	
Glycerin	5% v/v	
Jojoba oil	1 % v/v	
Grape seed oil		9% v/v
Soy lecithin		1% v/v
Emulsifying wax		4% v/v

   Mft lotion DTD 50 mL
   Sig: apply to hands q3-4h prn dryness

   You are preparing 3 orders of this prescription with no overage. How many mL of rose water are needed?

7. If the final preparation has a density of 0.91 g/mL how many grams will be dispensed?

8. The patient uses 2 grams per application. If the density of the formulation is 1.2 g/mL, how many full applications are dispensed to the patient?

9. How many microliters of glycerin are needed for 1 order of this prescription?

10. The amount of glycerin in this formulation weighs 3.1575 g. What is the specific gravity of glycerin?

11. What is the ratio of rose water to glycerin (smallest reduction)?

12. Assume the density of grape seed oil is 4.25 g/tsp. How many grams of grape seed oil will be needed to fill the prescription?

13. In anticipation of multiple orders for this prescription you decide to compound 400 mL of the formulation. How many mL of emulsifying wax will be needed to prepare this amount?

Gels

1. Example prescription order:

   Capsaicin 20 mg
   Methylparaben 50 mg
   Carbomer 934P 1.0 g
   Ethanol (95%) 40 mL
   Triethanolamine 4-5 gtts
   Water 60 mL
   Mft gel DTD 15 g
   Sig: Apply to hands qod prn arthritis pain

   What is the concentration of capsaicin in % w/w?

   A. 0.4%
   B. 0.133%
   C. 0.02%
   D. 0.05%
   E. 0.5%

2. If methylparaben is available as a 1.25% stock solution, in ethanol, how many milliliters are required?

   A. 5 mL
   B. 3 mL
   C. 4 mL
   D. 6 mL
   E. 8 mL

3. If the SAW on the balance used is 70 mg and a 10-mL graduated cylinder is available, which of the following procedures could be used to measure the capsaicin?

   A. Dissolve 80 mg capsaicin in 4 mL ethanol and take 2 mL of that solution to add to the preparation.
   B. Dissolve 60 mg capsaicin in 8 mL ethanol and take 3 mL of that solution to add to the preparation.
   C. Dissolve 100 mg capsaicin in 5 mL ethanol and take 3 mL of that solution to add to the preparation.
   D. Dissolve 100 mg capsaicin in 10 mL ethanol and take 2 mL of that solution to add to the preparation.
   E. Dissolve 50 mg capsaicin in 4 mL ethanol and take 0.5 mL of that solution to add to the preparation.

4. If the dropper used to add the TEA is calibrated to 20 drops/mL, how many milliliters are added if 5 drops are used?

   A. 2.5 mL
   B. 0.25 mL
   C. 4 mL
   D. 0.4 mL
   E. 25 mL

5. How often should this prescription be administered?

Compounding and Calculations Review

A. Four times daily as needed
B. Every other day as needed
C. Twice daily as needed
D. Three times daily
E. Once daily

6. Example prescription order:

   Scopolamine HBr 0.3% w/v
   Methylparaben 0.1% w/v
   Poloxamer (20% w/w) qs 10 mL
   Mft gel DTD 3 × 0.1 mL/syringe
   Sig: Apply contents of one syringe behind ear 1 h before travel ud.

   How many milligrams of scopolamine HBr are included in this preparation?

   A. 0.2 mg
   B. 1 mg
   C. 0.9 mg
   D. 0.25 mg
   E. 0.5 mg

7. If the specific gravity of the final preparation is 1.2, how many grams are applied behind the ear?

   A. 0.12 g
   B. 0.24 g
   C. 0.083 g
   D. 0.83 g
   E. 1.2 g

8. If poloxamer is available as a 30% solution, how many parts of poloxamer 30% and water are required to make the 20% poloxamer?

   A. 1 part water and 2 parts 30% poloxamer
   B. 1 part water and 3 parts 30% poloxamer
   C. 2 parts water and 5 parts 30% poloxamer
   D. 4 parts water and 2 parts 30% poloxamer
   E. 1 part water and 6 parts 30% poloxamer

9. How many milligrams of methylparaben are included in this preparation?

   A. 0.2 mg
   B. 0.4 mg
   C. 0.5 mg
   D. 0.3 mg
   E. 0.1 mg

10. What does "ud" mean, as stated in the patient directions?

    A. Both ears
    B. The left ear
    C. As directed
    D. Before lunch
    E. After dinner

11. Example prescription order:

    Lidocaine   4% w/v
    Methylparaben   25 mg

Propylparaben   2.5 mg
Carbomer 934P   0.5 g
Ethanol (95%)   20 mL
Triethanolamine   2–5 gtts
Water   30 mL
Mft gel
Sig: Apply to burns tid prn pain

Assuming the final volume is equal to that of the ethanol and water combined, how much lidocaine in grams is required to prepare this formulation?

12. The methylparaben and propylparaben come in a single ethanolic stock solution at a concentration of 12.5 mg/ mL methylparaben and 1.25 mg/ mL propylparaben. How many microliters of this stock solution are required to prepare this formulation?

13. The methylparaben and propylparaben come in a single ethanolic stock solution at a concentration of 12.5 mg/ mL methylparaben and 1.25 mg/mL propylparaben. How many additional mL of 95% ethanol will be required to prepare this formulation?

14. The dropper used to dispense the triethanolamine was calibrated such that 20 drops filled a 10 mL graduated cylinder to the 4 mL mark. If 4 drops are used to gel the formulation, how many mL will have been added?

15. The density of ethanol is 0.789 g/mL and that of water is 1 g/ mL. What is their combined weight, in grams, in this preparation?

16. If the patient uses 3.5% of their prescription during each application, how many full days will the prescription last?

17. How many parts methylparaben are required per part propylparaben?

Aqueous Nasal Sprays

1. Example prescription order:
   Dihydroergotamine mesylate 0.25 g
   Ethanol, 95% 2.00 mL
   Glycerin 5.00 mL
   Methylparaben 0.20 g
   Sterile water for injection qs 100 mL
   Mft metered nasal spray DTD 30 mL
   Sig: sprays 2 each nostril qd

   If ethanol is available in 100% and 50% solutions, how many milliliters of 50% ethanol solution must be mixed with 100% ethanol to make 1 L of the 95% ethanol?

   A. 100 mL
   B. 900 mL
   C. 300 mL
   D. 250 mL
   E. 500 mL

2. Methylparaben is available as a 3% stock solution in ethanol, how many milliliters are needed to complete the preparation?

    A. 2 mL
    B. 5 mL
    C. 2.4 mL
    D. 1 mL
    E. 8 mL

3. What is the percentage of dihydroergotamine, in w/v?

    A. 0.3%
    B. 0.2%
    C. 0.25%
    D. 0.15%
    E. 0.10%

4. If the density of glycerin is 0.92, how many grams of glycerin will be needed for this preparation?

    A. 1.38 g
    B. 1.4 g
    C. 3 g
    D. 2.5 g
    E. 2 g

5. If after 10 sprays using the nasal pump there is a loss in weight of 2.5 mg, what is the dose delivered through the valve (DDV), in mL (assuming a specific gravity of 1)?

    A. 25 mL
    B. 2.5 mL
    C. 0.25 mL
    D. 250 mL
    E. 0.025 mL

6. Using the DDV calculated in the question above (#5), how many mg of Dihydroergotamine mesylate are delivered with each dose?

    A. 0.01875 mg
    B. 1.875 mg
    C. 0.1875 mg
    D. 62.5 mg
    E. 0.0625 mg

7. Morphine sulfate 200 mg

    Naltrexone 2 mg

    0.9% sodium chloride injection qs 100 mL

    Nft: Nasal spray 20 mL

    Sig: 1 actuation each nostril q4h prn pain

    Before compounding the above prescription, 20 mL of water was added to the aqueous pump and primed. The weight of the primed nasal spray was 30 g. After 10 actuations of the nasal spray, the weight was 28.4 g. Based on this information, what is the dose of morphine delivered through the valve (density of water is 1)?

    A. 3.2 mg/actuation
    B. 320 mcg/actuation

    C. 640 mcg/actuation
    D. 32 mg/actuation
    E. 460 mcg/actuation

8. Before compounding of the above prescription, 20 mL of ethanol (density is 0.8 g/mL) was added to the aqueous pump and primed. The weight of the primed nasal spray was 30 g. After 10 actuations of the nasal spray, the weight was 29.1 g. Based on this information, what is the dose of naltrexone delivered through the valve?

    A. 2.25 mcg/actuation
    B. 2.25 mg/actuation
    C. 1.8 mcg/actuation
    D. 1.8 mg/actuation
    E. 225 mcg/actuation

9. Assuming that the volume of water delivered through the valve is 115 μL, what is the maximum dose of morphine that is delivered per day?

    A. 27.6 mg
    B. 2.76 mg
    C. 276 mcg
    D. 27.6 mcg
    E. 2.76 mcg

10. Example prescription order:

Oxymetazoline HCl	0.05% w/v
Ethanol (95%)	2% v/v
Glycerin	5% v/v
Methylparaben	0.1 % w/v
Sterile water for injection	qs 100 mL

    Mft metered nasal spray DTD 20 mL

    Sig: sprays 2 each nostril q 12 h prn nasal congestion. Discontinue if bleeding occurs.

    The density of ethanol is 0.789 g/mL. How many grams of ethanol will be used to prepare the formulation?

11. How many teaspoons of glycerin are needed for this formulation?

12. How many milligrams of oxymetazoline HCl will be used to prepare this formulation?

13. How many milligrams of oxymetazoline HCl will be dispensed to the patient?

14. How many micro grams of methylparaben are required to prepare this formulation?

15. If the methylparaben comes in a stock solution with a concentration of 20 mg/mL, how many mL are needed for the preparation?

16. Each spray emits 0.25 mL of the formulation. How many milligrams of oxymetazoline HCl is the patient receiving per dose?

Compounding and Calculations Review

17. Ethanol is available to you only as a 100% solution. How many mL of water are required to prepare 250 mL of 95% ethanol (assume no volume contraction)?

Rectal Suppositories

1. Example prescription order:

   Benzocaine 50 mg
   Menthol 20 mg
   Resorcin 10 mg
   Zinc oxide 300 mg
   Witepsol H35 qs 100%
   Mft: sup DTD VI
   Sig: 1 sup pr q 8 h prn hemorrhoid pain

   How often should the suppositories be administered?

   A. Every 4-6 hours as needed
   B. Every 8 hours as needed
   C. Four times per day
   D. As needed
   E. Every 6 hours as needed

2. If the SAW on the balance used is 100 mg, which of the following procedures could be used to measure the resorcin, assuming a two-suppository overage?

   A. Measure 100 mg resorcin and geometrically dilute to 200 mg with zinc oxide. Remove 120 mg of the mixture that contains 80 mg resorcin.
   B. Measure 90 mg resorcin and geometrically dilute to 180 mg zinc oxide. Remove 160 mg of the mixture that contains 80 mg resorcin.
   C. Measure 500 mg resorcin and geometrically dilute to 1000 mg with zinc oxide. Remove 250 mg of the mixture that contains 80 mg resorcin.
   D. Measure 50 mg resorcin and geometrically dilute to 200 mg with zinc oxide. Remove 10 mg of the mixture that contains 80 mg resorcin.
   E. Measure 60 mg resorcin and geometrically dilute to 300 mg with zinc oxide. Remove 150 mg of the mixture that contains 80 mg resorcin.

3. If the suppository mold used held 3 mL and the specific gravity of the molten mixture is 1.1, how many grams of Witepsol are required, assuming a two-suppository overage?

   A. 17.52 g
   B. 1.752 g
   C. 23.36 g
   D. 0.2336 g
   E. 2336 g

4. How many milligrams of benzocaine are required to fill this preparation assuming a two-suppository overage?

   A. 100 mg
   B. 200 mg
   C. 300 mg
   D. 400 mg
   E. 500 mg

5. How many grams of Witepsol are required to fill this prescription if each suppository weighs 2 grams and assuming no suppository overage?

   A. 6.48 grams
   B. 5.236 grams
   C. 2.35 grams
   D. 4.5 grams
   E. 8 grams

6. Example prescription order:

   Sumatriptan   25 mg
   Cocoa butter   QS 100%
   Mft: sup dtd #4
   Sig: i sup pr q 4-6 h prn migraine

   Each suppository mold holds 2 grams of the prepared formulation. How much cocoa butter, in milligrams, is required to prepare the 4 suppositories?

7. Each suppository mold holds 2 grams of the prepared formulation. What is the percent w/w of sumatriptan in each suppository?

8. If the density of cocoa butter is 0.9 g/mL, what volume, in milliliters, of preparation will be added to each suppository mold, which can hold 2 g of material? Assume sumatriptan does not influence the density.

9. If the density of cocoa butter is 0.9 g/ml, what volume, in fluid drams, of preparation will be added to each suppository mold, if each mold can hold 2 g?

10. How many grains of sumatriptan are required to fill this prescription if preparing 2 suppositories overage?

Vaginal Suppositories

1. Example prescription order:

   Metronidazole 40 mg
   Water 5%
   PEG base qs 100%
   Mft: sup DTD #4
   Sig: sup 1 pv qhs for infection

   What will be the total quantity of material needed if the mold makes suppositories that weigh 2 grams each (assume no overage)?

   A. 10 grams
   B. 7 grams
   C. 8 grams
   D. 6 grams
   E. 4 grams

2. When should the patient administer this medication?

   A. In the morning before breakfast
   B. Twice daily
   C. After dinner

D. At bedtime

E. Before lunchtime

3. What will be the total amount of PEG base needed for this prescription, if each suppository weighs 2 grams (assume no overage)?

   A. 7.44 grams

   B. 5.36 grams

   C. 6.34 grams

   D. 10.25 grams

   E. 11.34 grams

4. How many mL of water are needed for each suppository?

   A. 3 mL

   B. 5 mL

   C. 0.1 mL

   D. 3.2 mL

   E. 4.5 mL

Compounding and Calculations Review

Basic Principles of Pharmaceutical Calculations

The Metric System

The most widely used units of measure comprise the metric system. It is fundamental in all aspects of pharmacy, from production to dispensing. By convention, the metric system allows for interconversion between units by a factor of 10 (see Table 1). For example, 1 meter is 1/10 as large as 1 dekameter. The basic units of length, weight and volume are meters, grams, and liters, respectively. The multiples of these basic units are denoted by the addition of a prefix and are outlined in Table 1.

Table 1. The Metric System Convention

Prefix	Factor × Basic Unit
pico	10^{-12}
nano	10^{-9}
micro	10^{-6}
milli	10^{3}
centi	10^{-2}
deci	10^{-1}
deka	10^{1}
hecto	10^{2}
kilo	10^{3}

To convert grams to picograms, one would divide the value in grams by 10–12 grams. For example:

Example: Convert 3.65 grams to picograms.

Answer: 3.65 grams x 1 picogram/10^{-12} grams = 3.65 x 10^{12} picograms

Apothecaries

Common Systems

Although the metric system is the official system for weights and measures as stated in the United States Pharmacopoeia and National Formulary (USP/NF), the common systems of measurement are still used in pharmacy, and therefore should be recognized. Typically, suppliers and manufacturers of substances that are sold to individual pharmacies or pharmaceutical manufacturers use the avoirdupois system of measurement. Pharmacists when dispensing medications use the apothecaries' system.

Table 2. Apothecaries Fluid Measure

	Gallon (gal)	Quart (qt)	Pint (pt)	Fluid Ounce	Fluid Dram	Minim
Gallon	1	4	8	128	1024	61440
Quart		1	2	32	256	15360
Pint			1	16	128	7680
Fluid ounce				1	8	480
Fluid dram					1	60
Minim						1

Table 3. Apothecaries Weight Measure

	Pound(lb)	Ounce	Dram	Scruple	Grain (gr)
Pound(lb)	1	12	96	288	5760
Ounce		1	8	24	480
Dram			1	3	60
Scruple				1	20
Grain(gr)					1

Compounding and Calculations Review

Avoirdupois

Table 4. Avoirdupois System

Units of Weight	Pound (lb)	Ounce (oz)	Grain (gr)
Pound (lb)	1	16	7000
Ounce (oz)		1	437.5
Grain (gr)			1

Conversion Between Systems

Table 5. Conversion Between Systems

Volume:

mL =	16.23 minums
1 minum =	0.06 mL
1 fluid dram =	3.69 mL
1 fluid ounce =	29.57 mL
1 pt =	473 mL
1 gallon =	3785 mL

Weight:

g =	15.432 grains
1 kg =	2.20 lb (avoir.)
1 grain =	0.065 g or 65 mg
1 oz (avoir.) =	28.35 g
1 ounce (apothecary) =	31.1 g
1 lb (avoir.) =	454 g
1 lb (apoth.) =	373.2 g

Other:

oz (avoir.) =	437.5 gr
1 ounce (apoth.) =	480 gr
1 gallon =	128 fluid ounces

Density, Specific Gravity, and Specific Volume

Density

The density of a substance is its mass per unit volume, or the weight of a material required to fill a specific volume at a specific temperature. At 4°C the density of water is one, meaning there is 1 g for every milliliter of water. All other densities are based on this convention, using water as a reference point. To find the density of other substances, one would need to find what volume is taken up by a known mass of that substance and divide that mass by its volume. For example:

Example: Find the density of ethanol if 100 mL weighs 78.9 g
Answer: Density = 78.9 g/100 mL = 0.789 g/mL

Specific Gravity

The specific gravity of a substance is the ratio of its weight to the weight of a standard at a specific temperature, which is water for liquid and solid substances. The specific gravity may be calculated by dividing the weight of a substance by the weight of an equal amount of water. When given a specific gravity, it is assumed that it is in relation to water. For example:

Example: What is the specific gravity of 10 mL of ethanol that weighs 7.89 g and if 10 mL of water weighs 10 g?
Answer: Specific Gravity = 7.89/10 g = 0.789

Compounding and Calculations Review

Specific Volume

Unlike specific gravity, which is a ratio of weights of equal volume, specific volume is a ratio of volumes of equal weight at a specific temperature. Similar to specific gravity, water is used as the standard for liquids and solids. The specific volume is found by dividing the volume of a substance by the volume of water of an equal weight. For example:

Example: What is the specific volume of 10 g ethanol that has a volume of 12.67 mL?

Answer: Specific volume = 12.67 mL/10 mL = 1.267

Basic Pharmaceutical Calculations

Ratios

A ratio is the relation of two quantities expressed as the quotient of one divided by the other. Therefore, the ratio of 4 capsules to 5 capsules is 4/5, which is typically written as 4:5 to show the relationship as a ratio rather than a fraction. The ratio of 4 capsules to 2 capsules or 4/2 does not equal 2. Solvable fractions are left in the ratio form to show that it is a relationship, or operation, rather than a true fraction. However, ratios can be reduced, such that 4/2 equals 2/1 or 2:1.

Proportions

A proportion is a statement of equality between two ratios, typically written in one of the following ways:

a/b = c/d
a:b = c:d
a:b :: c:d

The proportions are read a is to b as c is to d, where a and d are known as the extremes and b and c are the means. The product of the means equals the product of the extremes, which allows one to find a missing term by algebraic means. The following example illustrates this point.

Example: If 6 liters of a sodium chloride solution contain 5 grams of sodium chloride, how many liters will contain 2 grams of sodium chloride?

Answer: 5 grams/6 liters = 2 grams/X liters, therefore, (2 grams)(6 liters)/5 grams = X liters = 2.4 liters

Aliquots

When the amount required for a prescription or compound exceeds the limit of precision for a measuring instrument or is below the smallest amount measurable, the method of aliquoting can be used to precisely weigh out and dispense the correct dose. The aliquot method involves weighing or measuring an amount above the smallest amount measurable and then diluting it down so as to achieve a measurable dilution containing the correct amount of drug.

Aliquots Involving Solid Dispersions

The following procedure can be used to satisfy the aliquot method:

1. First calculate the desired dilution by setting up a ratio as follows:

    a/c = b/d
    where:
    a = the amount of substance needed
    b = the smallest amount weighable (SAW)
    c = a × some multiple in order to get above the smallest amount weighable
    d = b × the same multiple in c

2. From this you will know that a is the amount needed and b is the amount weighed out. Then dilute b down to d and measure out c. The amount measured in c will contain the desired amount (a).

Example: How would you measure 30 mg of chlorpheniramine maleate (SAW for the balance you are using is 70 mg), and then dilute to 20 g with lactose?

Answer: 30 mg (amount needed)/90 mg (30 mg x 3)=70 mg (SAW)/210 mg (70 mg x 3)

Compounding and Calculations Review

Weigh out 70 mg of chlorpheniramine maleate, then dilute with lactose to 210 mg by geometrically mixing with 140 mg of lactose (210 mg–70 mg). From this dilution, measure out 90 mg of the powder, which contains 30 mg of chlorpheniramine maleate (the amount desired). To complete the question, dilute that to 20 g by adding 19.910 g lactose (20,000 mg–90 mg).

Aliquots Involving Solid-in-Liquid Dispersions

Aliquoting a solid using a liquid as the diluent requires that the solubility of the solid in that liquid be known. Because we must measure an amount greater than the SAW for the balance or measuring device used, the quantity of liquid used to dilute the solid must be sufficient to completely solubilize the drug. Furthermore, when using a graduated cylinder, there is also a limit of sensitivity for that measuring device. As a general rule, graduated cylinders can accurately measure volumes equal to 20% or greater than the total volume of the container. For example, a 50-mL graduated cylinder can accurately measure 10 mL or greater in volume. The following example shows one method for achieving a proper aliquot of a solid diluted with a liquid.

Example: Prepare the following prescription if the solubility of theophylline is 25 mg/mL and the SAW of the balance is 70 mg.

> Theophylline 50 mg
> Water qs 100 mL

Answer: First, measure enough theophylline to be above the SAW for the balance. This is achieved by measuring 100 mg. Since the solubility of theophylline is 25 mg/mL, use enough water to dilute the 100 mg of theophylline to be below this solubility limit, which could be 4 mL or more of water. So, the procedure is:

1. Weigh out 100 mg of theophylline
2. Dissolve in 4 mL of water
3. Take from this dispersion 2 mL, which will contain the desired 50 mg of theophylline. Note: use a 10-mL graduated cylinder to measure this volume.
4. Qs to 100 mL with water to complete the prescription.

The procedure for liquid-in-liquid dispersions is similar and requires knowing the miscibility of the two liquids used.

Dimensional Analysis

For most conversions or calculations involving units, the method of dimensional analysis is a useful tool for keeping track of the units involved in order to ensure proper calculations. This method involves setting up a calculation such that all of the units cancel except for the desired unit for the given calculation.

Example: Convert 50 μg/mL to g/L using dimensional analysis.

Answer: (50 μg/1 mL) x (1000 mL/1 L) x (1 mg/1000 μg) x (1 g/1000 mg) = 0.05 g/L

In this example, all of the units are canceled except for the grams and liters, which proves that the answer calculated is the correct conversion, assuming the ratios used are correct.

Dosage Calculations

When calculating doses for a patient, it is important to take into account the age, weight, sex, and surface area of the individual, as well as the delivery device. Various equations have been designed for calculating dosages based on age, weight, and body surface area.

Dosage Adjustment for Pediatric Patients

Because the pharmacokinetics and pharmacodynamics of medications delivered to pediatric patients differs from that of adults, the dose must be adjusted. Several equations have been developed to take into account the patient's age and/or weight in determining dosage adjustments.

Young's Rule: (Age/(age + 12)) x adult dose = dose for child

Cowling's Rule: (Age at next birthday (in years) x adult dose) /24 = dose for child

Fried's Rule for Infants: (Age (in months)/150) x adult dose = dose for child

Clark's Rule: (Weight (in lb)/150 (average weight of adults in lb)) x adult dose = dose for child

Dosage Adjustment Based on Body Weight

For drugs in which weight influences efficacy or toxicity, the dose must be adjusted for patients who do not meet the average adult weight of 70 kg. Typically, doses involving these drugs are on a per kg basis, such as 150 μg/kg. If the patient's weight is

Compounding and Calculations Review

given in lb, it must be converted to kilograms and the amount calculated from the given dose per kg. This convention is commonly used, especially for potent or toxic drugs that have a narrow therapeutic index, and is the most common dosing method.

Dosage Adjustment Based on Body Surface Area

Determination of body surface area (BSA) is more precise for dosage adjustments compared to adjustments based on age and body weight. Because several factors can effect the weight of a patient, it is more desirable to calculate a dose based on surface area rather than weight alone. For example, a 300-lb, 6-foot-tall male body builder would have significantly different drug distribution and pharmacokinetics when compared to a 300-lb, 5-foot-tall obese patient, which would be reflected in the surface area calculations. The most widely used nomogram for the calculation of surface area is shown in Figures 1 and 2, which take into account both weight and height.

Body Surface of Adults

Nomogram for determination of body surface from height and mass[1]

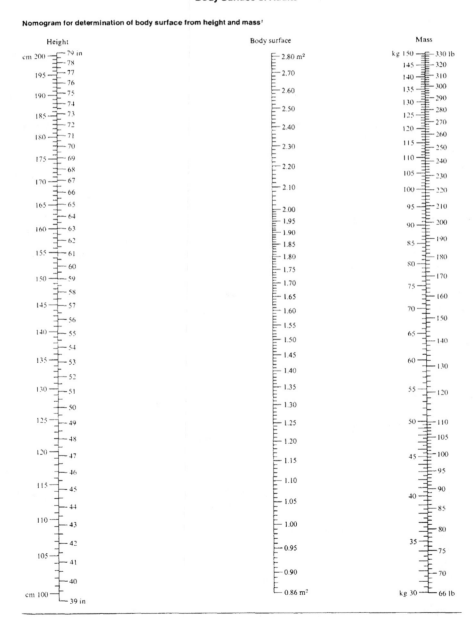

[1] From the formula of Du Bois and Du Bois, *Arch. intern. Med.*, **17**, 863 (1916): $S = M^{0.425} \times H^{0.725} \times 71.84$, or $\log S = \log M \times 0.425 + \log H \times 0.725 + 1.8564$ (S: body surface in cm^2, M: mass in kg, H: height in cm).

Figure 1. Body surface area nomogram for adults, from Geigy Scientific Tables, Eighth Edition, Vol. 1, C. Lentener (1981).

Compounding and Calculations Review

Body Surface of Children

Nomogram for determination of body surface from height and mass[1]

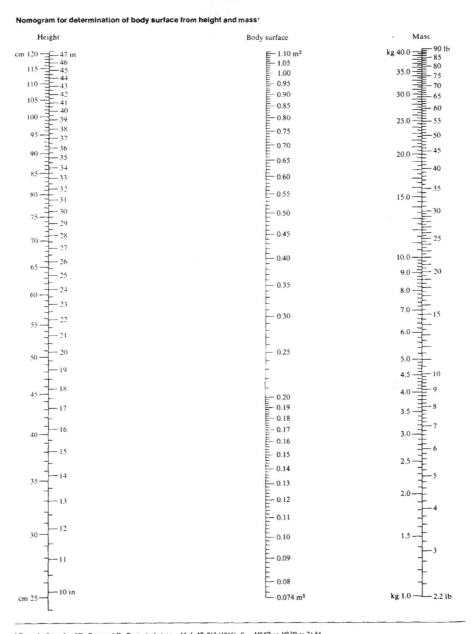

[1] From the formula of Du Bois and Du Bois, *Arch. intern. Med.*, **17**, 863 (1916): $S = M^{0.425} \times H^{0.725} \times 71.84$, or $\log S = \log M \times 0.425 + \log H \times 0.725 + 1.8564$ (*S*: body surface in cm², *M*: mass in kg, *H*: height in cm).

Figure 2. Body surface area nomogram for children, from Geigy Scientific Tables, Eighth Edition, Vol. 1, C. Lentener (1981).

Drawing a straight line from the known height to the known weight intersects the surface area column at the estimated surface area for that patient. Once the surface area is known, the following equation can be used to adjust the dose of a potent medication, based on the average adult surface area:

(BSA of patient (m²)/1.73 m² (average adult BSA)) x adult dose = approximate dose for the patient

Compounding and Calculations Review

Dosage Calculations Involving Various Delivery Devices

For the most part, directions for administration of medications to patients are given in a manner relative to the ability of the patient to understand. This is typically achieved by using tablespoons (tb) or teaspoons (tsp) for liquid preparations. One tablespoon corresponds to 15 mL, whereas one teaspoon corresponds to 5 mL. The accepted general practice is that the direction should be written in either tablespoons or teaspoons for ease of administration unless a measuring device is supplied to the patient for milliliter doses.

Example: How many teaspoons would the patient take if the prescription calls for 10 mL?
Answer: 10 mL x (1 tsp/5 mL) = 2 tsp

So, the directions are written so that the patient administers 2 teaspoonfuls per dose, rather than 10 mL.

Many times, pediatric patients receive prescriptions involving a certain number of drops per dose. For these prescriptions, a calibrated dropper is supplied and the number of drops/mL is known or determined such that the desired dose can be accurately administered. Although there are variations between droppers, most commercially available droppers are calibrated to deliver 20 drops of water per milliliter. Because water is not always used as the diluent and if the number of drops per milliliter is unknown, the pharmacist should determine the actual number of drops per milliliter for that given liquid prior to dispensing. A dropper can be calibrated by counting the number of drops needed to fill a given volume.

Example: If a pharmacist counted 30 drops of a medication while filling a 10-mL graduated cylinder to the 3-mL mark, how many drops per milliliter does this dropper dispense?
Answer: (30 drops/3 mL) = (x drops/1 mL) = 10 drops/mL

Example: If the prescription called for 0.8 mL of the drug product to be dispensed per dose, how many drops should be specified on the prescription label?
Answer: 0.8 mL x (10 drops/1 mL) = 8 drops

Concentration

Percentage of Strength

Many of the pharmaceutical preparations that are encountered during compounding or dispensing involve the use of percentages. The percentage sign (%) represents a ratio of 1 part of a substance to 100 parts of another substance or of the mixture. For example, in a 1% liquid preparation, this corresponds to 1 g of solute in 100 grams of total mixture, which in most cases is 1 gram per 100 mL of total mixture. There are three ways to express percentage strength, depending on the components.

Percent Weight-in-Volume (% w/v)

This corresponds to 1 gram of solute in 100 mL of total solution (solute and solvent) or the total volume regardless of the solvent type. In some instances, the term mg% is used to denote the number of milligrams of solute in 100 mL of total solution.

Example: What is the percentage strength w/v of 2.5 grams of a substance contained in 400 mL of an aqueous solution?
Answer: (2.5 g/400 mL) = (X g/100 mL) = 0.625% w/v

Percent Volume-in-Volume (% v/v)

This corresponds to the number of milliliters of liquid solute in 100 mL of the total volume (solute and solvent) of the preparation.

Example: What is the percentage strength v/v of 10 milliliters of a substance contained in 1000 mL of an aqueous solution?
Answer: (10 mL/1000 mL) = (X mL/100 mL) = 1% v/v

Percent Weight-in-Weight (% w/w)

This corresponds to the number of grams of solute or drug in 100 grams of the total weight (solute and diluent) of the preparation.

Example: What is the percentage strength w/w of 15 grams of a substance contained in 500 mg of a solid dispersion?
Answer: (15 g/500 g) = (X g/100 g) = 3% w/w

Compounding and Calculations Review

Ratio Strength

Ratio strength is a method of expressing concentration in the form of a ratio and is typically used to express concentration of dilute solutions or liquid preparations. Much like the percentage strength designations, the ratio strength is the ratio of parts of solute contained in some parts of a solvent or total mixture. For example, 2 parts of chlorpheniramine maleate contained in 100 parts of total solution is ratio strength and is written as 2:100. The first term is reduced to 1 such that the ratio in the previous example is 1:50 or 1 part chlorpheniramine maleate to 50 parts total solution. If the parts are liquid then one would use milliliters. Likewise, one would use grams for solid materials. So, in the previous example, the ratio 1:50 would be 1 gram of chlorpheniramine maleate contained in 50 mL of the total solution.

Dilutions

Dilutions involve taking a liquid or solid solution or dispersion of a known concentration and reducing the strength or concentration by adding a diluent of a known volume or weight. When making dilutions, it is easiest to convert ratio strength to percentage strength in order to perform the calculations. Dilutions of liquids, solids, alcoholic solutions, and the method of alligation will be discussed.

Dilution of Liquids and Solids

There are two methods to calculate the percentage strength of a diluted solution for both liquids and solids. The following examples illustrate dilution of liquids and solids.

Example: What is the percentage strength if 250 mL of a 5% (w/v) ciprofloxacin IV solution is diluted to 1 liter?

Answer:

> Method 1: Set up the proportion:
>
> (Initial quantity) x (initial concentration) = (final quantity) x (final concentration)
>
> (250 mL) x (5%) = (1000 mL) x (X %)
>
> X = 1.25% (w/v)
>
> Method 2: Knowing the quantity of dissolved solute, calculate the new concentration:
>
> From the question, 5 g are dissolved per 100 mL of solution. So, for 250 mL, there are 12.5 g of ciprofloxacin. Set up the following ratio:
>
> 12.5 g/1000 mL = X/100 mL
>
> X = 1.25 or 1.25% (w/v)

Example: What is the volume needed to dilute 300 mL of a 10% (w/v) lidocaine HCl solution in order to make a 2% solution?

Answer: (300 mL) x (10%) = (X mL) x (2%)

X = 1500 mL

Dilution of Alcohol

When water is used as a diluent for alcoholic solutions, there is an appreciable contraction in the volume. This complicates the methods previously described for the dilution of liquids. The same proportion method can be used. However, after calculating the final volume needed or the amount of water to add, one must qs to that amount rather than add the calculated volume of water. The following example illustrates this point.

Example: How many milliliters of water are needed to dilute 200 mL of 95% (v/v) ethanol to make a final concentration of 38%?

Answer: (200 mL) x (95%) = (X mL) x (38%)

X = 500 mL total solution

Therefore, use 200 mL of 95% (v/v) ethanol and enough water to make 500 mL.

Alligations

The method of alligation is used when solutions of different concentrations are mixed. The calculations allow one to make a solution of a given concentration or to find the concentration of the final mixture, each of which is calculated somewhat differently.

Finding the concentration of a mixture:

> This method is used when mixing two or more solutions of varying concentrations and known volumes, in order to determine the final concentration.

Compounding and Calculations Review

Example: What is the concentration of sodium chloride in percent strength of a mixture of 200 mL of 20% (w/v) sodium chloride, 300 mL of 15% (w/v) sodium chloride, and 400 mL of 30% sodium chloride?

Answer:

20 x 200 4000
15 x 300 4500
30 x 400 12000 +
Total: 900 20500 ÷ 900 mL = 22.8%

Making a solution of a known dilution with two or more solutions of known concentrations:

This type of alligation is termed alligation alternate and it allows one to calculate the relative number of parts of two or more components of known concentrations that can be mixed to form the desired dilution. The concentration of the desired solution must lie between the concentrations of the available solutions, meaning that it must be stronger than its weakest component and weaker than its strongest component. The following example illustrates this method.

Example: How much 15% dextrose and 2% dextrose solutions are needed to make a 5% dextrose solution?

Answer: To solve this problem, a ratio is set up between the known components and the difference between the known components and the desired mixture is calculated to form the final ratio to be mixed, as follows:

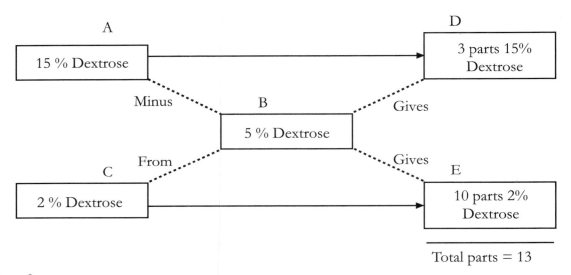

Figure 3.

In other words, % solution A minus % solution B (desired concentration) equals number of parts of solution C, which is given in E; and % solution B (desired concentration) minus % solution C equals number of parts of solution A, which is given in D. So, in this example, mixing 3 parts of the 15% dextrose solution and 10 parts of the 2% dextrose solution will make 13 parts of 5% dextrose solution.

Milliequivalents and Normality

Earlier in this chapter the units for concentration of solute dissolved in an aqueous solution were discussed. For the most part, the units of concentration are grams per liter or % (w/v). However, in the United States, solutions of electrolytes are almost exclusively discussed as milliequivalents (mEq). This unit of measure takes into account the chemical potential of the electrolyte solution and is related to the total number of ionic charges in solution. The normality of a solution is the number of equivalents per liter of solution. In order to convert from the unit of weight to the unit of mEq, the valence and molecular weight of the ionic substance must be known. The equation used for conversion is as follows:

mEq = (mg x valence)/MW and mg = (mEq x MW)/valence

Example: How many mEq of potassium are in 1 liter of a 1% (w/v) KCl solution?

Answer: Molecular weight of KCl = 74.5

mg of KCl = 1000 mL x (1 g/100 mL) x (1000 mg/1 g) = 10,000 mg

mEq = (10,000 mg x 1)/74.5 = 134.23 mEq KCl

Compounding and Calculations Review

Milliosmoles

For intravenous preparations, the osmotic pressure exerted by the solution is important for determining what effect it will have on biological membranes. The osmotic pressure is proportional to the total number of particles in solution. This is termed the osmolarity of the solution and has the unit of milliosmoles (mOsm). For non-electrolytes, 1 mmol of the substance corresponds to 1 mOsm. However, for electrolyte solutions, the degree of dissociation becomes important in calculating the total number of species in solution. Because of this, the calculated values of osmolarity may differ slightly from experimentally determined values. The osmolarity can be calculated using the following equation:

mOsm/L = (weight of substance (g/L)/MW(g)) x number of species x 1000

Example: If a 2-liter solution contains 3 grams of KCl, what does this correspond to in mOsm/L?

Answer: ((3 g/2 L)/74.5 g) x 2 (K and Cl) x 1000 = 40.3 mOsm/L

The term osmolality is occasionally used to describe the concentration of species in solution. Osmolality represents the number of mOsm per kilogram of solvent, versus per liter of solvent in the case of osmolarity. When using osmolality, the solvent must be weighed unless it is water, which has a specific gravity of 1. The equation used for osmolarity is applicable to osmolality, but rather than using g/L,

Tonicity

The tonicity of a solution is related to the osmotic pressure of the solution and how that pressure relates to the bodily fluids to which the solution is being compared. Solutions with equal osmolarities are termed iso-osmotic, while solutions that have the same osmolarities as body fluids to which they are being compared are termed isotonic. The tonicity or degree of difference between the osmolarities is a significant factor in the distribution of water between physiological membranes. When cells are exposed to hypertonic solutions, water will diffuse out of the cell according to the principle of osmosis and likewise, hypotonic solutions will cause the cell to swell as water diffuses into the cell. For most applications, 0.9% (w/v) sodium chloride is considered isotonic. For calculations involving other species, a sodium chloride equivalent is used to relate the tonicity of the other species to the tonicity of sodium chloride. For example, lidocaine HCl has a sodium chloride equivalent equal to 0.22, so 1 gram of lidocaine HCl exhibits the same tonicity as 0.22 g of sodium chloride in solution. This relationship allows for the calculation of isotonic solutions comprising various species. If a drug is added to the solution, the sodium chloride equivalent can be calculated and subtracted from the amount of tonicity adjusting agent (typically sodium chloride or dextrose) required to make an isotonic solution.

Example: How many grams of sodium chloride are required to make the following prescription?

Lidocaine HCl 100 mg

Purified water qs 100 mL

Sodium chloride qs to make an isotonic solution

Answer:

1. Calculate the sodium chloride equivalent for the lidocaine HCl (Table 2 gives the sodium chloride equivalent for lidocaine HCl):

Table 2. Sodium Chloride Equivalents

Substance	Molecular Weight	Ions	i	Sodium Chloride Equivalent
Atropine sulfate	695	3	2.6	0.12
Benzalkonium chloride	360	2	1.8	0.16
Boric Acid	61.8	1	1.0	0.52
Cocaine hydrochloride	340	2	1.8	0.16
Dextrose	180	1	1.0	0.18
Ephedrine hydrochloride	202	2	1.8	0.29
Glycerin	92	1	1.0	0.34
Lidocaine hydrochloride	289	2	1.8	0.22
Mannitol	182	1	1.0	0.18
Phenobarbital sodium	254	2	1.8	0.24
Phenylephrine hydrochloride	204	2	1.8	0.32
Pilocarpine hydrochloride	245	2	1.8	0.24
Potassium chloride	74.5	2	1.8	0.76

Table 2. Sodium Chloride Equivalents (cont'd)

Substance	Molecular Weight	Ions	i	Sodium Chloride Equivalent
Potassium penicillin G	372	2	1.8	0.18
Sodium chloride	58	2	1.8	1.00
Sodium iodide	150	2	1.8	0.39
Tetracaine hydrochloride	301	2	1.8	0.18
Tobramycin	468	1	1.0	0.07
Urea	60	1	1.0	0.59
Zinc chloride	136	3	2.6	0.62

Sodium chloride equivalent = 0.22×100 mg = 22 mg NaCl

2. Calculate the total amount of sodium chloride needed to make the solution isotonic:

$0.9\% = (0.9$ g/100 mL$) \times 100$ mL = 0.9 g or 900 mg

3. Subtract the lidocaine HCl sodium chloride equivalent from the total amount of sodium chloride needed to make the solution isotonic:

900 mg - 22 mg = 878 mg NaCl that must be added to the prescription to make it isotonic

Compounding and Calculations Review

Questions

Basic Principles of Pharmaceutical Calculations

1. Convert 1.45 mg to picograms.

    A. 1.45 picograms
    B. 1.45×10^{-4} picograms
    C. 3.45×10^{-7} picograms
    D. 1.45×10^{-9} picograms
    E. 1.45×10^{9} picograms

2. How many fluid ounces are contained in 5 quarts?

    A. 1.6 fluid ounces
    B. 16 fluid ounces
    C. 160 fluid ounces
    D. 1600 fluid ounces
    E. 0.16 fluid ounces

3. If a bulk powder purchased by a pharmacist weighs 3 lb, what is its corresponding weight in grains?

    A. 2.1×10^{4} gr
    B. 2.1×10^{3} gr
    C. 2.1×10^{2} gr
    D. 2.1×10^{-4} gr
    E. 2.1×10^{-3} gr

4. If a prescription calls for 2.5 mg/kg and the patient weighs 110 lb, what is the dose to be delivered for this patient?

    A. 75 mg
    B. 700 mg
    C. 125 mg
    D. 2.5 mg
    E. 25.2 mg

5. Substance A is poured into a graduated cylinder to the 100-mL mark and then weighed. What will the density be if the weight was 94 g for the 100 mL?

    A. 0.25 g/mL
    B. 0.5 g/mL
    C. 1.06 g/mL
    D. 0.94 g/mL
    E. 9.4 g/mL

6. A prescription calls for 2 g of a pharmaceutical liquid. If the density of the pharmaceutical liquid is 0.976 g/mL, what will be the corresponding amount in mL?

    A. 3.73 mL
    B. 5.2 mL
    C. 1.987 mL
    D. 1.952 mL
    E. 2.05 mL

7. A new pharmaceutical active substance has a specific gravity of 1.02. How many milliliters does 2 grams of this substance occupy?

    A. 2.78 mL
    B. 3.56 mL
    C. 1.96 mL
    D. 3.92 mL
    E. 3.05 mL

8. If the specific gravity of a substance is 0.956, what is the specific volume?

    A. 1.05
    B. 0.956
    C. 2.10
    D. 1.46
    E. 0.87

9. How many grains are contained in 1.5 kg of a raw material?

    A. 23149 gr
    B. 35648 gr
    C. 25785 gr
    D. 25468 gr
    E. 49845 gr

10. What is the specific gravity of 30 mL of mineral oil that weighs 6.5 g and if 10 mL of water weighs 10 g?

    A. 0.22
    B. 3.5
    C. 7.8
    D. 10.8
    E. 20.5

11. If the specific gravity of a liquid substance is 6.5, what is the volume occupied by 9 grams of the material?

    A. 5.2 mL
    B. 1.38 mL
    C. 230 mL
    D. 25.4 mL
    E. 45.2 mL

Basic Pharmaceutical Calculations

1. If a prescription calls for 5 g of sodium chloride, how many milliliters of a stock solution are needed if every 1000 mL contains 20 g?

    A. 300 mL
    B. 400 mL
    C. 250 mL
    D. 25 mL
    E. 40 mL

2. Using the aliquot method, how would a pharmacist measure 30 mg of pseudoephedrine HCl if the SAW for the balance he or she is using is 70 mg and the diluent is lactose?

    A. Weigh 80 mg pseudoephedrine HCl and dilute to 300 mg with lactose. From this mixture, remove 90 mg that will contain the necessary 30 mg pseudoephedrine HCl.

Compounding and Calculations Review

B. Weigh 60 mg pseudoephedrine HCl and dilute to 240 mg with lactose. From this mixture, remove 120 mg that will contain the necessary 30 mg pseudoephedrine HCl.

C. Weigh 70 mg pseudoephedrine HCl and dilute to 210 mg with lactose. From this dilution, remove 90 mg that will contain the necessary 30 mg pseudoephedrine HCl.

D. Both b and c are correct.

E. None of the above.

3. How would a pharmacist measure 15 mg of methylparaben using ethanol as a diluent, if the SAW for the balance is 80 mg and a 20 mL graduated cylinder is available?

A. Dissolve 60 mg methylparaben in 10 mL ethanol and take 2 mL from the solution, which will contain 15 mg methylparaben.

B. Dissolve 90 mg methylparaben in 12 mL ethanol and take 2 mL from the solution, which will contain 15 mg methylparaben.

C. Dissolve 120 mg methylparaben in 5 mL ethanol and take 3 mL from the solution which will contain 15 mg methylparaben.

D. Dissolve 0.5 g methylparaben in 100 mL ethanol and take 10 mL from the solution which will contain 15 mg methylparaben.

E. Dissolve 0.3 g methylparaben in 50 mL ethanol and take 20 mL from the solution, which will contain 15 mg methylparaben.

4. Convert 50 mg/mL to µg/L using dimensional analysis.

A. 5×10^{7} µg/L

B. 5×10^{5} µg/L

C. 5×10^{2} µg/L

D. 5×10^{-7} µg/L

E. 5×10^{2} µg/L

5. 750 mL of D_5W runs for 5 hours. Calculate the flow rate in mL/hr and mL/min.

A. 130 mL/hr, 3 mL/min

B. 160 mL/hr, 5 mL/min

C. 150 mL/hr, 2.5 mL/min

D. 155 mL/hr, 2.8 mL/min

E. 130 mL/hr, 2.5 mL/min

6. One liter of NS runs for 8 hours at 700 drops/hour. What is the drop factor?

A. 7.5 drops/mL

B. 2.5 drops/mL

C. 3 drops/mL

D. 5.6 drops/mL

E. 7 drops/mL

Dosage Calculations

1. Calculate the dose needed for a 3-month-old infant if the adult dose is 500 mg ciprofloxacin per dose.

A. 10 mg

B. 300 mg

C. 150 mg

D. 800 mg

E. 100 mg

2. What is the dose for a 15-kg child if the adult dose is 65 mg?

A. 25.2 mg

B. 30.4 mg

C. 65 mg

D. 58 mg

E. 14.3 mg

3. If the dose of a given drug is 2 mg/kg, what is the dose for a 200-lb adult male?

A. 182 mg

B. 204 mg

C. 15 mg

D. 84 mg

E. 18.2 mg

4. If a patient weighs 300 lb and is 5'11" tall, what is the dose, based on body surface area, if the normal dose for an adult is 300 mg?

A. 300 mg

B. 200 mg

C. 434 mg

D. 450 mg

E. 150 mg

5. A prescription is brought into the pharmacy directing that 30 mL is to be administered for each dose. What is the dose in teaspoons?

A. 6 tsp

B. 4 tsp

C. 2 tsp

D. 8 tsp

E. 5 tsp

6. If a prescription calls for 2 tablespoons per day, how many milliliters are required for a 30-day prescription?

A. 90 mL

B. 900 mL

C. 500 mL

D. 850 mL

E. 50 mL

7. If a pharmacist determines while calibrating a dropper bottle that 30 drops filled a 10-mL graduated cylinder to the 5-mL mark, what is the calibration in drops/mL?

A. 8 drops/mL

B. 6 drops/mL

C. 8.5 drops/mL

D. 4 drops/mL

E. 6.5 drops/mL

Compounding and Calculations Review

8. A prescription calls for 1.2 mL to be administered for each dose. If a dropper is calibrated to deliver 5 drops/mL, what is the required dose in drops?

   A. 6 drops
   B. 5 drops
   C. 10 drops
   D. 20 drops
   E. 3 drops

9. If a dropper bottle holds 30 mL and the dropper is calibrated to deliver 5 drops/mL, how many 15-drop doses can be administered?

   A. 15
   B. 10
   C. 4
   D. 20
   E. 8

10. You have an order for 1.5 mg of epinephrine. If your stock solution is 1:1000, how many mL should you dispense?

    A. 1.5 mL
    B. 2.5 mL
    C. 5 mL
    D. 0.5 mL
    E. 6 mL

11. You have an order for Lanoxin 0.8 mg I V. Your stock is available in 500 mcg/2 mL. How many mL should you dispense?

    A. 2.3 mL
    B. 3.2 mL
    C. 5 mL
    D. 1.6 mL
    E. 9 mL

Concentration

1. What is the percentage strength (w/v) of 50 mg of cefuroxime dissolved in water to make a 500 mL D_5W solution?

   A. 0.2%
   B. 0.1%
   C. 0.01%
   D. 2.5%
   E. 0.025%

2. What is the percentage strength (w/w) for zinc oxide if 20 grams are mixed with 80 grams petrolatum?

   A. 25%
   B. 20%
   C. 15%
   D. 30%
   E. 22.5%

3. Convert 50% w/v to ratio strength.

   A. 1:2
   B. 1:4
   C. 2:5
   D. 2:1
   E. 1:1

4. What is the percentage strength of the final solution if 250 mL of 1% lidocaine HCl is diluted to 500 mL?

   A. 2%
   B. 1%
   C. 0.5%
   D. 1.5%
   E. 10%

5. How many milliliters of water are needed to dilute 500 mL of 90% ethanol to a 50% concentration?

   A. 500 mL
   B. 800 mL
   C. 400 mL
   D. 900 mL
   E. 600 mL

6. What is the concentration of KCl in percentage strength of a mixture of 300 mL 5% KCl, 400 mL 2% KCl, 250 mL 8 % KCl, and 400 mL 7.5% KCl?

   A. 2.5%
   B. 5.4%
   C. 3.2%
   D. 8.5%
   E. 4.5%

7. How many mEq of KCl are in 200 mL of a 5% KCl solution?

   A. 100 mEq
   B. 200 mEq
   C. 1.34 mEq
   D. 13.4 mEq
   E. 134.23 mEq

8. How many mOsm/L of KCl are present in 1000 mL of a 5% solution?

   A. 1342 mOsm/L
   B. 342 mOsm/L
   C. 2345 mOsm/L
   D. 13.42 mOsm/L
   E. 134.2 mOsm/L

9. Which of the following is considered to be isotonic?

   A. 0.9% NaCl
   B. 0.45% NaCl
   C. 0.225% NaCl
   D. 1.8% NaCl
   E. 0.75% NaCl

10. How many grams of sodium chloride are required to make the following prescription?

Compounding and Calculations Review

Cocaine HCl 10 mg
Purified water qs 100 mL
Sodium chloride qs to make an isotonic solution

- A. 898.4 mg
- B. 89.84 mg
- C. 98.65 mg
- D. 8.98 mg
- E. 8.98 Kg

11. You have a vial of potassium solution that contains 20 mEq of potassium per 5 mL. You add 2.5 mL to a one liter IV bag. What is the final concentration of potassium in the bag?

- A. 0.41 mEq/mL
- B. 0.15 mEq/mL
- C. 0.30 mEq/mL
- D. 0.01 mEq/mL
- E. 0.09 mEq/mL

12. A one liter bag of ½ NS contains 22.5 mEq of sodium. The flow rate is 25 drops/min, with a drop factor of 15 drops/mL. What is the hourly dose of sodium?

- A. 2.45 mEq/hr
- B. 2.25 mEq/hr
- C. 2.33 mEq/hr
- D. 2.56 mEq/hr
- E. 2.16 mEq/hr

13. A 0.8% solution of lidocaine is flowing at 50 mL/hr. What is the hourly dose?

- A. 500 mg/hr
- B. 400 mg/hr
- C. 360 mg/hr
- D. 460 mg/hr
- E. 510 mg/hr

Calculations for Sterile Products

1. A physician orders atropine sulfate 0.8 mg. Using a stock atropine sulfate of 0.4 mg/mL, calculate the volume of atropine that is needed to complete the physician's order.

- A. 2.6 mL
- B. 3 mL
- C. 2 mL
- D. 1.8 mL
- E. 10 mL

2. An emergency room doctor orders 50 units of U100 insulin stat. Using a 1-cc syringe, how much insulin would you dispense?

- A. 0.5 mL
- B. 0.6 mL
- C. 0.25 mL
- D. 1 mL
- E. 0.3 mL

3. A hospital physician orders 100,000 Units of penicillin to be added to a 1 L bag of saline and infused over 4 hours. Your infusion is set at 8 drops/mL. What is the flow rate in drops/minute?

- A. 33.3 drops/minute
- B. 50 drops/minute
- C. 20 drops/minute
- D. 55 drops/minute
- E. 65 drops/minute

4. 500 mL of NS is infused at 55 mL/hr. How long will the infusion go?

- A. 3 hours
- B. 7.5 hours
- C. 10 hours
- D. 15 hours
- E. 9 hours

5. 450 mL of D_5W ½ NS is delivered in 100 minutes. Your drop factor is 10 drops/mL. Calculate the flow rate in drops/min.

- A. 49 drops/min
- B. 30 drops/min
- C. 25 drops/min
- D. 45 drops/min
- E. 52 drops/min

6. 250 mL of saline is infusing at 25 mL/hr. How much saline does the patient receive in 30 minutes?

- A. 13.6 mL
- B. 12.5 mL
- C. 10 mL
- D. 9.8 mL
- E. 15 mL

7. The label on a drug vial says to reconstitute with 8 mL of water to get 10 mL of a 400,000 Units/mL solution. You add 10 mL by mistake. What would the resulting concentration of the drug be?

- A. 333,333 Units/mL
- B. 450,300 Units/mL
- C. 500,100 Units/mL
- D. 300,000 Units/mL
- E. 555,555 Units/mL

8. An order for heparin is 1000 Units/hr in 1 L D_5W, to be infused for 4 hours. Calculate the amount of heparin to add to the I V.

- A. 4000 Units
- B. 5500 Units
- C. 3300 Units
- D. 4500 Units
- E. 3000 Units

9. You reconstitute a vial of drug with 4 mL of saline. The vial contains 500 mg of drug. What is the final concentration of drug in the vial?

Compounding and Calculations Review

A.   132 mg/mL
B.   160 mg/mL
C.   125 mg/mL
D.   100 mg/mL
E.   400 mg/mL

10. How much dextrose is contained in 450 mL of D$_5$W?

A.   22.5 g
B.   32.9 g
C.   43.6 g
D.   52.9 g
E.   20.3 g

11. You add 4 g of drug to 1 liter of NS. The hourly dose is to be 240 mg. Calculate the flow rate. How long will the IV run?

A.   18 hr
B.   15 hr
C.   17 hr
D.   13 hr
E.   12 hr

12. An IV solution of heparin contains 2500 Units in 250 mL and takes 2 hours to infuse. How much drug is infused in 30 minutes?

A.   625 Units
B.   700 Units
C.   550 Units
D.   330 Units
E.   600 Units

13. There is an order for lidocaine 15 mg subcutaneously. Stock is a 1% solution. How many mL of lidocaine are required?

A.   3.2 mL
B.   2.6 mL
C.   1.5 mL
D.   1.9 mL
E.   3.5 mL

14. You have an order for Depo-Provera 0.45 g. Stock is available in 500 mg/10 mL vial. How much volume should you dispense?

A.   5 mL
B.   8 mL
C.   6 mL
D.   9 mL
E.   3 mL

15. How many mEq of sodium are in 100 mL of saline? (MW = 23 (sodium) and 35 (chlorine))

A.   16.5 mEq
B.   15.5 mEq
C.   13.9 mEq
D.   23 mEq
E.   58 mEq

16. You add 1 g of aminophylline to 500 mL of NS. The patient is to receive 60 mg/hr. What is the flow rate?

A.   10 mL/hr
B.   15 mL/hr
C.   22 mL/hr
D.   39 mL/hr
E.   30 mL/hr

17. 30 mL of a 10% solution contains _____ g of drug.

A.   0.3
B.   30
C.   13
D.   300
E.   3

18. You have an order for 500 mL of NS to run for 3 hours. Your infusion rate is set at 8 drops/mL. The flow rate in drops/min would be:

A.   22 drops/min
B.   24 drops/min
C.   33 drops/min
D.   16 drops/min
E.   30 drops/min

19. A 6% solution would be:

A.   6 g/100 mL
B.   60 g/L
C.   60 g/100 mL
D.   A and B
E.   None

20. You add 4 mL of a 350 mg/mL solution of methotrexate to 500 mL saline. What is the final concentration in the bag?

A.   2.2 mg/mL
B.   3.3 mg/mL
C.   2.8 mg/mL
D.   2.0 mg/mL
E.   3.0 mg/mL

21. How many milligrams of drug are in 30 mL of a 1:10,000 solution?

A.   30 mg
B.   3 mg
C.   300 mg
D.   30 g
E.   0.3 mg

Appendixes

NAPLEX® Competency Statements

NAPLEX Blueprint

The NAPLEX Competency Statements

The NAPLEX Competency Statements provide a blueprint of the topics covered on the examination. They offer important information about the knowledge, judgment, and skills you are expected to demonstrate as an entry-level pharmacist. A strong understanding of the Competency Statements will aid in your preparation to take the examination.

Area 1

Assess Pharmacotherapy to Assure Safe and Effective Therapeutic Outcomes (Approximately 56% of Test)

1.1.0   *Identify, interpret, and evaluate patient information to determine the presence of a disease or medical condition, assess the need for treatment and/or referral, and identify patient-specific factors that affect health, pharmacotherapy, and/or disease management.*

    1.1.1   Identify and assess patient information including medication, laboratory, and disease state histories.

    1.1.2   Identify patient specific assessment and diagnostic methods, instruments, and techniques and interpret their results.

    1.1.3   Identify and define the etiology, terminology, signs, and symptoms associated with diseases and medical conditions and their causes and determine if medical referral is necessary.

    1.1.4   Identify and evaluate patient genetic, and biosocial factors, and concurrent drug therapy, relevant to the maintenance of wellness and the prevention or treatment of a disease or medical condition.

1.2.0   *Evaluate information about pharmacoeconomic factors, dosing regimen, dosage forms, delivery systems and routes of administration to identify and select optimal pharmacotherapeutic agents, for patients*

    1.2.1   Identify specific uses and indications for drug products and recommend drugs of choice for specific diseases or medical conditions.

    1.2.2   Identify the chemical/pharmacologic classes of therapeutic agents and describe their known or postulated sites and mechanisms of action.

    1.2.3   Evaluate drug therapy for the presence of pharmacotherapeutic duplications and interactions with other drugs, food, and diagnostic tests.

    1.2.4   Identify and evaluate potential contraindications and provide information about warnings and precautions associated with a drug product's active and inactive ingredients.

    1.2.5   Identify physicochemical properties of drug substances that affect their solubility, pharmacodynamic and pharmacokinetic properties, pharmacologic actions, and stability.

    1.2.6   Evaluate and interpret pharmacodynamic and pharmacokinetic principles to calculate and determine appropriate drug dosing regimens.

    1.2.7   Identify appropriate routes of administration, dosage forms, and pharmaceutical characteristics of drug dosage forms and delivery systems, to assure bioavailability and enhance therapeutic efficacy.

1.3.0   *Evaluate and manage drug regimens by monitoring and assessing the patient and/or patient information, collaborating with other health care professionals, and providing patient education to enhance safe, effective, and economic patient outcomes.*

    1.3.1   Identify pharmacotherapeutic outcomes and endpoints.

    1.3.2   Evaluate patient signs and symptoms, and the findings of monitoring tests and procedures to determine the safety and effectiveness of pharmacotherapy. Recommend needed follow-up evaluations or tests when appropriate.

    1.3.3   Identify, describe, and provide information regarding the mechanism of adverse reactions, allergies, side effects, iatrogenic, and drug-induced illness, including their management and prevention.

    1.3.4   Identify, prevent, and address methods to remedy medication non-adherence, misuse, or abuse.

    1.3.5   Evaluate current drug regimens and recommend pharmacotherapeutic alternatives or modifications.

Area 2

Assess Safe and Accurate Preparation and Dispensing of Medications (Approximately 33% of Test)

2.1.0   *Demonstrate the ability to perform calculations required to compound, dispense, and administer medication.*

    2.1.1   Calculate the quantity of medication to be compounded or dispensed; reduce and enlarge formulation quantities and calculate

Appendix A

NAPLEX® Competency Statements

the quantity or ingredients needed to compound the proper amount of the preparation.

2.1.2 Calculate nutritional needs and the caloric content of nutrient sources.

2.1.3 Calculate the rate of drug administration.

2.1.4 Calculate or convert drug concentrations, ratio strengths, and/or extent of ionization.

2.2.0 *Demonstrate the ability to select and dispense medications in a manner that promotes safe and effective use.*

2.2.1 Identify drug products by their generic, brand, and/or common names.

2.2.2 Identify whether a particular drug dosage strength or dosage form is commercially available and whether it is available on a nonprescription basis.

2.2.3 Identify commercially available drug products by their characteristic physical attributes.

2.2.4 Assess pharmacokinetic parameters and quality assurance data to determine equivalence among manufactured drug products, and identify products for which documented evidence of inequivalence exists.

2.2.5 Identify and provide information regarding appropriate packaging, storage, handling, administration, and disposal of medications.

2.2.6 Identify and provide information regarding the appropriate use of equipment and apparatus required to administer medications.

2.3.0 *Demonstrate the knowledge to prepare and compound extemporaneous preparations and sterile products.*

2.3.1 Identify techniques, procedures, and equipment related to drug preparation, compounding, and quality assurance.

2.3.2 Identify the important physicochemical properties of a preparation's active and inactive ingredients.

2.3.3 Identify the mechanism of and evidence for the incompatibility or degradation of a product or preparation and methods for achieving its stability.

3.1.1 Identify the typical content of specific sources of drug and health information for both health care providers and consumers, and recommend appropriate resources to address questions or needs.

3.1.2 Evaluate the suitability, accuracy, and reliability of clinical and pharmacoeconomic data by analyzing experimental design, statistical tests, interpreting results, and formulating conclusions.

3.2.0 *Recommend and provide information to educate the public and healthcare professionals regarding medical conditions, wellness, dietary supplements, and medical devices.*

3.2.1 Recommend and provide health care information regarding the prevention and treatment of diseases and medical conditions, including emergency patient care and vaccinations.

3.2.2 Recommend and provide health care information regarding nutrition, lifestyle, and other non-drug measures that promote health or prevent the progression of a disease or medical condition.

3.2.3 Recommend and provide information regarding the documented uses, adverse effects, and toxicities of dietary supplements.

3.2.4 Recommend and provide information regarding the selection, use, and care of medical/surgical appliances and devices, self-care products, and durable medical equipment, as well as products and techniques for self-monitoring of health status and medical conditions.

Area 3

Assess, Recommend, and Provide Health care Information that Promotes Public Health (Approximately 11% of Test)

3.1.0 *Identify, evaluate, and apply information to promote optimal health care.*

Abbreviations

A & O
Alert and oriented

A&P
Auscultation and percussion

A1
Abortus-1

AA
Alcoholics Anonymous

AAFP
American Academy of Family Physicians

AAP
American Academy of Pediatrics

ABD
Abdomen

ABG
Arterial blood gases

AC
Before meals

AC and HS
Before meals and at bedtime

AC & HS
Before meals and at bedtime

ACE
Angiotensin converting enzyme

ACIP
Advisory Committee on Immunization Practices (CDC)

Adj BW
Adjusted body weight

AHFS
American Hospital Formulary Service

AIDS
Acquired immunodeficiency syndrome

Alk Phos
Alkaline Phosphatase

ALL
Acute lymphocytic leukemia

ALP
Alkaline phosphatase

ALT
Alanine aminotransferase

AM
Morning

AMA
Against medical advice

ANA
Antinuclear antibody

Anti-ds DNA
Anti-double-stranded deoxyribonucleic acid

Anti-HAV
Antibody to hepatitis A virus

Anti-HBc
Antibody to the hepatitis B core antigen

Anti-Hbe
Antibody to the hepatitis 'e' antigen

Anti-HBs
Antibody to the hepatitis B surface antigen

Anti-HCV
Antibody to the hepatitis C virus

AP
Anterior-posterior

APAP
Acetaminophen

ARF
Acute renal failure

ASA
Aspirin

ASCVD
Atherosclerotic cardiovascular disease

AST
Aspartate aminotransferase

ATC
Around the clock

Appendix B

Abbreviations

AUC
Area under the concentration time curve

AV
Arteriovenous

Baso
Basophils

BCG
Bacille Calmette-Guérin

bid
Twice a day

BKA
Below knee amputation

BM
Total cells counted in bone marrow

BM
Bowel movement

BM-Bx
Bone marrow-biopsy

BP
Blood pressure

BPH
Benign prostatic hypertrophy

bpm
Beats per minute

BRBPR
Bright red blood per rectum

BS
Bowel sounds

BSA
Body surface area

BUN
Blood urea nitrogen

c/c/e
Clubbing/cyanosis/edema

C3
Complement component 3

C4
Complement component 4

Ca
Calcium

CA-125
Cancer antigen 125

CABG
Coronary artery bypass graft

CAD
Coronary artery disease

CAP
Community acquired pneumonia

CAPD
Continuous ambulatory peritoneal dialysis

CBC
Complete blood count

CC
Chief Complaint

CCE
Clubbing, cyanosis, edema

CDC
Centers for Disease Control and Prevention

CEA
Carcinoembryonic antigen

CHF
Congestive heart failure

CINV
Chemotherapy-induced nausea & vomiting

CK
Creatine kinase

CKMB
Creatine kinase myocardial band

Cl
Chloride

Cl_{cr}
Creatinine clearance

Abbreviations

CML
Chronic myelogenous leukemia

CMV
Cytomegalovirus

CN
Cranial nerves

CNS
Central nervous system

CO_2
Carbon dioxide (pCO_2 = peripheral or arterial carbon dioxide)

COMT
Catechol-O-methyltransferase

COPD
Chronic obstructive pulmonary disease

COX
Cyclooxygenase

COX-2
Cyclooxygenase-2

CrCl
Creatinine clearance

CSF
Cerebral spinal fluid

CT
Computed tomography

CTA
Clear to auscultation

CTX
Chemotherapy

CV
Cardiovascular

CVA
Cerebrovascular accident

CVA
Costovertebral angle

CVAT
Costovertebral angle tenderness

CVD
Cisplatin, vinblastine, dacarbazine

CXR
Chest x-ray

D. bili
Direct bilirubin

D_5W
Dextrose 5% in water

DBP
Diastolic blood pressure

DEXA
Dual energy x-ray absorptiometry

DIP
Distal interphalangeal

DM
Diabetes mellitus

DMARD
Disease-modifying antirheumatic drug

DNA
Deoxyribonucleic acid

DOE
Dyspnea on exertion

DTR
Deep tendon reflex

E.C.
Enteric coated

ECASA
Enteric coated aspirin

ECG
Electrocardiogram

ED
Emergency department

EGD
Esophagogastroduodenoscopy

EKG
Electrocardiogram

Appendix B

Abbreviations

ELISA
Enzyme linked immunosorbent assay

EMS
Emergency medical services

ENDO
Endocrine

EOMI
Extra-ocular movements (or muscles) intact

EOS
Eosinophils

ESR
Erythrocyte sedimentation rate

ESRD
End-stage renal disease

EtOH
Ethanol

EXT
Extremities

FAC
Fluorouracil, doxorubicin (Adriamycin), cyclophosphamide

FBG
Fasting blood glucose

FDA
Food and Drug Administration

FEV1
Forced expiratory volume in 1 second

FSH
Follicle stimulating hormone

FT$_3$
Free triiodothyronine

FT$_4$
Free thyroxine

FT$_4$I
Free thyroxine index

FTA-ABS
Fluorescent treponemal antibody absorption

FVC
Forced vital capacity

G-1
Gravida-1

G-4
Gravida-4

GAD
Generalized anxiety disorder

GBS
Guillain-Barré Syndrome

GC
Gonococci or gonococcal infection

GEN
General appearance or presentation

GERD
Gastroesophageal reflux disease

GI
Gastrointestinal

GPC
Gram-positive cocci

gtt
Drop

GU
Genitourinary

H/O
History of

H$_2$RA
Histamine-2 receptor antagonist

HA
Headache

HAART
Highly active antiretroviral therapy

HAV
Hepatitis A virus

HbA$_{1c}$
Hemoglobin A$_{1c}$

Abbreviations

HBc
Antigen hepatitis B core antigen

HbcAg
Hepatitis B core antigen

HBe
Antigen hepatitis B 'e' antigen

HBIG
Hepatitis B immune globulin

HBs
Antigen hepatitis B surface antigen

HbsAg
Hepatitis B surface antigen

HCG
Human chorionic gonadotropin

HCO$_3$
Bicarbonate

Hct
Hematocrit

HCTZ
Hydrochlorothiazide

HD
Hemodialysis

HEENT
Head, ear, eyes, nose, and throat

HER2
Human epidermal growth factor receptor-2

Hgb
Hemoglobin

HiB
Haemophilus Influenzae, type B

HIV
Human immunodeficiency virus

HJR
Hepatojugular reflux

HLA
Human leukocyte antigen

HPI
History of present illness

HR
Heart rate

HS
At bedtime

HSM
Hepatosplenomegaly

HSV
Herpes simplex virus

HTN
Hypertension

IBW
Ideal Body Weight

IgG
Immunoglobulin G

IgM
Immunoglobulin M

IL-2
Interleukin-2

IM
Intramuscular

INH
Isoniazid

Inorganic Phos
Inorganic phosphorus

INR
International normalized ratio

IP
Intraperitoneal

IU
International Units

IV
Intravenous

IVDA
Intravenous drug abuse

Appendix B

Abbreviations

IVP
Intravenous push

IVPB
Intravenous piggy back

JNC VI
Sixth report of the Joint National Committee on Prevention, Detection, Evaluation, and Treatment of High Blood Pressure

JVD
Jugular venous distention

K
Potassium

kcal
Kilocalorie

LDH
Lactate dehydrogenase

LDL
Low-density lipoprotein

LE
Lower extremity

LES
Lower esophageal sphincter

LFTs
Liver function tests

LH
Luteinizing hormone

LHRH
Luteinizing hormone releasing hormone

LLL
Left lower lobe

LLQ
Left lower quadrant

LMP
Last menstrual period

LPF
Low power field

LTC
Long-term care

Lymph
Lymphocytes

m/r/g
Murmurs/rubs/gallops

MAO-A
Monoamine oxidase type A

MAO-B
Monoamine oxidase type B

MCH
Mean corpuscular hemoglobin

MCHC
Mean corpuscular hemoglobin concentration

MCP
Metacarpophalangeal

MCV
Mean corpuscular volume

MDI
Metered dose inhaler

Mg
Magnesium

MI
Myocardial infarction

MIC
Minimum inhibitory concentration

MIU
Million international units

MMR
Mumps, Measles, and Rubella

MMSE
Mini-mental status exam

Monos
Monocytes

MRI
Magnetic resonance imaging

Abbreviations

MRSA
Methicillin resistant Staph aureus

MTP
Metatarsophalangeal

MU
Million units

MUGA
Multiple-gated acquisitions of data

MVA
Motor vehicle accident

MVI
Multivitamin

MWF
Monday, Wednesday, Friday

N/V
Nausea and vomiting

NA
Narcotics Anonymous

NA
Not applicable

Na
Sodium

NAD
No apparent (acute) distress

NC/AT
Normocephalic, atraumatic

NCAT
Normal cephalic, atraumatic

NEURO
Neurological

Neut
Neutrophils

NG
Nasogastric

NIH
National Institutes of Health

NKA
No known allergies

NKDA
No known drug allergies

NL
Normal

NPO
Nothing by mouth

NS
Nasal spray

NSAID
Nonsteroidal anti-inflammatory drug

NSR
Normal sinus rhythm

NT/ND
Nontender, nondistended

o/p
Ova or parasites

O_2
Oxygen (pO_2 = peripheral or arterial oxygen)

OA
Osteoarthritis

OB/GYN
Obstetrician/Gynecologist

OC
Oral contraceptive

OHSS
Ovarian hyperstimulation syndrome

OSHA
Occupational Safety and Health Administration

OTC
Over the counter

OU
Both eyes

P
Puffs

Appendix B

Abbreviations

P-1
> Para-1

P-4
> Para-4

PC
> After meals

PCA
> Patient controlled analgesia

PCN
> Penicillin

PCP
> Pneumocystis carinii *pneumonia*

PCP
> Primary care physician

PD
> Parkinson's disease

PERRLA
> Pupils equal, round, and reactive to light and accommodation

Ph-
> Philadelphia chromosome negative

Ph+
> Philadelphia chromosome positive

Phos
> Inorganic phosphorus

PIP
> Proximal interphalangeal

Plt
> Platelets

PMN
> Polymorphonuclear leukocyte

po
> By mouth (oral)

PO$_4$
> Phosphate

ppd
> Pack(s) (of cigarettes) per day

PPD
> Purified protein derivative

prn
> As needed

PSA
> Prostate specific antigen

PT
> Prothrombin time

PTT
> Partial thromboplastin time

PUD
> Peptic ulcer disease

PVD
> Peripheral vascular disease

q
> Every

q am
> Every morning

qd
> Once a day

q hs
> At bedtime

qid
> Four times a day

qod
> Every other day

q wk
> Every week

RA
> Rheumatoid arthritis

RBC
> Red blood cells

RDA
> Recommended daily allowance

RDW
> Red (cell) distribution width

Abbreviations

REM
Rapid eye movement

RF
Rheumatoid factor

ROM
Range of motion

RPR
Rapid plasma reagin

RR
Respiratory rate

RRR
Regular rate and rhythm

RSV
Respiratory syncytial virus

RUE
Right upper extremity

RUQ
Right upper quadrant

Rx
Prescription

S/P
Status post

S_1
First heart sound

S_2
Second heart sound

S_3
Third heart sound (abnormal)

S_4
Fourth heart sound (abnormal)

SBP
Systolic blood pressure

SCr
Serum creatinine

SE
Status epilepticus

Segs
Neutrophils

SEM
Systolic ejection murmur

Serum Cr
Serum creatinine

SGPT
Serum glutamic pyruvic transaminase

SHBG
Sex-hormone binding globulin

Sig
Directions

SL
Sublingual

SLE
Systemic lupus erythematosus

Sp
Species

SQ
Subcutaneous

SR
Sustained release

SSRI
Selective serotonin reuptake inhibitor

STD
Sexually transmitted disease

Subq
Subcutaneous

SULFAS
Sulfonylureas

Sx
Symptoms

T. bili
Total bilirubin

T_4
Levothyroxine

Appendix B

Abbreviations

Tart
Tartrate

TB
Tuberculosis

TDT
Terminal transferase

TG
Triglycerides

TIA
Transient ischemic attack

TIBC
Total iron binding capacity

tid
Three times a day

TM
Tympanic membrane

TMP/SMX
Trimethoprim/sulfamethoxazole

TNF
Tumor necrosis factor

TPHA
T. pallidum hemagglutination assay

TSH
Thyroid Stimulating Hormone

TT$_3$
Total triiodothyronine

TT$_4$
Total thyroxine

TTS
Transdermal therapeutic system

UC
Ulcerative colitis

ud
As directed

UE
Upper extremity

URI
Upper respiratory infection

USP DI
United States Pharmacopeia Drug Information

USP NF
United States Pharmacopeia National Formulary

UTI
Urinary tract infection

UV
Ultraviolet

UVA
Ultraviolet-A

UVB
Ultraviolet-B

UVC
Ultraviolet-C

VA
Veterans Affairs

Vd
Volume of distribution

VLDL
Very low-density lipoprotein

VS
Vital signs

WBC
White Blood Cells

WD
Well-developed

WD,WN
Well-developed, well-nourished

WNL
Within normal limits

yo
Years old

Nondrug Reference Ranges for Common Laboratory Tests in Traditional and SI Units[a]

Laboratory Test	Reference Range Traditional Units	Conversion Factor	Reference Range SI Units	Comment
Alanine aminotransferase (ALT)	0–30 IU/L	0.01667	0–0.50 μkat/L	SGPT
Albumin	3.5–5 g/dL	0.00	35–50 g/L	
Ammonia	30–70 μg/dL	0.587	17–41 μmol/L	
Aspartate aminotransferase (AST)	8–42 IU/L	0.01667	0.133–0.700 μkat/L	SGOT
Bilirubin (direct)	0.1–0.3 mg/dL	17.10	1.7–5 μmol/L	
Bilirubin (total)	0.3–1.0 mg/dL	17.10	5–17 μmol/L	
Calcium	8.5–10.8 mg/dL	0.25	2.1–2.7 mmol/L	
Carbon dioxide (CO_2)	24–30 mEq/L	1.000	24–30 mmol/L	Serum bicarbonate
Chloride	96–106 mEq/L	1.000	96–106 mmol/L	desirable
Cholesterol (HDL)	>10 mg/dL	0.026	>1.55 mmol/L	desirable
Cholesterol (LDL)	100 <130 mg/dL	0.026	<3.36 mmol/L	males
Creatine kinase (CK)	25–90 IU/L (males)	0.01667	0.42–1.50 μkat/L	females
	10–70 IU/L (females)		0.17–1.17 μkat/L	adults
Serum creatinine (SCr)	0.7–1.5 mg/dL	88.40	62–133 μmol/L	
Creatinine clearance (CrCl)	90–140 mL/min/1.73 m²	0.017	1.53–2.38 mL/sec/1.73 m²	
Folic acid	150–540 ng/mL	2.266	340–1020 nmol/L	GGTP
g-Glutamyl transpeptidase	0–30 U/L (but varies)	0.01667	0–0.50 μkat/L (but varies)	
Globulin	2–3 g/dL	10.00	20–30 g/L	fasting
Glucose (fasting)	<110 mg/dL	0.056	6.1 mmol/L	males
Hemoglobin (Hgb)	14–18 g/dL	0.622	8.7–11.2 mmol/L	females
	12–16 g/dL		7.4–9.9 mmol/L	
Iron	50–150 μg/dL	0.179	9–26.9 μmol/L	TIBC
Iron-binding capacity	250–410 μg/dL	0.179	45–73 μmol/L	LDH
Lactate dehydrogenase	100–210 IU/L	0.01667	1667–350 nmol/L, 1.7–3.2 μkat/L	Lactic acid
Serum lactate (venous)	0.5–1.5 mEq/L	1.000	0.5–1.5 mmol/L	
Serum lactate (arterial)	0.5–2.0 mEq/L	1.000	0.5–2.0 mmol/L	
Magnesium	1.5–2.2 mEq/L	0.500	0.75–1.1 mmol/L	
5´ Nucleotidase	1–11 U/L (but varies)		0.01667 0.02–0.18 μkat/L (but varies)	
Phosphate	2.6–4.5 mg/dL		0.85–1.48 mmol/L	
Potassium	3.5–5.0 mEq/L	1.000	3.5–5.0 mmol/L	
Sodium	136–145 mEq/L	1.000	136–145 mmol/L	
Total serum thyroxine (T_4)	4–12 μg/dL	12.86	51–154 nmol/L	Total T_4
Triglycerides	<150 mg/dL	0.0113	<1.26 mmol/L	Adults >20 yo
Total serum triiodothyronine (T_3)	78–195 ng/dL	0.0154	1.2–3.0 nmol/L	Total T_3
Urea nitrogen, blood	8–20 mg/dL	0.357	2.9–7.1 mmol/L	BUN
Uric acid (serum)	3.4–7 mg/dL	59.48	202–416 μmol/L	

[a]Some laboratories are maintaining traditional units for enzyme tests.

Answers

Case 1 Angina Pectoris

1. The answer is C (3.2.1)

Rupture of an atherosclerotic plaque with subsequent thrombus formation presenting as unstable angina may rapidly progress to acute MI if extension of the thrombus leads to total vessel occlusion. Therefore, in addition to therapies that correct imbalances between myocardial oxygen supply and demand, rapid initiation of one or more antiplatelet agents plus anticoagulation with UFH or LMWH is recommended. Organic nitrates and aspirin are recommended for both stable and unstable angina patients in the absence of contraindications.

2. The answer is A (1.2.0)

Thrombolytic therapy should be initiated only for patients with strong evidence of MI (ST segment elevation, new bundle branch block), which is not present in WK. Aspirin should be promptly initiated in all patients with unstable angina unless a contraindication to therapy exists. For hospitalized patients with unstable angina in whom PCI or an early noninterventional approach (as in WK) is planned, clopidogrel should be added to aspirin and continued for 1-9 months (ACC/AHA Guidelines). Although inotropic doses of dopamine (e.g., 4-6 μg/kg/min) have been shown to increase renal blood flow and GFR secondary to increased cardiac output in patients with CHF, low doses of 1-3 μg/kg/min have not been demonstrated to provide renal protection or alter the course of acute renal failure. Dobutamine is utilized in the short-term management of cardiac decompensation. Diltiazem should be considered if the patient continues to experience anginal episodes in the future.

3. The answer is E (1.2.4)

Bradycardia and first-degree AV block as seen in WK in conjunction with an elevated serum digoxin level (ACC/AHA 2005 Update to the Guidelines for the Evaluation and Management of Chronic Heart Failure recommend digoxin levels of 0.5-1 ng/mL) are consistent with possible digoxin toxicity. Potassium may significantly accumulate in patients with marked renal insufficiency (creatinine clearance less than 20-30 mL/min) due to decreased excretion, and it is evident in WK with a serum potassium level of 5.6 mEq/L and estimated creatinine clearance less than 30 mL/min. Treatment doses of enoxaparin should be reduced to 1 mg/kg q 24 h in patients with an estimated creatinine clearance less than 30 mL/min per the manufacturer's package insert.

4. The answer is C (1.2.6)

Digoxin is subject to accumulation in patients with renal impairment. Glyburide and lisinopril have not been shown to significantly decrease digoxin clearance. The serum level was obtained in the post-distribution phase (beyond 8 hours post-dose) and therefore should not be falsely elevated. Exercise prior to drawing levels may drive digoxin into the muscles, thus making the serum level appear falsely low.

5. The answer is D (1.1.1)

A 12-lead EKG should be obtained within 10 minutes in patients with ongoing chest discomfort. A cardiac-specific troponin and/or CPK-MB should be measured as well, per current ACC/AHA guidelines. Liver function tests are not useful for risk stratification. A lipid panel is useful in risk stratification and should be obtained during hospitalization. Lipids can appear falsely low in patients who present with ACS as LDL levels can decrease by as much as 50% from baseline within the first day following an ACS event. A period of 4 to 6 weeks is often needed before lipid levels return to baseline.

6. The answer is C (1.2.5)

LMWH does not appreciably affect the aPTT. Monitoring the level of anticoagulation with anti-Xa levels may be indicated in selected patients (e.g., pregnancy, morbid obesity, severe renal impairment).

7. The answer is C (1.2.2)

Because platelets play a major role in the propagation of an intracoronary thrombus, the benefit of aspirin in the acute coronary syndromes is secondary to its antiplatelet activity.

8. The answer is B (2.2.0)

The GUSTO IV-ACS trial demonstrated a lack of benefit with abciximab therapy in patients with UA/NSTEMI in whom early revascularization is not planned within 48 hours. Therefore, abciximab is indicated only in patients with UA/NSTEMI as an adjunct to PCI or when PCI is planned within 24 hours per current ACC/AHA guidelines. Eptifibatide and tirofiban are both cleared primarily via the kidney, and therefore they require dosing adjustment in the presence of significant renal impairment. No dose adjustments are necessary in hepatic dysfunction. Abciximab does not require dose adjustments for hepatic or renal impairment. One of the most common adverse reactions to abciximab is back pain.

9. The answer is E (2.2.0)

Plavix is the brand name for clopidogrel. Persantine (A) is the brand name for dipyridamole. Aggrenox (B) is the brand name for aspirin/dipyridamole. Pletal (C) is the brand name for cilostazol. Ticlid (D) is the brand name for ticlopidine.

10. The answer is C (3.2.1)

Ibuprofen, ketoprofen, naproxen, and other NSAIDs are associated with sodium retention, which may exacerbate CHF. They may also inhibit renal prostaglandins, resulting in decreased renal blood flow and renal function. NSAIDs also may antagonize the effect of diuretics. Diphenhydramine is an antihistamine with no significant analgesic activity.

Case 2 Hypertension

1. The answer is C (1.1.4)

Answers

Both ibuprofen and licorice can cause an inadequate response to antihypertensive therapy. NSAIDs may cause vasoconstriction of afferent arterioles in the kidney and therefore will increase the blood pressure. Glycyrrhetinic acid is the active component of licorice that causes inhibition of the peripheral metabolism of cortisol. Cortisol binds with aldosterone to the mineralocorticoid receptor, resulting in a hypermineralocorticoid condition. Acetaminophen and inhaled beclomethasone have no effect on efficacy of antihypertensive treatments. Furosemide may lower blood pressure, resulting from fluid overload.

2. The answer is A (1.1.4)

Both oral albuterol and corticosteroids can cause a problem with HTN control, but inhaled albuterol and corticosteroids are of less concern if used appropriately. Albuterol and corticosteroids administered by the inhaled route provide equivalent concentrations in the bronchia at lower doses than oral preparations with fewer systemic side effects.

3. The answer is E (1.1.4)

History of hypertension (2 elevated readings spanning 5 weeks), obesity (BMI >30), renal insufficiency (GFR <60 mL/min), and age (men older than 55) are all considered major risk factors for cardiovascular disease according to JNC 7. While a family history of premature cardiovascular disease is a major risk factor, PG's mother's history of a myocardial infarction at the age of 68 years is not considered premature cardiovascular disease.

4. The answer is C (1.1.4)

eGFR by MDRD (mL/min/1.72 m^2) = 186 x (S$_{cr}$)$^{-1.154}$ x (Age)$^{-0.203}$ x (0.742 if female) x (1.212 if African American). The MDRD equation was named after the Modification of Diet in Renal Disease study. The results are expressed relative to a standard body surface area of 1.73 m^2 to allow for different body sizes. The equation is only valid for persons 18 years of age or older and not reported in younger patients. MDRD has not been validated for drug dosing and alternative estimates of GFR, such as Cockcroft-Gault, should be used.

5. The answer is B (2.2.1)

Propranolol is a nonselective, beta-adrenergic-receptor-blocking agent that is contraindicated in patients with bronchial asthma.

6. The answer is A (3.2.1)

Compelling indications for treatment include heart failure, postmyocardial infarction, high coronary disease risk, diabetes, chronic kidney disease, and recurrent stroke prevention.

7. The answer is B (2.2.1)

Lotrel is the brand name for the combination of amlodipine and benazepril. Kerlone is the brand name for betaxolol. Coreg is the brand name for carvedilol. Altace is the brand name for ramipril. Norvasc is the brand name for amlodipine.

8. The answer is B (2.2.1)

Enalapril is an angiotensin-converting-enzyme inhibitor and hydrochlorothiazide is a thiazide-type diuretic.

9. The answer is C (3.2.1)

Alpha-1-blockers may have a favorable effect on prostatism and dyslipidemia. Alpha-1-blockers decrease LDL cholesterol and increase HDL cholesterol.

10. The answer is D (1.3.1)

JNC 7 blood pressure classification is as follows: normal, systolic BP <120 and diastolic BP <80; prehypertension, systolic BP 120-139 or diastolic BP 80-89; Stage 1 hypertension, systolic BP 140-159 or diastolic BP 90-99; and Stage 2 hypertension, systolic BP ≥160 or diastolic BP ≥100.

Case 3 Myocardial Infarction

1. The answer is C (1.2.4)

Severe uncontrolled hypertension (blood pressure >180/110 mmHg) is a relative contraindication to the use of thrombolytics. Alteplase can be used in this circumstance if it is determined that the potential benefit outweighs the risk. The only absolute contraindications to the use of thrombolytics are previous hemorrhagic stroke at any time, other strokes or CVA within 3 months, known intracranial neoplasm, active internal bleeding, known structural vascular lesions (e.g., AVM), significant closed head trauma or facial trauma within 3 months, and suspected aortic dissection.

2. The answer is E (1.2.0)

Choice of a specific thrombolytic agent does not appear to be a major determinate of outcome following acute MI. While a 1% mortality benefit was seen with an accelerated tPA compared to streptokinase, the additional cost ($2000) may offset this benefit.

3. The answer is B (1.1.4)

Thrombolytics are considered most beneficial in the treatment of acute transmural MI in terms of survival and LV function when administered within 3 hours after the onset of symptoms. However, significant survival benefit occurs up to at least 12 hours after the onset of symptoms.

4. The answer is C (1.3.0)

The degree of anticoagulation with heparin is most often monitored by the PTT. The PT, INR, and platelet aggregation time are not appreciably altered by therapeutic doses of heparin. Bleeding time can be used to monitor heparin effect, but is clinically burdensome and inconsistent.

5. The answer is E (1.1.1)

Troponin-I, CPK-MB, and ST segment elevation ≥1 mm are all relatively specific indicators of myocardial injury.

Answers

6. The answer is E (1.1.3)

Any, or all, of these agents can be given to KM post-MI. Late administration of beta-blocker therapy has been shown to prevent recurrent MI and death as well as improve left ventricular function. A number of studies have shown that the long-term use of ACE inhibitors following myocardial infarction reduces the incidence of recurrent MI, congestive heart failure, and death. Cholesterol-lowering drugs, like the statins, should be administered to all patients post-MI who have an LDL-cholesterol level of 100 mg/dL to prevent further endothelial damage and recurrent MI.

7. The answer is B (1.2.4)

Nifedipine, acetaminophen, and enoxaparin are devoid of any significant antiplatelet activity. While abciximab is a potent antiplatelet agent, it must be administered IV, and its cost and safety profile make it unsuitable for long-term outpatient use. Clopidogrel is a suitable alternative to aspirin for this indication.

8. The answer is D (1.1.0)

KM's diagnosis with hypertension and hypercholesterolemia place him at an increased risk of myocardial infarction. KM has a body mass index (BMI) of 41.2 and obese people (BMI >30) have an increased risk of AMI. Tobacco use increases the risk of many embolic events, including myocardial infarction. Men who are 45 or older and women who are 55 or older are more likely to have an AMI than younger men and women. KM is only 38 years old; therefore, his age does not put him at additional risk.

9. The answer is C (1.2.1)

Zocor is the brand name for simvastatin. Lipitor is the brand name for atorvastatin. Mevacor is the brand name for lovastatin. Pravachol is the brand name for pravastatin. Lopid is the brand name for gemfibrozil.

10. The answer is B (2.2.1)

Nicotine has very high first pass metabolism, therefore oral tablets are an ineffective means of delivery. Nicotine gum, transdermal patch, oral inhaler, and nasal spray products are all available for nicotine replacement therapy.

Case 4 Stroke

1. The answer is C (1.1.1)

While not a contraindication, clinicians are warned against using rt-PA in patients who have had major surgery or serious head trauma (excluding head trauma) in the previous 14 days. Evidence of intracranial hemorrhage, active internal bleeding, serious head trauma within the past 3 months, and known cerebral aneurysm are all contraindications to rt-PA use for the treatment of acute ischemic stroke.

2. The answer is D (1.1.2)

Systemic lupus is consistent with the development of hyper-coagulable disorders and is usually associated with venous thrombosis but may precipitate in arterial thrombosis in patients with underlying cardiovascular disease. Mechanical prosthetic cardiac valves have a higher propensity for thromboembolic events than do bioprosthetic valves. The three most common types of mechanical cardiac valves include the Starr-Edwards ball valve, the Bjork-Shiley disk valve, and the St. Jude medical valve. The first two have the highest propensity for thromboembolism. Valves in the mitral position tend to be far more thrombogenic than in the aortic positions. Diabetes is a well-recognized independent risk factor for stroke with a relative risk estimated at 1.5-3.0. The chance of having a stroke nearly doubles for each decade of life after age 55. A person who's had one or more TIAs is almost 10 times more likely to have a stroke than someone of the same age and sex who hasn't.

3. The answer is C (1.2.2)

Surgical intervention is the preferred treatment option for atheromatus lesions in the carotid arteries but since surgery is not an option for this patient, a number of medical modalities should occur. Since platelets are a key contributing factor to atheromatus lesions, aspirin should be initiated. A number of randomized trials have shown aspirin alone to be of significant benefit with up to a 24% relative risk reduction in incidence of nonfatal stroke. The angiotensin-receptor antagonist, candesartan, showed improved survival in phase II safety studies; HMG CoA reductase inhibitors have shown neuroprotective effects resulting from antiinflammatory properties.

4. The answer is C (1.2.2)

St. Jude mechanical heart valves are less thrombogenic in nature than the older mechanical heart valves (Starr-Edwards ball and Bjork-Shiley disk valves) but mechanical valves inserted in the mitral position are far more thrombogenic than in the aortic position. Since further anticoagulation may be required to treat other comorbidities, a repeat CT scan should be performed to rule out the likelihood of hemorrhage, whether thrombolytic therapy was used or not. Systemic embolization is nearly twice as likely to occur in patient with mechanical valves being treated with aspirin than those being treated with warfarin. The level of anticoagulation intensity varies based on the thrombogenicity of the valve, the presence of other risk factors for thrombus formation, and the site of valve replacement.

5. The answer is C (1.1.3)

The demonstrated risk reduction of coronary heart disease events by lipid-lowering agents is well documented. Less established are the same benefits extended to the effect on stroke. That is, until secondary statin prevention trials were completed where pravastatin demonstrated a total stroke incidence reduction when therapy was administered over 1 year. Diabetes is a well-recognized independent risk factor for stroke as well as

Answers

disorders of lipid/triglyceride metabolism. Although glycemic strict control has been shown to reduce diabetic complications, it is postulated that positive benefits may be seen related to the risk of stroke, though the evidence is less established. Benzodiazepines are first-line agents for treating seizures with lorazepam (1-4 mg over 2-10 minutes), being the preferred agent because of a shorter half-life over diazepam (5 mg over 2 minutes to a maximum of 10 mg).

6. The answer is E (1.3.2)

Patients may be admitted to a general medical unit, an intensive care unit, or to an integrated stroke unit. The health care team should be capable of performing frequent assessments of neurological and blood pressure measurements during the first 24-26 hours after the onset of stroke to allow for early detection of brain hemorrhage or recurrent stroke.

7. The answer is E (1.1.4)

Abnormalities in swallowing (dysphagia) are common in patients who have suffered a stroke. Patients must undergo a formal evaluation of swallowing to guide nutrition and avoid aspiration. Deaths are generally attributable to stroke as a result of medical complications such as pneumonia, sepsis, new cerebral infarction, cerebral edema, fever, and serious arrhythmias.

8. The answer is E (1.1.3)

The effects of aspirin on the treatment of acute ischemic stroke were evaluated in three trials. Two of the three, the International Stroke Trial and the Chinese Acute Stroke Trial, found that the use of early aspirin in patients treated within 48 hours of stroke onset reduced both the stroke recurrence risk and mortality. For every 1,000 acute strokes treated with aspirin, about 9 deaths or nonfatal stroke recurrences will be prevented in the first few weeks and approximately 13 fewer patients will be deceased or dependent at 6 months.

9. The answer is E (3.3.1)

Actos (pioglitazone) use has been associated with fluid retention and symptoms of heart failure, including edema and dyspnea. Plaquenil (hydroxychloroquine sulfate) is indicated for the treatment of SLE. Since the patient is taking warfarin, all major changes in diet and exercise should be discussed with the physician. Aspirin cannot be substituted for Tylenol (acetaminophen) if a patient is taking warfarin. Aspirin's antiplatelet effect can increase the likelihood of bleeding when used concomitantly with warfarin.

10. The answer is C (3.3.2)

The primary focus for primary and secondary stroke prevention is related in large part to modifiable risk factors for stroke. These factors include hypertension, diabetes mellitus, smoking, and various cardiac conditions. Nonmodifiable risk factors include older age, male sex, race, and genetic factors, such as SLE.

Case 5 Asthma

1. The answer is B (1.2.3)

Betagan® is an ophthalmic beta-blocking agent. Oral beta-blockers can precipitate asthma exacerbations in susceptible patients. Although not commonly observed, ophthalmic beta-blockers are systemically absorbed and can precipitate exacerbations. Although subtherapeutic theophylline levels (C) and nonadherence (E) might also precipitate exacerbations in some patients, SL's long-standing control and the timing of the exacerbation in relation to starting the new eye drops would suggest that they are not the most likely contributors. Acetaminophen (A) does not affect theophylline clearance.

2. The answer is B (1.1.3)

According to the guidelines, for patients with mild persistent asthma the preferred treatment is low-dose inhaled corticosteroids. Alternatively, patients may be treated with cromolyn, leukotriene modifiers (B), or sustained-release theophylline (serum concentration 5-15 mcg/mL). According to the guidelines, only patients with intermittent asthma do not require daily medication use (E). Oral prednisone (D) is reserved for acute exacerbations (short term) or for management of patients with severe persistent asthma. Serevent® (D) should only be used in conjunction with inhaled corticosteroids or leukotriene modifiers and would be used on a schedule rather than as needed.

3. The answer is B (1.2.1)

Xopenex (levalbuterol) is the R-enantiomer of racemic albuterol. Bronchodilation has been similar when equimolar doses of levalbuterol and racemic albuterol (1.25 mg and 2.5 mg) have been given.

4. The answer is C (1.1.3)

Cough (I) and chest tightness (II) may be present in a patient experiencing an acute asthma exacerbation. Fever (III) would be a sign of infection and not a presenting symptom of asthma.

5. The answer is C (1.1.2)

A peak flow meter measures the rate that air is forced out of a patient's lungs. A low measure of peak flow indicates obstruction. Peak flow does not measure air intake (A), total lung capacity (B), the rate of air exchange (D), or respiratory rate (E).

6. The answer is C (1.2.4)

Inhaled corticosteroids can cause thrush. After using a steroid inhaler, patients should be instructed to rinse their mouth to reduce this problem (C). Pulmicort® is a maintenance medication and it should not be taken orally to relieve symptoms of an acute exacerbation (B). It is metabolized in the liver and very little is excreted in the urine unchanged; therefore, routine renal assessment is unnecessary (A). It may take 4-8 weeks for the patient to see benefit from the Pulmicort® (D). In the United

States, Pulmicort® is only supplied as a dry powder inhaler, therefore is not used with a spacer device (E).

7. The answer is C (1.3.1)

A patient who is responding to albuterol will be able to breathe more comfortably (I) and, therefore, will have a lower respiratory rate (II). Albuterol may increase the heart rate and relief of symptoms may decrease the heart rate, making it a less than ideal monitoring parameter for response to treatment (III).

8. The answer is C (3.2.4)

Shaking container and priming the inhaler are important steps (A, B). The correct breathing process is slow and deep.

9. The answer is B (3.2.4)

Proper technique for peak flow monitoring includes several steps. Patients should first stand up if possible (B), take in as deep a breath as possible and place their mouth around the mouthpiece of the meter forming a tight seal. Blow out through the mouth as hard and fast as possible. Patients should do at least three readings, recording the date, time, and the highest flow achieved on a log. It typically takes 2 weeks during good asthma control to determine a personal best peak flow.

10. The answer is D (1.3.5)

According to the NIH guidelines for the treatment of asthma, the preferred treatment for moderate persistent asthma is a medium-dose inhaled corticosteroid (D) or a low-dose inhaled corticosteroid and long-acting inhaled beta $_2$ agonist. Alternatively, patients may be treated with low-dose inhaled corticosteroids and either a leukotriene modifier, theophylline or zileuton.

Since SL is already on theophylline, the addition of a medium-dose inhaled corticosteroid is a reasonable next step. Albuterol (A) is not a recommended maintenance medication and should be used for acute symptoms. Prednisone (B) should be reserved for those who do not respond to other recommended treatments. Cromolyn would not be expected to provide significant benefit and Foradil® should only be used in conjunction with inhaled corticosteroids or leukotriene modifiers.

Case 6 Asthma

1. The answer is C (1.1.4)

The maximum recommended dose of Advair® Diskus for all strengths is one puff twice daily. Two puffs twice daily increases the dose of salmeterol, which may cause WH's cardiovascular effects (C). There is no drug interaction between Advair® and Lasix® (A). The combination of Advair® and Flovent® (B) increases the fluticasone dose but would not lead to WH's cardiovascular symptoms. Noncompliance with an albuterol dosing regimen is not likely to cause these side effects (D) and while Advair® may cause hypertension, it is not a contraindication to therapy (E).

2. The answer is D (2.2.1)

Advair® is a combination product of fluticasone and salmeterol.

3. The answer is C (1.2.3)

The profile notes that WH's therapy was switched to Advair® due to WH forgetting which inhaler to take. The doctor intended for WH to use the Advair® (C) instead of using the Flovent® and Serevent® inhalers (E). Advair® is recommended for daily rather than as-needed use (A). Albuterol is typically used as needed for asthma exacerbations (B). The profile does not suggest that WH discontinue using the albuterol inhaler (D).

4. The answer is D (3.2.4)

NHLBI guidelines recommend that patients proceed to the ED when they experience a serious exacerbation characterized by PEF < 50% predicted or personal best that is unresponsive to treatment with beta agonists. This is usually characterized by marked wheezing and shortness of breath.

5. The answer is C (3.2.1)

According to NHLBI guidelines, patients with intermittent asthma should be limited to using short-acting inhaled beta$_2$-agonists (i.e., albuterol) to treat acute attacks, less than two times per week (B). No daily controller medication is indicated (A, D). If a patient uses a beta$_2$-agonist more frequently (three or more times per week), he or she may have more severe asthma, which requires daily use of a controller medication (B). Using a combination of both short- and long-acting beta$_2$-agonists along with inhaled corticosteroids is recommended for moderate persistent and severe persistent asthma therapy (C,E).

6. The answer is D (1.3.1)

Advair® is a combination product that is intended for daily use to maintain control of symptoms (D). Short-term beta-agonists are typically used for relief of acute exacerbations (A). Advair® is indicated for maintenance therapy in patients with persistent asthma, from moderate to severe (C). Since Advair® contains salmeterol, it is recommended that patients discontinue using the salmeterol inhaler when prescribed Advair® (B). Intermittent asthma is associated with acute attacks that can be treated with limited use of short-acting beta-2 agonists (E).

7. The answer is C (1.2.3)

Hepatic enzyme inducers enhance corticosteroid metabolism (I), while inhibitors may decrease corticosteroid metabolism (III). Rifampin is an inducer, and therefore may reduce corticosteroid efficacy by enhancing corticosteroid metabolism (II).

8. The answer is B (1.3.2)

Leukotriene modifiers (a.k.a., anti-leukotrienes) are indicated for daily use in the prevention and chronic treatment of asthma (A). Therefore, these agents should not be used in the treat-

Answers

ment of acute attacks (B). These medications are not recommended to treat acute exercise-induced bronchospasm or status asthmaticus, but can be used as preventative therapy (D). Headache, abdominal pain, and dizziness are all potential side effects of this class of medications (C). Some patients may benefit from both a leukotriene inhibitor and an inhaled corticosteroid (E).

9. The answer is C (1.2.1)

WH is taking 110 mcg, 2 puffs BID, which is equal to 440 mcg per day. The recommended initial dose and strength for patients currently taking fluticasone propionate (Flovent) 440 mcg per day is Advair 250/50 1 puff twice daily.

10. The answer is C (1.3.3)

Since Advair® contains salmeterol, WH should not use salmeterol concomitantly with the Advair® Diskus (B). WH should keep his albuterol inhaler as a reliever medication for acute asthma exacerbations, because Advair® will not stop these attacks once they have begun (A, D). WH should not exceed the recommended dose until he consults with his physician (E). It is also important that WH contact his physician immediately if he is experiencing any tachycardia or cardiovascular symptoms (C). This may be a serious sign of salmeterol overdose.

Case 7 Cystic Fibrosis

1. The answer is C (1.1.3)

The most prevalent pathogen to cause a pulmonary exacerbation of cystic fibrosis during childhood is *Staphylococcus aureus*. *Pseudomonas aeruginosa* becomes the most common organism in adolescents and adults. *Haemophilus influenza* is cultured more frequently early in life (2-5 years) and its frequency decreases with increasing age (C). Burkholderia *cepacia* and Stenotrophomonas maltophilia are less common pathogens found at any age (A, B, D, E).

2. The answer is B (1.2.1)

The standard approach to treatment of *Pseudomonas aeruginosa* in patients with cystic fibrosis is to use two medications with differing mechanisms (B) to enhance activity and reduce selection of resistant organisms. It is preferred that one of the agents be an aminoglycoside when possible. In this case, a medication effective for *staphylococcus aureus* is also recommended. Therefore, ticarcillin/clavulanate is a rational second agent that will be effective for both organisms. Monotherapy (A, D, E) is not recommended. Both meropenem and ceftazidime (C) share a mechanism of interfering with penicillin binding proteins.

3. The answer is E (2.1.1)

In the case of EF, she will require pancrelipase to cover her meals, nutrition at night, and her additional snack during the day. Each day, EF receives nine capsules for meals and four capsules for snacks or supplements. And therefore, she will need at least 390 pancrelipase capsules per 30 days. The pancrelipase usual dose does not exceed 10,000 lipase units/ kg/day. Her dose is equivalent to 156,000 lipase units/day or about 8,800 units/kg/day which falls below the maximum recommended dosage.

4. The answer is C (2.2.5)

Patients who are unable to swallow intact pancreatic enzyme product (PEP) capsules may sprinkle the contents on a small amount of acidic food such as apple sauce. PEPs must be taken with food (A). PEPs do not need to taken separately from calcium/aluminum products (B). PEP capsules should be swallowed whole and crushing/chewing may cause early release of enzymes and/or loss of activity (D). Drug retained in the mouth may cause irritation to the oral mucosa (E).

5. The answer is D (3.2.2)

Vitamin D3 is synthesized in the skin when it is exposed to ultraviolet-B rays from sunlight. Green vegetables are a source of vitamin K, organ meats are a source of vitamin A (B), and citrus fruits are a source of vitamin C (C). Carbonated beverage intake may increase calcium excretion (E).

6. The answer is B (2.2.5)

Dornase alpha should be stored under refrigeration and ampules should be protected from strong light. Unused ampules should be stored in their protective foil pouch under refrigeration.

7. The answer is A (1.2.2)

Macrolide antibiotics are thought to have a wide range of effects on different pathways of the inflammatory process and inhibit virulence factors produced by *Pseudomonas aeruginosa* (A). Hypertonic saline may work by increasing airway surface liquid volume (B). Inhaled steroids and prednisone are anti-inflammatories with no effect on *Pseudomonas aeruginosa* (C, D). Tobramycin inhaled (TOBI®) is an aminoglycoside antibiotic with activity against *Pseudomonas aeruginosa* and no direct anti-inflammatory properties (E).

8. The answer is E (2.2.2)

Tobramycin inhaled (TOBI®) 300 mg is available as a 5-mL single-dose ampule in a carton of 56 to complete the normal regimen of BID alternating months (E). Tobramycin injection is supplied at a concentration 40 mg/mL as both 2-mL or 30-mL vials, however given by the inhaled route would be considered off-label.

9. The answer is E (2.2.6)

According to the *Infection Control Recommendations for Patients With Cystic Fibrosis* and if the manufacturer's instruction allow, nebulizer parts need to be disinfected with either of those agents or boiling/microwaving. It is best to avoid mixing inhaled solutions as dornase alpha is incompatible (A) and the recommended sequence is bronchodilators, (hypertonic saline), dornase alpha, antibiotics (B). Bacterial contamination is possible with nebulizers that have been in contact with mucous membranes and/or sputum (C). Vinegar is not adequate for disinfection (D).

10. The answer is D (1.1.4)

Cystic fibrosis is a multi-system disease affecting the respiratory, digestive, endocrine, bone and joint, and reproductive systems. Faulty transport of salt leads to thick, sticky mucus that blocks the ducts in these organs. Other diseases to monitor patients with cystic fibrosis for included pansinusitis, hepatobiliary disease, diabetes, osteoporosis, infertility, and depression. Obesity and coronary heart disease are not commonly associated with cystic fibrosis.

Case 8 Rhinitis (Perennial)

1. The answer is C (1.2.4)

The FDA has requested that manufacturers cease marketing products containing phenylpropanolamine (PPA). An association between hemorrhagic stroke and the use of PPA contained in cough and cold products has been reported. Although the risk of hemorrhagic stroke is low, the FDA does not believe that the benefits warrant the risk of a serious stroke. Generally, if the product has been properly stored and has not reached its expiration date, it would be acceptable to use. As this patient does have uncontrolled allergy symptoms, many other therapies would most likely be more effective. However, the fact this product has been removed from the market is the primary reason that this patient should not use it.

2. The answer is A (1.1.1)

Offspring of parents with allergic disease have about a 25% risk of also developing allergic diseases. The patient's allergic history influences his son's risk factor for disease (B). The son's disease does not affect the father (C). The patient's asthma and sinus disease are comorbidities of allergic disease (D, E).

3. The answer is D (1.3.1)

Although maximum efficacy is typically seen after 3 to 14 days of consistent therapy, onset of action can occur after 12 hours.

4. The answer is A (2.2.5)

It is important to blow the nose prior to administering the spray. This allows a clearer passage for the spray to reach its target site as does tilting the head forward. Directing the spray away from the septum helps decrease the chances of damaging the septum and allows the medication to reach the turbinates. Blowing the nose after administration simply removes the medication from the nose.

5. The answer is D (1.3.3)

Epistaxis is the most commonly reported adverse effect of intranasal corticosteroids. Nasal septal perforation, nasal sores, and cataract formation are less common adverse effects, but they have been reported. Increased intraocular pressure, not decreased intraocular pressure, has also been reported as a rare adverse effect when using intranasal corticosteroids.

6. The answer is A (1.3.2)

If used correctly, intranasal corticosteroids are one of the most effective medications available to treat allergic rhinitis. Adding an antihistamine/decongestant, an intranasal or an ophthalmic antihistamine may be somewhat helpful (B, C, E). Because he still continues to have symptoms, this patient may be a candidate for immunotherapy (D). Doubling the dose of intranasal corticosteroids has not been proven to be effective (A).

7. The answer is D (3.2.1)

An ocular antihistamine, such as olopatadine, would be the most effective choice. It will help decrease ocular symptoms (D). Although effective, a mast cell stabilizer such as cromolyn requires more frequent dosing (E). A decongestant eye drop such as Visine® will suppress redness, but long-term use may result in a rebound effect (A). Ophthalmic corticosteroid use may lead to the development of glaucoma and cataracts (B). Artificial tears may be soothing in the short-term but will not help relieve the redness, itching, or tearing (C).

8. The answer is A (1.2.4)

For many years package inserts with antihistamines stated that the use of antihistamines in those with asthma was contraindicated. It was once thought the drying effects of the older antihistamines would worsen asthma symptoms. However, histamine is one of many mediators which contribute to asthma, and blocking histamine receptors may actually lead to a slight improvement in lung function. No dose modification, specific dose route, or use in combination with other medications is necessary for the use of antihistamines in those with asthma.

9. The answer is C (1.2.4)

Rebound congestion or rhinitis medicamentosa is a frequent adverse effect of using decongestant nasal sprays for more than 5 to 7 days. Nasal spray decongestants are ineffective for rhinorrhea and very effective for the short-term relief of congestion. The pollen season may be worse than previous seasons. However, his main complaint was the increased congestion, which is most likely a result of the oxymetazoline. He could be administering the nasal spray improperly, but it would not result in his symptoms being much worse. There is no drug reaction between the oxymetazoline and the antihistamine he is using.

10. The answer is D (3.2.4)

To avoid seasonal outdoor pollens, patients should try to stay

Answers

indoors with the air conditioner on if possible. Windows should remain closed, including car windows, to help minimize pollen exposure. Windy days promote the dissemination of pollen and patients should try to avoid outdoor activities during windy days.

Case 9 PUD NSAID

1. The answer is D (1.3.3)

Nonselective NSAIDs, e.g., ibuprofen and naproxen, cause ulcers primarily by the systemic inhibition of the COX-1 enzyme (D). Anti-inflammatory effects result from the inhibition of COX-2 (E). Nonselective NSAIDs do not cause ulcers by increasing gastric acid secretion (A) or by directly damaging the GI mucosa (B). Although nonselective NSAIDs cause superficial damage to the GI mucosa (a topical effect), the primary mechanism for ulcer formation is related to their systemic effects (inhibition of COX-1), which results in the inhibition of mucosal prostaglandins (C) and impairment of the mucosal barrier.

2. The answer is C (1.1.4)

The risk associated with psychological stress and NSAID-induced ulcers/complications has not been established (C). However, age >65 years (A), history of PUD or an ulcer complication (B), concomitant anticoagulation (D), and multiple NSAID use (E) are all well-established risk factors for NSAID ulcers and related complications.

3. The answer is B (3.2.1)

Enteric-coated aspirin may protect against the topical mucosal damage in the stomach and minimize dyspepsia associated with aspirin, but the enteric coating does not prevent ulcer formation, because aspirin is released in the duodenum and then absorbed systemically (A). Buffering aspirin may cause less dyspepsia, but buffering does not protect ulcers from forming because of its systemic effects (B). Lower dosages of aspirin, e.g., 81 mg/day, may also cause peptic ulcers, but ulcer risk is less than with higher aspirin dosages (C). Taking food, milk (D), or an antacid (E) with aspirin may minimize dyspepsia associated with aspirin but does not prevent peptic ulcers.

4. The answer is D (1.1.4)

Ulcer risk associated with nonselective NSAIDs is related to the relative inhibition of COX-1 versus COX-2. Although all of the listed NSAIDs inhibit both COX-1 and COX-2 and may cause ulcers, nabumetone (D) is associated with the lowest ulcer risk because of its greater inhibition of COX-2 than COX-1. In contrast to the nonselective NSAIDs, e.g., ibuprofen (A), naproxen (B), diclofenac (C), and aspirin (E), nabumetone (as well as etodolac and meloxicam) is considered to be partially COX-2 selective NSAIDs and, therefore, is associated with less ulcer risk.

5. The answer is D (1.1.3)

Upper GI bleeding is the most frequent serious complication associated with nonselective NSAIDs (D). Gastric outlet obstruction (A) and ulcer perforation (C) and penetration (E) are also serious complications of NSAIDs, but they occur much less frequently than bleeding. Gastric cancer is not a complication of NSAID treatment (B).

6. The answer is B (1.2.0)

The recommended regimen to heal an NSAID-induced ulcer (whether the NSAID is continued or discontinued) is a PPI, e.g., pantoprazole 40 mg qd (B). Although an H_2RA, e.g. famotidine (C, D) or sucralfate (E), may be used to heal the ulcer, substantial evidence indicates that PPIs provide more rapid relief of symptoms and the most rapid rate of ulcer healing. When the NSAID is continued, however, the ulcer heals at a slower rate (8-12 weeks) than when the NSAID is discontinued (4-8 weeks). Misoprostol, although effective, is not labeled for ulcer healing in the United States (only indicated as cotherapy for reducing ulcer risk in patients taking NSAIDs) (A). Misoprostol (in the dose indicated) requires four times a day dosing versus once daily for a PPI and its side effects are more troublesome for the patient.

7. The answer is C (1.2.0)

The preferred cotherapy for reducing the risk of NSAID ulcers is a standard dose of a PPI, as there is sufficient evidence to support this indication at this daily dosage (C). There is insufficient evidence to support the use of H_2RAs (A, B), even at higher dosages, when used as prophylactic cotherapy for the reduction of ulcer risk. Cotherapy with misoprostol is effective, but the minimum effective daily dose is 400 mcg/day (D). Misoprostol 600 and 800 mcg/day are more effective than the 400 mcg/day dosage but are associated with increased adverse effects. Misoprostol 600 mcg/day provides similar efficacy to the 800 mcg/day with fewer adverse effects. There is insufficient evidence to support the efficacy of sucralfate cotherapy for this indication (E).

8. The answer is A (1.3.3)

The most important side effects associated with misoprostol are abdominal cramping and diarrhea, as they are often troublesome and may lead to discontinuation of the medication (A). The abdominal cramping and diarrhea are dose-related and occur more frequently at higher misoprostol dosages. Although other side effects may occur, they occur less frequently and usually are not as troublesome (B, C, D, E).

9. The answer is E (1.2.3)

Low-dose aspirin is often used in patients who require the cardioprotective effects of aspirin because celecoxib is devoid of antiplatelet activity. However, there is evidence to indicate that when low-dose aspirin is combined with celecoxib, the aspirin is likely to negate the ulcer-sparing effects of celecoxib (E). Low-dose aspirin does not alter the anti-inflammatory effects of celecoxib (A). Celecoxib does not alter the antiplatelet effects of low-dose aspirin (B, D). Although aspirin and celecoxib have the potential to impair renal function, combining these agents does not cause nephrotoxicity, per se (C).

10. The answer is C (2.2.1)

Misoprostol is contraindicated during pregnancy as it induces uterine contractions (C). It is not contraindicated in patients with liver disease (A), asthma (B), diabetes (D) or SLE (E).

Case 10 GERD OTC

1. The answer is C (1.1.3)

Heartburn is typically described as a burning sensation that arises from the chest (or sternum) and moves upward toward the neck (C). Typical heartburn does not arise from the epigastrium (A, B) or the umbilicus (E). Typical heartburn that arises from the chest does not move downward toward the stomach (D). Heartburn is the most common typical symptom of gastroesophageal reflux disease, but it may be part of a symptom complex that accompanies other acid-related disorders such as indigestion or dyspepsia and peptic ulcer disease.

2. The answer is E (1.1.0)

Patients with heartburn occurring 3-4 days/week that persists for 3 months or longer should be excluded from self-treatment and referred to their primary care provider for further medical evaluation because of the frequency and duration of their symptoms (E). Patients with heartburn occurring 3-4 days/week of less than 3 months duration (A), heartburn which is characterized as mild to moderate (D), heartburn accompanied by a sour taste (B), or heartburn unresponsive to a trial of nonprescription H_2RAs are generally all self-treatable (C).

3. The answer is C (1.2.1)

The FDA has specifically defined "frequent" heartburn related to the nonprescription use of omeprazole as heartburn that occurs two or more days a week (C). All other definitions are incorrect (A, B, D, E).

4. The answer is A (3.2.0)

All of the nonpharmacologic modifications listed are recommended for JC to reduce her heartburn (B, C, D, E) except elevation of the foot of the bed (A). JC should be counseled to elevate the head of the bed by using 6-inch blocks or a 10-inch foam wedge. Elevating the head of the bed enables gravity to facilitate the return of refluxate from the esophagus to the stomach thereby limiting contact time between the refluxate and the esophageal mucosa. Elevating the foot of the bed reverses the effect of gravity and increases contact time between the refluxate and the esophageal mucosa. The longer the contact time between the refluxate and the esophageal mucosa, the greater the chance for esophageal injury.

5. The answer is B (1.2.0)

The preferred management of this woman's frequent heartburn is Prilosec OTC 20 mg daily for 14 days (B). Nonprescription omeprazole is the drug of choice for frequent heartburn (heartburn that occurs two or more days a week). Scheduled dosages of an antacid (E) or an H_2RA (regardless of strength) (C, D) are intended for mild, infrequent, or occasional heartburn. This patient is a candidate for self-treatment with nonprescription omeprazole so it is not necessary to refer her to her primary care provider at this time (A).

6. The answer is E (1.1.0)

Patients who self-treat heartburn with nonprescription omeprazole and have recurrent symptoms on completion of the 14-day regimen should contact their primary care provider to determine if they should continue taking the medication (E). Self-treatment with nonprescription omeprazole is limited to 14 days and no more than every 4 months. The patient should not be advised to continue taking the regimen (A), increase the daily dosage (B), or add an H_2RA (D). Although these may be viable options for the physician, they are not appropriate for self-care. Nonprescription omeprazole is indicated for frequent heartburn (daily for 14 days) and should not be used on a prn basis (C).

7. The answer is A (1.3.3)

The most common side effects associated with the short-term use of nonprescription omeprazole are headache and diarrhea (A). Constipation, intestinal gas (B), nausea (C), itching, and skin rash (E) occur less frequently. Vomiting is uncommon (C). Dry mouth and cough (D) are usually not associated with the administration of nonprescription omeprazole.

8. The answer is C (1.2.1)

An H_2RA 1 hour prior to eating (A) is the preferred management of an individual who wishes to prevent anticipated heartburn after eating certain foods or meals (C). The onset of symptom relief with an H_2RA requires about 45 minutes to an hour. Taking an H_2RA immediately prior to eating does not allow adequate time for onset of the H_2RA antisecretory effect (B). Taking the H_2RA twice daily is unnecessary for this indication (D). Taking the H_2RA at bedtime will not prevent heartburn after the dinner meal the next day (E), as the duration of the H_2RA antisecretory effect lasts for up to 8-10 hours.

9. The answer is D (1.3.3)

In patients with normal renal function, about 15%-30% of magnesium is absorbed from magnesium-containing salts and then renally eliminated. Renal failure decreases the elimination of magnesium, which may lead to accumulation and toxicity (D). Renal failure does not increase the absorption (B), distribution (C), or elimination (A) of magnesium. Renal failure does not decrease magnesium absorption (E).

Answers

10. The answer is B (1.3.0)

The preferred initial management of this woman's heartburn is to begin with nonpharmacologic measures (A). Dietary and lifestyle modifications (B) will most likely prevent her mild and infrequent heartburn, especially if she ate smaller and more frequent meals and avoided lying down for several hours after eating. If these measures are not effective, then a calcium-containing antacid may be recommended prn heartburn and not on a scheduled basis (C). The use of nonprescription H_2RAs (D) or omeprazole (E) is not warranted at this time and should not be recommended as initial treatment for this woman. Although a H_2RA or PPI may be used during pregnancy, the woman should discuss use of these agents with her primary care provider to determine the risk versus the benefits of such use.

Case 11 Constipation (Temporary)

1. The answer is B (1.1.3)

Constipation is a symptom and not a disease. Patients (not physicians) typically characterize constipation subjectively as hard stools (A), straining when passing stool (C), incomplete evaluation (D), and infrequent bowel movements (E), all of which may be accompanied by abdominal bloating. A change in stool color (B) is not descriptive of constipation.

2. The answer is A (1.1.0)

Constipation can affect individuals of all ages and both sexes. However, the prevalence of constipation in the United States is higher in women than men and higher in the elderly (greater than 65 years of age) (A). IBD (B) (inflammatory bowel disease) is associated with diarrhea, not constipation. Men (C) have a lower prevalence of constipation than women. Patients with IBS (C) (irritable bowel syndrome) may have either constipation or diarrhea. Women who are pregnant have a higher prevalence than women who are not (E). Constipation is not as prevalent in children under 18 years of age (D, E).

3. The answer is D (1.1.0)

Individuals who describe a change in the caliber of the stool (A), especially "pencil-thin," marked or severe abdominal pain (B), distention or cramping, blood in the stool (C), unexplained weight loss, fever, nausea and vomiting, or constipation that persists after 1 week of self-treatment (E) should be referred for further medical evaluation, as these may be indicative of a more serious problem. A recommendation of self-treatment is appropriate for patients with mild-to-moderate symptoms less than 2 weeks in duration (D).

4. The answer is E (3.2.2)

Nonpharmacologic measures that include specific dietary and lifestyle changes constitute the initial step in preventing or mini-mizing constipation and should be included in the treatment plan of all patients who complain of constipation. Lifestyle and dietary changes, however, usually do not provide a sufficiently rapid response in symptomatic patients such as AW. Increasing dietary fiber (A), fluids (especially water) (B), and physical activity (C) are all important for good health but also serve to decrease the risk of constipation. This is particularly important during travel (D) as individuals sit or are immobile for long times and eating habits are often disrupted. Sleeping more may be important to an individual, but it decreases mobility and physician activity (E).

5. The answer is C (3.2.2)

Bran-containing foods (A), prunes (B), legumes (D), and vegetables (E) such as broccoli provide higher amounts of fiber per serving than "white" foods such as pasta (C), bread, or rice.

6. The answer is D (1.2.0)

Nonprescription pharmacologic treatment is indicated (A) because this individual is symptomatic, uncomfortable, and requesting assistance. Because symptoms are mild and less than 2 weeks in duration, and the patient does not have any exclusions to self-care, treatment with a nonprescription medication is appropriate (E). Similar to dietary fiber, fiber supplements (e.g., psyllium, polycarbophil) usually require at least 1-3 days to soften the stool and are usually associated with some degree of bloating or flatulence (B). Emollients such as docusate are effective stool softeners when the goal of therapy is to avoid straining/constipation. However, there is insufficient evidence to support their use as a laxative to "treat" constipation (C). A single dose of Milk of Magnesia (magnesium hydroxide) will provide a more rapid evacuation of stool than fiber or docusate and will relieve her symptoms (D). The patient does not have any exclusions for the use of magnesium-containing laxatives.

7. The answer is C (1.3.1)

Saline laxatives such as magnesium hydroxide (Milk of Magnesia) usually provide watery evacuation of the bowel in about 6-8 hours (C). Drinking 8 ounces of water following the dose usually facilitates the laxative action and helps to prevent dehydration. All of the other timeframes listed are incorrect (A, B, D, E).

8. The answer is B (1.2.5)

Docusate salts (sodium or calcium) are anionic detergents (surfactants) that promote the mixture of water with fecal matter, thereby softening the stool (B). Fiber supplements (bulk laxatives) (A) act similar to dietary fiber, i.e., increasing stool bulk by retaining water. Saline laxatives such as magnesium hydroxide (D), bisacodyl (C), and PEG 3350 (E) work by other mechanisms.

9. The answer is A (1.3.0)

Senna is considered a stimulant laxative. Anthraquinone glycosides such as senna are prodrugs that are converted by colonic bacteria to their active form (aglycons) and then stimulate colonic motility (A). Stimulant laxatives may also act by increasing the secretion of fluid into the bowel lumen, releasing kinins that stimulate chloride secretion in the colon. Senna laxatives (as with other anthraquinones) usually act within 6-12 hours (D), may cause abdominal cramping (C), and discolor the urine (from pink to red or brown to black) (B). Long-term use is associated with a darkening of the colonic mucosa (melanosi coli) (E).

10. The answer is D (1.3.3)

Aluminum salts such as aluminum-containing antacids or sucralfate (B), medications that contain anticholinergic properties such as amitriptyline (A), diuretics such as hydrochlorothiazide (C), and some calcium-channel blockers such as verapamil (E) may cause constipation. Misoprostol is associated with a dose-dependent diarrhea (D).

Case 12 NV (Not Chemo Related)

1. The answer is C (1.1.3)

The classic symptoms of motion sickness are nausea and vomiting (C). Other common symptoms include pallor, cold sweat, excessive salivation, dizziness, and restlessness. Headache, loss of appetite (A), belching and flatulence (D) occur less frequently. Difficulty in breathing (B) and increased heart rate (E) are uncommon.

2. The answer is E (1.1.4)

Motion sickness occurs when the body is subjected to accelerations of movement in different directions or under conditions where visual contact with the outside horizon is lost. The balance center of the inner ear sends messages to the brain that conflict with visual clues. Looking outside the window of a car, plane, train, or boat helps reconcile visual input with vestibular input to overcome the neuronal mismatch (E). Reading and playing hand-held games (D), smoking or being in close proximity to smokers (B), as well as fear, stress, and anxiety (A) in anticipation of an upcoming trip may contribute to motion sickness. The duration or length of the trip (C) is important because the longer motion is sustained, the greater the risk of developing motion sickness.

3. The answer is B (3.2.2)

The best treatment for motion sickness is to prevent it. Preventing motion sickness can best be accomplished by nondrug measures such as avoiding strong odors or aromas (A), avoiding excessive food or alcohol (D) before and during travel, sitting facing forward in a slightly reclined position (C), sitting where motion is felt the least such as over the wing in an airplane and in the front seat of a car (E), and keeping your eyes on the horizon or another distant, unmoving object. Individuals should be advised to keep their head and body as still as possible and not to get up and move around (B).

4. The answer is D (1.2.1)

The antihistamines (central cholinergic blockers) are first-line therapy for motion sickness because they have been proven to be effective and have an acceptable safety profile (D). None of the other classes listed are considered first-line therapy (A, B, C, E).

5. The answer is E (1.3.1)

Most medications used to prevent motion sickness must be taken at least 1 hour before travel in order to allow sufficient time for onset of effect (D). Antihistamines such as Bonine are considered first-line therapy for motion sickness (A). Use should be continued during travel. Since this patient took Bonine "when she got sick" it is not surprising that the drug was not effective (E). Anticholinergic medications work best by blocking the cholinergic receptors before they are stimulated. In addition, gastric motility decreases following the onset of motion sickness. The dosage form and dose were likely appropriate (B, C).

6. The answer is B (2.2.2)

Nonprescription motion sickness products include Dramamine (dimenhyrinate) (A), Bonine (meclizine) (C), Antivert (meclizine) (D), and Marezine (cyclizine) (E). Phenergan (promethazine) (B) is the only phenothiazine that is effective against motion sickness, but it is only available by prescription.

7. The answer is A (1.3.3)

The most common side effects associated with nonprescription dosages of motion sickness medication are dry mouth and drowsiness (A). Blurred vision (C) and constipation (not diarrhea) (E) may occur but are less frequent with these dosages. Dizziness (B) and fatigue (D) are uncommon.

8. The answer is C (1.2.0)

Scopolamine is effective for motion sickness involving car, air, train, or sea travel regardless of the dosage form that is used (B). Oral scopolamine tablets are better suited for travel of short duration (C) than the transdermal dosage form as anti-motion sickness effects last 6-8 hours after an oral dose of the tablets versus up to 72 hours after application of the transdermal patch (A). The onset of effect with the oral dosage form is about 1 hour (D). The tablets are usually less costly than the transdermal dosage form (E).

9. The answer is D (1.2.0)

The individual should be instructed to apply the transdermal scopolamine patch (which is about the size of a dime) to a hairless area behind the ear, not the upper arm or chest (D). The patch should only be applied to skin in the post-auricular area. All other teaching points are correct (A, B, C, E).

10. The answer is A (3.2.2)

Sea-Band is a knitted elastic wrist band which works by applying pressure on the Nei Kuan acupressure point on each wrist by means of a plastic stud (A). Although these bands serve as

Answers

an alternative to medications, their effectiveness in specifically preventing motion sickness is uncertain. The wrist band uses the ancient Eastern concept of acupressure to control nausea and vomiting. Pressure is applied to Chi energy, which travels along meridians known as "acu" points. The Sea-Band may be washed up to five times with a mild detergent in warm water without losing its elasticity. Acustimulation (C) bands (Relief Band) use electrical stimulation on the P6 acupuncture point. The acupressure band is worn on both wrists, but the acustimulation band is worn on only one wrist. Acupuncture involves stimulation of certain points and meridians with needles inserted into the skin (B). Acupoint therapy involves stimulation of certain points and meridians with a therapy stick (D). Acutherm (E) is not medically relevant.

Case 13 ADEs

1. The answer is A (1.3.3)

All five of the listed agents have been associated with hepatotoxicity in the clinical literature. Only amiodarone (A), however, is associated with enhanced toxicity with longer duration of exposure (i.e., increased cumulative dose).

2. The answer is E (1.3.3)

Although it can be difficult to determine the causative agent, JG's clinical presentation and liver biopsy are characteristic of warfarin-induced (E) hepatotoxicity. Transaminases are elevated approximately threefold with no jaundice, and the liver biopsy results are classic, especially the presence of steatohepatitis. The symptoms are similar to the hepatotoxicity caused by amiodarone (A) but the biopsy results are not as amiodarone causes phospholipidosis. Lisinopril (B), allopurinol (C), and furosemide (D) are only rarely associated with hepatotoxicity and may cause either cytotoxic or cholestatic findings.

3. The answer is D (3.1.2)

JG likely has a component of chronic liver disease that has been exacerbated by a drug-induced injury. Therefore, the etiology of his liver disease does not match the type of liver disease that was required of subjects in the pilot study. In addition, the study did not find any meaningful clinical benefits of using milk thistle. Therefore, JG should not receive milk thistle based on the fact that the study lacks evidence of clinical benefits in patients like JG.

4. The answer is A (1.2.4)

The (-)-S- and (+)-R-enantiomers of warfarin are metabolized by the CYP1A2 and CYP2C9 hepatic isozymes, respectively. Amiodarone (A) decreases the activity of both of these cytochrome P450 enzymes to reduce warfarin metabolism and increase its anticoagulation effect. INR should be closely monitored. Lisinopril (B), furosemide (D), and digoxin (E) do not interfere with warfarin metabolism. ECASA (C) may enhance the anticoagulation activity of warfarin but not by a mechanism that involves altered metabolism.

5. The answer is D (1.2.6)

Digoxin (D) doses should be empirically decreased by approximately 50% if amiodarone is added to the regimen. Digoxin concentration usually increases by approximately 40% due to decreased tubular secretion and displacement of digoxin from tissue-binding sites. Amiodarone has no clinically important interaction with lisinopril (A), ECASA (C), or KCL (E). Amiodarone decreases warfarin (B) metabolism so the dose of warfarin should be decreased (not increased). If the decision is made to discontinue amiodarone therapy (which is likely in this patient), the doses of warfarin and digoxin will need to be increased with care because amiodarone has an extremely long half-life and will continue to be present in the patient's body for some time.

6. The answer is E (1.2.4)

Amiodarone has no clinically important effect on renal function, nor is it cleared by the kidneys (E). Amiodarone does commonly cause elevations in serum transaminase concentrations that may or may not be symptomatic (B). It also commonly causes pulmonary toxicity that requires discontinuation of the drug and, possibly, steroid therapy (C). Thyroid dysfunction (either hypothyroidism or hyperthyroidism) may also occur (D), as well as bradycardia, hypotension, and cardiac dysrhythmias (A). Periodic eye examinations should also be performed to detect corneal microdeposits.

7. The answer is C (2.3.1)

When amiodarone is diluted in saline solutions it may form a visibly apparent cloudy precipitation due to the salting out effect of amiodarone. This is especially evident with dilute amiodarone solutions (<1 mg/mL). Provided it is not mixed in a polyvinyl chloride (PVC) container, amiodarone is stable in dextrose 5% water. Its stability in Ringer's lactate or sterile water in not known.

8. The answer is A (3.2.2)

Hypercholesterolemia is a known risk factor for liver disease from drug-induced steatohepatitis (A). Since JG is experiencing this type of liver toxicity, JG should be counseled about measures to lower his cholesterol.

9. The answer is C (2.1.3)

There are several ways to approach this calculation. Perhaps the easiest is to determine that 15 mEq of KCl is contained in 187.5 mL of normal saline, based on the KCl concentration in the bag (20 mEq KCl in 500 mL normal saline or 0.08 mEq/mL). 187.5 mL divided by 60 minutes equals 3.125 mL/min.

10. The answer is C (1.2.1)

Lovastatin (A), atorvastatin (B), simvastatin (D), and rosuvastatin (E) all undergo metabolism via the CYP enzymes.

Pravastatin (C) is primarily conjugated with no CYP metabolism. Therefore, it is the statin least likely to be affected by JG's liver dysfunction.

Case 14 Cirrhosis

1. The answer is D (3.2.1)

Esomeprazole (D) by continuous infusion administration is used to treat nonvariceal upper gastrointestinal hemorrhage. The gastroenterologist has performed an endoscopy and determined the cause of hemorrhage to be esophageal varices. Therefore, esomeprazole may be stepped down to ranitidine for the purpose of providing stress ulcer prophylaxis while EK remains critically ill on the ventilator. Therapy with octreotide (A) reduces the likelihood of rebleeding from varices and should be continued for a total of 3–5 days of treatment. Oral propranolol should be initiated once EK is stable. Lorazepam (B) should be used as needed to provide symptom-triggered therapy of alcohol withdrawal. Enteral administration of nutrition (E) or medications (C) should not occur until the recent variceal hemorrhage is stable and should not replace vitamin supplementation.

2. The answer is B (1.1.2)

The Child-Pugh score does not use serum creatinine (B) when it is calculated. It is calculated based on the presence and extent of ascites, the presence and extent of encephalopathy, and serum values of total bilirubin, albumin, and either prothrombin time or INR. This is unlike the Model for End-stage Liver Disease (MELD) that does use serum creatinine when it is calculated by the formula $9.57 \times \log_e$ (creatinine, mg/dL) + $3.78 \times \log_e$ (bilirubin, mg/dL) + $11.20 \times \log_e$ (INR) + 6.43.

3. The answer is C (2.1.3)

Fifty units per hour of octreotide are to be administered. If 200 mL delivers 400 units, then 25 mL each hour will deliver the required 50 U.

4. The answer is D (1.2.1)

Albumin, when administered as 1.5 g/kg followed by 1 g/kg 3 days later in patients with spontaneous bacterial peritonitis, has been shown in a randomized study to reduce the incidence of renal dysfunction (D) and short-term mortality. It is commonly administered as a method to increase vascular oncotic pressure in an attempt to reduce ascitic fluid volume but this has never been proven effective in studies.

5. The answer is A (3.1.2)

Cost effectiveness is calculated as change in cost divided by the change in effect. The high cost of rFVIIa relative to the low savings associated with reduced use of blood products means that it would not be cost-effective at the studied dosage regimen if the only beneficial outcome is reduced blood product usage.

6. The answer is C (1.2.1)

This patient has a prolonged prothrombin time most likely due the inability to produce clotting factors secondary to liver failure. Desmopressin (A) causes the release of von Willebrand's factor to enhance platelet adhesiveness. This is not beneficial in coagulopathy associated with liver dysfunction. Vitamin K (B) is frequently administered when liver failure is present because many clotting factors require vitamin K for activity and some patients may be nutritionally deficient. However, vitamin K alone has minimal effect on prothrombin time when used for this indication. Fresh frozen plasma (C) contains clotting factors that will replace those deficient in EK due to his inability to synthesize adequate amounts in the liver. It is an appropriate treatment to attempt to restore a prolonged PT toward normal in EK. Cryoprecipitate (D) contains large amounts of fibrinogen and Amicar (E) inactivates proteases that break down clots but neither is currently warranted.

7. The answer is D (1.3.3)

EK's hyponatremia is likely caused by excessive production of ADH and aldosterone leading to hypervolemic hyponatremia. Therefore, EK's total body sodium stores are actually high but the serum concentration appears low due too much fluid retention. Replacing sodium with saline (A) or hypertonic saline (B) is not warranted as EK is not suffering adverse consequences from hyponatremia and his total body sodium is elevated. The administration of a thiazide diuretic (C) will cause the loss of more sodium than water and may worsen hyponatremia. A loop diuretic would be a better choice as it should cause the excretion of more water than sodium. Fluid restriction (D) will help lessen the extent of hypervolemia to aid in the reversal of hyponatremia. Demeclocycline (E) is used to inhibit ADH during isolated states of too much ADH.

8. The answer is C (1.3.3)

IV vasopressin at doses exceeding 0.04 U/min may cause excessive vasoconstriction and induce ischemia or hypertension. Ischemia may occur in the skin and soft tissue (necrotic digits), gastrointestinal tract (elevated lactate), or heart (infarction). Therefore, monitoring should frequently evaluate for cardiac ischemia (C) by assessing cardiac enzymes and ECG.

9. The answer is C (2.1.2)

Based on EK's weight of 77 kg, a caloric intake of 25 kcal/kg/day requires 962.5 mL of Nutren 2.0 per day. This volume of Nutren 2.0 provides 77 g of protein, which is equivalent to 1 g/kg of protein daily.

10. The answer is E (1.3.1)

EK is not diagnosed with community-acquired pneumonia. EK's has end-stage liver disease and is diagnosed with spontaneous bacterial peritonitis (SBP). According to several expert recommendations, EK requires lifelong prophylaxis to prevent reoccurrence of SBP. Prophylaxis is usually provided with sulfamethoxazole-trimethoprim but EK has a history of de-

Answers

veloping a maculopapular rash to sulfa. Therefore, the best option is to provide prophylaxis with an oral quinolone.

Case 15 Pancreatitis

1. The answer is C (1.3.3)

Thiazide diuretics (C) are strongly associated with acute pancreatitis. Rare reports of acetaminophen (A), amlodipine (B), ibuprofen (D), and lansoprazole (E) have appeared in the literature but most contain other possible etiologies.

2. The answer is A (1.2.1)

Meperidine is generally recommended to control the pain of acute pancreatitis because it may cause less spasm of Oddi's sphincter than morphine and its derivatives. Because the clinical significance of opioid-induced sphincter spasm is unknown, it is reasonable to select a more potent opioid if adequate pain relief is not achieved with meperidine.

3. The answer is B (1.1.2)

Serum lipase (B) is the most sensitive and specific marker of acute pancreatitis. It peaks within 24 hours and normalizes within a week. Serum amylase (A) peaks within hours but may rise in response to other disease states and bodily sources. While alcohol use is a risk factor for developing pancreatitis, blood alcohol content (C) does not correlate with onset. C-reactive protein (D) is indicative of nonspecific inflammation. Lactate (E) is indicative of nonspecific tissue hypoperfusion.

4. The answer is E (1.3.3)

Flumazenil is a benzodiazepine antagonist used for the reversal of benzodiazepine-induced sedation or the management of benzodiazepine overdose. Physostigmine and its salts are reversible acetylcholinesterase inhibitors that can be used to reverse the effects produced by the overdose of anticholinergic drugs or plants. Naloxone and naltrexone are pure opiate antagonists. Acetylcysteine is a derivative of L-cysteine that is used as a mucolytic agent and in the treatment of acetaminophen overdose.

5. The answer is A (3.2.2)

While parenteral nutrition should be initiated in patients unable to tolerate enteral nutrition, it is associated with increased risk of infection compared to enteral nutrition. Whether parenteral nutrition increases infection risk compared with no nutrition is unknown in acute pancreatitis. Current guidelines from the American Society of Parenteral and Enteral Nutrition recommend initiating parenteral nutrition in patients with acute pancreatitis after 5 days if enteral nutrition is not sufficient. Parenteral nutrition is also associated with prolonged hospital stay and mortality compared with enteral nutrition. It has not been shown to alter pain or analgesic requirements.

6. The answer is A (1.1.1)

BW's low hemoglobin/hematocrit suggests that he is anemic. His mean cell volume (MCV) is increased, suggesting macrocytic red blood cells. His mean cell hemoglobin concentration (MCHC) is within normal limits, indicating a normal concentration of hemoglobin or normochromic red blood cells. A normochromic, macrocytic anemia is often found in alcoholic patients who are likely to have a dietary folic acid deficiency.

7. The answer is D (2.1.2)

Kcal/day = 66.47 + (13.75 x 68.2 kg) + (5.0 x 177.8 cm) - (6.76 x 52 years) = 1541.7 kcal/day Additional calories would be required for BW based on stress and physical activity factors.

8. The answer is C (2.1.1)

BW requires 1500 kcal from dextrose. IV dextrose provides 3.4 kcal/g. Grams of dextrose = 1500 kcal / 3.4 kcal/g = 441 g mL of 70% dextrose = 441 g / 0.7 g/mL = 630 mL

9. The answer is E (1.2.1)

Although imipenem-cilastatin (E) is an antibiotic with a broad spectrum of activity, it is the best choice provided. The flora of infected pancreatic necrosis is often polymicrobial. Pathogens that are commonly isolated from infected necrosis include *Escherichia coli*, *Klebsiella pneumoniae*, *Enterococcus* species, *Staphylococcus aureus*, *Proteus mirabilis*, *Pseudomonas aeruginosa*, *Enterobacter aerogenes*, *Bacteroides fragilis*, and other anaerobes. Thus, aztreonam (A) and gentamicin (B) are not the best choices for BW's empiric therapy due to their predominantly gram-negative spectrum of activity. Vancomycin (C) and cefazolin (D) are limited by their predominantly gram-positive spectrum of activity.

10. The answer is A (3.2.3)

Pancreatic enzyme products are dosed according to lipase content. Therefore, this product likely contains 12,000 units of lipase per capsule. The label should indicate the quantity of amylase and protease contained within each capsule. The "MS" stands for microsphere.

Case 16 Gout

1. The answer is B (1.1.3)

Uric acid is produced from the breakdown of purine from the diet and from conversion of tissue nucleic acid to purine nucleotides. Red cells have no nucleus that would release nucleic acids upon breakdown with age (A). Anaerobic metabolism and parathyroid hormone activity are unrelated to uric acid synthesis (C, E). Purine metabolism is regulated by several enzyme systems, and the liver is not involved in uric acid synthesis (D).

2. The answer is C (3.2.2)

Patients that are obese can have increased production of uric acid (A). Alcohol intake increases the production of uric acid and decreases renal clearance of uric acid (B). Although smoking cessation should be advocated for this patient, it has no impact on uric acid production or clearance (C). During an acute attack of gouty arthritis, application of ice to the affected joint decreases pain and swelling (D). Heat application can be detrimental and should be avoided. Immobilization of the affected joint may speed recovery (E).

3. The answer is B (1.1.4)

Two thirds of uric acid produced each day is excreted in the urine. Thiazide diuretics (B) decrease renal clearance of uric acid by decreasing tubular secretion and/or increasing uric acid reabsorption secondary to decreased ECF volume. The other medications have no impact on uric acid levels (A, C, D, E).

4. The answer is D (3.1.2)

Pain was scored on a visual analogue scale from 0 mm (no pain) to 100 mm (most severe pain ever), a validated method for the assessment of pain. Pain reduction observed in this trial is clinically significant and shows that the treatments are effective (C). Results from this trial indicate that naproxen and prednisolone are equally effective for the treatment of acute gout (D).[1] The slight difference in reduction in pain scores is not statistically significant as indicated by the wide confidence interval (CI), which includes 0. A p value is not needed to interpret the results since a confidence interval is provided (E).

1. Janssens H, Janssen M, van de Lisdonk EH, van Riel P, van Weel C. Use of oral prednisolone or naproxen for the treatment of gout arthritis: a double-blind, randomized equivalence trial. *Lancet* 2008; 371:1854-60.

5. The answer is D (1.2.1)

Allopurinol (I) is an antihyperuricemic agent indicated for long-term prophylactic therapy. It is not effective for acute treatment and may actually worsen acute gouty arthritis. For this reason, it is standard practice to avoid initiating allopurinol therapy during the inflammatory phase of acute gout. Colchicine (II) is effective for acute gouty arthritis but is associated with more significant toxicity compared to NSAIDs. Corticosteroids (III) are also effective for acute gouty arthritis but are reserved for patients with contraindications or cases resistant to NSAIDs or colchicine. Intra-articular corticosteroid injections are useful when only one or two joints are affected. Systemic corticosteroids are generally used in patients with renal insufficiency (contraindication to NSAID and colchicine use) and polyarticular attacks.

6. The answer is A (1.2.4)

Patients with heart failure should avoid NSAIDs because of the possible adverse effect of sodium and fluid retention, resulting in worsening of heart failure (A). Patients with GERD can use NSAIDs but should be advised to take the medication with food and to report any worsening of GERD symptoms to their provider (D). Patients with COPD, hyperlipidemia, and Parkinson's disease can safely take NSAIDs (B, C, E).

7. The answer is C (1.1.3)

Gout is characterized by rapid onset (B) of excruciating pain, swelling, and inflammation. It is typically monoarticular (D), with the first metatarsophalangeal joint (big toe) being the most commonly affected joint (C). Other joints commonly affected include instep, ankle, heel, knee, wrist, and fingers. Hyperuricemia is often, but not always, present (A). A definitive diagnosis can only be made by visualizing urate crystals in synovial fluid aspirated from the affected joint (E).

8. The answer is C (1.2.0)

Colchicine may be useful when sodium and water retention caused by either NSAIDs or corticosteroids may worsen disease states such as congestive heart failure (CHF) (C). It is also used as an alternative to NSAID therapy in patients with peptic ulcer risk. It does not enhance renal elimination of uric acid (A), but works by decreasing neutrophil chemotaxis and enzyme release. Traditional colchicine dosing for treatment of an acute attack was usually 0.6 mg to 1.2 mg initially followed by 0.6 mg every 1 to 2 hours until relief of symptoms, diarrhea develops, or a total dose of 4-8 mg has been reached. This dosing regimen is no longer recommended. Current dosing recommendations are 1.2 mg (2 tablets) at the first sign of a gout flare followed by 0.6 mg one hour later (B).[1] This dosing regimen is the FDA-approved dosage for Colcrys, the only approved colchicine product in the United States, and is supported by a randomized, placebo-controlled trial comparing high-dose colchicine and low-dose colchicine. The trial demonstrated equal efficacy between the different dosing schedules with substantially fewer adverse effects in the low-dose group. Traditional high-dose colchicine dosing regimens should no longer be used for treatment of acute gout. The likelihood of success with colchicine is greatly reduced if treatment is delayed beyond 48 hours after the onset of symptoms (D). Colchicine is most beneficial when given in the first 12-36 hours of an attack. Colchicine can be administered intravenously, but it is associated with significant toxicity and death and should be avoided (E).

1. US Food and Drug Administration. Information for Healthcare Professionals: New Safety Information for Colchicine (marketed as Colcrys). www.fda.gov/Drugs/DrugSafety/Postmarket DrugSafetyInformationforPatientsandProviders/DrugSafetyInformationforHeathcareProfessionals/ucm174315.htm

9. The answer is E (1.2.3)

Data reviewed during the approval process for Colcrys revealed the importance of drug interactions in the development of colchicine toxicity. Life-threatening and fatal drug interactions have been reported in patients treated with colchicine when P-glycoprotein (P-gp) and/or hepatic cytochrome P450 3A4 (CYP3A4) inhibitors are used concomitantly.[1] Current prescribing information states that colchicine should not be used with P-gp or strong CYP3A4 inhibitors in patients with renal or

Answers

hepatic impairment.[2] In patients with normal renal and hepatic function, clinicians should consult the prescribing information for specific dosage adjustments recommended if a potentially interacting drug is required. Fatal colchicine toxicity has been reported with clarithromycin (A), a strong CYP3A4 inhibitor, and with cyclosporine (C), a P-gp inhibitor. Neuromuscular toxicity has been reported with diltiazem (B) and verapamil, moderate CYP3A4 inhibitors. Colchicine-induced neuromuscular toxicity and rhabdomyolysis have been reported in patients using HMG-CoA reductase inhibitors, including atorvastatin (D). Clinicians should carefully weigh the potential benefits and risks and advise patients to promptly report any signs or symptoms of muscle pain, tenderness, or weakness. Losartan (E) is not a P-gp or CYP3A4 inhibitor and should not interact with colchicine.

1. US Food and Drug Administration. Information for Healthcare Professionals: New Safety Information for Colchicine (marketed as Colcrys). www.fda.gov/Drugs/DrugSafety/PostmarketDrugSafetyInformationforPatientsandProviders/DrugSafetyInformationforHeathcareProfessionals/ucm174315.htm

2. Colcrys [package insert]. Philadelphia, PA: Mutual Pharmaceutical Company, Inc.; 2010.

10. The answer is A (1.2.7)

Immediate-release products should be used for treatment of acute gouty arthritis (I). Enteric-coated and delayed-release NSAIDs are not recommended for the treatment of acute gouty arthritis because of their delayed onset of action (II, III).

Case 17 Osteoarthritis

1. The answer is A (1.2.1)

The American College of Rheumatology recommends acetaminophen up to 1 gram QID as initial therapy for osteoarthritis (A). Acetaminophen is effective and safe. Recent studies have indicated that acetaminophen is not as effective as NSAIDs but remains the initial drug of choice due to superior safety. If the response is inadequate, then NSAIDs, tramadol, or opioids should be considered (B, C, D). Of these, NSAIDs are preferred unless a contraindication is present. Opioids are helpful for acute pain exacerbations but are not recommended for long-term use due to the potential for tolerance and dependence. Hyaluronic acid is indicated only for OA of the knee when other treatments have failed (E).

2. The answer is E (1.3.2)

Hepatic enzymes (AST and ALT) should be checked at baseline then periodically (annually) (I). For diclofenac it is recommended to also check AST and ALT within 4 weeks after initiating therapy. Increased liver enzymes and drug-induced hepatitis are rare adverse effects associated with NSAID therapy. A CBC should be checked periodically to detect hematologic adverse effects (II). NSAIDs can cause nephrotoxicity due to effects on renal prostaglandins. Serum creatinine should be checked within a few days to a week after initiating therapy, then periodically, especially in patients at risk (III). Other adverse effects include GI upset, photosensitivity (instruct patients to avoid the sun or wear sunscreen), inhibition of platelet aggregation, fluid retention and peripheral edema, rarely CNS effects (drowsiness, dizziness, headache, depression, confusion, tinnitus), and hypersensitivity reactions (bronchospasm, urticaria). NSAIDs also cause GI ulcers and increase cardiovascular risk.

3. The answer is B (2.1.1)

Small studies have shown that topical NSAIDs are effective for treatment of OA. Topical diclofenac products are available but no topical ibuprofen product is commercially available in the U.S. at this time. To compound 50 grams of 5% ibuprofen cream, you would need 2500 mg of ibuprofen (B). A 5% cream would contain 5 grams of ibuprofen per 100 grams of cream; therefore, to make 50 grams of cream it would take 2.5 grams, or 2500 mg.

4. The answer is B (2.2.1)

The generic name of Celebrex is celecoxib; the brand name for piroxicam is Feldene (A). Lodine is the brand name for etodolac; Mobic is the brand name for meloxicam (C). Relafen is the brand name for nabumetone; Naprosyn is the brand name for naproxen (D). Voltaren is the brand name for diclofenac (E).

5. The answer is E (1.2.3)

NSAIDs inhibit platelet aggregation and can increase the effects of warfarin (A). The INR should be monitored closely and patients should watch for signs/symptoms of bleeding. NSAIDs can increase the serum levels of lithium and phenytoin; use caution and monitor drug levels closely (B, C). NSAIDs reduce the renal clearance of lithium. Ibuprofen, and possibly other NSAIDs, may inhibit the hepatic microsomal enzymes responsible for phenytoin metabolism, leading to increased phenytoin levels. NSAIDs can decrease the effects of antihypertensives, especially ACE inhibitors (lisinopril) and diuretics; monitor blood pressure closely (D). Various mechanisms are involved in this interaction. NSAIDs do not interact with ranitidine or other H_2-receptor antagonists (E).

6. The answer is A (1.1.3)

Crepitus is a crackling noise heard when the joint is moved (A). It results from the rubbing of bone fragments. Swelling and joint enlargement may also be noted on physical exam and are findings consistent with OA (B, E).

7. The answer is C (2.2.2)

The only NSAIDs available without a prescription in the United States are ibuprofen 200 mg and naproxen 220 mg (C). Ketoprofen 12.5 mg is FDA approved for nonprescription use but is currently not being marketed. All other NSAIDs are prescription only.

8. The answer is C (1.3.5)

Treatment algorithms for osteoarthritis generally follow the following steps: 1) lifestyle modification; 2) acetaminophen; 3) NSAID; 4) intra-articular injection; 5) tramadol; 6) opioid; 7) surgery. Patient response to NSAIDs is highly variable and unpredictable. For this reason, a patient who does not respond to the first NSAID chosen should be given a trial of another agent from either the same or a different NSAID chemical class. This process may need to be repeated for a given patient before an agent is found that produces satisfactory benefits with tolerable side effects. Therapy should be continued for at least 2 to 3 weeks before determining efficacy, or lack thereof. This patient has been taking ibuprofen for a sufficient time period. Switching to naproxen would be appropriate at this time (C). Tramadol and opioids are reserved for patients who do not achieve adequate pain relief with NSAIDs, cannot tolerate NSAIDs, or have contraindications to NSAID use (D, E). Intra-articular injections are generally reserved for patients unresponsive to oral analgesics and are especially helpful for OA of the knee (A, B).

9. The answer is C (3.2.3)

The main adverse effect with glucosamine is GI discomfort (C). Other adverse effects include drowsiness and headache. In clinical trials, adverse effects were not significantly different from placebo. Results from clinical trials vary. Some studies, including a 3-year, randomized, placebo-controlled study in adults with OA of the knee have found glucosamine to be effective for the symptoms of OA (B). One study has suggested that it may have disease-modifying properties. The GAIT trial conducted by the NIH found glucosamine, chondroitin, and their combination to be no more effective than placebo. Studies evaluated different salts. It appears that glucosamine hydrochloride is likely not effective for OA but that glucosamine sulfate may have beneficial effects in OA. Research suggests that glucosamine must be taken for at least 1 month before improvement in symptoms can be expected (A). It is not effective for acute pain. Conflicting reports exist regarding glucosamine's effects on blood glucose levels. Patients with diabetes can use glucosamine for OA but should closely monitor their blood glucose levels (D). Glucosamine is a dietary supplement and, therefore, not regulated by the FDA (E). A reputable manufacturer should be recommended to help ensure product reliability.

10. The answer is D (3.2.2)

The American College of Rheumatology recommends a number of non-drug measures, including education, self-management programs, support groups, physical therapy, occupational therapy, exercise programs (aerobic, stretching, strengthening, and range-of-motion exercises), assistive devices (wedge insoles, cane, brace, orthotic shoes), heat or cold treatment, and weight loss. Weight loss decreases symptoms and disability and is important in reducing the biomechanical force on weight-bearing joints. Even a 5-lb weight loss can be beneficial (II). Exercise is important to improve or maintain joint mobility

(III). Exercises should be taught and then observed before the patient exercises at home to ensure safety and effectiveness. Inactivity or rest can worsen symptoms and disability by leading to further deconditioning and weight gain (I).

Case 18 Rheumatoid Arthritis

1. The answer is C (1.3.3)

If a patient with RA develops intolerable toxicity to the first DMARD chosen, that drug should be discontinued and another DMARD started (C). Adding systemic corticosteroids to the regimen while continuing the DMARD may not mask its adverse effects (e.g., hepatotoxicity from methotrexate) and may lead to even more severe DMARD toxicity (A). Immunosuppressive agents should be reserved until patients have had adequate trials of multiple DMARDs (B). If the patient responded well to the first DMARD, others should be attempted before considering surgical options (D). Tolerance to the serious toxicities of DMARDs (e.g., hepatotoxicity, bone marrow suppression) does not occur, and continuation of the present regimen only risks more severe toxicity (E).

2. The answer is D (3.2.2)

Cardiovascular disease (CVD), infections, malignancy, and osteoporosis are the comorbidities with the greatest impact on morbidity and mortality associated with rheumatoid arthritis. Patients should be routinely assessed for these comorbidities and measures implemented to help reduce risk. Strategies to help reduce cardiovascular disease include stopping smoking (A); following a low-fat, low-cholesterol diet (C); engaging in regular exercise (E); using aspirin, statins, and blood pressure medications when needed; and keeping NSAID and glucocorticoid doses low. This patient has elevated blood pressure that could potentially be lowered with the DASH diet (B). Aggressive treatment with antihypertensive medications is also warranted to help reduce CV risk. Reducing carbohydrate intake (D) will not impact risk of the major comorbidities.

3. The answer is B (1.3.2)

Laboratory monitoring of ANA and rheumatoid factor is expensive and does little to assess the patient's clinical response to therapy (B). More useful outcome-monitoring parameters include joint swelling, warmth, and tenderness assessed on physical exam (A); degree of pain using visual analog scale; patient's perception of symptoms, morning stiffness, afternoon fatigue, ability to perform activities of daily living (C, E); quality of life measured using standardized questionnaires (D); and joint radiographs to assess progression of joint damage. The 2008 ACR Guidelines recommend a number of instruments to measure disease activity including the Disease Activity Score in 28 joints (DAS 28).[1] Components used in the calculation are number of swollen and tender joints, erythrocyte sedimentation rate (ESR) or C-reactive protein (CRP), and a

Answers

subjective measure of the patient's general health. A score of 3.2 or less indicates low disease activity. The DAS 28 and other similar instruments can be used to guide initial treatment decisions, assess response to therapy, and monitor disease progression.

1. Saag KG, Teng GG, Patkar NM, et al. American College of Rheumatology 2008 recommendations for the use of nonbiologic and biologic disease-modifying antirheumatic drugs in rheumatoid arthritis. *Arthritis Rheum.* 2008; 59:762-784.

4. The answer is C (3.2.1)

The 2008 ACR Guidelines recommend periodic pneumococcal vaccinations and annual influenza vaccinations for all patients receiving biologic DMARDs (C).[1] Hepatitis B vaccination is recommended if hepatitis risk factors are present (e.g., intravenous drug abuse, multiple sex partners in the previous 6 months, health care personnel). This patient does not have any risk factors for hepatitis B, therefore this vaccination is not needed (D). Live vaccines (e.g., varicella-zoster vaccine [B], intranasal influenza vaccine [A, E], oral polio, rabies) are contraindicated in patients taking biologic DMARDs.

1. Saag KG, Teng GG, Patkar NM, et al. American College of Rheumatology 2008 recommendations for the use of nonbiologic and biologic disease-modifying antirheumatic drugs in rheumatoid arthritis. *Arthritis Rheum.* 2008; 59:762-784.

5. The answer is D (2.2.5)

Adalimumab must be stored in the refrigerator (36°F to 46°F). Do not store at room temperature (D). Do not freeze (C). The injection site should be rotated (A). The recommended sites for injection include the front of the middle thighs or the abdomen (except for the 2-inch area right around the navel). Each new injection should be given at least 1 inch from the previous site. Do not inject through clothing and do not inject where skin is tender, bruised, red, or hard, or where there are scars or stretch marks (B). Used pens should be disposed of in a puncture-resistant container, either a Sharps container or a can with a secure lid (E). The container should be labeled "used needles and syringes" and disposed of according to state and local laws. Used pens should not be disposed of in household trash nor should the puncture-resistant container be placed in recycle bins.

6. The answer is E (1.2.2)

Adalimumab is a recombinant human IgG1 monoclonal antibody that binds to soluble and bound tumor necrosis factor (TNF), making it biologically inactive (E). Tumor necrosis factor is a pro-inflammatory cytokine that appears to play a key role in the inflammation of rheumatoid arthritis. Other TNF antagonists include etanercept, infliximab, golimumab, and certolizumab. Anakinra is an interleukin-1-receptor antagonist (A). NSAIDs inhibit cyclooxygenase (B). Leflunomide inhibits pyrimidine synthesis (C). Methotrexate and other DMARDs inhibit cytokine production (D).

7. The answer is B (1.3.3)

Leflunomide can cause hepatotoxicity (B). Rare cases of severe liver injury, including cases with fatal outcome, have been reported with leflunomide. Most cases of severe liver injury occur within 6 months of therapy in patients with multiple risk factors for hepatotoxicity. Routine monitoring of liver transaminases is recommended. Methotrexate rarely causes pulmonary fibrosis; this adverse effect is not associated with etanercept (A). Use of biologic DMARDs is associated with an increased risk of infection and malignancy, specifically lymphoma and skin cancer. Sulfasalazine is a nonbiologic DMARD and is not associated with an increased risk of lymphoma (C). Hydroxychloroquine is a nonbiologic DMARD; it does not increase the risk of infection but may cause retinal toxicity (D). Methotrexate is not associated with retinal toxicity (E).

8. The answer is D (1.3.3)

Leflunomide is pregnancy category X (D). Both men and women must follow a washout protocol following discontinuation of leflunomide before trying to conceive. The washout protocol consists of taking cholestyramine 8 gm TID for 11 days. Plasma levels of the metabolite should be measured to confirm success. Without the washout protocol it may take 2 years to reach undetectable plasma concentration levels.

9. The answer is B (2.1.1)

The correct dose for this patient is 273 mg, so 3 vials would need to be reconstituted (B). To convert the patient's weight to kilograms, divide weight in pounds by 2.2 (200/2.2 = 90.9 kg). Multiply weight in kilograms by 3 to calculate the dose (90.9 x 3 = 272.7 mg). This dose can be rounded up to 273 mg. Each vial should be reconstituted with 10 mL of sterile water to provide a 10 mg/mL solution. This solution must be diluted prior to administration.

10. The answer is C (2.1.4)

To determine the final concentration, divide the dose in mg by the volume in mL (273 mg/250 mL = 1.09 mg/mL) (C). The total volume should be 250 mL. Therefore, if a 250-mL bottle or bag of 0.9% sodium chloride injection is used, a volume of the diluent equal to the volume of reconstituted infliximab should be removed prior to adding the infliximab solution. In this example, 27.3 mL of the diluent would need to be removed before adding the 273 mg of infliximab (the concentration of the reconstituted infliximab is 10 mg/mL). The final concentration of reconstituted and diluted infliximab solutions should be 0.4-4 mg/mL and should be administered by IV infusion over at least 2 hours.

Case 19 SLE

1. The answer is E (1.1.3)

SLE is associated with excessive and abnormal autoantibody production and the formation of immune complexes. These autoantibodies may be directed against nuclear, cytoplasmic, and surface components of many organs' systems, and the immune complexes will deposit in these organs. Subsequent immune activation by the complexes causes release of mediators that cause constitutional symptoms (fatigue, fever, malaise). Immune activation also accounts for the involvement of not only the skin and joints (II), but also the kidneys, bone marrow, pulmonary system, heart, central nervous system, and/or GI tract in many patients (III).

2. The answer is D (1.1.4)

The classic presentation of SLE is in a female of child-bearing age (B). African Americans (C) have a higher incidence of SLE than Caucasians, as do Hispanics, Asians, and Native Americans. The etiology of the disease remains poorly understood, but it appears to include both a genetic predisposition (E) and exposure to environmental triggers. Suspected environmental triggers include UV light (A), viral infections, certain chemicals such as hydrazine and aromatic amines, or estrogens.

3. The answer is A (1.2.4)

Use of hydroxychloroquine is associated with a small risk of developing retinal toxicity. Thus, ophthalmic exams are recommended every 6-12 months while using it. It can also rarely cause blood dyscrasias, so monitoring of CBC may be appropriate, though rarely is it required on a scheduled basis. Hydroxychloroquine does not appear to alter electrolytes or kidney function (B, C), nor does it appear to cause hepatotoxicity (D). Lastly, it does not appear to have any adverse effect on endocrine function or insulin resistance (E). In fact, some evidence exists suggesting a modest improvement in glycemic control.

4. The answer is D (3.1.2)

This appears to be a short, uncontrolled case series. There was no mention of randomization, or of a placebo or comparator drug (A). Likewise, there was no comparison group of patients (B, E). This also appears to be a single trial, rather than a compilation of several trials (C). A further criticism of this trial would be the lack of objective endpoints.

5. The answer is D (1.3.5)

Proliferative forms of lupus nephritis are often progressive and require use of some form of immunosuppressive therapy (A). While discontinuation of naproxen (B) may offer short-term improvement of renal function due to improved renal blood flow, such action would not alter the progression of the disease. Hydroxychloroquine, regardless of dose (C), is not a potent enough immunosuppressant to control lupus nephritis. Steroids are potent enough to limit progression by themselves in many cases. However, if the disease is severe or rapidly progressing, higher doses and additional potent immunosuppressants may be required (E).

6. The answer is B (2.2.2)

Prednisone is not utilized in anything but oral formulations

(B), as it requires first-pass conversion to its active metabolite, prednisolone, for activity.

7. The answer is E (3.2.2)

Appropriate rest and exercise (without overexertion) is crucial in managing the fatigue associated with SLE (A). Avoidance of smoking (B) is important because hydrazines in tobacco smoke may serve as an environmental trigger for a flare-up of SLE. Limitation of exposure to sunlight when outdoors (along with use of sunscreens) will block much of the ultraviolet light that may exacerbate the skin manifestations of SLE (C). Consumption of moderate dose omega-3 fatty acids (3 g daily) has been shown to have modest anti-inflammatory effects not only in SLE, but in RA and OA as well (D). Conversely, consumption of a micronutrient supplement designed to provide extra copper did not show any clinical benefit in SLE patients.

8. The answer is D (1.2.4)

Hepatotoxicity has been observed rarely in selected NSAIDs, such as diclofenac and indomethacin, but has not been deemed a class effect meriting a blanket warning. Concern was raised about cardiovascular events with rofecoxib, a COX-2 specific inhibitor, and has been subsequently observed in both specific and nonspecific cyclooxygenase inhibitors. While the evidence base is somewhat contradictory at points, the FDA felt that the gravity of the event was sufficient to merit a warning. GI bleeds are an undisputed class effect of NSAIDs, as reduction in prostaglandin synthesis results in a decrease in the protective mucus layer of the GI tract.

9. The answer is A (2.2.2)

The OTC forms for naproxen are all 220 mg per tablet (A), measured as its sodium salt. All of the other strengths listed are available, but only by prescription.

10. The answer is D (1.3.3)

Procainamide, along with hydralazine, are the two drugs most commonly associated with drug-induced lupus. Procainamide has greater risk with longer duration, while hydralazine has greater risk with increasing dose. The remaining drugs are only very rarely associated with drug-induced lupus.

Case 20 Acid/Base Disorders

1. The answer is C (1.1.1)

Total body water is approximately 60% of total body weight for males and 50% for females. Based on a total body weight of 60 kg, SG's calculated total body is 36 kg. A, B, D and E are incorrect because they represent greater than or less than 60% of the total body weight.

2. The answer is A (1.1.1)

The intravascular fluid compartment is 5% of the total body

Answers

weight, and based on a weight of 60 kg, the calculated intravascular fluid compartment is 3 kg.

3. The answer is A (1.1.1)

Extracellular volume deficit induces a drop in blood pressure and increased heart rate. These symptoms are observed when a 4%-6% total body weight loss is the result of extracellular volume loss.

4. The answer is E (1.1.2)

Typical presenting features of extracellular fluid deficit include hypotension (E), tachycardia, and hemoconcentration reflected by hypernatremia, not (A) hypertension, (B) bradycardia, (C) hyponatremia, or (D) hypocalcemia.

5. The answer is C (1.2.6)

Fluid deficit can be calculated using the formula: ((current serum sodium concentration - 140)/140)) x total body water in kg. Total body water = wt in kg x 0.6 (males) or 0.5 (females). Based on serum sodium concentration of 149 and a total body water of 36 kg, the fluid deficit is calculated to be 2.3 L.

6. The answer is D (1.2.6)

The initial fluid requirement is a maintenance requirement of approximately 1.8 L (30 mL/kg/day) plus the deficit of 2.3 L, or approximately 4 L.

7. The answer is C (1.1.1)

The 2% of the total body potassium (B) is in the extracellular compartment and the highest potassium concentration is in the intracellular fluid compartment or 150 mEq/L (A) are true statements. The interstitial and intravascular concentration of potassium is 4-5 mEq/L, therefore (C) the highest potassium concentration is in the intracellular fluid compartment is the false statement. Metabolic acidosis (D) does result in a shifting of potassium to the extracellular space, and insulin (E) does cause a shifting of potassium into the intracellular compartment. Therefore D and E statements are true.

8. The answer is A (3.2.2)

Prazosin is indicated as an agent that may precipitate depression.

9. The answer is D (3.2.2)

Alpha blockers are known to cause first dose syncope, and common side effects include palpitations, headache, and drowsiness. NSAIDs decrease the effect of alpha blockers. NSAIDs, especially indomethacin, may antagonize the antihypertensive effect by inhibiting renal prostaglandin synthesis and/or by causing sodium and fluid retention.

10. The answer is C (1.1.1)

SG's hypochloremia is the result of vomiting (C) and resulted from loss of hydrogen and chloride. Severe vomiting is usually associated with metabolic alkalosis, therefore, metabolic acido-

sis (A) is incorrect. SG has not been on diuretics, therefore (B) is incorrect. Excessive use of intravenous saline (D) usually causes hypernatremia. SG does not have hypoaldosteronism (E) listed in his medical history, therefore (E) is also incorrect.

Case 21 Dietary Supplements

1. The answer is B (1.1.3)

When used in conjunction with darkness, melatonin has been shown to improve sleep onset insomnia. Patients reported falling asleep faster. HP should be advised to turn bedroom lights off prior to taking melatonin to trigger endogenous melatonin release and increase the possibility of sleep onset. Melatonin has not been studied for the treatment of anxiety (A). Melatonin has not been shown to improve early morning awakenings, especially in the elderly (C). Melatonin helps cause sedation rather than preventing sedation. It is not expected to help patients with narcolepsy (D). The role of melatonin for preventing jet lag symptoms is unclear. In one well-designed clinical trial, melatonin did not improve symptoms of jet lag when compared to placebo. Melatonin may help patients with jet lag simply by allowing them to fall asleep at the appropriate time upon arriving at the new time zone. Currently, exogenous melatonin does not appear to change or shift the circadian release pattern of melatonin (E).

2. The answer is E (1.3.3)

Melatonin has not been associated with hyperpigmentation. Melanin, which is a pigment in the skin and not related to melatonin, can affect skin pigmentation. Daytime drowsiness has rarely been reported with melatonin. Melatonin, however, is considered to cause much less daytime drowsiness as compared to other OTC antihistamines such as diphenhydramine (Sominex). Levels of melatonin peak within 45 minutes of taking a nighttime dose and levels decline rapidly by morning (A). In clinical trials, tachycardia or palpitations has been observed infrequently (B). Patients taking melatonin have reported transient feelings of dysthymia or depressed mood (C). Melatonin at high doses of 75-300 mg, when used in conjunction with a progestin, has been shown to partially inhibit ovulation. HP is attempting to conceive, and while HP is not taking high doses of melatonin, it is reasonable to recommend HP withhold melatonin as well as any other OTC drugs for now. She should be instructed on nondrug measures for her insomnia (D).

3. The answer is D (1.2.2)

Endogenous melatonin is released between 9 p.m. and 4 a.m. These times correspond to natural sleep circadian patterns. The lowest effective melatonin dose should be used for insomnia. In clinical trials, the lowest effective dose used was 0.3 mg. Other doses up to 10 mg have also been effective. If HP does not fall asleep with these doses, doses greater than 10 mg will not likely be effective (A). Since natural melatonin release is triggered by darkness, exogenous melatonin should be taken just prior to bedtime with reading lights off (B). Clinical studies have shown that sleep onset occurs between 30 and 45 minutes following a dose of melatonin (C). Melatonin is considered a less potent hypnotic than benzodiazepines. Patients who have taken benzodiazepines for insomnia in the past should be informed that melatonin may not result in a similar degree of sedation (E).

4. The answer is E (1.2.3)

There are no drug interaction studies between zolpidem and melatonin. When zolpidem was given to healthy adults, it did not alter endogenous melatonin levels. In general, melatonin is considered a less potent hypnotic than zolpidem. Patients taking zolpidem should not require melatonin for sleep. Taking both agents concomitantly may increase sedation. Melatonin has been studied as an adjunct to cancer chemotherapy. Many of these trials were small and lacked a placebo control, making the results difficult to interpret. More research is needed on the role of exogenous melatonin in cancer (A). Melatonin may be useful in people suffering from jet lag since it may help them fall asleep at the new bedtime hour (B). Melatonin has been associated with causing dysphoria and has led to the development of mania in some people. For this reason, it is best that patients with depression or mania avoid taking melatonin supplements (C). Fluvoxamine has been shown to increase peak melatonin levels. Further research is needed to assess the role of melatonin supplementation on serotonergic drugs. Melatonin is an end-product of serotonin (D).

5. The answer is E (1.2.2)

Melatonin is an end-product of serotonin and in some cases has led to a worsening of depressive symptoms. In patients with depression, melatonin was beneficial in helping induce sleep, but it was also associated with dysphoria. Until more is known about melatonin, patients with depressive symptoms should not use melatonin. Melatonin has been shown to affect prolactin levels in women. If HP becomes pregnant and chooses to nurse her infant, she should avoid melatonin while nursing since prolactin is essential in regulating milk production (A). Children are abundant producers of melatonin. Children who suffer from insomnia should be evaluated by a physician and should not be treated with OTC drug products (B). There is no evidence to suggest melatonin will work for chronic insomnia, and it has not been studied for this indication. In clinical practice, however, melatonin is often used for chronic insomnia in the elderly. Melatonin is selected because it is associated with fewer side effects than other OTC and prescription drugs (C). Melatonin may increase the sedating effects of alcohol and should be avoided as alcohol should not be used as a hypnotic. Patients taking both should be extra careful and should avoid driving or performing tasks that require full attention (D).

6. The answer is D (1.2.7)

Multivitamins containing zinc are not effective in shortening the symptoms of the common cold. Zinc lozenges are thought to release Zn++ ions that circulate in the oropharyngeal cavities. Multivitamins containing zinc are taken orally and are absorbed by the gastrointestinal tract and are unable to release zinc ions. There is some controversy as to which formulation is best; however, all three zinc formulations have been shown to have a benefit in relieving the symptoms of the common cold (A). Zinc lozenges are most effective if started within the first 48 hours of the first cold symptom (B). The common cold typically lasts for 7-10 days. Zinc lozenges have been shown to decrease symptoms by 1-2 days at best (C). Zinc lozenges must be taken every 2 hours while awake to maintain the flow of Zn++ ions and prevent rhinovirus from docking in the respiratory passages (E).

7. The answer is E (1.2.7)

Zinc lozenges are effective on the basis of their ability to release zinc ions; therefore, they should not be chewed or crushed. Zinc lozenges have not been proven to be effective in children. In one clinical trial, there was no benefit in children taking zinc lozenges (A). Zinc lozenges have not been studied during pregnancy, and therefore, safety is unknown. HP should avoid taking zinc lozenges while pregnant or while trying to conceive (B). The amount of elemental zinc that is absorbed during a course of zinc lozenges has not been quantified but appears to be within a safe range when the lozenges are taken for up to 10 days. For this reason, zinc lozenges should not be taken beyond 10 days or on a continuous basis. Instead, an oral multivitamin containing zinc is a better and more reliable option for zinc supplementation (C). Zinc lozenges have not been studied in treating influenza. Zn++ ions have been studied in vitro for their effects on rhinoviral capsid proteins. If symptoms of the common cold do not respond within 7-10 days, zinc lozenges should be discontinued (D).

8. The answer is D (3.2.1)

Numbness is not a recognized side effect of zinc lozenges. Nausea is a common side effect of zinc lozenges. To minimize nausea, zinc lozenges may be taken on a full stomach (A). Mouth sores have been reported in clinical trials and may be related to the astringent effects of zinc lozenges. Newer formulations of zinc are much more palatable and are associated with fewer mouth sores (B). Taste disturbances are common. Flavoring ingredients vary among the various zinc lozenge manufacturers. Patients should select a product that is most palatable (C). Some zinc lozenges have astringent-like properties in the mouth (E).

9. The answer is E (2.2.1)

Although most zinc lozenge trials show a benefit, not all show reductions in symptom severity or duration. For this reason, zinc lozenges may not work in everyone, including HP. The zinc lozenge trials involved both people with naturally acquired colds and healthy volunteers who agreed to be injected with the rhinovirus (A). Ingredients like mannitol-sorbitol combinations, tartrate, and citrate are thought to inactivate the release of Zn++ from the lozenge. As a result, manufacturers have

Answers

removed these excipients from their products (B). Researchers do not quite know which zinc lozenge dose is best, and therefore, they have studied various doses. Zinc gluconate-glycine 13.3 mg, zinc gluconate 23 mg, and zinc acetate 10 mg have all been used and seem to be associated with some beneficial effects (C). Many of the zinc lozenge trials had difficulty masking the flavor of the zinc lozenges as compared to placebo pills, and this may have affected the study outcomes (D).

10. The answer is C (1.1.2)

Fever is not considered a symptom of the common cold. Typically, a fever is a sign of the flu or a bacterial infection. HP is afebrile and does not appear to have the symptoms of the flu such as fatigue and malaise. Watery eyes are a common symptom of the common cold. HP is exhibiting watery eyes, possibly related to her sneezing (A). Sneezing is a common finding related to the common cold. HP is complaining of sneezing (B). Nasal stuffiness is common during a cold. This is also associated with a runny nose (D). Runny nose is a common symptom of the common cold. Typically, it is associated with watery eyes and sneezing (E).

Case 22 Fluids & Electrolytes

1. The answer is D (1.1.2)

Typical signs and symptoms of hypomagnesemia include positive Chvostek's (facial twitch) and Trousseau's (hand spasm) signs (A), tremor (B), generalized convulsions (C), cardiac manifestations including increased QT interval and prolonged QRS complex (E), and refractory hypokalemia. Hypomagnesemia lowers the threshold for nerve stimulation.

2. The answer is A (1.1.1)

Patients that lose fluids based on diarrhea, sweat, and diuretics may have significant sodium and water losses. If these losses continue, more ADH (antidiuretic hormone) is released, and water is retained, resulting in hypovolemic hyponatremia (A). There is a decreased extracellular volume, and urine sodium is usually <10 mEq/L.

3. The answer is C (1.1.1)

Sodium deficit can be calculated using the following formula: volume of distribution of Na (desired - current Na concentration) = (0.5 L/kg) (70 kg) (140 - 129 mEq/L) = 385 mEq

4. The answer is D (1.1.1)

The amount of maintenance fluid needed to replace normal insensible losses and maintain adequate perfusion varies in a nonlinear manner. The first 10 kg of body weight needs 100 mL/kg, the next 10 kg need 50 mL/kg, and each kilogram beyond 20 kg needs 20 mL/kg. As a 70-kg woman, JJ needs 1000 mL for the first 10 kg, 500 mL for the second 10 kg, and 1000 mL for the remaining 50 kg. The total is 2500 mL (D).

5. The answer is C (1.1.2)

Acidosis (A), potassium-sparing diuretics (B), sickle cell disease (D), and chronic renal failure (E) are all associated with hyperkalemia. The GI tract is a site of potassium loss through vomiting and diarrhea. This patient is experiencing chronic diarrhea (C).

6. The answer is D (1.2.0)

All therapies except parenteral potassium replacement (D) are used to treat hyperkalemia. Sodium polystyrene sulfonate (Kayexalate) (A) is a cationic-anionic exchange resin used to treat hyperkalemia. It works by binding itself to potassium and exchanging with sodium in the gastrointestinal tract. Sodium bicarbonate (B) can produce a temporary alkalosis and will lower potassium as it lowers pH. Dextrose and insulin (C) cause potassium ions to move from the intravascular to intracellular space. Furosemide, a loop diuretic (E), can cause hypokalemia by inhibiting reabsorption in the ascending Loop of Henle and distal renal tubules.

7. The answer is C (1.1.0)

The most common cardiovascular signs and symptoms of hypokalemia are hypertension, arrhythmias (C), ST segment depression, presence of U waves, and flattened T waves.

8. The answer is C (1.2.0)

Hypomagnesemia can cause potassium wasting, and the resulting hypokalemia is usually refractory to potassium repletion. The hypomagnesemia should be corrected first, then hypokalemia (C).

9. The answer is A (3.2.3)

Liquid potassium supplements should be diluted in 3-4 oz of water or juice to mask the bitter taste and reduce the gastrointestinal side effects (nausea, vomiting, and diarrhea) (A). Sustained-release products should be swallowed whole. Extended-release wax tablets should be swallowed whole and not allowed to dissolve in the mouth. Patients should be counseled to take potassium supplements with food and to not double up doses if they miss a dose.

10. The answer is D (3.2.3)

Magnesium is primarily intracellular and serum magnesium is a poor reflection of repletion status. It may take 24-72 hours to reflect serum levels after magnesium therapy. Use magnesium supplements with caution in digitalized patients (choice III) and in patients with renal impairment (II) because of possible magnesium accumulation, which can result in alterations in cardiac conduction, leading to possible heart block.

Case 23 Enteral Nutrition

1. The answer is C (1.2.4)

Enteral nutrition, although not always necessary, for patients with mild to moderate diarrhea is not contraindicated. Enteral feedings may be administered in conjunction with appropriate medical management, such as antidiarrheal medications, the addition of fiber to diet, and antibiotics when appropriate. Answers A, B, D and E are absolute contraindications to the use of enteral nutrition.

2. The answer is D (1.1.4)

Patients must give consent for enteral feedings and cannot be forced to eat.

3. The answer is B (1.2.4)

JC is a candidate for enteral nutrition. Though cancer may be the underlying problem, it is not an indication. Likewise, nausea and vomiting can play an important role but may be a reason to avoid enteral feedings.

4. The answer is B (2.2.6)

Surgically placed gastrostomies and jejunostomies are both invasive and generally reserved for long-term use. PEG tubes are less invasive than surgically placed enteral tubes, however they are also for long-term use. Nasogastric tubes are the least invasive of those listed, and can be removed as soon as they are no longer needed. They do not require surgery or incisions and are indicated for short-term feeding.

5. The answer is C (1.2.5)

Though all statements regarding fiber are true, the patient does not display any signs of constipation. In fact, the patient has been experiencing "diarrhea all the time." Therefore, the benefit of reduced intestinal transit time does not apply.

6. The answer is E (1.2.1)

All of the statements with the exception of ovarian cancer are factors indicative of malnutrition. The patient lost 12 kg (estimated) within a 3- to 4-week time period. This equates to around 14% of usual body weight. Her current weight of 82 kg is 150% of her ideal body weight of 54.7kg. She also states she has a poor appetite.

7. The answer is C (1.2.7)

The amount of bacterial translocation cannot be estimated or calculated. Bacterial translocation has been observed in animal studies only; it does not have any influence on the formula one would select.

8. The answer is D (1.2.5)

Thus far, and with information given, JC has not demonstrated a need for the specialized formulas. The laboratory values and patient description do not support the use of these formulas at this time.

9. The answer is D (1.3.2)

Severe sepsis is extremely uncommon, which is a major advan-

tage of enteral feedings over parenteral nutrition. Mechanical and metabolic complications listed are commonly associated with enteral feedings.

10. The answer is B (1.2.4)

This statement is false, as the continuous feeding methods do not allow the patient to move around freely because of the continuous feedings via pump. The other statements are true.

Case 24 Iron Deficiency Anemia

1. The answer is C (1.2.3)

Food decreases iron bioavailability, though some patients may take it with food to decrease gastrointestinal side effects (C). Fluoroquinolones (A) form a ferric ion-quinolone complex, therefore decreasing the absorption of the fluoroquinolone. Iron requires an acidic environment for optimal absorption; therefore, H_2 blockers (B) and antacids (D) will decrease the absorption. Iron decreases the absorption of levothyroxine, which may result in symptoms of hypothyroidism (E).

2. The answer is E (1.1.1)

Decreased mean corpuscular volume (MCV) (I) is indicative of a microcytic anemia and often is decreased in iron deficiency anemia before decreases in hemoglobin/hematocrit are seen. MCV is the average volume of a red blood cell. High total iron binding capacity (TIBC) (II) and low serum iron and ferritin (III) are characteristic of iron deficiency anemia. TIBC represents the capacity to bind iron to transferrin. Ferritin represents stored iron and is representative of total iron stores.

3. The answer is D (1.1.4)

Chronic administration of nonsteroidal anti-inflammatory drugs (D) may decrease the acidity of the stomach, which prevents the conversion of dietary iron to the reduced Fe^{2+} form that is absorbed by the small intestine. GH's other medications do not decrease the absorption of dietary iron and therefore will not contribute to the development of iron deficiency anemia (A, B, C, E).

4. The answer is C (1.3.1)

Hemoglobin/hematocrit levels will typically return to normal before iron stores (B); therefore, discontinuation should not be considered until ferritin levels return to normal (C). Duration of treatment of iron deficiency varies based on cause and other patient-specific factors, but it is typically at least 3 to 6 months in duration (A, D). Only if patients have recurrent negative iron balances should they be considered for long-term treatment. In this case, patients are often continued on 30 mg to 60 mg elemental iron daily once deficiency is corrected (E).

5. The answer is E (1.1.3)

Pica (E) is a craving for and compulsive eating of non-food

Answers

items and is a result, although rare, of iron deficiency anemia, not a cause. Inadequate intake (A), especially in underdeveloped countries, is a common cause of iron deficiency anemia. Blood loss (B) by various causes that include but are not limited to gastrointestinal bleed, trauma, arteriovenous malformations, and heavy menstruation can lead to iron deficiency. Erythropoiesis-stimulating agents (C) increase the body's demand for iron in the formation of red blood cells, resulting in iron deficiency if not adequately supplemented during treatment. Malabsorptive syndromes (D) can also cause iron deficiency anemia.

6. The answer is C (1.3.2)

Ferritin (C) represents stored iron and is representative of total iron stores. It is the best indicator of iron overload. A strict iron deficiency anemia is a microcytic anemia, which can cause a decreased MCV (A). Correction of the iron deficiency will correct the MCV but iron overload will not result in an MCV > normal. Transferrin (B) is the protein that carries iron in the blood. Transferrin saturation indicates the amount of iron that is ready for use to make red blood cells. It is not indicative of total body iron. Red blood cell distribution width (RDW) (D) is elevated in iron deficiency anemia because the bone marrow is releasing large, immature red blood cells to compensate for the anemia. Correction of the iron deficiency will correct the RDW but iron overload will not result in a RDW < normal. Serum iron (E) is the concentration of iron bound to transferrin. Because this does not take into account stored iron, it is not a good indicator of iron overload. The serum iron level may remain normal or even low despite high levels of stored iron.

7. The answer is C (2.2.2)

All ferrous sulfate products are available over-the-counter (I). They include tablets, slow-release tablets, elixir, drops (II), and liquid.

8. The answer is B (1.3.3)

Iron sucrose (B) is an appropriate choice. It has been shown to have the fewer anaphylactic reactions than iron dextran (A). While recommending iron dextran would be appropriate, it has been associated with more risk for adverse reactions compared to the other 3 IV iron formulations, with a black-box warning for risk of anaphylactic reactions. A 25 mg test dose is required prior to administration of the first therapeutic dose. While ferric gluconate (C) would be appropriate, all of the IV iron products have the potential to cause hypotensive reactions. Iron sucrose (D) cannot be administered IM, only IV. Iron dextran may be delivered IM, though this is not typically done because of the complex Z-track administration technique and staining of the skin. Ferric gluconate (E) must be administered in separate 125-250 mg infusions.

9. The answer is C (3.1.2)

P values of > 0.05 (C) are not considered statistically significant. Because ferritin values are continuous data, a confidence interval that does not contain "0" (D, E) is considered statistically significant.

10. The answer is D (3.2.3)

Dark stools (A), constipation or diarrhea, nausea, and vomiting are common side effects of iron. These side effects are dose-dependent and giving smaller doses more frequently may improve side effects (B, D). Administering with food (C) may also help to decrease side effects; however, absorption may be decreased as much as 50%. Oral iron products contain different amounts of elemental iron (E). Side effects are similar when equivalent doses of elemental iron are taken.

Case 25 Anticoagulation

1. The answer is E (1.3.3)

Although variable depending on the specific NSAID and individual dose, potential mechanisms for increased risk of bleeding with warfarin therapy include pharmacokinetic interactions (I) (i.e. decreased metabolism via CYP interactions and decreased plasma protein binding), antiplatelet effects (III), and inhibition of GI protective prostaglandins and direct irritation to the GI mucosa (II).

2. The answer is D (1.3.3)

Amiodarone (D) increases INR levels by decreasing warfarin metabolism within 1 week and may last for 1-3 months after amiodarone has been discontinued. Carbamazepine (A) is an enzyme inducer and will increase the metabolism of warfarin therefore decreasing INR levels. Green leafy vegetables (B) are high in vitamin K, which antagonizes the effects of warfarin therefore decreasing INR levels. Nonadherence (C) can decrease the INR. The net effect of hypothyroidism (E) is a decrease in the metabolism of clotting factors, resulting in a decrease in the INR.

3. The answer is B (1.3.2)

Hemoptysis (B) is the medical term for coughing up blood from the respiratory tract and may indicate a supratherapeutic INR. The others are signs and symptoms of stroke, which would be more likely to occur with a subtherapeutic INR.

4. The answer is E (1.3.2)

Increasing the dose by 5% and rechecking the INR in one week (E) is the best answer. Decreasing the dose (A) and/or holding doses (C) would only further decrease the INR. Increasing the dose by 25% (B) would be too much of an adjustment in this situation (a patient who was previously therapeutic and no reason for the change in INR can be identified). Waiting 4 weeks to recheck after an adjustment (B) would also be too long to wait. Although in certain situations (with INR values slightly out of the goal range in individuals who were previously therapeutic) dose adjustments are not always necessary, waiting 1 month to recheck would not be appropriate (D).

5. The answer is C (1.3.2)

The best answer is C. For INR values greater than 5 but less than 9, CHEST guidelines recommend holding 1-2 doses and reinitiating therapy at a lower dose once the INR is within goal OR hold ing1 dose while administering low-dose oral vitamin K. Simply decreasing the dose (A) in this situation would not be appropriate. Instructing the patient to decrease their intake of green leafy vegetables (B) would further increase the INR if any affect. Administering aspirin (D) or increasing the warfarin dose (E) in a patient with a supratherapeutic INR would only further increase their risk of bleeding.

6. The answer is A (1.2.7)

In the absence of bleeding, low-dose vitamin K administered orally (A) is effective in reversing the INR within 24 hours without overcorrecting or resulting in warfarin resistance. SQ (B) is not recommended due to the unpredictable and sometimes delayed response. IM (C) is not recommended due to the increased risk of hematoma formation. The potential for anaphylaxis is increased with the IV route (D); however, this would be the preferred route in the presence of serious or life-threatening bleeding. Sublingual (E) vitamin K is not an available dosage form.

7. The answer is E (3.2.2)

Broccoli (E) has high amounts of vitamin K in a typical serving. Green leafy vegetables are also high in vitamin K. Mayonnaise (B) is also high in vitamin K, but a person would need to consume 7 tablespoons in one serving, which is not a typical serving. All other options have low or moderate amounts of vitamin K. (Coumadin Patient Education Booklet)

8. The answer is B (3.2.3)

Garlic can increase fibrinolytic activity, decrease platelet aggregation, and increase prothrombin time, all of which may increase the risk of bleeding if taken with warfarin. (Natural Medicines Comprehensive Database 2000)

9. The answer is A (1.2.3)

It is well documented that Bactrim will increase the anticoagulant effects of warfarin. Bactrim inhibits the metabolism of warfarin in addition to decreasing the plasma protein binding of warfarin. Bactrim should either be avoiding in combination with warfarin or if no alternative therapy is available, the dose of warfarin should be decreased with close monitoring of the INR while receiving Bactrim and for several weeks after therapy is discontinued.

10. The answer is C (2.2.3)

The 4-mg tablet of Coumadin is blue (C) in color. The remaining strengths and colors are as follows: 1-mg tablet is pink, 2-mg tablet is lavender, 2.5-mg tablet is green, 3-mg tablet is tan, 5-mg tablet is peach, 6-mg tablet is teal, 7.5-mg tablet is yellow, and 10-mg tablet is white.

Case 26 Drug-Induced Hema Disorders

1. The answer is A (1.3.3)

Compared to other antipsychotics, clozapine has about a 10-fold higher incidence of agranulocytosis (A). Monitoring of white blood cell (WBC) counts and absolute neutrophil counts (ANC) need to occur weekly, not monthly (B), for the first 6 months and then if counts are acceptable, WBC counts and ANC can be monitored every other week for the next 6 months. If counts remain acceptable, WBC counts and ANC can be monitored every 4 weeks. Duration of treatment (C) is not a reliable predictor for the development of agranulocytosis. About 88% of cases have occurred in the first 26 weeks of treatment, but some cases have developed after years of use. If WBC counts are < 2000/mm³ and/or ANC is < 1000/mm³, clozapine should be discontinued and not re-challenged (D). WBC counts and ANC should be monitored weekly for at least 4 weeks after the drug is discontinued or until WBC is e•3500/mm³ and ANC is e•2000/mm³ (E).

2. The answer is E (1.3.3)

It is imperative to counsel patients on clozapine to report any flu-like symptoms (I), since fatalities from clozapine-induced agranulocytosis have generally occurred secondary to infections in compromised immune systems. Clozapine may cause drowsiness (II), especially upon initiation of the medication. Clozapine should not be stopped abruptly (III) as psychosis and cholinergic rebound (headache, nausea, vomiting, diarrhea) may occur. Clozapine should be tapered over 1-2 weeks.

3. The answer is D (3.1.1)

USP DI (D) has a volume geared towards the patient and has drug information written at an appropriate level for patients to understand. Choices A, B, and C are sources of drug information for health care professionals. The Red Book (E) is a resource for prescription, OTC, and herbal price and product information.

4. The answer is B (1.2.4)

Clozapine does not have any effect on the bones (B). The risk of agranulocytosis (A) with clozapine is significant and therefore warrants monitoring of WBC counts and ANC weekly for the first 6 months and if acceptable, every other week for the next 6 months; if still acceptable, monitoring may then occur every 4 weeks. Clozapine has the highest risk of seizures (C) as compared to all available antipsychotic agents. Myocarditis (D) is rare but serious and has been reported in association of clozapine. Orthostatic hypotension with or without syncope can occur and rarely, respiratory and/or cardiac arrest may occur (E).

5. The answer is E (3.2.1)

The first goal of treatment is to remove the drug that is caus-

Answers

ing the agranulocytosis. In most cases, the neutropenia will resolve on its own 1-3 weeks after the offending drug is discontinued (I). However, if an infection has resulted secondary to neutropenia, it must be treated with the appropriate antibiotics (II). Although success rates have been questionable, granulocyte or granulocyte-macrophage colony stimulating factor (G-CSF or GM-CSF) have been shown to decrease recovery time, result in less use of antibiotics, and shorten hospitalizations (III).

6. The answer is C (1.3.3)

There have been no reported cases of agranulocytosis with metformin (C). During clinical trials, approximately 7% of patients receiving metformin developed asymptomatic subnormal serum vitamin B_{12} levels. Antithyroid medications cause agranulocytosis in about 0.3%-0.6% of patients (A). Ticlopidine generally causes neutropenia within the first 3 months of treatment at a rate of approximately 2.4% (B). Between 1992-1997, 116 cases of agranulocytosis with 22 deaths were reported to the FDA MedWatch program for ticlopidine. Sulfasalazine can result in life-threatening agranulocytosis at a rate of about 0.6% in patients with arthritis (D). Generally, these episodes occur within the first 3 months and often within the first 6 weeks of therapy. Dapsone has been known to cause drug-induced agranulocytosis and the patient usually has a rapid, progressive deterioration due to sepsis (E).

7. The answer is D (1.3.3)

There have been no reports of hypothyroidism associated with clozapine (D). Among the atypical antipsychotics, clozapine is associated with a greater weight gain (A) than olanzapine, risperidone, or ziprasidone. The mean weight gain with clozapine after 10 weeks is 8.9 lb. The weight gain associated with clozapine increases the risk for diabetes (B). However, clozapine has been associated with the development of diabetes early in therapy even without significant weight gain. Clozapine can result in insulin resistance, leading to secondary hyperinsulinemia. Clozapine treatment has resulted in significant increases in triglycerides (C) and total cholesterol (E), although the mechanism has not been defined.

8. The answer is B (1.3.2)

Doses should be reduced over 1 to 2 weeks if possible when discontinuing therapy (B). Clozapine needs to be discontinued immediately if total WBC decrease to below 2000/mm³ (A) or if ANC drops to below 1000/mm³ (C). The patient needs to be monitored and clozapine should not be resumed. If total WBC decrease to below 3000/mm³ but above 2000/mm³ and/or ANC drops to below 1500/mm³ but above 1000/mm³, therapy should be discontinued; may rechallenge the patient when WBC > 3500/mm³ and ANC > 2000/mm³. If therapy is interrupted for e•48 hours, the dose should be reinitiated at 12.5-25 mg/day (D). Abrupt discontinuation may lead to psychosis or cholinergic effects (headache, nausea, vomiting, diarrhea) (E).

9. The answer is D (2.2.1)

The trade name for clozapine is Clozaril (D). Clinoril (A) is the trade name for sulindac, which is a nonsteroidal anti-inflammatory drug. Klonopin (B) is the trade name for clonazepam, and it is a benzodiazepine. Catapres (C) is the trade name for clonidine and its labeled use is for hypertension. Cogentin (E) is the trade name for benztropine, which is an anticholinergic agent utilized in Parkinson's disease or for the relief of extrapyramidal signs and symptoms induced by antipsychotic agents.

10. The answer is C (1.3.3)

Clozapine does not cause bradycardia, but rather has the potential to cause tachycardia (C). Weight gain (A), drowsiness (B), and hypersalivation (or sialorrhea) (D) are common side effects to be monitored. Drowsiness or sedation are most prominent on initiation or titration of therapy but tend to decrease with continued therapy or dose reduction. If it is problematic, the larger part of the daily dose can be administered at bedtime. Clozapine has potent anticholinergic effects that often result in constipation (E).

Case 27 Diabetes

1. The answer is B (1.2.1)

Regular insulin is the recommended for intravenous (IV) use in the treatment of DKA because of the documented efficacy and safety of the product. Until the advent of the rapid-acting insulin analogs, it was the only short-acting insulin solution. The rapid-acting analogs have been used subcutaneously in the treatment of mild DKA but until recently they had not been evaluated for intravenous administration. A recent study (*Diabetes Care* 2009; 32:1164) did evaluate the use of glulisine IV in the treatment of DKA. Efficacy was similar when compared to Regular insulin. More studies need to be conducted to determine the safety of the IV administration of the rapid-acting analogs in the treatment of DKA and the cost of replacing the less-expensive Regular. Levemir should not be used because it is a long-acting insulin. Humalog 75/25 is a suspension that should not be given intravenously.

Source: Kitabchi AE, Umpierrez GE, Miles JM, Fisher JN. Hyperglycemic crises in adult patients with diabetes. *Diabetes Care.* 2009; 32:1335.

2. The answer is B (2.1.1)

Two-thirds of 40 mEq is 26.6 mEq, which you round down to 26 mEq for accuracy in measurement. Since the stock bottle is 2 mEq/mL, you would add 13 mL of potassium chloride to the IV bag. The other 14 mEq would be added as potassium phosphate.

3. The answer is A (3.2.1)

Many cases of DKA are preventable. Identifying the cause of

the diabetes is important. Educating patients and their family on the appropriate management of sick days should be conducted during the hospitalization or soon thereafter. All of these topics should be reviewed with the patient. Illness makes blood glucose more difficult to control. The stress of the illness increases the release of counter-regulatory hormones that cause blood sugar to rise. It is most important to cover the use of insulin during illness. Many patients have a tendency to stop taking their insulin when they are ill because of nausea/vomiting or a decrease in appetite, however, the body often needs more insulin during illness. Discontinuing insulin or an interruption in insulin therapy for economic reasons is a common cause of diabetic ketoacidosis. Patients should be given information on sick day management, which includes how often to monitor blood sugar, use of supplemental insulin, and the intake of carbohydrates to replace fluids and calories lost to fever, nausea, and vomiting. For patients who have had repeated episodes of DKA, monitoring blood ketones at home may help to detect early ketoacidosis. Self-treatment of fever, nausea, and diarrhea is important as well as reviewing when to contact the health care team.

4. The answer is E (2.2.1)

Choice E is correct. The rest of the answers are generic names for other insulins: glargine, Lantus (long-acting insulin analog that serves as a basal insulin administered once or twice daily); lispro, Humalog (rapid-acting insulin analog given before meals); aspart, NovoLog (rapid-acting insulin analog given before meals); and glulisine, Apidra (rapid-acting insulin analog given before meals).

5. The answer is B (1.3.3)

NovoLog is a rapid-acting insulin with an average onset of 15 minutes, a peak in 1 hour, and a duration of action of 2-3 hours. Lantus is a long-acting insulin with a duration of action of almost 24 hours. It provides a constant serum concentration of insulin throughout the day without a peak. Most likely the symptoms JW is experiencing are hypoglycemia secondary to the noontime NovoLog. While JW is advised to take one unit of NovoLog for every 10 grams of carbohydrates for each meal, insulin sensitivity can vary throughout the day. His insulin to carbohydrate ratio may need to be adjusted for lunch time (e.g., one unit for every 12 grams of carbohydrate). Another cause of the hypoglycemia may be that JW is overestimating the amount of carbohydrate that he is eating, leading to an incorrect dose of insulin (too high). Finally, his use of the insulin pen should be observed to rule out incorrect dosing. His activity or exercise routine prior to these episodes should also be evaluated for its contribution to hypoglycemia.

6. The answer is C (1.3.1)

Based on the Diabetes Control and Complications Trial (DCCT 1993), the hemoglobin A1c goal is less than 7%. In the DCCT, patients who achieved this goal were less likely to develop microvascular complications or experience progression in microvascular complications that were already established. The

American College of Endocrinology (ACE) recommends a more stringent A1c goal of less than 6.5%. While the lowest tolerated A1c should be achieved in each patient, the lower the A1c the greater the risk of severe hypoglycemia. A1c values greater than 7% put the patient at greater risk for developing microvascular complications. In some patients, the recommended A1c goal may not be achievable for a variety of reasons and may place them at risk for severe hypoglycemia (especially patients with hypoglycemic unawareness). As always, the balance between the two must be in the best interest of the patient for safety and efficacy while minimizing adverse effects.

7. The answer is C (2.2.5)

According to the manufacturer, unopened (not punctured) NovoLog FlexPens should be stored in the refrigerator (36 to 46°F). Patients may get several pens at one time and may not use them for long periods of time. If they are stored in the refrigerator, then they should retain potency until the manufacturer's expiration date. The date they are dispensed does not effect the expiration or discard date. Excessive heat (temperature <80°F) may lead to a decrease in insulin potency. FlexPens that have been exposed to excessive heat (>37°C) or have been frozen should not be used. Once punctured, FlexPens should be stored at room temperature, avoiding sunlight and heat, and not refrigerated. Discard punctured FlexPens after 28 days.

8. The answer is D (3.2.3)

Vitamin D deficiency is considered widespread among adults with more than 50% at risk. Vitamin D deficiency may play a role in the pathogenesis of autoimmune diseases in type 1 diabetes, cardiovascular disease, bone health, decline in cognitive function, and cancers such as breast and colon. Sources of vitamin D are fortified foods, oily fish, and sunshine. The American Academy of Dermatology recommends that adequate vitamin D be obtained through diet and supplements but not from unprotected exposure to UV light due to the increased risk of skin cancer. Vitamin D status is determined by measuring 25 hydroxyvitamin D levels. Levels less than 20 ng/mL indicate deficiency and levels between 21 and 29 ng/mL indicate vitamin D insufficiency. Current recommendations by the American Academy of Pediatrics are 400 IU daily for children and adolescents. For adults, the daily maintenance dose is 800 to 1000 IU but this may be inadequate for replenishing depleted stores. The best recommendations is for JW to have a 25-hydroxyvitamin D level drawn and supplementation dose based on maintaining level at or above 30 ng/mL.

9. The answer is C (1.2.2)

Choice A describes the mechanism of action of Byetta (exenatide). Choice B describes the glucose-lowering effects of Glucophage (metformin). Choice C describes the mechanism of Symlin (pramlintide). Amylin, a peptide produced by the beta cell in equimolar amounts with insulin, is greatly diminished in type 1 diabetes. Administration of this drug in combination with insulin prior to a meal results in a significant reduction in the postprandial glucose AUC. It usually results in

Answers

a reduction in the amount of insulin needed. However, it is very expensive and should be considered a second-line approach to improving glycemic control. Choice D describes the mechanism of action of the sulfonylureas. Choice E describes the action of the thiazolidinediones (pioglitazone and rosiglitazone).

10. The answer is E (1.1.4)

A foot examination should be performed at least annually to evaluate pulses, sensation, and vascular status. Risk factors that predict ulcers or amputation should be identified during the exam. Given JW's age and lack of cardiovascular disease, there is insufficient evidence to support the use of aspirin for primary prevention. Retinopathy screening should be repeated 1 year after the last screen. Less frequent screening could be done at 2 to 3 years if he has had more than one consecutive normal screening. Microalbumin screening should be repeated once a year since patient was negative for microalbumin and has normal blood pressure. Since the last lipid profile was low risk in terms of values, then another assessment should be repeated in 2 years (ADA Standards of Care Recommendations, 2010)

Case 28 Dyslipidemia

1. The answer is C (1.3.2)

The primary target for individuals that suffer from hyperlipidemia is lowering LDL-C to goal. However, the target changes for individuals that have triglyceride concentrations e•500 mg/dL. In the setting of significant hypertriglyceridemia, lowering triglyceride concentrations then becomes the primary objective because individuals that have triglyceride concentrations e•500 mg/dL are at risk for developing pancreatitis.

2. The answer is B (1.2.6)

Lovaza is the only prescription strength omega-3 fish oil that has been approved by the FDA for the treatment of elevated triglyceride concentrations. Zetia (ezetimibe) is a lipid medication that inhibits cholesterol absorption at the small intestine brush border that is used primarily to lower LDL-C and has very little effect on triglyceride concentrations. Metformin is a biguanide that is used as a first-line agent in diabetes. Welchol (colesevelam) and cholestyramine are bile acid sequestrants that are primarily used to decrease LDL-C concentrations and can as a side effect cause increased triglycerides.

3. The answer is D (1.3.3)

All four of these agents can lower triglyceride concentrations with some overlap in reduction ranges. Fibrates lower triglyceride concentrations the most with typical decreases ranging from 40%–50%. Niacin in typically used doses can lower triglycerides an average of 25%–45% and Lovaza can reduce triglyceride concentrations up to 45%. Statins can lower concentrations of triglycerides from 7%–30%. Statins' ability to lower triglycer-

ides is directly proportional to their LDL-C-lowering effects. Therefore, higher doses of statins would be expected to lower triglycerides to a greater extent, but even with the highest doses, their triglyceride-lowering potential still is not as great as the aforementioned medications.

4. The answer is D (3.2.3)

Fish oil supplements can lower triglyceride concentrations if used in appropriate doses. Prescription omega-3 fatty acids (Lovaza) are approved by the U.S. Food and Drug Administration for use an adjunct to diet in adults with very high triglyceride concentrations. Lovaza is derived from natural sources (fish) and is composed of approximately 90% omega-3 fatty acids. Lovaza comes in 1-gram capsules that contain 465 mg and 375 mg of EPA and DHA, respectively, that are responsible for lowering triglyceride concentrations. Most studies have looked at doses up to 4 grams of EPA and DHA with very good results in their ability to lower triglyceride concentrations. Fish oil is not approved to lower blood glucose and does not treat gout or erectile dysfunction.

5. The answer is C (2.2.1)

Elevated triglyceride concentrations can arise from several different factors. Primary hypertriglyceridemia is genetically based. Secondary hypertriglyceridemia can arise from poorly controlled disease states and some medications such as oral contraceptives with high-dose estrogens, glucocorticoids, and atypical antipsychotics. Diabetes is one of the most common causes of hypertriglyceridemia. Tighter glycemic control can often help to reduce triglycerides. Obesity and poorly controlled hypothyroidism can also contribute to elevated triglyceride concentrations. Individuals that consume excessive amounts of sugars and starches tend to have elevated triglyceride concentrations as well as individuals who drink excessive amounts of alcohol.

6. The answer is A (2.2.4)

If Niaspan is added to a patient's medication regimen for the management of the lipid profile, the patient should understand some basic fundamentals with the use of nicotinic acid in general. Niaspan is typically used to modify the cholesterol profile by increasing HDL-C concentrations and lowering elevated triglycerides. While it lowers LDL-C, it does so to a lesser extent than statins. Patients should also know some of the potential side effects that can be seen with the use of this agent: flushing may occur and increases in serum glucose concentrations can be seen, particularly in higher doses in those with underlying diabetes. Niacin can also increase serum uric acid concentrations. Patients may also experience some upper GI distress while on Niaspan. The extended-release (ER) formulation (Niaspan) is associated with less hepatotoxicity than when compared to the sustained-release (SR) or immediate-release (IR) formulations. Combination therapy with statins has been associated with increased risk of myalgias.

7. The answer is B (1.1.4)

Advicor is the trade name for niacin and lovastatin. Pravigard is the trade name for pravastatin and aspirin. Vytorin is the trade name for simvastatin and ezetimibe. Caduet is the trade name for atorvastatin and amlodipine. There is currently no commercially available product that contains both simvastatin and fenofibrate.

8. The answer is D (1.2.4)

Some potential side effects that can be seen with the use of niacin are hyperuricemia, hyperglycemia, flushing, and hepatotoxicity. For this patient case, the gout may be exacerbated by the use of Niaspan by potentially elevating serum uric acid concentrations. His control with his diabetes may be worsened as well, particularly with doses >1 gm. Niaspan can cause insulin resistance in some individuals, resulting in increased concentrations of blood glucose. Niacin does not affect patient weight.

9. The answer is D (1.3.1)

The combination of a statin and fibrate is commonly employed to help the patient with a mixed dyslipidemia to attain his/her lipid goals. However, it is important to recognize that there is an increased risk of myopathy with this combination. According to the packet insert, doses of simvastatin >10 mg/day plus Lopid are associated with an increased risk of adverse effects such as myopathy. If combination therapy is deemed necessary with a statin and fibrate, substituting TriCor for gemfibrozil will lessen the risk of myopathy as compared to the gemfibrozil/statin combination. All patients should be counseled on risk/benefits of combination therapy with a statin and fibrate, including myopathy.

10. The answer is D (1.1.4)

Simvastatin 80 mg daily would be expected to lower LDL-C by approximately 47%. Atorvastatin is a more potent statin but 10 mg daily would be expected to lower LDL-C by 39%. Lovastatin is one of the least potent statins and 40 mg daily would likely yield LDL-C lowering of approximately 32%. Pravastatin is slightly more potent than lovastatin but has less LDL-C-lowering ability than atorvastatin and 80 mg of pravastatin would likely yield a average 37% decrease in LDL-C. Rosuvastatin is the most potent statin currently marketed and 10 mg daily is associated with an average 52% decrease in LDL-C.

Case 29 Obesity

1. The answer is A (3.3.2)

The NHLBI lifestyle change recommendation for weight loss includes a 500-1000 kcal/day reduction containing 30% or less total kcal from fat, 15% total kcal from protein, and >55% of total kcal from CHO.

2. The answer is C (3.2.1)

Orlistat has been shown to reduce the absorption of some fat-soluble vitamins and beta-carotene (C). For this reason, patients using orlistat should be encouraged to take a daily multivitamin supplement. The supplement should be taken at least 2 hours before or after the administration of orlistat, such as bedtime. There are no reports of orlistat-induced hypomagnesemia (B). A low-fat diet does not induce a deficiency in liposoluble vitamins (E). Under physician supervision, the use of a potassium supplement is recommended for very low calorie diets (<500 kcal/d) but not for low-calorie diets (A).

3. The answer is A (1.3.3)

Side effects of orlistat include oily spotting; flatus and discharge; fecal urgency; a fatty, oily stool; and oily evacuation. In most cases these effects are mild and transient and decrease in frequency with ongoing treatment. Patients should be advised about these GI-related effects, and that these side effects will increase if the daily fat content of food is greater than 30% of total calories or if a single meal has a very high fat content (B, E). Furthermore, the daily fat content should be spread out as evenly as possible over three meals. The addition of fiber to the diet (with psyllium) has been shown to decrease GI events with orlistat without decreasing efficacy (A). Because of orlistat's mechanism of action, if a meal does not contain fat, the dose may be skipped (D). No significant interaction has been noted with pravastatin (C).

4. The answer is B (1.2.4)

The safety and efficacy of orlistat in obese adolescents was evaluated in a randomized, placebo-controlled, double-blind study that enrolled 539 patients aged 12 to 16 assigned to 120 mg of orlistat or placebo three times a day with meals in addition to a low calorie diet (no more than 30% of calories from fat) for 54 weeks. Adolescents treated with orlistat plus diet had a significantly reduced BMI compared with the ones receiving placebo plus diet. Tolerability was good and reported adverse events were generally similar to those seen in adults treated with orlistat such as fatty/oily stool, oily spotting and oily evacuation consistent with the drug's mechanism of action. Both groups showed a similar increase in fat free mass and bone mineral content (reflecting normal growth). (B)

All other compounds have not been tested (A,C,E) or FDA approved for this population (D).

5. The answer is A (1.3.5)

The most significant potential drug interaction with orlistat relates to cyclosporine. (A) No formal drug interaction studies between the two agents have been conducted, but reports have been made of changes in cyclosporine absorption with variations in dietary intake. For this reason, and because of the critical nature of maintaining appropriate cyclosporine levels in transplant patients, the recommendation is that orlistat and cyclosporine not be taken within 2 hours of each other. To date no significant interactions have been reported with phenytoin and digoxin or other drugs such as glyburide, nifedipine, and pravastatin.(B,C,D,E)

Answers

6. The answer is D (1.2.2)

Unlike sibutramine or phentermine, orlistat does not have CNS activity. Orlistat acts locally by inhibiting lipases within the gastrointestinal tract. Orlistat binds to lipase enzymes and prevents them from breaking down the triglyceride molecules. The intact triglycerides cannot be absorbed and are passed out of the body. Weight loss results because the amount of dietary fat absorbed is substantially reduced by approximately 30%.

7. The answer is D (1.2.4)

Diethylpropion (Tenuate) is a noradrenergic drug similar to phentermine (A). Diethylpropion is approved by the FDA for short-term use only for the treatment of obesity and can be administered once a day with the extended release formulation (B, D). Because of its side effect/noradrenergic profile, diethylpropion should not be used in patients with high blood pressure or ischemic heart disease (E). Diethylpropion should be taken in the morning or midmorning; if taken too late, it may cause insomnia (C).

8. The answer is C (1.1.3)

Obesity is a chronic disease for which no drug therapy offers a cure. As soon as drug therapy is discontinued, weight gain occurs. Clinical trials with both orlistat and sibutramine have shown a weight loss nadir at 6 months after which no further weight loss is achieved. The comprehensive weight management described by the APhA weight loss management guideline always includes a low calorie diet in addition to increased exercise and behavioral modification with or without pharmacotherapy.

9. The answer is D (1.2.4)

Chitosan is derived from the polysaccharide chitin, which is found in the exoskeleton of shellfish. Chitosan acts as a fiber and has similar properties to cellulose (C). It reportedly binds to fat and may prevent its absorption. At least two studies have raised questions about whether chitosan effectively absorbs fat. Compared to orlistat, chitosan blocked a negligible amount of fat absorption (A). No randomized controlled trials to date have shown the superiority of chitosan over low-calorie, low-fat diets (D). The FDA does not regulate labeling of herbal or dietary supplements (B). There have been reports of unpredictable amounts of active ingredients in OTC herbal preparations.

10. The answer is C (1.2.1)

Brand names for Phentermine include Fastin, Ionamin, Adipex-P and others. Brand name for orlistat is Xenical, sibutramine is Meridia. Mazindol is available under Sanorex, and Mazanor, while diethylpropion is available under Tenuate or Tenuate Dospan.

Case 30 Dialysis Therapy

1. The answer is C (1.3.5)

Ampicillin (A), which primarily covers gram-positive organisms, is not a good alternative to gentamicin. Ceftazidime (C) and cefepime are recommended because they cover a broad spectrum of gram-negative organisms. As part of empiric therapy for peritonitis, ceftazidime and cefepime are less likely to cause nephrotoxicity than gentamicin. Cefoxitin (B), linezolid (D), and azithromycin (E) offer limited coverage against the common organisms that cause CAPD peritonitis.

2. The answer is C (1.2.0)

Specific to the case, the patient should receive antibiotic therapy for his peritonitis intraperitoneally (IP) via his CAPD bags. The goal of IP therapy is to maintain good drug levels in the dialysate and at site of infection. In the case of vancomycin, since the elimination half-life is prolonged in ESRD, it can be dosed every 3-5 days in most patients on CAPD and still maintain adequate concentrations. Intravenous administration of antibiotics can be used as an alternative to IP administration of antibiotics to treat CAPD-related peritonitis if necessary.

3. The answer is C (1.2.3)

Cipro is known to interact with calcium, magnesium, zinc, iron, and sevelamer. Tums (A), which contains calcium carbonate, and Niferex (B), which is an iron complex, can significantly reduce the absorption of Cipro and should not be taken together. It is recommended that the Cipro dose be taken at least 2 hours before calcium, magnesium, zinc, and/or iron preparations or sevelamer (D) or 6 hours afterwards (E). Nexium (C), which increases stomach pH, should not have an effect on Cipro absorption.

4. The answer is D (1.1.2)

In CAPD-related peritonitis, bacteria are isolated in 80%-90% of cases. *S. epidermidis* is the most common at 30%-45%. *S. aureus* follows at 10%-20%. The gram-negative range is 5%-10%. *Candida* approximates 1%-10%. Five percent to 20% of peritoneal cultures are culture negative. Cefazolin is recommended in place of drugs like vancomycin and ampicillin because of the prevalence of *S. epidermidis* and sensitivity to cefazolin and concern of either frequency of existing resistance or developing resistance of other gram-positive organisms (*S.aureus, Enteroccoci*) to these other agents.

5. The answer is C (1.3.0)

EPO and Aranesp are not recommended to be given IM (A or D). EPO can be given IP (B) but its bioavailability via this route is poor. The best alternative to IV administration is to give EPO SQ (C). Subcutaneous administration of EPO is especially useful in patients who are on peritoneal dialysis. Blood levels are more constant and EPO has been shown to be more effective when given SQ as compared to IV. In many patients,

SQ doses are often lower than IV doses. Aranesp could also be given IV or SQ. SQ administration would be appropriate in a patient on CAPD.
Competency Statement:

6. The answer is E (1.3.5)

Iron deficiency is common in ESRD. In many patients, IV iron administration is required as replacement therapy to correct this deficiency. In the past, the standard of therapy has been IV iron dextran. However, anaphylaxis, although rare, can occur with this agent. Iron dextran (A) should not be given again to a patient who has this serious reaction. Desensitization (B) is no longer used or test dose given after reaction (C). Fortunately, there are other IV iron products available and can be given to a patient who has had a reaction to iron dextran. Iron sucrose (E) is one such product that be given to this type of patient. Oral iron products (D) are poorly absorbed, not well tolerated, and do not provide enough iron in most patients to correct a significant iron deficiency. Although in some patients on CAPD, oral iron if tolerated, may be used as maintenance therapy after adequate replacement.

7. The answer is A (1.3.1)

Epoetin (EPO) acts like endogenous erythropoietin to stimulate erythropoiesis in patients with anemia from renal failure. Target levels for dosing are Hgb 11-12 g/dL and Hct 33%-36%. These levels should be monitored at least weekly initially then every 3 to 4 weeks. An appropriate response to a specific dose would be an increase in Hgb of 1g/dL after 2 to 4 weeks and Hct of 1 to 2 points per week but no more than 4 points in 2 weeks. Since JC has had an appropriate response since his previous Hgb and Hct, his dose should be kept the same and reassessed in 4 weeks.

8. The answer is B (1.1.1)

The most common cause for epoetin resistance is iron deficiency. For epoetin to stimulate erythropoiesis, iron must be present to be incorporated into the heme portion of hemoglobin. Ideally, iron deficiency should be corrected before initiating epoetin therapy and if necessary during therapy with iron supplementation. Assessment includes determining transferrin saturation (TSat) and serum ferritin and these should be determined every 3 months. Target ranges are 20%-50% for TSat and 100-800 ng/mL for serum ferritin. The other lab tests do not apply to the monitoring of epoetin therapy.

9. The answer is A (1.3.5)

Both Aranesp and Epogen are erythropoietin products. Doses of Aranesp are in mcg/kg and doses of EPO are in units/kg. The starting dose of Aranesp is 0.45 mcg/kg/week whereas the starting dose of EPO is 150 units/kg/week (A). Aranesp has a three-fold longer half-life (C), which allows for less frequent dosing compared to EPO (B). Aranesp also provides more sustained EPO concentrations. Both can be given IV or SC. The target goals and side effect profile are similar for both agents D and E.

10. The answer is A (1.3.4)

JC may get more benefit if he took his Neurontin (A) on a regular schedule, such as every night and during the day if needed but on a regular schedule. Neurontin is effective for both neuropathy and restless leg syndrome. However, since Neurontin is eliminated renally, a low-dose regimen would be appropriate to start. This regimen should be titrated based on response and tolerability. Common side effects of Neurontin include somnolence, ataxia, nystagmus, and headaches. Another option would be to increase his clonazepam (B) dose for restless leg syndrome but clonazepam is not effective for peripheral neuropathy. Phenytoin (C) may also be used for neuropathies and sometimes restless leg syndrome but dosing is more complicated based on the fact that protein binding is altered in ESRD, serum drug concentration monitoring is required, and liver metabolism of other drugs (e.g., Lipitor, diltiazem) is increased. Ropinirole (D) has been used in restless leg syndrome, but there are very little data in dialysis patients and this would be adding another drug. Quinine (E) is associated with significant hematologic toxicity. The use of quinine to treat leg cramps is off label and is highly discouraged.

Case 31 Dosing of Drugs in Renal Failure

1. The answer is D (1.2.0)

The total clearance of enoxaparin is lower and the elimination is delayed in patients with renal failure. Most beta blockers are metabolized by the liver. However, the clearance of atenolol is dependent on renal function. Amlodipine, like most calcium channel blockers, is metabolized by the liver.

2. The answer is D (1.2.4)

Integrilin is contraindicated for use in dialysis patients. Aggrastat is another glycoprotein IIb/IIIa inhibitor that may be used in patients with ESRD at 50% of the normal recommended dose.

3. The answer is A (1.3.0)

ACE inhibitors are good agents to add to JM's current regimen. The prevalence of left ventricular hypertrophy (LVH) is greatly increased in patients with ESRD (>60%) and ACE inhibitors have been shown to reverse LVH. ARBs have also been shown to be effective and may have similar benefits as ACE inhibitors in patients with renal failure. Thiazide diuretics (C) are not effective in patients with renal failure for control of hypertension. Clonidine (B), hydralazine (D), and minoxidil (E) are not considered first-line agents in this type of patient. However, they may be used if other classes were ineffective or not tolerated.

4. The answer is A (1.3.2)

Like most ACE inhibitors, the dosage of lisinopril should be reduced in patients with renal failure since it is eliminated pri-

Answers

marily by the kidneys. Spironolactone (B) is a weak diuretic and is not effective at this level of renal function. The use of spironolactone is problematic in patients with renal failure due to the risk of hyperkalemia. Unlike most diuretics, furosemide can be used in patients with renal failure if the patient has some urine output. At this level of renal impairment, furosemide is used primarily for fluid management. The dosage of metoprolol (C), like most beta blockers, does not have to be reduced since its elimination is dependent on liver function. Clonidine (D) doses in patients with ESRD are similar to doses used in other populations. Angiotensin-receptor blockers (E) can be used in patients with renal failure.

5. The answer is C (1.3.0)

Dialysis has little effect on phenytoin since it is highly protein bound and primarily metabolized by the liver. However, since it is highly protein bound, albumin and level of renal function have a significant effect on the ratio of free drug to bound drug (free fraction). In patients like this, the free fraction is increased. Since measured phenytoin levels represent the total drug concentration of unbound phenytoin and phenytoin bound to albumin, the phenytoin level should be adjusted to reflect the altered plasma binding seen with hypoalbuminemia and ESRD. Therefore the following equation can be used in patients with ESRD who are receiving dialysis regularly to indicate what the measured phenytoin level may be when corrected for albumin and renal failure:

Adjusted Phenytoin level = measured total phenytoin level/ [(0.1 x albumin) + 0.1]

Adjusted phenytoin level = 6.4/ [(0.1 x 3.1) + 0.1] = 15.6
The type of dialysis (A), PT/INR (B), calcium level (D), and phosphorus level (E) are not needed in order to interpret phenytoin levels.

6. The answer is D (1.2.6)

Digoxin has a large Vd, is extensively distributed into tissues, and is minimally removed by HD. Despite this there is a significant reduction in the Vd of digoxin in patients with renal failure and if a loading dose is given the total amount must be reduced. Drugs with a large Vd are distributed widely throughout tissues and are present in only small amounts in the blood, so they are not easily removed by HD. However, digoxin is primarily eliminated by the kidneys and therefore, the maintenance dose must be adjusted for renal dysfunction. For many drugs, including digoxin, peritoneal dialysis has less of an effect on drug clearance compared to hemodialysis. Digoxin is typically given every other day or three times weekly in HD patients.

7. The answer is A (1.2.6)

Piperacillin/tazobactam (A) is eliminated primarily by the kidneys and requires dose adjustment in patients with ESRD. All other answers (B, C, D, E) do not require dose adjustment in ESRD.

8. The answer is B (2.1.3)

The physician ordered 0.05 mcg/kg/min. Based on a weight of 75.3 kg, that equals 225.9 mcg/h. The concentration of the drip is 0.05 mg or 50 mcg/mL. So, if you divide 225.9 mcg/h by the concentration of 50 mcg/mL, the resulting rate is 4.5 mL/h.

9. The answer is E (1.2.5)

The extent to which a drug is affected by dialysis is determined by several characteristics of the drug, including molecular size, protein binding, volume of distribution, water solubility, route of elimination, and clearance. Dialysis is dependent on the use of a membrane in which the movement of drugs is largely determined by the size of the molecule in relation to the size of the membrane pore. As a general rule, smaller drug molecules pass more easily across the membranes and, therefore, are more dialyzable. Drugs with a high degree of protein binding have a small plasma concentration of unbound drug available for dialysis, and the bound molecule is too large to cross the dialysis membrane. A drug with a large Vd is present in only small amounts in the blood and is minimally dialyzed. The dialysate for HD is an aqueous solution, so drugs with high water solubility will be dialyzed to a greater extent than lipid-soluble drugs. The plasma clearance or metabolic clearance of a drug is the sum of the renal and nonrenal clearance. If a drug has a large nonrenal clearance, the contribution of HD is low. But if a drug has a high renal clearance, or significantly cleared by the kidney, HD affects the plasma clearance and is considered clinically important.

10. The answer is C (3.2.3)

Like beta blockers and ACE inhibitors, aspirin (C) has been shown to reduce cardiovascular events and prevent subsequent AMIs. On the other hand, the use of agents such as vitamin E (B), vitamin D (D), and folic acid (E) and have not been proven to decrease cardiovascular events. Also, digoxin (A) has no proven benefit in this setting.

Case 32 Renal Failure (Chronic)

1. The answer is D (1.1.1)

The most common causes of chronic renal failure (CRF) are diabetes (A) and HTN (B). Hyperlipidemia (C) is a major risk factor for CRF. All three play a role in the progression of renal disease. One's risk of chronic renal disease can be increased based on family history (E). Hyperkalemia (D) is a result of chronic renal disease not a cause.

2. The answer is B (1.3.3)

Zestril (lisinopril) is an ACE inhibitor. Diovan (valsartan) is an ARB. Both can lead to increased serum potassium, especially with worsening renal function. Furosemide is a loop diuretic that is often used in combination with an ACE inhibitor or an

ARB to help decrease serum potassium in chronic renal failure patients. Atorvastatin is an HMG-CoA reductase inhibitor, metoprolol is a beta blocker, and amlodipine is a calcium channel blocker. None of these latter three agents would be expected to affect potassium.

3. The answer is E (1.2.7)

Kayexalate (sodium polystyrene sulfonate) is an example of a cation exchange resin. Sodium polystyrene sulfonate removes potassium by exchanging sodium ions for potassium ions in the GI tract before the resin is excreted from the body.

4. The answer is B (2.2.5)

Sanofi Aventis recommends that once a pen is in use (punctured) that it be discarded after 28 days.

5. The answer is D (1.1.2)

DW has stage 4 CKD. GFR (mL/min/1.73 m^2) = 175 x (S$_{cr}$)$^{-1.154}$ x (Age)$^{-0.203}$ x (0.742 if female) x (1.212 if African American) = 18. This is the MDRD equation that uses the standardized serum creatinine assay calibrated by isotope dilution mass spectroscopy (IDMS).

If the lab does not use a standardized serum creatinine assay method, then the MDRD equation is GFR (mL/min/1.73 m^2) = 186 x (S$_{cr}$)$^{-1.154}$ x (Age)$^{-0.203}$ x (0.742 if female) x (1.212 if African-American). The original MDRD equation also included albumin and BUN: 170 x SCr$^{-0.999}$ x age$^{-0.176}$ x SUN$^{-0.170}$ x SAlb$^{+0.318}$ (0.762 female) x (1.180 black).

CrCl associated with various stages of CKD is as follows:
Stage 1 = kidney damage with normal or increased GFR (greater than 90 mL/min)
Stage 2 = kidney damage with mild decrease in GFR (60-89 mL/min)
Stage 3 = moderate decrease in GFR (30-59 mL/min)
Stage 4 = severe decrease in GFR (15-29 mL/min)
Stage 5 = kidney failure (GFR less than 15 mL/min or dialysis)

6. The answer is A (3.1.1)

Identidex (I), Clinical Pharmacology, Physicians' Desk Reference (PDR), Drug Facts & Comparisons, Mosby's GenRx, and Ident-A-Drug Reference can be used to help identify medications. Goodman and Gillman's (II) contains basic pharmacologic and therapeutic information, but nothing to help identify medications. Applied Therapeutics (III) is a good source for drug treatment information but is not helpful in identifying medications.

7. The answer is D (1.1.3)

Renal osteodystrophy (bone disease) is a common manifestation of chronic renal failure (CRF). It is a complex disorder initiated by decreased elimination of phosphorus by the kidneys. This results in the inhibition of renal activation of vitamin D, which in turn decreases gut absorption of calcium. Low blood calcium concentration stimulates parathyroid hormone (PTH) secretion. As renal function declines, chronic PTH stimulation results in increased mobilization of calcium from bone. The anemia of CRF is characteristically normochromic and normocytic. It is attributable mainly to decreased erythropoietin secretion from damaged kidneys. As renal failure progresses, HTN usually develops from salt and water retention. Hyperkalemia, not hypokalemia, is more likely in patients with CRF.

8. The answer is D (3.1.1)

UpToDate (D) is likely to have information about recent studies and trends in drug therapy. The Handbook of Nonprescription Drugs (B) has only OTC information. Lexi-Comp (E) drug information provides much information about drugs, but not necessarily about the rationale behind the use of specific drug combinations. There is no such publication as Bruce's guide (C).

9. The answer is D (1.2.2)

Diuretics with a different mechanism of action can be given with furosemide to help overcome diuretic resistance. Most thiazide diuretics including hydrochlorothiazide (HCTZ) (A) are not effective with a low GFR. Zaroxolyn (metolazone) (D) is an exception to this rule. Combining metolazone with furosemide is effective in patients with decreased GFRs. Diamox (acetazolamide) (B), a carbonic anhydrase inhibitor, is ineffective in patients with a low GFR and may worsen acidosis associated with CRF. Bumex (bumetanide) (C) and Demadex (torsemide) (E) are both loop diuretics like furosemide.

10. The answer is D (1.2.1)

ACE inhibitors and beta blockers have been shown to improve outcomes post-MI, but beta blockers may mask signs and symptoms of hypoglycemia. Calcium channel blockers have not been shown to improve outcomes and should not routinely be used to reduce cardiovascular risk after an MI.

Case 33 Anxiety

1. The answer is A (1.2.1)

Venlafaxine is an antidepressant that is FDA-indicated for the treatment of GAD. The others have been used to treat generalized anxiety disorder but it is considered off-label because they lack FDA indications for this treatment.

2. The answer is E (1.1.2)

All three disease states have symptoms (i.e., shortness of breath, racing heart, decreased concentration, worry, chest pain) that mimic generalized anxiety disorder.

3. The answer is A (1.2.2)

Benzodiazepines facilitate the action of GABA by allowing an influx of chloride ions into the cell.

Answers

4. The answer is B (3.2.2)

Cognitive behavioral therapy has substantial data to support its use in anxiety disorders, in particular GAD. The other therapies have little or no evidence to support efficacy.

5. The answer is B (1.2.4)

JD is allergic to salicylates, so he is most likely to have an allergic reaction to St. Joseph's aspirin. The active ingredient in this product is in the salicylate class and could cause cross-sensitivity. JD should revisit his idea to start ASA therapy with his physician.

6. The answer is E (1.1.1)

Vitamin B_{12} deficiency (pernicious anemia) commonly results in a secondary intracellular deficiency of folate by the concept of "methylfolate trapping." Decreased levels of vitamin B_{12} and/or folic acid may indicate a megaloblastic anemia. On the basis of JD's laboratory profile, folate 2.5 ng/mL (2.5-20 ng/mL), vitamin B_{12} 200 pg/mL (200-900 pg/mL), and hematocrit 32% (37%-47%), he should be evaluated for both types of anemias.

7. The answer is C (2.2.2)

Effexor XR is available as 37.5 mg, 75 mg and 150 mg capsules. Answer C is the only available combination.

8. The answer is C (1.1.0)

The DSM-IV diagnostic criteria for GAD require that symptoms occur more days than not for a period of at least 6 months.

9. The answer is B (2.2.3)

Mirtazapine and venlafaxine are not SSRIs. Fluoxetine comes in capsule form. Citalopram is either orange or white. Sertraline is the only one available in a blue oblong tablet form.

10. The answer is A (3.1.1)

The NIMH (National Institute of Mental Health) (A) has the most current disease state information and is vetted by experts in the field. It has consumer-friendly information on a variety of disease states, including treatment options. Library books (B) may be useful, but may contain outdated information. The DSM-IV-TR (C) will provide diagnostic information, but does not discuss treatment. It may also be too complex for the patient's understanding. Wikipedia (D) and support groups (E) may have some useful information, but are not peer-reviewed and may provide incomplete or inaccurate information.

Case 34 ADHD & Schizophrenia

1. The answer is C (1.2.2)

Psychostimulants (methylphenidate, amphetamine), atomoxetine, and some antidepressants (tricyclics, bupropion, venlafaxine) affect the presynaptic neurons in the prefrontal cortex and frontal-subcortical pathways by inhibiting the reuptake and/or enhancing the release of dopamine and/or norepinephrine. The other neurotransmitters mentioned in the question currently are not thought to have any clinically significant role in mediating ADHD symptoms.

2. The answer is D (2.2.1)

Adderall tablets contain a fixed ratio combination of l-amphetamine aspartate, l-amphetamine sulfate, dextroamphetamine saccharate, and dextroamphetamine sulfate. The tablets are also available in an extended-release capsule form. The other answers are either immediate- or sustained-release preparations of methylphenidate.

3. The answer is E (1.3.3)

Both methylphenidate and amphetamine preparations can cause anorexia, insomnia, jitteriness, upper abdominal pain, and headache; and worsened motor hyperactivity and behavior dyscontrol as the shorter-acting stimulants wear off.

4. The answer is E (3.2.2)

Although core symptoms can be improved with drug therapy for ADHD, learning disorders such as dyslexia need to be addressed with educational interventions and specific remedial therapies. Detoxification and chemical dependency treatment along with 12-step peer support groups are indicated to treat substance abuse. Family interventions and individual and group psychotherapies can help with conduct problems and oppositional defiant behaviors.

5. The answer is C (1.2.4)

Postmarketing surveillance of pemoline has shown association with cases of jaundice, hepatitis, and acute liver failure. Although the number of cases reported is not high, it is significantly higher than in the general population. The other side effects listed have not been associated with pemoline therapy.

6. The answer is B (1.2.4)

Neoplastic disease is the decoy answer and is not associated with ADHD. People with untreated ADHD have significantly elevated rates of and corresponding morbidity from all the others listed, including 50% greater risk of bicycle accidents, 33% more emergency room visits, 3-4 times greater risk of motor vehicle accidents, more absenteeism and lower productivity in school or at work, and higher incidence of domestic violence, relationship problems, and divorce in adults. There is also the individual and societal morbidity associated with the increase in delinquent behavior including disorderly conduct, vandalism, assault, fighting, theft, minor in possession of tobacco or alcohol, and possession of controlled substance. An estimated 25% of prison inmates have untreated ADHD.

7. The answer is D (2.2.2)

Concerta uses an osmotic controlled-release delivery system of methylphenidate and is available in 18 mg, 27 mg, 36 mg, and 54 mg strengths. They are all CII-controlled substances.

8. The answer is A (1.2.1)

Strattera is the brand name for atomoxetine, a selective norepinephrine reuptake inhibitor approved by the FDA for treatment of ADHD. Vyvanse, Daytrana, and Focalin are different forms of methylphenidate and Dextrostat is dextroamphetamine—all stimulant medications indicated for ADHD.

9. The answer is D (1.3.4)

Abuse of prescribed stimulants in adults and teenagers with ADHD, even those with a strong history of substance abuse/dependence, is very low. Fully one-third to one-half of adults and adolescents referred for treatment of ADHD also have a psychoactive substance use disorder, with marijuana abuse being three times more prevalent than abuse of cocaine or methamphetamine. Concern remains for diversion or abuse of prescribed stimulant medication by others, for example patient's friends, siblings, parents, other relatives, or acquaintances.

10. The answer is B (2.2.3)

Provigil is available only in tablet form, although caplet shaped. Even though it is FDA approved to treat excessive daytime sleepiness in patients with narcolepsy, obstructive sleep apnea, and shiftwork sleep disorder, it is finding some off-label efficacy in treating ADHD symptoms. The others are all available only in capsule form.

Case 35 Depression & Bi-Polar Disorders

1. The answer is D (1.3.3)

Given that JM is experiencing symptoms consistent with major depression, which is common following an MI. It's unclear whether the previous and current use of amitriptyline was for chronic back pain, depression, or both, but it does appear that antidepressants are indicated for symptoms of depression. SSRI are usually considered first in patients with ACS and in patients experiencing depression and HF. Statement I is incorrect. Statements II and III are true statements about amitriptyline's side effects thus making a change of medication necessary.

2. The answer is C (1.1.4)

Of the medications listed, alprazolam is the most correct answer. Alprazolam and other benzodiazepines are associated with increased falls and increased morbidity and mortality in older persons, especially in nursing homes. Antihypertensive agents, including diuretics and ACE inhibitors, can lead to falls particularly in patients with low blood pressure. Agents with a greater risk for postural hypotension (e.g., alpha-1 antagonists) and medications that possess this pharmacologic property (e.g., amitriptyline) are also significantly problematic.

3. The answer is B (1.2.4)

Although tricyclic antidepressants have this antiarrhythmic effect, their other cardiovascular effects (e.g., alpha-1 antagonism thus can exhibit postural hypotension and has pro-arrhythmic effects) make them difficult to tolerate for patients with cardiac disease; thus, A and D are false. Statement B is correct and is an area of ongoing research. Although controversial in all cardiac illness, sertraline (SADHART study), has been shown to be somewhat effective and a safe antidepressant in many patients post-MI. No medications have an FDA approval for depression in heart disease.

4. The answer is B (1.1.4)

Response to antidepressant medication in older adults is associated with an increased (slower) time to response and a lower rate of remission. Older patients can experience remission at rates greater than previously thought but continuous use over several years is probably necessary for this remission to occur at those rates.

5. The answer is B (1.2.6)

Choice A is incorrect. This describes a linear dose-response curve. Choice B is the correct answer signifying a flat dose-response curve. Choice C is incorrect. This describes a curve linear dose-response curve. Choice D is incorrect. This describes an inverse curve linear dose-response curve. Choice E is incorrect. Most side effects associated with serotonin antidepressants are dose-dependent and predictable rather than idiosyncratic

6. The answer is A (2.2.1)

Choice A is correct since sertraline is available in a liquid formulation at an equivalent dose. It is unavailable in a disintegrating or chewable tablet, so choices B and D are incorrect. Choice C is incorrect since citalopram, fluoxetine, paroxetine, and sertraline are all available in a liquid formulation. Choice E is incorrect. Although aripiprazole is an atypical antipsychotic indicated as an augmentation strategy in depression, it is ineffective as antidepressant in monotherapy.

7. The answer is C (3.1.2)

The mean dose is the average dose given per patient. The mode indicates the dose used more often. Therefore, statements I and II are correct. Given that no further information is provided about efficacy, there is no basis to support statement III.

8. The answer is D (1.2.6)

Concurrent use of an MAOI antidepressant with another antidepressant is contraindicated (with few exceptions) due to risk of serotonin syndrome. Abrupt discontinuation of phenelzine can lead to a significant discontinuation syndrome, so it is best to institute a gradual taper. Since phenelzine binds irreversibly to MAO-A and MAO-B, a 2-week period is necessary to allow for enzyme turnover prior to starting another antidepressant.

Answers

9. The answer is B (1.3.3)

Sertraline may also be associated with GI discomfort at this much higher dose. JM has shown some treatment response to venlafaxine, so changing to a sustained-release formulation may decrease GI effects and allow the use of a drug that appears to be effective for treatment of depression in JM. On the basis of this information, choice B is correct. Once-daily dosing of immediate-release venlafaxine is not associated with less side effects and it also is not indicated for once-daily dosing at higher doses.

10. The answer is C (3.1.1)

Choices A, B, D, and E primarily provide information for health professionals. However, the USP-DI has a volume specifically devoted to drug information written so consumers can understand it.

Case 36 Drug Abuse & Alcoholism

1. The answer is C (3.2.2)

Contraindications to naltrexone use include acute hepatitis, liver failure (C), concomitant opioid analgesics or a positive urine screen for opioids, hypersensitivity to naltrexone, current opioid dependency or withdrawal, and failure of a naloxone challenge.

Patients with depression (A), heart failure (B), renal failure (D), and hypertension (E) can safely take naltrexone.

2. The answer is D (1.1.3)

All selections (A, B, C, E) are FDA approved for alcoholism except topiramate, which is only approved for migraine and epilepsy. Although studies have been done indicating this drug may be a possible agent to use in the future.

3. The answer is B (1.2.3)

Naltrexone, an opiate antagonist, should not be given with Suboxone (B) (buprenorphine plus naloxone). When Suboxone is given by mouth, it acts as an opiate agonist, since the naloxone, an opiate antagonist, is not absorbed from the GI tract. Naltrexone is contraindicated in people taking opiates agonists because it will precipitate an opiate withdrawal syndrome. Antabuse (disulfiram) and Campral (acamprosate) can be safely given with naltrexone since they do not interact with naltrexone mechanism of action.

4. The answer is D (1.3.3)

Disinhibition is an uncommon adverse effect of benzodiazepines, however it can occasionally occur, but is usually in the elderly patient. Anterograde amnesia (A), bradycardia (B), lightheadedness (C), and somnolence (E) are common adverse effects of benzodiazepines.

5. The answer is D (1.1.1)

The CAGE is a four-item screening tool to identify patients in need of further work-up for alcoholism. It is an acronym for asking the following questions: Have you ever felt you ought to CUT down on your drinking? Have people ANNOYED you by criticizing your drinking? Have you ever felt bad or GUILTY about your drinking? Have you ever had a drink first thing in the morning (EYE opener) to steady your nerves or get rid of a hangover? The SF-36 (A) rates quality of life. The GAF (Global Assessment of Functioning, C) is a general scale rating functional capacity. The BPRS (Brief Psychiatric Rating Scale, B) is used primarily to rate symptoms of psychotic disorders. The Beck-A (E) rates anxiety symptoms/disorders.

6. The answer is A (3.2.1)

It is acceptable to use Zyban (bupropion) and nicotine replacement therapy concurrently (C), though it is not clear that this improves outcomes over bupropion monotherapy. All of the other statements are false. Not all health-related problems will always be linked to smoking (B) and a patient does not need to have a smoking-related problem to consider smoking cessation (D). Patients with psychiatric disorders often have a higher rate of nicotine dependence and should be offered smoking cessation therapy (E).

7. The answer is A (1.2.4)

Listerine antiseptic mouthwash contains alcohol. Antabuse is disulfiram. Disulfiram's clinical effect results from an adverse reaction due to blocking the oxidation of alcohol at the acetaldehyde stage by inhibiting aldehyde dehydrogenase, which would cause a reaction in a patient ingesting alcohol. Campral is acamprosate, a GABA agonist/glutamate antagonist, and would not cause an adverse reaction with alcohol. Revia (B) is naltrexone, an opiate antagonist, and would not cause an adverse reaction with alcohol.

8. The answer is A (2.2.1)

A Nicotrol 21-mg patch is available OTC for smoking cessation. Nicorette gum (B) is not available in a 10-mg dosage form (only 2 mg and 4 mg). Zyban 150 mg (C) is available by prescription only, and Chantix (D) and Nicotrol (E) are prescription-only products.

9. The answer is C (1.3.3)

The most common side effects with bupropion include: dizziness (11%), headache (25%), insomnia (16%), nausea (18%), pharyngitis (11%), and xerostomia (24%). Sexual dysfunction (A) is not common with bupropion, as it is with antidepressants that inhibit serotonin reuptake and bupropion is often used to help treat antidepressant sexual dysfunction. Arthralgias (A) and hypertension (E) are side effects that should not be expected.

10. The answer is D (1.1.2)

Anhedonia (loss of interest), insomnia, avolition (reduction in goal-directed activities), poor concentration, insomnia/hypersomnia, weight changes, and mood reactivity and amotivation are all signs of depression (A, B, C, E) and occasionally can occur in substance use disorder. Confusion (do not confuse with poor concentration) and dysphoria (a change in mood where anxiety, irritability, depression (or mania), and insomnia occur together) are more common in substance use disorders such as alcoholism (E).

Case 37 Bipolar Disorder

1. The answer is E (3.2.2)

Inadherence to her medication regimen and stress from family and financial problems are likely contributors to this episode of depression in DL. Although alcohol use can contribute to depression, DL's history of current alcohol intake is not clear so it needs to be considered only as a possible contributing factor.

2. The answer is A (2.2.2)

The Depakene is the most likely medication to cause GI irritation. In many cases, changing to the extended-released divalproex will relieve GI irritation. Sodium valproate liquid is not a delayed-release formulation, so it is unlikely to decrease GI irritation. Increasing the dose of Depakene or taking the entire dose at bedtime could increase GI irritation. Changing to a generic valproic acid capsule would have little impact on improving symptoms of dyspepsia since it is also an immediate-release formulation.

3. The answer is E (1.1.4)

The use of antidepressants in bipolar I disorder increases the potential risks associated with destabilizing mood, even when mood stabilizers are a part of the medication regimen. This destabilization of mood may take place acutely or upon chronic use of antidepressants. Thus all of the answers are correct statements.

4. The answer is C (1.3.2)

Statements I and II are correct because monitoring serum concentration provides information that can be used to determine if dosing is adequate to achieve a serum concentration likely to result in therapeutic response to valproic acid. Valproic acid can cause hepatotoxicity, so liver enzymes should be monitored periodically. Statement III is incorrect because valproic acid is not associated with pulmonary toxicity.

5. The answer is C (1.3.3)

Sedation is a side effect of benzodiazepines, valproic acid, and beta blockers. Depression, both unipolar and bipolar, can be associated with somnolence. Hypomania is associated with a decreased need for sleep with less potential of secondary somnolence. Therefore, C is the correct answer.

6. The answer is E (1.3.5)

Statements I, II, and III all provide drugs or drug classes than can be used in bipolar disorder. Olanzapine, as well as some other antipsychotics, are indicated for use in bipolar disorder. Lithium and lamotrigine are both indicated for use in the maintenance phase of bipolar disorder.

7. The answer is C (1.2.6)

A gradual titration schedule is used for lamotrigine in order to decrease the incidence of rash. Valproic acid increases plasma levels of lamotrigine. When used in combination, the titration of lamotrigine must occur more slowly with a lower starting dose in order to reduce the risk of rash. Abruptly reducing the dose of valproic acid by 50% could lead to an exacerbation of symptoms and would still require the use of the slower lamotrigine titration schedule.

8. The answer is B (3.2.2)

Choice A is unlikely to improve adherence and could decrease likelihood of adherence. Choice C is incorrect because it is not possible to make these changes to DL's medication regimen and meet her therapeutic needs. Choices D and E are incorrect because they are impractical in a regimen containing five medications, especially because DL lives 50 miles from the clinic. Choice B uses a technique known as behavioral tailoring to tie medication-taking behaviors with other routine activities.

9. The answer is C (1.2.5)

Choice C would provide a trough serum concentration of valproic acid. Most clinicians monitor trough serum concentrations of 50-125 g/mL in acute phase of mania in bipolar disorder patients with higher concentrations providing better response particularly in monotherapy. It is less clear of the best concentration for response in combination therapy. Plasma level determination is always a consideration for patients where there is known inadherence in patients.

10. The answer is B (1.3.5)

Although all of the agents mentioned have some potential for weight gain, lamotrigine appears to be the most weight neutral.

Case 38 ADHD & Schizophrenia

1. The answer is A (1.3.3)

Pseudo-Parkinsonian side effects of first-generation antipsychotic medication is due to blockade of postsynaptic dopamine receptors resulting in imbalance between dopaminergic and cholinergic systems on which normal motor function depends, resulting in relative functional dopamine deficiency and cholinergic excess in the area of the striatum. Histamine H_1 blockade causes sedation and increased appetite and blockade of alpha-1 adrenergic receptors leads to orthostatic hypotension and reflex tachycardia. Anticholinergic side effects include dry mouth,

Answers

blurred vision, constipation, tachycardia, urinary retention, memory impairment, and ejaculatory dysfunction. Serotonergic blockade results in sedation, weight gain, and orthostasis.

2. The answer is D (2.2.3)

Risperdal M-Tabs, Zyprexa Zydis, and Saphris are orally disintegrating tablets of the second-generation antipsychotic medications risperidone, olanzapine, and asenapine, respectively. The others are either solid tablets or capsules of first- or second-generation antipsychotic medications that need to be swallowed for GI absorption. Saphris is not swallowed, but absorbed sublingually and has negligible GI absorption if swallowed.

3. The answer is B (1.2.4)

The first-generation antipsychotic medications are associated with the potential for disorders of movement and muscle tone including acute and tardive dyskinesia, which can become irreversible; acute and tardive dystonia; akathisia; tremor; and pseudo-Parkinsonism. They are not associated with alopecia or autoimmune disorders and are frequently associated with weight gain and constipation. Patients should also be warned about postural hypotension, effects of increased prolactin secretion, dry mouth and associated dental problems, cardiac arrhythmia, urinary retention, blurred vision, sedation and need to avoid alcohol due to additive sedating effect, increase in skin sensitivity to the sun, decrease in sweating and potential for heat stroke, and neuroleptic malignant syndrome.

4. The answer is C (1.1.3)

Thought insertion is a delusion that certain thoughts are not one's own but put into one's mind from someone else. Thought broadcasting is a delusion that one's thoughts are being transmitted out loud that others can hear. Delusions of being controlled are feelings, impulses, thoughts, or actions that are experienced as being under the control of some outside force. Erotomanic delusions are firm, fixed beliefs with no basis in reality that another person (usually of higher status, rank, or wealth) is in love with the individual. Ideas of reference is the correct answer.

5. The answer is E (1.3.5)

Statement I is correct because pre- and post-marketing experience has shown that second-generation antipsychotic medications are much less prone to cause extrapyramidal side effects, orthostatic hypotension, hyperprolactinemia (except risperidone), less weight gain, sedation, and abnormalities of glucose and lipid metabolism (except olanzapine and quetiapine), less cognitive slowing and better effect on negative symptoms, and less risk of tardive dyskinesia than the first-generation antipsychotics. Because patients don't feel as uncomfortable, it is thought that second-generation antipsychotics may then have the advantage of better medication adherence and improved level of daily functioning. Large and well-controlled studies conclude that these medications are as effective as first-generation antipsychotic medications for controlling positive symptoms of schizophrenia. Statements I, II, and III are true, thus E is the correct answer.

6. The answer is A (1.3.3)

Antipsychotic medications can cause movement disorders due to postsynaptic dopaminergic blockade in the basal ganglia, particularly the dopamine D_2 receptor.

7. The answer is C (1.1.3)

Both choice I and II are diagnostic criteria for schizophrenia, but mood symptoms are either not present or present only briefly during the active phase of psychotic symptoms. In addition, the symptoms are not due to a medical condition, medication effect, or substance abuse.

8. The answer is B (3.2.2)

Regular monitoring of vital signs is a medically related measure but the others are designed to assist a patient to integrate successfully in the general community, maintain independent living in a personal home environment, attain self-support with steady employment, and develop interests and social life outside of home and family—all of which can be impaired by symptoms of schizophrenia.

9. The answer is A (1.2.4)

Although all antipsychotics can cause transient leukopenia, there is a 0.8%-0.9% risk of developing agranulocytosis with clozapine. Because deaths have been associated with agranulocytosis in patients who did not have their white blood cell count monitored while receiving clozapine in Europe prior to its availability in the U.S., the FDA requires routine monitoring of WBC in patients receiving clozapine and reporting to a national registry.

10. The answer is A (1.3.3)

A result of dopamine activity in the hypothalamic-pituitary axis is inhibition of prolactin secretion. Blockade of dopamine receptors removes some degree of this inhibition, resulting in increased secretion of prolactin, which is associated with all the first-generation antipsychotic medications and risperidone. Among the second-generation antipsychotics, quetiapine and clozapine use does not lead to elevation of prolactin levels, equal to placebo. At low doses, olanzapine does not elevate prolactin secretion; however, at higher doses, prolactin secretion is more significant. Prolactin levels are only mildly elevated at very high doses of ziprasidone. Risperidone is associated with elevated prolactin at low, moderate, and high doses. Clinically some patients with high prolactin levels show very little or no symptoms, while others with only mild prolactin elevation have very troubling effects. Symptoms of hyperprolactinemia can include diminished libido, erectile dysfunction, gynecomastia, galactorrhea, osteoporosis, and amenorrhea. Typically, one would expect worsening sexual dysfunction as prolactin levels rise.

Answers

Case 39 Headache

1. The answer is E (1.1.3)

Migraine symptoms can vary, but at minimum involve headache pain (A) to some degree. Other migrainous features include photophobia (B), phonophobia, nausea (C), vomiting (D), and cutaneous allodynia (when innocuous stimulation of normal skin is perceived as painful). Diarrhea (E) is not typically associated with migrainous symptoms.

2. The answer is C (1.1.4)

Evidence suggests that triptans are most effective in treating acute migraine attacks when given at the start of the headache (C), when the pain is still perceived as mild; therefore, choices B, D, and E are incorrect. Additionally, it appears that larger single doses of triptans are more effective than smaller, divided doses given over time. Currently, triptans are not indicated for migraine prophylaxis, so choice A is false.

3. The answer is E (2.2.2)

Triptans are currently available as injectables, nasal inhalations, oral tablets, and rapidly disintegrating oral tablets. The wide variety of dosage forms allows patients to have more flexibility when treating an acute migraine. All triptans are available as oral tablets. Sumatriptan is also available as a subcutaneous solution and nasal inhalation, making choice A incorrect. Both naratriptan and almotriptan are only available as oral tablets, so choices B and D are incorrect. Rizatriptan is also available as a rapidly disintegrating oral tablet, not as a subcutaneous injection (C). Zolmitriptan is available as a nasal inhalation (E) and rapidly disintegrating oral tablet.

4. The answer is E (1.2.2)

Triptans are serotonin 5-HT 1B/1D receptor agonists (E). It is believed that these agents work by vasoconstriction of cerebral arteries and reduction in neural inflammation associated with migraines. Therefore, choices A, B, C, and D are incorrect.

5. The answer is E (1.3.3)

Rhinitis (A) has been reported with Migranal (dihydroergotamine nasal spray) in up to 26% of patients. Other adverse effects include taste disturbances, GI effects (nausea, vomiting, and diarrhea [B]), dizziness (D), rash (C), and vasospasm to a lesser degree. Dihydroergotamine has been reported to elevate blood pressure significantly in patients with and without a history of hypertension so hypotension (E) is unlikely.

6. The answer is B (3.2.3)

Melatonin is also commonly used to treat circadian rhythm disorders (B). Because there is some evidence that cluster headaches are circadian in nature, it is postulated that melatonin would help regulate and prevent the development of cluster headaches. The recommended dose of melatonin for prophy-laxis of cluster headaches is 10 mg orally at bedtime. Melatonin is not commonly used for liver toxicity or depression, so choices A, C, D, and E are incorrect.

7. The answer is A (1.1.4)

Beta blockers have proven to be effective for prophylaxis against migraine headaches. Propranolol, timolol, atenolol (A), and metoprolol are commonly used for migraine prophylaxis. To date, only propranolol and timolol have received FDA approval for this indication. These agents may take a few weeks before becoming effective in prevention of migraine, so it is recommended that the trial period last at least 3 months before determining failure of therapy. Calcium carbonate (B), dexamethasone (C), and vitamin E (E) have not been shown to be effective prophylactic therapies. Use of opioids (D) for migraine prophylaxis is not recommended due to the risk of dependency with long-term use and therefore is not considered first-line for migraine prophylaxis.

8. The answer is C (3.2.2)

In addition to medication, there are numerous nonpharmacologic approaches that can assist in the prevention of migraines. Limiting caffeine intake is helpful to minimize headache occurrence; however abrupt withdrawal from chronic caffeine consumption (C) may result in caffeine-withdrawal headaches in CG who drinks 4-5 cups of coffee daily and would be the least appropriate recommendation. Caffeine intake should be reduced gradually. Other patient counseling points may include recommendations on avoiding alcohol (A), smoking cessation (B), keeping a diary to track migraine patterns (D), avoiding large amounts of monosodium glutamate (MSG) (E), and using of relaxation techniques. Each patient has individual triggers, so the patient should be encouraged to identify potential triggers and avoid them if possible. Other triggers can include menstruation, use of oral contraceptives, and changes in altitude/weather.

9. The answer is C (2.2.1)

The trade names of sumatriptan include Imitrex (C), Sumavel, and Alsuma. The other choices are incorrect because Amerge (A) is the trade name for naratriptan, Axert (B) is the trade name for almotriptan, Maxalt (D) is the trade name for rizatriptan, and Migranal (E) is the trade name for dihydroergotamine.

10. The answer is C (1.2.4)

Dihydroergotamine (C) is FDA pregnancy category X. It should not be administered during pregnancy due to its oxytocic and uterine-stimulating effects. Aspirin (A) is pregnancy category C during the first and second trimesters and is contraindicated during the third trimester. Butorphanol (B), Midrin (D), and Naratriptan (E) are pregnancy category C.

Answers

Case 40 Pain Management

1. The answer is C (1.1.0)

The use of morphine patient-controlled analgesia (PCA), choice C, is the most appropriate of all choices. The fentanyl patch should not be used as initial therapy for acute surgical pain in opioid-naïve patients (B). The intramuscular route of administration results in erratic and unpredictable absorption of pain medications. Additionally, the onset of pain relief is slower compared to the IV route, resulting in variable effects of analgesia, so choice A is not the most appropriate choice. This patient is expected to be in pain for the majority of a 24-hour period due to his recent surgery; therefore, around-the-clock analgesia is more appropriate compared to intermittent pain coverage. Meperidine (E) is not a good option for TS due to his kidney disease. The acetaminophen daily dose in the Darvocet dosing regimen exceeds recommended daily dose, so choice D is not appropriate.

2. The answer is E (1.2.6)

Choice A is incorrect because no correlation exists between a patient's body weight and dosage requirements. Likewise, no maximum dose of morphine exists, so choice B is also incorrect. The effective treatment dose with morphine must be balanced with presence of adverse effects. The correct answer is choice E. Drug allergies should always be considered prior to initiating any drug therapy and PCA morphine parameters must be specified prior to initiating PCA use.

3. The answer is A (1.2.0)

Because of TS' kidney disease, meperidine (A) is not a good option due to the accumulation of its active neurotoxic metabolite in patients with renal dysfunction. All other options are reasonable and may be tried for TS' pain. Tramadol's opioid and non-opioid mechanisms of action are effective in treating pain (B). Although morphine may cause nausea and vomiting, these are expected and transient side effects, so choice C is still an acceptable treatment option. Acetaminophen is often used as an adjunct in opioid therapy, so choice E is also an acceptable option.

4. The answer is C (1.2.6)

Typical conversion of IV to oral morphine is 1:3. Thus, 60 mg IV morphine is approximately equal to 180 mg oral morphine, Dilaudid (45 mg PO or 9 mg IV). Doses for choices A, D, and E are too low. The dose for choice B is too high.

5. The answer is E (2.2.1)

All choices are available as sustained tablets (of the same opioid as the listed regimen) in which the total dose may be given once or twice daily. Regimen I equals 60 mg of morphine daily, regimen II equals 20 mg oxycodone daily, and regimen III equals 120 mg of morphine daily. Morphine is available as 60 mg and 120 mg sustained-release tablets and oxycodone is available as a 20 mg sustained-release tablet.

6. The answer is A (3.2.2)

Choice C is incorrect because promethazine will help with nausea associated with opioid use, but has not been shown to enhance analgesia. Acetaminophen may be used in conjunction with opioid analgesics as long as the maximum daily dose is not exceeded (B). Increased risk of severe adverse effects may result if doses are doubled; therefore, it should not be done by the patient at home (D). Choice E is incorrect because sustained-release pain medications should be taken around-the-clock and not as prn basis. The correct answer is choice A; constipation is a side effect of opioid analgesic for which many people do not develop tolerance; therefore, laxatives are often needed.

7. The answer is C (1.2.2)

The correct answer is choice C because opioid receptors, located both in the brain and spinal cord, are responsible for analgesia. Opioid effect on the GI tract is responsible for the adverse effects of opioids, not for analgesia; therefore, choices B and E are incorrect.

8. The answer is A (2.1.1)

Calculation: 0.6 mL x 50 mg/mL = 30 mg of morphine. A total volume of the morphine and normal saline was prepared (30 mg/30 mL), so the final concentration is 1 mg/mL.

9. The answer is E (3.2.2)

The correct answer is choice E; when acute pain patients were evaluated for their risk of addiction when using opioid analgesics for treatment of their pain, the risk is very low (<1%). Choices A, B, C, and D are incorrect.

10. The answer is C (1.1.3)

A physical exam and proper evaluation of the patient's monitoring parameters should be first completed prior to continuing with all other options, so choice C is correct. Administering naloxone reverses analgesia and should be given only if respiratory depression occurs (B). Choices A, D, E should be considered only after proper assessment of the situation has been done and only when additional therapies are warranted.

Case 41 Parkinson's Disease

1. The answer is C (3.2.0)

As a class, the dopamine agonists share similar side effects, with nausea and drowsiness being very common and should be discussed with the patient. Therefore, choice C is correct. If patients experience nausea, administration with food may help. Other side effects include confusion, constipation, edema, orthostatic hypotension, visual hallucinations, and psychosis. Iron preparations do not interact with dopamine agonists. However, iron preparations can bind to other antiparkinson medications, such as carbidopa/levodopa and COMT inhibitors (e.g., entacapone).

2. The answer is E (1.2.4)

This patient has a history of benign prostatic hypertrophy (BPH), causing bladder outlet obstruction. Acute complete urinary retention may be precipitated by anticholinergic medications (e.g., benztropine, trihexyphenidyl). Therefore, the use of trihexyphenidyl (E) should be avoided or used with caution. The dopamine agonists pramipexole (A) and ropinirole (C), as well as the monoamine oxidase type B inhibitors, rasagiline (B), and selegiline (D) will not exacerbate BPH.

3. The answer is E (1.2.0)

General dosing for entacapone is 200 mg administered with each dose of carbidopa/levodopa (standard release or sustained release) up to a total of 1600 mg/d (or eight doses). This is also referred to as flexible dosing. Therefore, if the carbidopa/levodopa is changed to 5 times per day, the entacapone administration should also be changed similarly to 5 times per day. Therefore, choice E is correct; and choices A, B, C, and D are incorrect. Another COMT inhibitor, tolcapone (Tasmar), is administered on a fixed dosing interval of 100 mg or 200 mg tid at 6-hour intervals, with the first dose taken with the first daily dose of carbidopa/levodopa. However, tolcapone has been associated with liver impairment and is not routinely prescribed.

4. The answer is C (3.2.1)

In Parkinson's disease, the development of hallucinations or delusions is commonly drug-induced and is associated with antiparkinson agents. Therefore, adding or increasing the dose of any antiparkinson drug will make the hallucinations and delusion worse. Therefore, choices A, B, D, and E are incorrect. The most appropriate option is to reduce the pramipexole dose (C) until symptoms are improved or resolved. When the dose is reduced, MF may experience a significant worsening of the parkinsonism symptoms; however, a slight worsening is acceptable to most caregivers and patients if the hallucinations/delusions are significantly eliminated.

5. The answer is E (1.1.3)

The primary concern associated with administering antipsychotic agents to patients with Parkinson's disease is the risk of significantly worsening the parkinsonism. Traditional antipsychotic agents such as haloperidol and phenothiazine agents (e.g., chlorpromazine) will block striatal dopamine receptors and have significant potential to worsen pre-existing parkinsonism; therefore choices B and D are incorrect. Of all antipsychotic agents, clozapine and quetiapine are least likely to worsen parkinsonism. Therefore, choice E is the correct answer. Amitriptyline (A) and citalopram (C) are incorrect because these drugs are antidepressants and are not effective for managing hallucinations/psychosis in Parkinson's disease.

6. The answer is A (1.2.6)

Approximately 90% of pramipexole is excreted unchanged in the urine. Therefore, renal function impairment (A) will in-crease plasma pramipexole concentrations. Pramipexole dosage adjustments may be required to avoid excessive plasma accumulation and associated toxicities. The enzyme dopa decarboxylase is responsible for metabolizing levodopa but has no activity on pramipexole or the other dopamine agonists; therefore choice C is incorrect. Inhibition of cathechol-O-methyltransferase or monoamine oxidase does not affect pramipexole pharmacokinetics; therefore choices D and E are incorrect.

7. The answer is C (1.2.4)

Administration of COMT inhibitors, entacapone and tolcapone, is commonly associated with an intensification of urine color (dark yellow or amber); therefore choice C is correct. The discoloration is the result of urinary excretion of entacapone/tolcapone metabolites. Although the condition is benign, it can result in discoloration of undergarments and bedding, especially in patients with urinary incontinence. When dispensing COMT inhibitors, it is appropriate to affix an auxiliary prescription label that reminds the patient of the potential occurrence of urine discoloration. Urine discoloration (dark amber or brown) may also occur with levodopa due to the urinary excretion of oxidized levodopa and metabolites; but this is uncommon and choice B is incorrect. Choices A, D, and E are incorrect because urine discoloration is not a side effect of anticholinergics (benztropine, trihexyphenidyl), dopamine agonists (pramipexole, ropinirole), or monoamine oxidase type B inhibitors (rasagiline, selegiline).

8. The answer is A (3.2.1)

The correct answer is choice A because each Stalevo tablet already contains entacapone 200 mg, and it would be inappropriate to administer Comtan (entacapone) concurrently. Choices B, C, D, and E are all true statements. Stalevo is a branded product formulation that contains three drugs (carbidopa, levodopa, entacapone) in one tablet. Carbidopa inhibits dopa decarboxylase and entacapone inhibits catechol-O-methyltransferase (COMT). Dopa decarboxylase and COMT are the major enzymes involved in the metabolism of levodopa. Inhibition of both these enzymes extends the half-life of levodopa and results in an extended duration of levodopa activity. Stalevo is used to manage wearing off or end of dose failure. Each Stalevo tablet contains a 1:4 ratio of carbidopa/levodopa + 200 mg of entacapone. Five dosages are available: 12.5/50/200, 18.75/75/200, 25/100/200, 31.25/125/200, and 37.5/150/200. The first number is the dose (mg) of carbidopa, the second of levodopa, and the third of entacapone. The maximum single dose of entacapone is 200 mg and, therefore, only one Stalevo tablet should be administered at each dosing interval. The maximum total daily dose of Stalevo is eight tablets (up to 1600 mg entacapone per day). MF is currently on carbidopa/levodopa 25/100 mg po QID and entacapone 200 mg po QID. If desired, he may be switched to Stalevo 25/100/200 po QID for convenience.

Answers

9. The answer is A (3.2.1)

Levodopa-induced dyskinesias are abnormal, involuntary, choreiform or writhing-like movements that can affect the upper and lower extremities, trunk, neck, and jaw. The most common type of dyskinesias occurs 30 to 60 minutes after a dose of carbidopa/levodopa and is associated with peak levels of levodopa (B). An enhancement of levodopa or dopaminergic activity can exacerbate dyskinesias (A). Management of levodopa peak-dose dyskinesias may consist of reducing the dose levodopa and/or other dopaminergic agents or a trial of amantadine, which has antidyskinesia effects (C). Adding an anticholinergic agent is ineffective (D). It is important to understand that abnormal rigidity or dystonia induced by dopamine receptor blockers (e.g., phenothiazine-induced dystonia) is responsive to anticholinergic agents (e.g., benztropine, diphenhydramine) and that this condition is distinct from levodopa-induced dyskinesias. Choice E is incorrect because addition of an atypical antipsychotic in a patient with Parkinson's disease is usually intended to manage hallucinations or psychosis.

10. The answer is A (1.3.2)

Citalopram is not contraindicated with any of the patient's current medications. Although the concurrent use of selective serotonin reuptake inhibitors (SSRIs) with rasagiline or selegiline is associated with a risk of serotonin syndrome as per the package labeling, this drug combination is not contraindicated and the combination is frequently used; therefore choice A is correct. Nonselective monoamine oxidase inhibitors (e.g., phenelzine, tranylcypromine) are contraindicated with carbidopa/levodopa and rasagiline/selegiline due to risk of hypertensive crisis. Amitriptyline possesses potent anticholinergic properties that can worsen MF's symptoms of benign prostatic hypertrophy and is therefore a poor antidepressant choice.

Case 42 Neonatal Therapy, Seizure Disorder

1. The answer is E (1.2.7)

Carbamazepine has a chew tablet, extended-release capsule, extended-release tablet, and suspension. The suspension must be shaken well and administered three to four times a day to ensure stable concentrations (B). The extended-release capsule may be swallowed whole or opened and placed on a small amount of applesauce for the patient to swallow, not chew (C). The patient should drink fluids after administration to make sure the mixture is completely swallowed. The extended-release tablet should be swallowed whole and not chewed or broken (A). It may be administered twice a day (D).

2. The answer is D (3.1.1)

FDA's Orange Book (D) would be the appropriate answer is it provides lists of approved generic versions of brand medication. It is titled: "Orange Book: Approved Drug Products

with Therapeutic Equivalence Evaluations" and is available free on the FDA's website for searching. The Drug Information Handbook (B) and AHFS (C) are general drug information resources. The Neofax (E) is a drug resource that provides dosing information for neonates specifically. The package insert (A) does not provide generic equivalency information.

3. The answer is A (2.1.1)

The nurse has the 4 mg/mL vial. Therefore, she should administer 0.5 mL to the patient to provide a dose of 2 mg. If the nurse had the 2 mg/mL vial, she could administer 1 mL to the patient. The other choices are incorrect.

4. The answer is D (1.2.6)

The half-life of carbamazepine during therapy initiation or after single doses is approximately 21-28 hours. As carbamazepine is an autoinducer, the half-life decreases dramatically to an average of 15 hours. Carbamazepine levels should be obtained 21-28 days after initiation.

5. The answer is C (1.3.3)

Carbamazepine is not associated with an increase in kidney stone formation (C). Topiramate and zonisamide are the two anticonvulsants with this adverse effect. Carbamazepine may cause a rash during therapy (A). A patient should stop the medication and call the physician immediately. Dizziness and drowsiness may occur at drug initiation and dose escalations (B). This usually resolves after continued therapy. Other adverse effects of carbamazepine include leukopenia, thrombocytopenia, and anemia. Hyponatremia may also be seen but this usually occurs more often in the elderly. Carbamazepine may be taken with food if needed (D). Due to concerns with drug interactions, he should notify his neurologist and pharmacist if he starts any other medication (E).

6. The answer is B (1.2.6)

The therapeutic concentration range for carbamazepine is 4-12 mcg/mL. Phenytoin's therapeutic range is 10-20 mcg/mL. Phenobarbital's therapeutic range is 10-40 mcg/mL. Therapeutic concentrations have not been well defined for the newer generation anticonvulsants as clinical outcome has not shown to correlate with specific concentration ranges.

7. The answer is D (1.1.3)

SB would be displaying signs of absence seizures (D), which are characteristic of staring or trance like state spells. Complex partial seizures (A) are seizures with one side of the body involved but there is a loss of consciousness. Simple partial seizures (B) involve one side of the body but no loss of consciousness. Myoclonic seizures (D) are characterized with sudden muscle jerks and atonic seizures (E) are called "drop attacks" with a fall due to loss of muscle tone.

8. The answer is E (1.1.1)

As SB has a sulfa allergy, he should not be prescribed

zonisamide (E). Zonisamide is structurally related to the sulfonamides. Lamotrigine (A) and topiramate (B) may be used as an adjunct therapy. Phenytoin (C) and valproic acid (D) may be used as monotherapy for generalized tonic-clonic seizures.

9. The answer is B (3.2.1)

Vitamin D (B) and calcium should be supplemented in patients on anticonvulsants, especially growing children to help prevent bone loss. Bone mineral density decreases have been seen in patients on carbamazepine, phenobarbital, phenytoin, and valproic acid. It is postulated that anticonvulsants may increase the catabolism of vitamin D, impair bone resorption and formation, and impair calcium absorption. Vitamin C (A), B (C, D), and E (E) may be supplemented in SB but he is not at risk for these deficiencies because of anticonvulsant therapy.

10. The answer is D (1.3.1)

The American Academy of Neurology has guidelines for discontinuing anticonvulsants in seizure-free patients. They recommend that discontinuation may be considered if the patient has been seizure free for 2-5 years (A), has a single seizure type (C), has a normal neurologic exam and IQ (E), and the EEG normalized (B) while on treatment. There is no reference regarding dose of medication for a specified time for discontinuing an anticonvulsant (D).

Case 43 Skin Cancers & Melanomas, Bone Marrow Transplantation

1. The answer is A (1.2.1)

Filgrastim stimulates production and proliferation of myeloid white blood cells (A). Darbepoetin stimulates production of red blood cells (B) and oprelvekin stimulates platelet production (C). Rituximab and vancomycin do not have stimulatory effects upon blood cell production (D, E).

2. The answer is A (1.1.3)

The definition of neutropenic fever is any fever >38.3°C or sustained fever of 38.1°C for at least an hour in the setting of white blood cell count <0.5 k/µL (A). Both the melphalan and acyclovir were initiated over 7 days earlier, decreasing the likelihood of a drug reaction from those agents (B, E). The total white blood cell count is still too low to cause an engraftment fever (D). Febrile seizures are seizures resulting from fevers, which generally occurs in young children. The situation in this question is not seizures arising from fevers (C).

3. The answer is C (2.1.1)

Step 1: Determine body surface area (BSA) of patient. BSA = sq rt ((ht [cm] x wt [kg])/3600). This gives an answer of: sq rt (182.8 cm x 80.9 kg)/3600 ! sq rt (4.11) = 2.02 m².
Step 2: The correct interpretation of this order is "100 mg/m²

IV every 24 hours on days -3 and -2 for total of 2 doses." Therefore, dose is 200 mg IV once daily on days -3 and -2 (C). Melphalan is never given twice daily (A, E). Answers B and D are not correct due to the mathematic calculation of daily dose.

4. The answer is E (1.2.1)

High-dose melphalan has a moderate-high emetic risk. Proper pre-medication requires serotonin antagonist, dexamethasone, and benzodiazepine (E). Prochlorperazine and haloperidol are both dopamine antagonists and not used concurrently (A). Diphenhydramine and ranitidine are not needed as melphalan does not release histamine or cause allergic reaction and neither have a role in decreasing nausea and vomiting (B). Prednisone can be used as antiemetic pre-medication in rare cases, but does not have potency of dexamethasone and requires higher dose for anti-emetic indication (C). Due to emetogenic potency, serotonin antagonist is required (D).

5. The answer is E (1.2.1)

Due to extremely low white blood cell counts, patients with neutropenic fevers need broad spectrum antibacterial coverage, which is provided with cefepime, a fourth-generation cephalosporin, and vancomycin (E). As such, ceftriaxone provides too narrow of coverage (A). Gentamicin may be considered, but only as addition to another broad-spectrum antibacterial, which dicloxacillin is not (B). The addition of cefazolin adds little to bacterial coverage, since most susceptible gram-positive organisms covered by cefazolin will be covered by levofloxacin that was started on day -2 (C). Antifungal therapy is only considered after several days of broad-spectrum antibacterial therapy with no abatement of fevers (D).

6. The answer is B (2.2.5)

Melphalan must be delivered to floor and infused completely within 1 hour of reconstitution (B). All other medications have longer stability.

7. The answer is D (1.2.1)

Palifermin is a keratinocyte growth factor that helps build the epithelium thereby mitigating mucositis commonly seen with high-dose melphalan. Palifermin must be initiated prior to chemotherapy (D). Viscous lidocaine simply treats the pain of mucositis and does not reduce incidence or duration (A). Becaplermin is topical indicated for diabetic foot ulcers (B). Mesna and dexamethasone have no role in mucositis (C, E).

8. The answer is C (3.2.1)

High-dose melphalan causes some degree of mucositis in virtually all patients (C). Rash may occur, but rarely (A). Hemorrhagic cystitis, constipation, and tinnitus are not associated with melphalan (B, D, E).

9. The answer is E (3.2.1)

Bone pain is thought to occur due to increased bone marrow activity and release of cytokines within bone marrow space.

Answers

This process irritates periosteum to cause pain. Elevation of any body part will have no effect (A). Same is true of cold compresses (B). Lidocaine patches are not effective due to extent of bone pain and inability to reach site of action (C). Diphenhydramine has minimal effect (D). Oxycodone is the most effective therapy for bone pain (E).

10. The answer is B (1.2.4)

Depressive symptoms may last long after stem cell transplantation procedure and he should continue and be reevaluated after recovery of blood counts at least (A). Zolpidem has no effect upon antiemetic activity (C). Terazosin has no interaction with melphalan (E). Acetaminophen should be discontinued because of potential to mask fevers—an important early warning sign of infection—rather than the effect of transplantation procedure on joint damage (B, D).

1. Rajkumar SV, Jacobus S, Callander NS, et al. Lenalidomide plus high-dose dexamethasone versus lenalidomide plus low-dose dexamethasone as initial therapy for newly diagnosed multiple myeloma: an open-label randomized controlled trial. *Lancet.* 2010; 11:29 – 37.

2. Antiemesis. NCCN Clinical Practice Guidelines in Oncology. V.2.2010. www.nccn.org (accessed 2010 Jul 3).

Case 44 Breast Cancer

1. The answer is D (1.2.6)

Anastrozole is the most appropriate choice. Since the patient has already received tamoxifen (A) and she is post-menopausal, the aromatase inhibitors would be the most appropriate treatment option. Aromatase inhibitors are indicated to treat advanced disease following progression on tamoxifen therapy. Faslodex is an anti-estrogen used for treatment in postmenopausal women with disease progression following antiestrogen therapy (B). Zoladex is a LHRH agonist used for palliative treatment of breast cancer (C). Megestrol Acetate is a progestin used as a third-line agent for palliative hormonal treatment (E). These three hormonal therapy options would not be first-line treatment agents.

2. The answer is C (1.2.1)

Zometa and Aredia are both bisphosphonates indicated for treatment of bone metastasis. Fosamax is only indicated for treatment of osteoporosis and Paget's disease.

3. The answer is E (1.3.3)

Ototoxicity (E) is not an adverse effect of Zometa therapy. All other symptoms listed are adverse effects of Zometa. While patients are on Zometa therapy, renal toxicity (B) is a common adverse effect that could occur. It is recommended that patients have a serum creatinine assessed prior to each treatment. Treatment should be withheld for renal deterioration (increase of 0.5 mg/dL in patients with normal baseline creatinine or an increase of 1 mg/dL in patients with abnormal baseline creati-

nine) and should be resumed only when creatinine returns to within 10% of baseline. Osteonecrosis of the jaw (C) can also occur in patient taking Zometa. Patients should have a dental examination with appropriate preventative dentistry prior to treatment with bisphosphonates. Finally, hypomagnesemia and hypophosphatemia (D) can occur shortly after administration of an IV bisphosphonate. Labs should be monitored closely.

4. The answer is C (3.2.2)

Bisphosphonates work to prevent osteoporosis by reducing bone resorption via inhibition of osteoclast activity. Elemental calcium and vitamin D supplementation are recommended when initiating bisphosphonate therapy (C). While Centrum Silver may contain calcium and vitamin D, the amounts are low and the other elements in the tablet have no relationship to bisphosphonate activity (A). Aspirin does not augment bisphosphonate therapy (D). Vitamin D (B) or calcium (E) alone would be less desirable than the two agents combined.

5. The answer is C (2.1.1)

Herceptin's FDA-approved dosage is 4 mg/kg loading dose the first week over 90 minutes. Subsequent maintenance doses of 2 mg/kg weekly are administered over 30 minutes. The maintenance dose of 2 mg/kg given every 3 weeks is incorrect. Giving a weekly maintenance dose of 2 mg/kg without first loading the patient with 4 mg/kg is also incorrect. An alternate dosing regimen commonly used for patients on Herceptin is 8 mg/kg loading dose the first week over 90 minutes with a maintenance dose of 6 mg/kg over 90 minutes every 3 weeks. However, this was not an option. The choice to give a loading dose of 8 mg/kg every 3 weeks (A) is incorrect as is the option to give a maintenance dose of 6 mg/kg weekly (B). Answer D is incorrect as it gives the weekly maintenance (2 mg/kg) dose every 3 weeks and E is incorrect for giving the 4 mg/kg loading dose every week.

6. The answer is C (1.2.4)

Because of the cardiac complications associated with Herceptin, patients with class III heart failure would not be good candidates for this treatment. The tumor must be Her2/neu positive to benefit from trastuzumab therapy (A). Herceptin targets the tumor cells that overexpress the Her2/neu protein. It is indicated for treatment in combination with Taxol or as a single agent in treatment of metastatic breast cancer (B). It can also be used as adjuvant treatment in Her2/neu overexpressing node-positive patients (D). Renal failure has no bearing on the use of Herceptin for treatment of breast cancer (E).

7. The answer is A (3.2.1)

Patients should contact clinic immediately if they have diarrhea or nausea and vomiting not responsive to antiemetics (A). All of the other answers are appropriate neutropenia precautions patients should take to avoid infection. Patients should also engage in frequent hand-washing as should all people who come into contact with them.

8. The answer is D (1.3.5)

NSAIDs and corticosteroids both have analgesic activity in the treatment of cancer-related bone pain. Neurontin is an anticonvulsant that is efficacious in treating neuropathic pain, not bone pain, making selections with III in them incorrect.

9. The answer is B (1.3.3)

Urinary retention is a common problem that can be treated. The patient does not have to discontinue opioids if they develop urinary retention.

All of the other answers are valid counseling points to use when a patient is beginning an opioid regimen.

10. The answer is C (1.2.1)

Cytarabine is a chemotherapy agent used in the hematological setting for the treatment of AML, ALL, CML, or in salvage regimens for NHL. It is not used to treat breast cancer. Taxol, Gemzar, Taxotere, and Xeloda would all be viable chemotherapy options for treatment of metastatic breast cancer (A, B, D, E).

Case 45 Lung Cancer

1. The answer is C (2.1.1)

The patient's BSA is 1.88 m ^{2} and the dose of cisplatin is 75 mg/m ^{2}. Therefore, the calculation of the dose EA should receive is 1.88 m ^{2} x 75 mg/m ^{2} = 141 mg.

2. The answer is C (2.1.4)

The final concentration of etoposide should not exceed 0.4 mg/mL to maintain stability for 48 hours (C). A final concentration of 0.6 mg/mL may also be prepared; however, stability is shortened to 8 hours (B). A concentration of 0.2 mg/mL is stable for 96 hours however per USP 797 guidelines would present an unacceptable risk to the patient for becoming contaminated (D). In addition, at final concentrations greater than 0.4 mg/mL, precipitation may occur. The dose of etoposide EA will receive is 188 mg. Therefore, the calculation of the volume of normal saline needed is (188 mg/0.4 mg/mL) = 470 mL. All other volumes result in concentrations too great or too small to meet stability criteria (A, E).

3. The answer is B (1.2.4)

Carboplatin is generally better tolerated than cisplatin and although substitution is fairly common its use has not been adequately studied, therefore it is not clear if a substitution leads to increased survival (A). Use of carboplatin does not decrease the number of cycles or allow for single agent use (C), as Etoposide in conjunction with either carboplatin or cisplatin is still a standard of treatment. Nausea/ vomiting, neurotoxicity, and ototoxicity are reduced compared to cisplatin (B). Myelosuppression is actually increased (D), especially thrombocytopenia rather than decreased.

4. The answer is C (1.3.3)

Etoposide is diluted in solubilizing agents that may contribute to hypotension (C), and thus limits the rate over which it can be safely administered. It is recommended that etoposide be infused over 30 minutes or longer. It is suggested that larger doses may be infused over a longer period of time to avoid fluid overload. Etoposide should not be given as a rapid intravenous infusion. Etoposide is not associated with abdominal cramps, cardiotoxicity, palmar-plantar erythrodysesthesia, or hemorrhagic cystitis, making the rest of these answers incorrect.

5. The answer is C (2.2.1)

Compazine is the brand name for prochlorperazine (C). Kytril is the brand name for granisetron (A); Zofran is the brand name for ondansetron (B); Phenergan is the brand name for promethazine (D); and Ativan is the brand name for lorazepam (E).

6. The answer is D (1.3.3)

Relaxation training, cognitive distraction, and counseling offering reassurance are all appropriate modalities to try to prevent emesis (D). Patients with nausea and vomiting should be counseled on eating small but frequent meals that have high nutritional content (C). Additionally, they should be advised to eat bland foods or stay with clear liquids. Cold items can be utilized to help prevent nausea and vomiting (B), while spicy foods should be avoided since they tend to aggravate nausea.

7. The answer is D (1.2.5)

Etoposide is cleared via renal and nonrenal processes, such as biliary excretion. In addition, it is highly protein bound, with 97% of the total drug bound to serum proteins (D). The disposition of etoposide is biphasic rather than triphasic (A, C, E). Answer B is incorrect because it only includes the fact that Etoposide is protein-bound, making it a less complete answer.

8. The answer is B (1.2.2)

Ondansetron works by competing for the binding sites of the serotonin receptors (B). Agents such as prochlorperazine, haloperidol, and promethazine act by competing for the binding sites of dopamine receptors (A). Diphenhydramine blocks histamine H_1 (C) and lorazepam facilitates the neurotransmitter gamma-aminobutyric acid (D). Alpha$_2$ receptors do not play a role in either stimulating or inducing emesis (E).

9. The answer is C (3.2.1)

Cisplatin is a potent renal tubular toxin. Sodium thiosulfate, an organic thiol donor, may diminish cisplatin-induced toxicity by donating a protective thiol group (A). However this agent has been used primarily as a rescue agent for high dose cisplatin given into the peritoneum (IP). Thus, unless a high-dose IP chemotherapeutic regimen is required, alternative strategies to lessen platinum-induced nephrotoxicity include ensuring adequate hydration (C), using lower doses of cisplatin, and/or switching to carboplatin. Leucovorin is a rescue medication used for methotrexate toxicity (B). Vitamin B_{12} is used

Answers

to treat pernicious anemia and vitamin B_{12} deficiencies (D). Pegfilgrastim stimulates the production neutrophils (E).

10. The answer is C (3.2.4)

Decreased rates of smoking over the last 30 years have lead to declines in mortality for both men and woman (C). Screening tools such as radiographic imaging are not recommended as they have not lead to enhanced survival (B). Three drug regimens have not been found to be superior compared to two drug regimens (A). Utilization of radiation have helped improve survival, but has not had the same impact on public health compared to smoking cessation (E). Surgical intervention is more a treatment of choice in non-small-cell lung cancer (D).

Case 46 Bacteremia & Sepsis

1. The answer is D (1.1.2)

Staphylococcus species account for approximately 50% of nosocomial bacteremia.

2. The answer is A (1.2.6)

Using this patient's IBW: Equation for Female: $[((140 - age) \times IBW \text{ in kg})/(72 \times SCr)] \times 0.85$
$((140 - 67)(54.7)(0.85))/((72)(1.2)) = 39$ mL/min.

3. The answer is A (3.2.1)

The CDC's Guidelines for the Prevention of Intravascular Catheter-Related Infections (*MMWR.* August 9, 2002) outlines many strategies for preventing IV catheter-related infections. Under the section on central venous catheters and catheter site care, the first recommendation is to designate one port exclusively for TPN if a multiport catheter is used (A). Choice B is incorrect as dressings should NOT be changed on tunneled or implanted catheters more than once a week until the insertion site has healed. Choice C is incorrect as pre-insertion prophylactic antibiotics are not recommended to be given routinely. Choice D is incorrect as CVC catheters are NOT routinely replaced. Choice E is incorrect as antibiotic lock solutions should only be used in special circumstances.

4. The answer is C (1.3.2)

A consensus statement from IDSA, ASHP, and SIDP, published in the January 1, 2009 AJHP (*Am J Health-Syst Pharm.* 2009; 66:82-98), recommend vancomycin dosing based on target serum trough levels no less than 10 μ/mL for less serious infections and 15-20 μ/mL for more serious infections such as bacteremia, osteomyelitis, meningitis, hospital-acquired pneumonia

5. The answer is C (3.2.1)

The 1995 CDC guidelines (CDC/HICPAC guidelines on vancomycin use. *MMWR.* 1995; 44:RR-12) do not recommend vancomycin as empiric therapy for the treatment of antibiotic-associated enterocolitis. Patients should first receive a course of treatment with metronidazole unless the colitis is severe and life threatening. The other choices all are appropriate recommendations for vancomycin use.

6. The answer is D (2.2.5)

All parenteral solutions should be inspected for particulate matter before final dispensing to the unit. Vancomycin should not be infused over less than 60 minutes to prevent infusion-related reactions. A label warning can help prevent too rapid an infusion.

7. The answer is C (1.3.3)

This type of reaction is not usually an allergic reaction, but a reaction related to the rate of infusion. The best advice is to slow down the rate of the infusion.

8. The answer is D (1.2.2)

Vancomycin is a glycopeptide antibiotic.

9. The answer is D (1.3.0)

Meperidine is metabolized to normeperidine, a metabolite that is renally eliminated and can cause CNS side effects, including seizure at high concentrations.

10. The answer is E (2.2.2)

There are both oral capsule and oral solution forms of vancomycin available. However, due to its poor absorption and very limited bioavailability outside the GI tract, it cannot be used to treat systemic infections. It's only use is in the treatment of *C. difficile* pseudomembranous colitis.

Case 47 Bone & Joint Infections

1. The answer is A (1.1.1)

Elevated C-reactive protein (CRP) (B) along with local tenderness (C) and erythema are all seen with osteomyelitis. In addition, patients will have fever (D), elevated ESR, and an elevated WBC count (E). Decreased platelets (A) are not consistent with osteomyelitis.

2. The answer is B (1.2.5)

The most important antibiotic parameter for effective treatment of osteomyelitis is that the antibiotic must penetrate the bone sufficiently in order to successfully eradicate the infecting bacteria.

3. The answer is C (1.1.3)

This patient probably developed osteomyelitis because he sustained a deep, open injury to his left lower leg, which was then contaminated by soil at the accident site. This allowed bacteria to easily gain entry into the bone. This is known as osteomyelitis due to a contiguous focus of infection, meaning the organism reached the bone from his infected wound site. JD's age (40 years) was not a risk factor for developing the osteomyelitis. As a point of interest, another less common way the bone can be infected is from the spread of bacteria through the bloodstream, known as hematogenous osteomyelitis. This occurs primarily in children and most commonly involves the long bones, such as the femur and tibia. Hematogenous osteomyelitis less commonly occurs in adults, with the exception of vertebral osteomyelitis, which occurs more frequently in older adults (over 50 years of age) and involves the vertebrae.

4. The answer is A (1.2.1)

The patient had an infection due to Pseudomonas aeruginosa, which is not covered by cephalexin therapy (A). The dose of cephalexin (B), patient compliance (C, D), or method of administration (E) is not an issue in this case. The important point is that the cephalexin does not treat the type of bacteria present in the wound drainage, thus making it ineffective in this patient.

5. The answer is C (1.3.2)

Initial aggressive treatment of pseudomonal osteomyelitis often includes combination therapy with an aminoglycoside plus a second agent active against Pseudomonas, such as piperacillin/tazobactam, ceftazidime, cefepime, or ciprofloxacin (A, D, E). An antipseudomonal beta-lactam antibiotic plus ciprofloxacin (B) have also been used to avoid the complications of aminoglycosides. Alternatively, monotherapy with an antipseudomonal beta-lactam or ciprofloxacin may also be appropriate, as long as the isolate is sensitive to the antibiotic and the patient's clinical response is monitored. If the patient is not responding to monotherapy, then a second agent may be added. The combination of cefazolin plus clindamycin (C), however, has no activity against Pseudomonas aeruginosa and would not be an appropriate regimen. For further information regarding the management of osteomyelitis, refer to: *Lancet.* 2004; 364:369-379.

6. The answer is D (1.3.1)

The appropriate duration of antibiotic therapy for the treatment of acute osteomyelitis is usually 4 to 6 weeks. Failure rates are greater when treated for shorter periods of time.

7. The answer is B (2.1.1)

Available product strengths of piperacillin/tazobactam include 2 g piperacillin/0.25 g tazobactam, 3 g piperacillin/0.375 g tazobactam, and 4 g piperacillin/0.5 g tazobactam. All are available as an 8:1 ratio of piperacillin to tazobactam. In order to compound 4 g of piperacillin and 0.5 g of tazobactam from the pharmacy bulk package, 20 mL of the solution containing 200 mg/mL of piperacillin and 25 mg/mL of tazobactam should be added to a compatible IV solution. Piperacillin: 4000 mg (or 4 g) / 200 mg/mL = 20 mL; Tazobactam: 500 mg (or 0.5 g) / 25 mg/mL = 20 mL.

8. The answer is E (3.2.1)

Based on the susceptibility report, the patient should be changed to the regimen of IV ceftazidime plus IV tobramycin (E). Combination therapy is often preferable initially for serious pseudomonal infections. However, there is some controversy regarding the value and necessity of combination therapy for Pseudomonas aeruginosa osteomyelitis, so single-drug therapy with an antipseudomonal beta-lactam antibiotic or ciprofloxacin may also be appropriate, as long as the isolate is sensitive to the antibiotic. Although oral moxifloxacin (C) has some antipseudomonal activity, ciprofloxacin traditionally has better coverage against this organism and is the preferred antipseudomonal fluoroquinolone in bone infections. Addition of oral rifampin to piperacillin/tazobactam (B) does not provide synergy against Pseudomonas, and discontinuing antibiotics (A) is not an option because they are needed to treat the infection. For further information regarding combination antibiotic therapy for Pseudomonas aeruginosa infections, refer to: *Lancet Infect Dis.* 2004; 4:519-527.

9. The answer is C (2.2.2)

Only ciprofloxacin (C) is available in an oral formulation. Therefore, the fluoroquinolones are the only class of antibiotics available orally for the treatment of Pseudomonas aeruginosa infections. Data that support the patient is improving clinically include that he is afebrile; clinical signs of inflammation (redness, pain, and purulent discharge) have resolved; and elevated laboratory parameters (WBC count, CRP, and ESR) are reduced or back to normal.

10. The answer is C (3.2.2)

Excessive alcohol consumption (e.g., JD's history of a six-pack of beer daily) may cause immune dysfunction and alter the capacity of the body to stave off infection. Compliance with outpatient oral antibiotic therapy is critical for successful treatment of acute osteomyelitis. Finally, the dietary supplement saw palmetto does not stimulate the immune system or promote wound healing but, rather, is used for benign prostatic hyperplasia. Another important point that the pharmacist should counsel JD is to avoid concomitant administration of dairy products, iron, calcium, multivitamins, or antacids with oral fluoroquinolone therapy as this may decrease absorption of ciprofloxacin. Additionally, excessive caffeine intake with ciprofloxacin may cause cardiac or CNS stimulation.

Case 48 Superficial Fungal Infections

1. The answer is B (1.1.0)

Candida albicans (B) accounts for 80%-90% of cases of vaginal candidiasis. The remainder of cases is caused by *Candida tropicalis* (C) and *Candida glabrata* (E). *Gardnerella vaginalis* (A) is a com-

Answers

mon cause of bacterial vaginosis. *Trichomonas vaginalis* (D), a protozoa, also is a cause of vaginosis.

2. The answer is E (1.1.4)

Risk factors for vaginal candidiasis include pregnancy, use of broad-spectrum antibiotics, use of high estrogen-containing oral contraceptives, corticosteroids or other agents that are immunosuppressive, an immunosuppressed host (for reasons other than medications), diabetes mellitus (especially if poorly controlled), sexual activity (especially with use of a diaphragm), and poor hygiene. Condom use is not associated with an increased risk of vaginal candidiasis.

3. The answer is A (1.2.0)

Over-the-counter products are recommended for individuals who have been previously diagnosed with vaginal candidiasis. Symptoms should be similar to past episodes as vaginal candidiasis may be mistaken for bacterial vaginosis or a sexually transmitted disease. A pregnant woman should be referred to her physician for treatment of vaginal candidiasis. Clotrimazole is classified as category B. Terconazole, butoconazole, miconazole, tioconazole, and fluconazole are classified as category C. The Centers for Disease Control and Prevention (CDC) Sexually Transmitted Diseases Guidelines 2006 recommends the use of topical azole therapy only for 7 days in pregnancy. Recurrent vaginal candidiasis may indicate a more serious problem that needs to be evaluated by a physician. Recurrences may be secondary to HIV, uncontrolled diabetes, immunosuppression, oral contraceptives, or hormone replacement therapy.

4. The answer is A (1.2.1)

Metronidazole is recommended for the treatment of bacterial vaginosis and vaginal trichomoniasis. It does not have activity against *Candida* spp. Butoconazole, terconazole, and clotrimazole are available as topical agents. Terconazole is available by prescription only. Topical nonprescription therapy is recommended for most patients as initial therapy. Fluconazole is available as an oral prescription only. See the CDC Sexually Transmitted Diseases Treatment Guidelines 2006.

5. The answer is D (2.2.1)

The active ingredient in Terazol 3 is terconazole. The brand names for clotrimazole are Gyne-Lotrimin, Mycelex, and Sweet'n'Fresh Clotrimazole. The brand names for nystatin are Mycostatin and Nystatin. The brand names for miconazole are Monistat, Femizol, and M-Zole. The brand name for butoconazole is Femstat.

6. The answer is C (1.2.0)

From clinical trials for acute vaginal candidiasis, it appears that both oral and topical therapies are equally efficacious. Fluconazole is approved for the treatment of vaginal candidiasis at a single dose of 150 mg. Fluconazole may improve patient compliance as the topical preparations are recommended to be used for 3-7 days (although single-dose therapy can be

used). Fluconazole is a generally more costly treatment option than the OTC topically administered products because a physician office visit is usually necessary to obtain a prescription.

7. The answer is B (1.2.3)

The systemic azole antifungal agents do not interact with hydrochlorothiazide as it is not metabolized via the cytochrome P450 (CYP450) system. Atorvastatin, phenytoin, warfarin, and cyclosporine all interact with the systemic azoles as they all have extensive CYP450 metabolism.

8. The answer is C (3.2.1)

Itraconazole capsules require an acidic environment and are best absorbed when taken with or immediately following a meal. Itraconazole suspension is best absorbed when given on an empty stomach. As absorption requires an acidic environment, the H_2 blockers, proton pump inhibitors, and antacids reduce the absorption of itraconazole capsules (the suspension is well absorbed regardless of gastric pH).

9. The answer is D (3.2.0)

LD should continue using the topical antifungal preparation even if menstruation begins. She needs to complete the entire course of therapy even if symptoms subside prior to completing therapy. Symptoms should improve within 48-72 hours and resolve within a week. If symptoms persist, she should contact her physician. It is important to advise LD that certain products are oil-based and may weaken latex condoms and diaphragms. If she uses latex condoms or a diaphragm for contraception, a nonoil-based product may be necessary.

10. The answer is A (1.1.3)

The vaginal discharge associated with vaginal candidiasis is nonodorous. A foul-smelling (fishy) vaginal discharge is often associated with bacterial vaginosis. Common signs and symptoms include itching, burning, irritation, dyspareunia (painful intercourse), non-odorous discharge that may be watery to thick, and erythema of the labia/vulva.

Case 49 Drug Resistance

1. The answer is D (1.2.2)

Since the primary resistance mechanism of MSSA is penicillinase production, addition of tazobactam, a ⬚lactamase inhibitor, to piperacillin will expand coverage to ⬚lactamase-producing bacteria. Choice B is incorrect because *Staphylococci* do not produce ESBLs. Choice C is incorrect because MRSA is resistant to all ⬚lactams and choice E is incorrect because VRE will not be covered due the addition of tazobactam.

2. The answer is A (1.2.2)

An oxacillin-susceptible, penicillin-resistant *S. aureus* isolate can be labeled as MSSA. Choice B is incorrect because *S. aureus* does not produce efflux pumps and choice E is incorrect because gram-positive organisms do not have an outer membrane. Choice C is the mechanism of resistance for MRSA.

3. The answer is B (1.2.2)

Choice A is the VRE mechanism of resistance. *Staphylococci* do not produce ESBLs and do not produce efflux pumps. An alteration of the 50S subunit only affects the activity of protein synthesis inhibitors. More than 50% of *S. aureus* isolates have an alteration in PBP2, which prevents ☐lactam antibiotics from binding to the site of action.

4. The answer is E (1.1.2)

MLS resistance is an inducible mechanism that emerges when the 50S ribosomal subunit of *S. aureus* is methylated (ermB). As a result of this alteration, antibiotics that bind to this subunit should be considered resistant. These antibiotics include **M**acrolides (e.g., erythromycin), **L**incosamides (e.g., clindamycin) and **S**treptogramins (e.g., quinupristin-dalfopristin) (MLS resistance). A D-test is routinely performed by microbiology labs to screen for MLS resistance.

5. The answer is E (1.2.6)

According to the 2009 ASHP/IDSA/SIDP Consensus Review on Therapeutic Drug Monitoring of Vancomycin, a loading dose of 25-30 mg/kg (based on actual body weight) can be used to facilitate rapid attainment of target troughs in seriously ill patients. In addition, doses of 15-20 mg/kg (based on actual body weight) given every 8-12 hours are recommended for most patients. Loading dose = 25 mg/kg x 102 kg = 2550 mg. Maintenance dose = 15 mg/kg x 102 kg = 1530 mg.

6. The answer is A (1.3.5)

According to the 2009 IDSA Clinical Practice Guidelines for the Management of Intravascular Catheter-Related Infections, vancomycin is the preferred agent despite the fact that CA-MRSA may be susceptible to drugs such as ciprofloxacin, clindamycin, and erythromycin. Choice C is incorrect because MRSA is resistant to piperacillin-tazobactam.

7. The answer is A (2.1.3)

The rate of infusion should be at least 500 mg/30 minutes or 16.7 mg/min. To convert mg/min to mL/min, 16.7 mg/min is divided by 5 mg/mL. The rate of infusion should be no faster than 3.3 mL/min.

8. The answer is E (2.1.1)

MR's current vancomycin dose of 1000 mg is divided by the max concentration of 5 mg/mL to give 200 mL. Thus, 1000 mg should be placed in at least 200 mL of D5W.

9. The answer is C (3.2.0)

A nasal swab with MRSA indicates colonization, not active infection. According to 2006 CDC Guidelines on the Management of Multidrug-Resistant Organisms in Healthcare Set-

tings, contact precautions should be implemented routinely for patients in acute care hospitals who are infected with MRSA and for those identified as having been colonized with MRSA. Routine use of topical mupirocin for MRSA decolonization is not recommended.

10. The answer is E (3.2.4)

According to the 2002 Guidelines for the Prevention of Intravascular Catheter-Related Infections, using a 2% chlorhexidine preparation for skin antisepsis is one of several strategies for preventing catheter-related infections. Catheters inserted in the internal jugular vein have been associated with a higher risk of infection compared to subclavian sites. Systemic vancomycin is an independent risk factor for acquiring VRE and has not been shown to reduce catheter-related infections in adults. Heparin reduces the rate of thrombosis and inline filters may reduce the rate of infusion-related phlebitis.

Case 50 Septic Shock

1. The answer is E (1.1.3)

The ACCP/SCCM consensus conference identified the need for a standard definition for sepsis and severe sepsis. This standardization of definition helps in evaluating future therapeutic strategies for managing patients with sepsis. Severe sepsis is defined as sepsis in the presence of organ dysfunction, hypoperfusion, or hypotension.

Dellinger RP, Carlet JM, Masur H et al. Surviving Sepsis Campaign guidelines for management of severe sepsis and septic shock. *Crit Care Med.* 2004; 32:858-73.

Institute for Healthcare Improvement.www.ihi.org and www.survivingsepsis.org (accessed 2010 Sept 13).

2. The answer is C (1.1.3)

Severe sepsis is a complex disease process that involves inflammation, coagulation, and impaired fibrinolysis. Bacterial endotoxin and exotoxins initiate an inflammatory process involving the release of TNF-alpha and interleukins in addition to other pro-inflammatory cytokines. The release of the inflammatory cytokines damages endothelial cells and causes a release of tissue factor. Tissue factor subsequently activates the clotting process, resulting in the production of thrombin and reduced levels of protein C. The production of thrombin causes a down regulation in the enzyme thrombomodulin, which is responsible for activation of protein C. Finally, inflammation causes an increase rather than a decrease in the production of PAI-1, which inactivates endogenous tissue plasminogen inhibitor, resulting in an impairment of fibrinolysis.

3. The answer is B (1.2.1)

Randomized controlled trials using moderate doses of corticosteroids (hydrocortisone 200 to 300 IVPB mg/day, for 7 days in three to four divided doses) have shown a reduction in mortality in patients' refractory to fluid replacement and vaso-

Answers

pressor therapy. This is true particularly in patients with relative adrenal insufficiency. As a result, the 2004 consensus conference recommends the use of corticosteroids in patients who remain in septic shock despite adequate fluid replacement and vasopressor therapy.

4. The answer is E (3.2.1)

The PROWESS trial was a randomized, double-blind, placebo-controlled trial that evaluated the use of recombinant human activated protein C, drotrecogin alfa, in the treatment of severe sepsis. Patients enrolled in the study had to have three or greater SIRS criteria and at least one organ dysfunction of no greater than 24-hour duration. Patients enrolled in the study were relatively sick as demonstrated by the fact that 75% had two or more organs that had failed at the time of enrollment. The results showed an absolute 6% reduction in mortality in the group that received drotrecogin alfa. When the results were stratified by the APACHE II scores at entry, only patients in the third and fourth quartile, those with APACHE II scores greater than 25, appeared to benefit. As a result, the FDA approved the use of the drug only in patients at high risk of death (i.e., APACHE II scores over 25). In addition, the FDA required that a study be completed to assess impact in patients at lower risk. The ADDRESS trial was initiated in response. It examined patients with severe sepsis at lower risk of death as defined by a single organ dysfunction and an APACHE II score of less than 25. The results showed no benefit in reduction of mortality with the use of drotrecogin alfa in these lower-risk patients.

5. The answer is E (1.2.2)

Drotrecogin alfa has been shown to have an effect on the inflammatory, coagulation, and impaired fibrinolysis process that occurs in severe sepsis. Its antiinflammatory properties are demonstrated by prevention of the release of TNF-alpha and interleukin-6 (A). Its anticoagulation properties are a result of the inactivation of factors Va and VIIIa, resulting in a reduction in the production of thrombin (B). Its actions on the fibrinolysis system (C) are a result of its inactivation of PAI-1 and prevention of activation of thrombin activatable fibrinolysis inhibitor (TAFI). Lastly, it inhibits leukocyte adhesion (D). Drotrecogin alfa, however, increases bleeding time, not decreases (E).

6. The answer is E (1.2.1)

While earlier trials of intensive glycemic control in critically ill patients demonstrated improvements in morbidity and mortality, more recent trials have demonstrated conflicting results. Despite these conflicting results, tight glucose control is often the goal in critically ill patients. The Normoglycemia in Intensive Care Evaluation Survival Using Glucose Algorithm Regulation (NICE-SUGAR) trial was designed to test the hypothesis that intensive glucose control improves 90-day mortality. This large, international, randomized trial reported that a blood glucose target of 180 mg or less per deciliter resulted in lower mortality than did a target of 81 to 108 per deciliter. Thus, for critically ill patients, the ADA recommends a goal glucose range of 140 to 180 mg/dL.

7. The answer is B (1.2.4)

The fact that JJ has severe sepsis significantly impacts the ability to effectively treat her myocardial infarction (A). She is not a candidate for undergoing a percutaneous coronary intervention (PCI) until her blood pressure stabilizes. In addition, implementation of beta blockers and ACE inhibitors need to be held until the blood pressure stabilizes (E). The drotrecogin alfa therapy also prevents concurrent administration of fibrinolytics (B, C). While not contraindicated, low-dose aspirin may increase the risk of bleeding if used concurrently with drotrecogin alfa (D).

8. The answer is B (1.2.1)

The rationale for using clindamycin in combination with beta-lactam antibiotics, such as penicillin, in streptococcal and staphylococcal toxic shock syndromes comes from laboratory evidence, suggesting the clindamycin may suppress the production of bacterial toxin production. Clindamycin is metabolized in the liver and does not need dosage adjustment in renal dysfunction.

9. The answer is D (2.2.1)

Zosyn is the trade name for piperacillin/tazobactam, a penicillin antibiotic. Cleocin is the trade name for clindamycin, a lincosamide antibiotic. Keppra is the name for levetiracetam, an anticonvulsant. Doribax is the name for doripenem, a carbapenem antibiotic.

10. The answer is A (3.1.2)

The NNT can be an effective way of displaying the absolute difference in a study. In a study which examines mortality as an outcome, it will tell you how many patients need to be treated with the study group compared to the control in order to save one life. In the PROWESS study, the NNT value of 16 tells you that for every 16 patients treated with drotrecogin alfa, one life is saved compared to treating these same patients with the placebo. The NNT can be calculated by dividing the absolute difference into one (A). In the case of the PROWESS trial, this can be displayed mathematically by the following equation: $1/0.06 = 16$. The NNT is different from the relative risk reduction. The relative risk reduction is the ratio between the decrease in risk in the treatment group and the risk in the control group. Using the PROWESS results as an example, the incidence of death was 30.8% in the placebo group and 24.7% in the drotrecogin alfa group. The relative risk reduction with drotrecogin alfa compared to placebo can be calculated by the following equation: $(30.8 - 24.7) / 30.8$. This amounts to an approximate 20% reduction in relative risk.

Case 51 STDs

1. The answer is A (1.2.1)

According to the 2006 treatment guidelines, penicillin IV remains the drug of choice for treatment of neurosyphilis. A penicillin-allergic patient will require penicillin desensitization.

2. The answer is D (1.3.5)

According to the 2006 CDC treatment guidelines, doxycycline 100 mg po bid or tetracycline 500 mg po bid for 14 days or azithromycin 2 g po x 1 are alternative treatments for primary syphilis in a patient with a penicillin allergy. Doxycycline 100 mg po bid x 7 days and azithromycin 1 g x 1 dose may treat chlamydia, but not syphilis. Tetracycline is dosed four times daily, rather than two times daily. Minocycline is not recommended for the treatment of syphilis.

3. The answer is A (2.2.1)

Bicillin L-A (I) contains penicillin G benzathine. Bicillin C-R (II) contains a mixture of penicillin G benzathine and penicillin G procaine, which would inadequately treat syphilis and thus is not recommended. Bicillin G (III) does not exist.

4. The answer is A (1.1.3)

A rash on the palms of the hands and soles of the feet (A) is a characteristic presentation of secondary syphilis. Meningitis (D) is characteristic of neurosyphilis. A penile chancre (E) is characteristic of primary syphilis. Gummas (C) are characteristic of tertiary syphilis. Mucopurulent discharge (B) is not a specific distinguishing feature of any stage of syphilis.

5. The answer is A (3.2.1)

The Jarisch-Herxheimer reaction occurs shortly after administration of an effective antibiotic, most frequently penicillin, in patients with spirochetal infections. The reaction is thought to be due to pyrogen release after spirochetal lysis. The infection is most frequently associated with initial treatment of syphilis but can occur in patients with other spirochetal infections, including leptospirosis, relapsing fever, and Lyme disease, or bacterial infections, including anthrax, tularemia, brucellosis, and rat-bite fever. The reaction is generally self-limiting, characterized by fever, headache, and myalgias, and is usually treated with NSAID therapy. Since the patient tolerated Augmentin (amoxicillin-clavulanate) well in the past, there is no allergic reaction to penicillin.

6. The answer is C (1.2.0)

According to the 2006 CDC treatment guidelines, pregnant patients with syphilis should receive a penicillin product for the treatment of syphilis at any stage. If the patient has a penicillin allergy, she should be desensitized.

7. The answer is B (1.1.3)

Genital HSV and primary syphilis are characterized by the presence of a lesion. However, genital HSV usually presents with multiple painful ulcers, while primary syphilis usually presents with a single, painless ulcer. Presentation of gonorrhea and chlamydia is characterized by discharge. The most common presentation of pelvic inflammatory disease is abdominal pain.

8. The answer is A (1.3.2)

Titers of nontreponemal tests (e.g., RPR) are monitored for efficacy for the treatment of syphilis. A four-fold reduction in RPR is a marker indicating efficacy of treatment. FTA-ABS is a treponemal test that is qualitative only and used to confirm the diagnosis of syphilis.

9. The answer is C (1.1.2)

By definition, latent syphilis is sero-reactivity without clinical evidence of disease. The RPR is a nontreponemal test and thus a screen. The FTA-ABS is a treponemal test and thus confirmatory for the diagnosis of syphilis.

10. The answer is E (3.2.0)

Sexually transmitted diseases are associated with all of these complications.

Case 52 Skin & Soft Tissue Infections

1. The answer is C (1.1.1)

Impetigo is caused by *Staphylococcus aureus* including methicillin-resistant strains or *Streptococcus pyogenes* (Group A *Streptococcus*). Bullous impetigo is generally associated with *S. aureus*, whereas the non-bullous form of the disease can be associated with either *Staphylococcus* or *Streptococcus*. *Propionibacterium acnes* is associated with the development of acne and not impetigo.

2. The answer is D (1.2.4)

The beta-lactamase stable penicillin dicloxacillin and the first-generation cephalosporin cephalexin are good choices for the treatment of impetigo, as is the topical antibiotic mupirocin. Erythromycin has also been used to treat impetigo; however, many strains of *Staphylococcus aureus* and *Streptococcus pyogenes* have recently become resistant. Though not listed as a possible answer, clindamycin retains activity against most macrolide-resistant strains and is an effective impetigo treatment. While levofloxacin possesses good activity against *Staphylococcus aureus* and *Streptococcus pyogenes*, the antibiotic has a relative contraindication for use in pediatric patients due to potential for arthropathy and possesses overly broad antimicrobial activity compared to the alternative answers. Impetigo caused by methicil-

Answers

lin-resistant *Staphylococcus aureus* can be problematic as these strains are increasingly resistant to many common impetigo treatments. Of the options listed, clindamycin and mupirocin are most likely to retain activity against MRSA.

3. The answer is C (1.2.1)

While all three of the antibiotics have been used to treat impetigo, DJ has a documented allergy to penicillin and should not receive dicloxacillin. There is a 3%-5% incidence of cross-reactivity between cephalosporins and penicillins, and DJ should not receive a cephalosporin without further confirmation of the type of allergic reaction. Cephalosporins should not be administered if DJ has a history of IGE-mediated hypersensitivity that might manifest as anaphylaxis, shortness of breath, hives, or urticaria. Both clindamycin and mupirocin would be good alternatives.

4. The answer is C (1.2.1)

Mupirocin has been shown to be an effective treatment for mild-to-moderate cases of impetigo where patients did not exhibit signs of systemic involvement. Mupirocin is less effective than oral alternatives in extensive cases. Because mupirocin is administered topically, it is associated with fewer adverse effects than systemically administered antibiotics. New lesions in the treated area should cease within 24 hours and existing lesions should heal within 5-7 days.

5. The answer is B (1.1.3)

The combination of vesicles with golden crusted lesions found in impetigo most resemble a herpes simplex infection. Acne generally is associated with hair follicles and comedones. Shingles may present with vesicles, but the lesions are usually expressed along the dermatosomes. Atopic dermatitis presents as erythematous papules or vesicles but generally is not associated with golden-crusted lesions. Erysipelas generally presents as bright-red, clearly demarcated lesions with raised margins.

6. The answer is A (1.3.1)

Topical therapy is the preferred first-line therapy for mild disease. Mupirocin and a newer topical antibiotic retapamulin are effective against MRSA; however, MRSA isolates are increasingly becoming resistant to mupirocin due to its widespread use for nasal decolonization of MRSA carriers. Adverse effects are generally less common with topical therapy that systemic therapy. Bacitracin-containing products tend to have lower response rates than alternative agents. Studies do not demonstrate superiority of either topical or systemic therapy in the clinical response in impetigo.

7. The answer is C (1.3.3)

Contact dermatitis is an adverse effect of Neosporin that can occur frequently (e"10%). The potential causative agent is neomycin. Dermatomycosis or superficial fungal infection is unlikely to occur with short-term application. Systemic absorption resulting in ototoxicity is also uncommon with short-term use unless large surface areas are treated. Diarrhea is unlikely for the same reason. Acne is not a side effect of Neosporin and in some cases is treated with topical antimicrobials.

8. The answer is B (3.2.1)

Generally impetigo lesions are painless and long-term skin changes or scarring are uncommon. As the prevention of impetigo is related to hygiene and exposure to pathogenic strains of *Streptococcus pyogenes*, reoccurrence of impetigo is common. A less common (1%-5%) but serious complication associated with streptococcal infections is post-streptococcal glomerular nephritis. Circulating bacterial-immune complexes are filtered and clog glomeruli, resulting in renal damage. This usually occurs several weeks after the infection, and antibiotics do not prevent this complication. Signs and symptoms include edema and facial swelling, decreased or bloody urination, and arthralgias. Rarely, systemic infectious complications can include sepsis, toxic shock syndrome, and sepsis.

9. The answer is E (3.2.1)

Impetigo is highly contagious, and all of the above may help prevent the spread of impetigo. DJ should not come into contact with other siblings or children until he has been on antibiotic therapy for at least 24 hours. His lesions should be washed with warm soapy water, which may lessen the pruritus while cleansing the infectious drainage. Covering the lesions may prevent scratching. Other household members should not come into contact with bed linens, washcloths, or towels that may contain infectious materials.

10. The answer is C (1.2.1)

Mupirocin possesses good activity against *Staphylococcus* and *Streptococcus* species, including MRSA, whereas it has little activity against other common skin flora such as *Propionibacterium*. Bacitracin also possesses good activity against *Staphylococcus* and *Streptococcus* species. Polymyxin has excellent gram-negative activity, including *Pseudomonas*, but possesses virtually no activity against gram-positive organisms. Retapamulin possesses excellent gram-positive activity including *Staphylococcus* and *Streptococcus* species and variable activity against gram-negative species, including some anaerobic organisms. Chlorhexidine has activity against both gram-positive and gram-negative organisms.

Case 53 Endocarditis

1. The answer is A (1.1.3)

Treatment of TB in patients with HIV infection follows the same general principles as treatment of non-HIV-infected patients. However, there are two major differences: (1) the increased risk of drug interactions, particularly when rifampin is used; and (2) paradoxical reactions that can be interpreted as clinical worsening. Nevertheless, the initial regimen should include isoniazid and rifampin, pyrazinamide, and ethambutol.

The regimen should contain four drugs prior to study results. Pyridoxine is not a TB medication.

2. The answer is B (1.3.2)

Do not use two drugs with the same mechanism of action (streptomycin and amikacin). Because the organism is resistant to rifampin, treatment with at least four agents will be required. Rifapentine and rifabutin are not active against rifampin-resistant strains. Several fluoroquinolones have significant antimycobacterial activities, including ciprofloxacin and moxifloxacin. Pyridoxine is not a TB medication.

3. The answer is D (1.3.1)

reatment of organisms with resistance to rifampin requires extended treatment period. Six months is the time period for treatment of nonresistant TB (short-course). TB does not require lifelong therapy. Current treatment guidelines recommend treating a rifampin-resistant strain of TB for 12-18 months of continuous therapy with a regimen of three to four active agents. For further information on duration of therapy and tuberculosis in general see the "Treatment of Tuberculosis" in MMWR 6/20/03 52(RR11); 1-77 by the American Thoracic Society, CDC, and Infectious Diseases Society of America.

4. The answer is C (1.2.0)

The usual adult dose of ciprofloxacin for treating TB is 1000-1500 mg orally daily.

5. The answer is A (1.3.3)

Ethambutol can cause optic neuritis. Risk for eye toxicity increases when the daily dose is raised above 15 mg/kg for longer than 4-6 weeks.

6. The answer is A (1.2.6)

Moxifloxacin, rifampin, and INH are metabolized by the liver. Ethambutol requires dosage modifications in patients with renal insufficiency to prevent toxicity.

7. The answer is C (1.1.3)

The definition of "multidrug-resistant TB" refers to isolates of *Mycobacterium tuberculosis* that are resistant to at least INH and rifampin, and possibly other agents as well.

8. The answer is E (3.3.2)

MR should be reminded continually to take his medications as instructed. Since he is still on INH, he does need to have strict restrictions on alcohol consumption. Moxifloxacin can lead to insomnia, nightmares, headaches, or other CNS side effects. If any of these side effects are noted, MR's physician should be notified.

9. The answer is C (1.3.0)

DOT is the most effective method for controlling adherence to antituberculosis therapy. Two drugs should never be discontinued prior to treatment conclusion. There are no twice-weekly

dosage regimens for ciprofloxacin or amikacin. Giving the total daily dose in the morning has not been shown to increase adherence. Four drugs are needed to treat this drug-resistant organism. Treatment of drug-resistant organisms requires continued treatment past sputum conversion to negative results.

10. The answer is C (3.3.0)

Tuberculosis, especially resistant TB, is a major health concern, and all cases of TB should be reported to the state health department. The police department is not the appropriate agency to notify for this type of public health concern. The state department of health will notify the CDC as appropriate. The Health Insurance Portability and Accountability Act (HIPAA) protects the privacy of health information but provides provisions to protect the health of the general public and therefore allows disclosures to public health entities for the purpose of preventing or controlling disease. However, HIPAA does not allow disclosure of this information to others such as employers. It is up to the patient to disclose this information to his employer.

Case 54 Upper & Lower Respiratory Tract Infections

1. The answer is D (1.1.3)

Based on studies, facial pain (A) or pressure, maxillary tooth pain (A), and purulent nasal discharge (C) are findings that may be associated with a higher likelihood of bacterial infection. Other symptoms associated with acute sinusitis include nasal congestion, nasal obstruction, hyposmia/anosmia, fever (B), cough, headache (E), halitosis, and malaise. These findings are not associated with convincing evidence that distinguishes viral from bacterial infection. Symptoms persisting for greater than 7-10 days are more likely to be associated with bacterial infections rather than viral infection (the average duration of the common cold, which is caused by viruses, is 7-10 days). Studies have shown that a duration of symptoms >7 days is a moderate predictor of acute bacterial sinusitis.

2. The answer is D (1.1.1)

Streptococcus pneumoniae accounts for 20%-40% of acute sinusitis. *Streptococcus pneumoniae*, *Haemophilus influenza*, and *Moraxella catarrhalis* are the most common pathogens recovered in acute sinusitis. Viruses account for 3%-15% of cases and *Staphylococcus aureus* accounts for <10% of cases of acute sinusitis. Anaerobes, such as *Bacteroides* species, are more common in chronic sinusitis. *Pseudomonas aeruginosa* and other gram-negative bacilli are common in nosocomial sinusitis. Acute bacterial sinusitis is suggested by worsening of symptoms after 5 days, persistence of symptoms >7-10 days, or symptoms that are more severe than those associated with a viral sinusitis. During the first 5-10 days, it may be difficult to distinguish between a viral upper respiratory tract infection and acute bacterial sinusitis.

Answers

3. The answer is A (1.1.4)

The goal is to establish a more normal nasal environment through moisturization, humidification, and a reduction in viscosity of mucus membranes and in local swelling. Nasal saline sprays and hydration help thin and clear secretions. There is no evidence to support the use of topical decongestants although they are widely used to alleviate nasal symptoms and promote mucus clearance. They rapidly shrink nasal tissue and help relieve obstruction but do not necessarily have an effect on draining the sinus itself. Evidence does not support the routine use of steroids for acute sinusitis. Antihistamines are also not recommended for routine use but may be beneficial in patients with underlying allergies.

4. The answer is A (1.3.5)

Initial antibiotic therapy should be with narrow-spectrum agents. Such agents would include amoxicillin, trimethoprim-sulfamethoxazole, and doxycycline. SN is sulfa allergic; therefore, amoxicillin would be the most appropriate first-line agent. Studies have shown that the benefits of antimicrobial therapy are small and that most patients improve with no antibiotic. Only patients with persistent, moderate-to-severe signs and symptoms should receive therapy. Therapy should be directed at the most likely pathogens. The emergence of antibiotic-resistant organisms such as *Streptococcus pneumoniae*, *Haemophilus influenzae*, and *Moraxella catarrhalis* has increased the frequency of use of the broader spectrum antibiotics; however, most still consider narrower spectrum agents first-line therapy due to cost, tolerance, and relatively benign course of most cases of acute sinusitis. If SN fails therapy, has had recent antibiotic use, or drug-resistant pathogens are suspected, broader spectrum antibiotics should be considered. These include amoxicillin/clavulanate, second- or third-generation oral cephalosporins, or respiratory quinolones (e.g., levofloxacin, gatifloxacin, moxifloxacin). SN had no risk factors for sinusitis secondary to methicillin-resistant *Staphylococcus aureus* and vancomycin-resistant *Enterococcus*, therefore, linezolid is inappropriate therapy.

5. The answer is E (2.2.1)

Augmentin is the brand name for amoxicillin/clavulanate. Levaquin is the brand name for levofloxacin. Ketek is the brand name for telithromycin. Ceftin is the brand name for cefuroxime. Zithromax is the brand name for azithromycin.

6. The answer is D (1.3.1)

A 10- to 14-day course is usually appropriate duration of therapy for acute sinusitis.

7. The answer is B (1.2.2)

Clavulanate is a beta-lactamase inhibitor; therefore, it will inhibit the bacterial enzyme that will inactivate or breakdown the amoxicillin.

8. The answer is D (3.2.2)

NSAIDs such as ibuprofen may cause gastrointestinal irritation and are recommended to be taken with food. Topical decongestants should not be used for more than 3 days and should be used as directed. If used for more than 3 days or more frequently, nasal congestion may recur or worsen. Rhinitis medicamentosa is a condition in which the nasal mucosa rebounds to a more congested and edematous state. In response, the patient tends to use the product more often. Tachyphylaxis may also occur with topical decongestants. Decongestants should not be used in individuals with heart disease, high blood pressure, thyroid disease, diabetes, or difficulty urinating secondary to an enlarged prostate.

9. The answer is C (3.2.2)

Quinolones chelate with cations such as aluminum, magnesium, calcium, iron, and zinc. This interaction significantly reduces absorption and bioavailability of orally administered quinolones. These products should be given at least 2 hours before or after the dose of levofloxacin to minimize this interaction. Central nervous system adverse effects are frequent with quinolones and may include headache, dizziness, confusion, drowsiness, insomnia, fatigue, malaise, lightheadedness, and restlessness. SN should finish the entire course of therapy even if she is feeling better.

10. The answer is A (1.1.4)

Streptococcus pneumoniae penicillin resistance occurs via alteration of the penicillin-binding protein.

Case 55 Urinary Tract Infections

1. The answer is E (1.1.4)

There are a number of risk factors that may contribute to the development of urinary tract infections, including female gender, age, pregnancy, spermicide and/or diaphragm use, urinary catheter use, structural or functional abnormalities of the urinary tract, and the presence of neurologic dysfunction. The most frequent cause of complicated urinary tract infections in male patients is instrumentation of the urinary tract, including the use of intermittent or indwelling urinary catheters or by undergoing a procedure such as a transurethral resection of the prostate (TURP). Urinary catheters increase the risk of infection by altering normal host defenses and promoting access of uropathogens into the bladder. As men age, the most frequent cause of infection is bladder obstruction due to benign prostatic hypertrophy (BPH). Urinary tract obstruction may lead to incomplete bladder emptying and may inhibit the normal flow of urine, disrupting the natural removal of bacteria from the bladder. This patient was admitted with a urinary catheter in place and has a PMH significant for a stroke with residual hemiparesis and BPH, which may both contribute to incomplete bladder emptying and the development of urinary tract infections. This patient is not currently receiving any medications that may suppress the immune system.

2. The answer is C (1.1.3)

The bacterial etiology of complicated urinary tract infections, such as urosepsis and pyelonephritis, is more variable than uncomplicated urinary tract infections due to the numerous factors that may contribute to their development (e.g., urinary catheter use, previous antibiotic use, presence of obstruction, etc). The common causative bacteria in complicated urinary tract infections include *Escherichia coli* (most common, 50% of cases), *Klebsiella pneumoniae, Proteus mirabilis, Pseudomonas aeruginosa, Enterobacter* species, *Serratia marcescens,* other gram-negative bacteria, *Enterococcus faecalis,* and *Candida* species. *Streptococcus pneumoniae,* a gram-positive cocci, is not a causative pathogen in the urinary tract, but is a primary cause of community-acquired respiratory tract infections. Since the preliminary results from this patient's urine and blood cultures are revealing the presence of a gram-negative rod, the causative organism is most likely *Escherichia coli, Klebsiella pneumoniae, Proteus mirabilis, Pseudomonas aeruginosa,* or *Enterobacter* species.

3. The answer is B (2.1.0, 1.2.6)

To estimate the creatinine clearance (mL/min) for antimicrobial dosing, the Cockroft-Gault equation for males can be used:
$CrCl_{males} = [(140\text{-Age}) \times IBW (kg)]/(72 \times serum\ creatinine)$ [(140-78) $\times$ 66]/(72 $\times$ 1.5) = 38mL/min

4. The answer is C (1.1.3)

All of the choices, with the exception of low serum glucose concentrations, are suggestive of the presence of a complicated urinary tract infection including urosepsis and pyelonephritis in this patient. The presence of costovertebral tenderness is suggestive of an upper urinary tract infection or pyelonephritis. Clinical symptoms such as fever and altered mental status (especially in the elderly) are indicators of the presence of systemic infection. Lastly, the presence of 20-25 white blood cells/hpf in the urine with the growth of gram-negative bacteria in the urine and the bloodstream are indicators of urosepsis or pyelonephritis. Serum glucose concentrations are not typically altered in the presence of infection, except in patients with diabetes mellitus, where the presence of infection may lead to an increase in serum glucose concentrations.

5. The answer is A (1.2.0)

Given the nature of his clinical presentation, aggressive management with parenteral antimicrobials is warranted, so that oral TMP/SMX or doxycycline are not the best empiric therapy options for initial treatment in this patient. And, based on his clinical presentation and residence in a skilled nursing facility, empiric antibiotic therapy should provide coverage against gram-negative bacteria including *Pseudomonas aeruginosa.* Therefore, parenteral ampicillin and ertapenem would not be appropriate choices for this patient since they are inactive against *Pseudomonas aeruginosa.* Therefore, the most appropriate empiric antibiotic for this patient would be parenteral cefepime, due to its excellent activity against gram-negative bacteria including *Pseudomonas aeruginosa.* This patient has a history of developing a rash to penicillin, but appears to have received cephalosporins (IM ceftriaxone) in the past without reaction.

6. The answer is C (1.3.2, 1.3.5)

The results of the patient's urine and blood culture reveal the presence of *Escherichia coli* that is susceptible to a number of different antimicrobials. While the clinician could consider maintaining the patient on cefepime therapy, it is prudent to switch the patient to an antimicrobial that offers more directed coverage against the infecting bacteria (streamline or direct antimicrobial therapy against the infecting pathogen) to limit the effect of the broad-spectrum antibiotic on the patient's normal flora as well as to decrease the emergence of resistance. Since the infecting organism is a susceptible *Escherichia coli,* cefepime, meropenem, aztreonam, and gentamicin are not necessary to treat this patient's infection since they are fairly broad-spectrum agents with antipseudomonal activity. And, the dose listed for gentamicin is also too high for his level of renal function, and it is a potential nephrotoxic agent. Therefore, parenteral cefazolin would be the most appropriate choice for continued antibiotic therapy in this patient due to its low cost and fairly narrow, directed spectrum of activity. It can be used parenterally until the patient stabilizes, at which time he can be converted to oral fluoroquinolone therapy for the remaining duration for his infection.

7. The answer is B (1.2.5, 2.2.3, 2.3.2)

Patients with congestive heart failure, hypertension, or renal dysfunction are often restricted in their sodium intake. Therefore, it is important to recognize which medications have large amounts of sodium in their preparations to avoid potential exacerbation of the conditions listed above. Certain anti-infectives have a large amount of sodium in their parenteral formulations, including penicillin G sodium, carbenicillin, ticarcillin (which has the most, 5.4 mEq/g), ticarcillin/clavulanate, piperacillin, and piperacillin/tazobactam. Therefore, if an alternative antibiotic is available, ticarcillin and ticarcillin/clavulanate should be avoided in patients with hypertension, congestive heart failure, or renal dysfunction. Parenteral fluoroquinolones, carbapenems, cephalosporins, and monobactams do not have a high amount of sodium in their preparations and can be considered for the treatment of infection in patients with hypertension, congestive heart failure, or renal dysfunction (although, dosage adjustment with renal insufficiency may be necessary, depending on the agent).

8. The answer is D (1.2.1)

The recommended duration of therapy for the treatment of patients with complicated urinary tract infections is 7-14 days, depending on the infection type and severity of infection. Patients with infections such as pyelonephritis or urosepsis (especially with concomitant documented bacteremia) are typically treated for a total duration of 14 days, which can include both intravenous and oral therapy.

Answers

9. The answer is A (3.2.1, 3.2.2)

The use of urinary catheters is frequently associated with the development of infection in the urinary tract due to alterations in normal host defenses and introduction of bacteria into the bladder. Bacteria can be introduced into the bladder during catheterization or by ascension up the outside lumen of the catheter along the mucosal border, or intraluminally via a contaminated collecting tube or drainage bag. The longer the patient has a urinary catheter, the greater the risk of developing a urinary tract infection. In patients with long-term (>2 weeks) urinary catheters who develop symptomatic urinary tract infections, the urinary catheter should be replaced to facilitate the resolution of symptoms and decrease the incidence of reinfection. Last, routine antibiotic prophylaxis is not recommended in patients with short-term or long-term indwelling urinary catheters to prevent the development of urinary tract infections because they may postpone the development of bacteriuria and lead to the emergence of resistant bacteria.

10. The answer is B (1.2.1)

Chronic bacterial prostatitis is a bacterial infection of the prostate gland and surrounding tissue, which is often the result of incomplete eradication of bacteria from the prostate. The most common causative organisms of chronic bacterial prostatitis include gram-negative aerobic bacilli such as *E. coli* (in 50-80% of cases). The treatment of chronic bacterial prostatitis often requires a long duration of therapy to ensure eradication of the organism from prostatic tissue and to prevent reinfection. The duration of therapy for chronic bacterial prostatitis is typically 4 to 6 weeks, although some patients may require a longer duration of therapy (up to 12 weeks). Therefore, of the treatment choices listed, TMP/SMX is the most appropriate because of its activity against the most common infecting pathogens and the correct duration of therapy. While levofloxacin is an excellent choice for the treatment of chronic bacterial prostatitis, the treatment duration is too short. Azithromycin does not have activity against common bacteria that cause chronic bacterial prostatitis. Ampicillin should not be used in JS due to his history of penicillin allergy, and is no longer recommended for the treatment of prostatitis. Parenteral therapy (ceftriaxone) is not typically employed for the treatment of chronic prostatitis unless the infecting organism is resistant to available oral antibiotics.

Hooten TM, Bradley SF, Cardenas DD, Colgan R, Geerlings SE. Diagnosis, prevention, and treatment of catheter-associated urinary tract infection in adults: 2009 international clinical practice guidelines from the Infectious Diseases Society of America. *Clin Infect Dis.* 2010; 50:625–63.

Lipsky BA, Byren I, Hoey CT. Treatment of bacterial prostatitis. *Clin Infect Dis.* 2010, 50:1641-52.

Case 56 Contraception & Infertility

1. The answer is C (2.2.2)

Only the diaphragm (C) requires a prescription (although the spermicidal gels are available without a prescription). Although it is a barrier method, the diaphragm requires measurement to prescribe the correct size. Male (A) and female (B) condoms are available without a prescription. Several forms of spermicidal agents (nonoxynol-9) (E) are available without a prescription. These include vaginal foams, jellies, and suppositories. The spermicidal (D) products are less effective than oral contraceptives and must be reapplied before each act of intercourse.

2. The answer is A (1.2.4)

Oral contraceptive tablets should be taken at the same time every day (B). This not only maximizes the contraceptive efficacy but also decreases the occurrence of spotting and breakthrough bleeding. Patients should be instructed on what to do if they miss a tablet. Pointing out the section in the patient package information is helpful as the patient knows where to look if this situation arises. Oral contraceptives do not provide protection from sexually transmitted diseases (A); a condom is required to decrease (but does not fully prevent) transmission. Oral contraceptives decrease the risk of ovarian and uterine cancer, especially with long-term use (E). Answer choices C and D are also true statements.

3. The answer is C (1.2.4)

Women who are known to be HIV-positive (C) may take oral contraceptives. The fact that oral contraceptives do not decrease their ability to transmit the virus should be emphasized to these patients. Oral contraceptives are often taken for menstruation-related problems. All other choices are contraindications stated in the package insert. Present or past history of venous thromboembolism (VTE) (B) is a contraindication due to estrogens increasing the risk of VTE. Oral contraceptives appear to induce a resistance to protein C and may lead to the development of deep VTE. The incidence of VTE is estimated to be 10–15 per 100,000 women-years for second-generation agents and 20–30 per 100,000 women-years for third-generation agents. Smoking increases the risk of serious side effects with oral contraceptives. Women who smoke more than 15 cigarettes per day and are over age 35 should not take oral contraceptives.

4. The answer is E (1.2.5)

Levonorgestrel (C) is considered to be the most androgenic, while the new progestins (desogestrel and norgestimate) are considered the least (E). Desogestrel has a small amount of androgenic activity. Androgenic effects account for the side effects such as acne, oily hair, and hirsutism. However, in clinical use most women are not affected by these problems.

5. The answer is E (3.2.1)

A decrease in glucose tolerance may occur (C), especially with the older progestins. Clinically, this is rarely a problem unless a patient has diabetes mellitus or is already known to have impaired glucose tolerance (IGT) or impaired fasting glucose (IFG).

A few women have increased blood pressure (B) due to the estrogenic component. In clinical trials, some women gained weight (A) and some experienced weight loss. It is difficult to establish a cause-and-effect relationship to the oral contraceptives. Oral contraceptives increase the risk of hepatic tumors but not pancreatic tumors (E). Breakthrough bleeding (D) may be experienced by some women starting hormonal contraception, but this tends to subside with continued use.

6. The answer is B (1.3.3)

Nausea and breast tenderness are most commonly associated with a combined oral contraceptive that contains too much estrogen (B) while a deficiency in estrogen (A) may cause vaginal dryness, light menses, or breakthrough bleeding early in the menstrual cycle. A combined oral contraceptive that contains too much progestin (D) may cause acne, hirsutism, and depression. A deficiency in progestin (C) should be considered if a female taking a combined oral contraceptive complains of heavy menses or breakthrough bleeding towards the end of her menstrual cycle.

7. The answer is D (3.2.2)

All are common adverse effects or considerations of the contraceptive method except that depot medroxyprogesterone acetate in fact has a low failure rate (D) when injections are repeated within 14 weeks (but the recommended interval between doses is 12 weeks). The pregnancy rate for depot medroxyprogesterone acetate is 0.3%. The return of fertility can be delayed with depot medroxyprogesterone acetate. The median time to conception for those women who do become pregnant is 10 months from the last injection. The range is 4–31 months. The levonorgestrel intrauterine system (Mirena) can cause irregular bleeding in the first 3–6 months of therapy (E). Some women cease bleeding after the first year of therapy and this is often a desired effect.

8. The answer is C (3.2.1)

Nausea and vomiting are most likely attributed to the estrogen component rather than the progestin component (C). Currently, over 20 combined oral contraceptive products can be used as emergency contraception in the United States (B). Even though the precise mechanism of EC is somewhat controversial, recent studies suggest levonorgestrel-only EC works by inhibiting ovulation (D). Both males and females 16 years and younger currently require a prescription for EC (A). There appear to be no known long-term complications secondary to levonorgestrel-only EC (E).

9. The answer is B (1.1.3)

Although combined oral contraceptives such as Yaz, Ortho Tri-Cyclen, and Estrostep Fe have FDA indications for acne (A), other oral contraceptives are also effective. The estrogen increases sex-hormone binding globulin (SHBG). SHBG binds free testosterone, thus decreasing the development of acne. The regulation of hormonal fluctuations may improve premenstrual symp-

toms (C) and irregular bleeding (E). Oral contraceptives decrease the amount of endometrial tissue and, thus the prostaglandins produced in endometrial cells. Dysmenorrhea is caused by the release of the prostaglandins that stimulate uterine contractions during menses. The contractions increase intrauterine pressure and cause pain. Oral contraceptives are very effective in many women in improving dysmenorrhea symptoms (D). Yeast vaginitis is not affected by oral contraceptives (B).

10. The answer is B (1.2.3)

Phenytoin increases the metabolism of many drugs that are hepatically metabolized, including estrogens (B). Progestins are not significantly affected. The other choices are potential mechanisms of drug interactions, but are not the cause of this interaction. There is no absolute solution to the drug interaction between oral contraceptives and phenytoin. Some clinicians would argue for a different contraceptive method, but if oral contraceptives were strongly desired, a product that contains 50 µg of ethinyl estradiol may be considered. When a woman is receiving a short course of a medication that decreases the effectiveness of an oral contraceptive, she should be advised to use a backup method of contraception. A condom or spermicidal agent is the most common choice. If a woman is using the agent only for non-menstrual reasons, this is not an issue. As this is becoming increasingly common, a woman should be questioned on this issue before assuming she needs backup contraception.

Case 57 Drugs in Pregnancy & Lactation

1. The answer is B (1.2.5)

After 40 minutes, five half-lives should have passed and the drug is expected to be at steady state (answer option III). Because the half-life is so short and the drug effect is almost immediate, no bolus is needed. Response to therapy must be monitored very closely.

2. The answer is B (1.2.2)

Vasopressin (B), or antidiuretic hormone, is similar in amino acid sequence to oxytocin. Oxytocin is capable of binding to vasopressin and oxytocin receptors in both the brain and kidney and possibly exerting an antidiuretic effect at high doses. The other hormones are pituitary in origin but are not similar in effects on fluid status.

3. The answer is C (1.2.5)

Multiple factors affect the placental transfer of drugs and the subsequent effect on the fetus. Some effects may not be observable for several years, such as those on development. Drugs with small molecular weights (under 500 daltons) are more likely to cross the placenta to the fetal circulation (C). A drug that is taken only once will be less likely to have an effect than chronic dosing (E). A peak serum concentration is usually lower

Answers

with one dose than chronic dosing. Thus, less drug is available to cross the placenta. Teratogens are weak acids and not bases (D). It has been hypothesized that acidic drugs alter the pH of the embryonic cell. By the thirty-second week after conception, all major organ systems are formed and integrated (A). Drugs that are ionized cannot cross into the placenta (B).

4. The answer is D (1.3.3)

Neonatal cataracts (D) have not been identified as a negative neonatal effect. The most common indication for long-term corticosteroid use is asthma and the effects attributed to the drug may be partially caused by the underlying condition. Mild intrauterine growth restriction (B) has been documented with the use of systemic corticosteroids throughout pregnancy. Suppression of the fetal adrenal axis is not unexpected (A). This may lead to an increased risk of infection and sepsis (C). Mothers on corticosteroids may have worsened glycemic control and develop gestational diabetes (E).

5. The answer is C (1.2.5)

Drugs that are not highly protein bound transfer more easily into breast milk (C). The other listed properties promote transfer into breast milk. The milk to plasma ratio of weak bases is 1, while the ratio is <1 for weak acids. The relative infant dose (RID) is a calculation which estimates infant exposure to maternal exposure on a dose/weight basis. The RID percentage is calculated by dividing the absolute infant dose (in mg/kg/day) in milk by the maternal dose (in mg/kg/day). It has been accepted that a RID of less than 10% is generally considered to be safe.

6. The answer is D (3.1.1)

Although most package inserts (answer option I) contain a statement on using the drug in breastfeeding, this information is usually somewhat vague. The latter two sources (answer options II and III, respectively) evaluate the information available from various studies and databases. Many drugs are designated as compatible or not with breastfeeding by the American Academy of Pediatrics in their publication. Although drugs may cross into breast milk, the negative effects on an infant may be far outweighed by the benefits of breast milk.

7. The answer is B (1.1.2)

Gravida stands for the number of pregnancies while Para stands for the number of deliveries. If only one number follows the P, then all births were term. CL has been pregnant three times as she is G 3 (A). She appears to be in her third pregnancy, as there is two deliveries noted (B). Multiple births are still designated as one pregnancy (C) Without additional information, one cannot tell if the child is living (D). This system does not refer to route of delivery (E).

8. The answer is E (1.1.4)

While any of the scenarios might possibly happen, Choice E is the most likely cause-and-effect scenario. CL describes what

sounds like mastitis. She appears to believe that antibiotics are relatively interchangeable. She is also somewhat modest and does not want to call her obstetrician's office and describe what has happened. Since she has not sought any professional help from a lactation consultant or nurse at her obstetrician's office, she may think she should give up breastfeeding and switch to formula feeding With your intervention, you can guide her to get an appropriate diagnosis and treatment so that she may resume breastfeeding her infant.

9. The answer is C (1.1.4)

The usual cause of mastitis is *Staphylococcus aureus* (C). The drug therapy of choice is dicloxacillin or clindamycin. Note that this patient is allergic to penicillin. It is important for the clinician to also consider methicillin-resistant *Staphylococcus aureus* (MRSA) since the incidence of MRSA infections has been increasing, even in patients who lack traditional risk factors for MRSA infection.

10. The answer is C (3.2.2)

The balance and type of carbohydrates, protein, and fats in breast milk is considered to be ideal (A). Additional benefits such as passage of antibodies from mother to infant are found in breast milk. Soy protein is usually not used initially (B). Children who were breastfed have shown a trend of less obesity in the future (C). Low-iron formulations should not be routinely used (D). The assumption that iron contributes to gastrointestinal problems such as constipation is largely unfounded. Formula should not be diluted more than what is listed in the package labeling since such dilution may change the correct fluid and nutrition balance as well as create stability issues (E).

Case 58 Menopause

1. The answer is B (1.2.2)

All of the listed agents are estrogens except Evista (raloxifene), which is a mixed estrogen agonist/antagonist. Climara (C) is a transdermal estrogen preparation and the other three estrogen products are oral. Raloxifene may increase or cause vasomotor symptoms in asymptomatic women.

2. The answer is C (3.2.1)

Although there is limited data that progestins may improve bone mineral density over estrogen use alone, it is not well-accepted data. Also, the doses are higher than many women tolerate. Estrogens have positive effects (e.g., increase HDL and decrease LDL) on lipoproteins. Most menopausal women would rather not have menstrual bleeding, so the progestin actually decreases the acceptance of the regimen for some women. Estrogens may slightly increase the risk of breast cancer.

3. The answer is C (1.2.5)

Ethinyl estradiol is a synthetic estrogen. 17☐estradiol is the primary and most potent endogenous estrogen. Equilin sulfate is a component of conjugated equine estrogens. The estrogenic compound is extracted from horse urine. Answer (E) gives the natural estrogens in reverse order of potency.

4. The answer is D (2.2.3)

Estring (D) is a vaginal ring used for local effects (vaginal dryness) while choice B is a vaginal ring used for systemic effects. Choice A is an OTC vaginal lubricant that may be used alone or in addition to a vaginal estrogen. There are multiple products available. Choice C is an injectable estrogen for moderate to severe vasomotor symptoms. It is rarely used in clinical practice today. Choice E is a topical estrogen that is systemically absorbed and used for vasomotor symptoms.

5. The answer is B (3.1.2)

Results from the Women's Health Initiative (WHI) conjugated equine estrogens/medroxyprogesterone acetate clinical trial arm showed an increased risk (attributable risk) of adverse cardiovascular events, strokes, invasive breast cancer, and pulmonary embolism. This challenged what was historically believed to be the benefits of hormone therapy, though much of this benefit was based on observational data. However, the WHI study population was an older population. Approximately two thirds of study participants were 60 years old or older at study initiation (A). Women with severe vasomotor symptoms were discouraged from entry into the study as they would be more likely to withdraw if randomized to placebo (C). Women who are symptomatic in menopause are most effectively treated with estrogen therapy. In February 2004, the estrogen-only arm of the WHI was halted due to no benefit on coronary heart disease and an increase risk of adverse events. Risk reduction for colon cancer has been shown in the WHI and an earlier study. The benefits on bone (by decreasing bone loss) are well documented. This study found a decreased risk of fractures in the 29%–38% range (for various sites) for both study arms. However, other targeted therapies with safer side effect profiles for osteopenia/osteoporosis exist. In cohort studies, many of the women were taking conjugated equine estrogens.

6. The answer is E (1.3.3)

Duloxetine is used to treat urinary incontinence. Therefore, retention of urine would be a possible adverse effect of duloxetine use. Clinical trials have shown that duloxetine 40 mg twice daily was effective at decreasing frequency of stress urinary incontinence episodes. The other options are all correct.

7. The answer is A (1.2.2)

Estropipate (A) is an estrogen and stimulates estrogen receptors in breast tissue. Raloxifene (B) is a mixed estrogen agonist/antagonist that does not stimulate breast tissue but has some benefit on lipoproteins. Tamoxifen (D) and toremifene (E) are used for their antagonistic properties on the breast but do not have well-documented positive effects on other sys-

tems. Alendronate (C) is a bisphosphonate that is used for osteoporosis prevention and treatment and does not affect breast tissue.

8. The answer is E (1.2.7)

Vivelle-Dot (A), EstroGel (B), Alora (D), and Climara (E) all contain estradiol. Climara is a transdermal patch and is changed once weekly. Vivelle-Dot and Alora are transdermal patches that are applied twice a week. EstroGel is a topical gel that is applied to both the inside and outside of the arm from wrist to shoulder. CombiPatch (C) is a combination estrogen/progestin (estradiol and norethindrone acetate) patch.

9. The answer is A (1.2.1)

Estratest (A) is esterified estrogens with low-dose methyltestosterone. Although indicated for difficult-to-treat vasomotor symptoms, it is often prescribed to increase libido. Methyltestosterone tablets (B) that are presently available are too potent to be prescribed for sexual desire improvement in women and would cause severe androgenic adverse effects. Fluoxymesterone (D) is another potent oral androgen used in men. AndroGel 1% (C) is a topical testosterone that has only been tested in men and is packaged to deliver a dose for males. Estradiol valerate (E) is long-acting injectable estrogen-only product.

10. The answer is D (2.2.2)

Both products are available in immediate-release tablets and extended-release formulations. Oxybutynin is also available as a syrup. Since oxybutynin, but not tolterodine, is available as a transdermal system (Oxytrol), answer option I is incorrect. The mechanisms of action are as stated in choice II, but both agents have anticholinergic properties that can be additive with anticholinergic properties of other drugs. Tolterodine is metabolized primarily by CPY2D6 and by CYP3A4 in persons who lack CYP2D6. Although oxybutynin is metabolized by CYP3A4 in the intestinal wall and liver, drug interactions with other CYP-active agents have not been identified.

Case 59 Neonatal Therapy

1. The answer is B (1.1.1)

A neonate is defined as age 0-30 days. An infant is defined as age 1 month to 1 year. A toddler is defined as age 1-3 years. A child is defined as age 3-12 years. An adolescent is defined as age 12-18 years.

2. The answer is A (1.1.1)

Normal AST, ALT, and alkaline phosphate levels for a neonate are 25-75 U/L, 13-45 U/L, and 150-420 U/L, respectively. Potassium levels in a newborn range from 3.7-5.9 mEq/L. Chloride levels in a newborn range from 98-113 mEq/L. BG Hill's hepatic enzymes, potassium, and chloride levels are normal.

Answers

3. The answer is C (1.1.3)

Early-onset sepsis is defined as blood or cerebrospinal fluid culture-proven infection occurring in the newborn who is younger than 7 days of age, and is usually acquired from the mother. Group B *Streptococcus* (A), the primary pathogen causing early-onset sepsis, is a gram-positive cocci organism in pairs or chains. *Listeria monocytogenes* (B) is a gram-positive bacilli organism. *Escherichia coli* (C) is a gram-negative rod organism that is a common cause of early-onset sepsis. *Staphylococcus epidermidis* (D), or coagulase-negative *Staphylococcus,* is a gram-positive organism that is a common cause of late-onset sepsis in the newborn. *Bacteroides* (E) is an anaerobic gram-negative bacilli. In addition to Group B *Streptococcus* and *Escherichia coli,* common causes of early-onset sepsis include *Haemophilus influenzae, Klebsiella* sp., *Enterobacter* sp., and *Listeria monocytogenes.*

4. The answer is E (2.1.1)

BG Hill weighs 3 lb 14 oz, which equals 1.76 kg. Ampicillin 176 mg IV q12h = 352 mg/day divided by 1.76 kg = 200 mg/kg/d. The standard dose for rule out sepsis in a neonate is 100 to 200 mg/kg/d divided q12 h.

5. The answer is C (1.2.6)

The goal trough is less than 2 μg/mL. A goal peak is 4-8 μg/mL. No change is needed for the current dose.

6. The answer is A (2.2.2)

Ampicillin sodium is the only intravenous formulation. Ampicillin trihydrate is available as a capsule and powder for suspension. There is no sulfate formulation available.

7. The answer is C (2.1.2)

6 mL/hr = 144 mL/day x 10% dextrose = 14.4 grams of dextrose. Each gram of dextrose contains 3.4 kcal, so 14.4 grams x 3.4 kcal = 49 kcal/day divided by 1.76 kg = 28 kcal/kg/day.

8. The answer is A (3.2.1)

Infants born at < 32 weeks gestation who are d•6 months at the beginning of RSV season are at high risk of severe RSV infection even if no other risk factors are present. Risk factors are considered when determining prophylaxis for infants born between 32 and 35 weeks gestation. Routine prophylaxis for full-term neonates is not recommended. American Academy of Pediatrics, Committee on Infectious Diseases. Policy Statement—Modified Recommendations for Use of Palivizumab for Prevention of Respiratory Syncytial Virus Infections. *Pediatrics.* 2009; 124(6):1694-1701.

9. The answer is C (1.2.2)

Gentamicin is an aminoglycoside antibiotic and binds to the 30S and 50S ribosomal subunit. This causes an inhibition of protein synthesis and results in a faulty cell wall membrane (I, II). Ampicillin is a penicillin antibiotic and causes cell death by binding to penicillin-binding proteins and affecting the cell wall (III).

10. The answer is C (3.1.2)

A case series (A) does not reliably establish a causal relationship, but suggests a potential hypothesis to be further studied. Because of the known potential risk of kernicterus (bilirubin deposits in the brain) related to sulfonamide use in the neonatal period, a randomized controlled trial (B) or crossover trial (D) design would be difficult due to ethical considerations. A retrospective cohort would be most appropriate to establish a causal relationship in this example.

Case 60 Pediatric Infectious Diseases

1. The answer is D (1.1.3)

Dizziness is not commonly reported in acute otitis media. It may be a symptom of middle ear problems. Balance and, thus, dizziness are coordinated through movement of fluid through the labyrinth, whereas movement of fluid through the cochlea is responsible for hearing. Otalgia (A), or ear pain, is almost universal in acute otitis media. It is not a good indicator in chronic otitis media because many of these patients do not experience pain or cannot express their pain. Otorrhea (B), or ear discharge, is also very common. The inflammatory and infectious processes produce excess fluid and mucous that the body attempts to drain. Temporary holes in the tympanic membrane are common during acute otitis media. Partial deafness (C) is very common as fluid accumulates behind the tympanic membrane. The membrane itself becomes unable to vibrate and initiate the process of hearing. Fever (E) is very common. If children are too young to let their parents or caregivers know that their ear hurts, fever, anorexia, and nausea/vomiting are such generic symptoms that acute otitis media may not be suspected.

2. The answer is E (1.2.1)

TMP/SMX has a high degree of cross-resistance with penicillins and beta-lactams in general. Therefore, if the patient has an infection caused by nonpenicillin-susceptible *Streptococcus pneumoniae,* TMP/SMX is most likely an ineffective alternative. It was useful in the past and was often a second-line agent, or first-line agent in penicillin-allergic patients (A). Its use is dramatically lower in pediatrics as safer and more efficacious agents have become available. Not only is cross-resistance a problem, but also the incidence of resistance to TMP/SMX itself is very high and increasing (B). Most recent studies do not recommend TMP/SMX for treating acute otitis media. Skin reactions have always been a serious complication of sulfa-containing medications (C). The incidence in children is low, but with many antibiotics that are more efficacious and safer, TMP/SMX should be avoided. *Haemophilus influenzae,* nontypable is the second most common organism causing acute otitis media (D). At least 10% of the isolates are resistant, giving further support to avoiding this drug in acute otitis media.

3. The answer is C (1.1.3)

Of bacterial causes of acute otitis media, *Streptococcus pneumoniae* currently accounts for approximately 40% of all cases of otitis media. Nontypable *Haemophilus influenzae* accounts for approximately 25%-30%, and *Moraxella catarrhalis* accounts for about 10%-15%. Other organisms found in otitis media (~5%) include Group A *Streptococcus*, *Staphylococcus aureus*, and anaerobes.

4. The answer is A (1.2.1)

Vancomycin is currently the only alternative when a patient has a highly penicillin-resistant *Streptococcus pneumoniae* infection. Clinicians fear that organisms will develop resistance to vancomycin if it is used indiscriminately. Clindamycin, although bacteriostatic, is used frequently for moderately resistant *Streptococcus pneumoniae* and in those with a penicillin allergy. It is often ineffective for highly resistant organisms. As mentioned, the two most common organisms are often resistant to TMP/SMX (B). Macrolide resistance is becoming a problem with Streptococcus pneumoniae and Haemophilus influenzae (C). Cefprozil may be active against some moderately resistant strains of *Streptococcus pneumoniae*, but the more resistant strains will be resistant to cefprozil and the drug is not active against many strains of *Haemophilus influenzae* (D).

5. The answer is C (1.2.2)

Streptococcus pneumoniae's resistance to beta-lactam antibiotics develops due to alterations in the PCN-binding protein. By increasing the dose (of amoxicillin, for example) this type of resistance can be overcome. Thus 90 mg/kg/day of amoxicillin is the appropriate therapeutic dose for otitis media today. *Streptococcus pneumoniae*'s resistance to macrolides is due to alterations of the ribosomal binding site and by efflux pumps (B/D). *Staphylococcus aureus* develops resistance to all beta-lactams by altering the mec A binding site (E). *Streptococcus pneumoniae* does not cause beta-lactamases to develop nor change the mec A binding site. One mechanism of resistance of gram-negative organisms is beta-lactamases (A).

6. The answer is B (3.2.2)

Breastfeeding has been shown to provide protection from developing acute otitis media. Infants who are breastfed until at least 4 months of age have significantly fewer episodes of acute otitis media than children who are bottle fed. Eustachian tube dysfunction is the most important factor leading to acute otitis media (A). Numerous etiologies exist for Eustachian tube dysfunction; however, when it does not function properly, otitis media and/or sinusitis often develop. Eustachian tube dysfunction prevents removal of inflammatory and infectious material from the middle ear and infection may ensue. Patient age at first occasion of acute otitis media is important

(C). If the infant develops acute otitis media before 6 months of age, the chances of recurring episodes are 50% more likely than in those infants/children whose first episode occurs after 6 months of age. Infants with allergies, atopy, or immunoglobulin G (IgG) deficiencies have a greater risk of developing acute otitis media (D). Infants and children exposed to secondhand smoke have a several-fold higher chance of developing acute otitis media and of developing recurrent infections (E). Day care attendance seems to increase the risk dramatically.

7. The answer is D (1.1.4)

The other four factors may affect the incidence of acute otitis media in children. The Eustachian tube in infants/children is angled only 10 degrees from horizontal compared with 45 degrees in adults (C). Nasal secretions draining into the Eustachian tube and the middle ear are sometimes a contributing factor to the development of acute otitis media. This drainage may occur more easily due to the decreased angle from nares to Eustachian tube. More important is the opposite process. Given the decreased angle, the body cannot remove inflammatory and infectious material from the middle ear; gravity is against us. The infectious material accumulates and leads to further inflammation and infection. The tensor veli palatini muscle in children is less efficient at opening the Eustachian tube (A). This again hinders removal of infectious and inflammatory material. In infants and young children, it does not. It also explains why infants cry when exposed to changes in altitude. It takes the physiological force involved in crying to open this muscle and allow the infant to normalize air pressure in the middle ear with atmospheric pressure. The shorter tube length simply makes it easier for infectious material to be inspired into the middle ear (B). As the Eustachian tube grows in length, an increased quantity of muscle aids in preventing retrograde inspiration of foreign material into the middle ear. Another physiological difference is that the cilia involved in expelling material from the middle ear do not function efficiently (E). Their movement may also be impaired during infection.

8. The answer is C (2.1.1)

KT is prescribed 90.9 mg/kg/day of amoxicillin. She takes 400 mg twice daily: 800 mg/day divided by her weight of 8.8 kg = 90 mg/kg/day. The majority of antibiotics dosed for pediatric patients are in mg/kg/day. 90 mg/kg/day of amoxicillin is the appropriate dose for otitis media today.

9. The answer is A (1.2.1)

High dose amoxicillin therapy (90 mg/kg/day) is the initial treatment and now standard treatment dose for acute otitis media (AOM) because of the increased prevalence of nonpenicillin-susceptible *Streptococcus pneumoniae*. This is recommended by the American Academy of Pediatrics for nonpenicillin allergic patients. If a patient fails this therapy, amoxicillin/clavulanic acid is recommended next at a dose of 90 mg/kg/day of amoxicillin. TMP/SMX is not recommended for AOM due to a high rate of resistance (B). If the patient has a non-type 1 penicillin allergy, a cephalosporin can be tried for

Answers

AOM, such as cefdinir, cefpodoxime, or cefuroxime (C). Ceftriaxone is an injectable cephalosporin that can be administered IM (D). A 1 or 3-day therapy of ceftriaxone is recommended for patients who cannot tolerate oral medications or fail amoxicillin/clavulanic acid therapy. Three-day treatment is recommended for nonpenicillin-susceptible *Streptococcus pneumoniae* strains. Azithromycin is recommended for patients with type 1 allergic reactions to PCN (E). Concerns of resistance also exist with the macrolide class. Antibiotics should be changed if the patient is still symptomatic after 48-72 hours of antibiotics, and the diagnosis should be re-examined. Since KT has no allergies, amoxicillin/clavulanic acid should be recommended.

10. The answer is D (3.2.1)

Prevnar 13 (D) is the vaccination for *Streptococcus pneumoniae*. Menactra (A) is meningococcal vaccine. Fluvirin (B) is an influenza vaccine. Varivax (C) is a varicella vaccine. Adacel (E) is a tetanus toxoid, reduced diphtheria toxoid and acellular pertussis vaccine.

Case 61 Pediatric Nutrition

1. The answer is B (3.2.1)

Since this patient is greater than 11 years old, he would receive 10 mL of an adult multivitamin formulation. If the pediatric preparation was administered in his PN solution, he may be under-dosed on the water-soluble vitamins and potentially overdosed on the fat-soluble vitamins. Adult multivitamin solutions are now available with phytonadione (vitamin K), so using one with vitamin K should be used. It is difficult to determine the length of PN therapy he will require, so addition of multivitamins is recommended. Since he is somewhat underweight, he may also have some vitamin deficiencies. Supplementation with folic acid and thiamine may also be required to meet his nutritional goals.

It is never appropriate to prepare a parenteral nutrition solution without vitamins. In fall 1988, 3 of 59 patients receiving PN at one university medical center died of refractory lactic acidosis. Each died within 5 weeks of receiving PN without thiamine and had had a clinical course strongly suggestive of acute beriberi. Thiamine was absent from the PN fluids given these patients as a result of a nationwide shortage of intravenous (IV) multivitamins. Thiamine, one of the components in the multivitamin products, is essential for two enzymes needed for aerobic metabolism: pyruvate dehydrogenase and œga-ketoglutarate dehydrogenase. In the absence of thiamine, pyruvate cannot enter the Krebs cycle, resulting in pyruvate accumulation and conversion to lactate. Furthermore, generation of NADH within the Krebs cycles is prevented, stimulating anaerobic glycolysis and further lactate production. Unlike the fat-soluble vitamins, the body stores of thiamine are minimal; the duration of availability of thiamine reserves is unknown.

2. The answer is C (2.1.3)

Using the standard formula: 20 kg = 1500 mL + 20 mL/kg for each kg greater than 20 kg 50 kg = 1500 mL + (20 mL/kg x 30 kg) = 2100 mL, then adding 10% for blood loss, the correct answer is 2310 mL/24 h. As the hourly rate of 96.25 ml/hr would be difficult to infuse with most infusion pumps, most physicians would adjust the rate to 96 mL/hour = 2304 mL/day.

3. The answer is B (3.2.1)

According to the FDA safety alert, "Hazards of Precipitation Associated with Parenteral Nutrition," the best way to avoid calcium phosphorus precipitation is to:

- determine the solubility of the calcium and phosphorus at the volume at the time the calcium is added and not at the final volume of the admixture;
- add the phosphorus salts first, calcium salts last;
- take amount of phosphorus present in the amino acid source (if any) when calculating the solubility of the calcium and phosphorus salts;
- flush the line between the addition of any incompatible ingredients;
- agitate the solution and check for precipitates during the compounding process; and
- use an inline filter to infuse the parenteral nutrition.

4. The answer is B (2.2.0)

Using the Holiday-Segar formula for calculating fluid requirements involves the following: 0-10 kg: 100 mL/kg/day; 10-20 kg: 1000 mL + 50 mL/kg for each kg > 10 kg; 20 kg: 1500 mL + 20 mL/kg for each kg > 20 kg. For this patient it would be 1500 mL + 600 = 2100 mL.

Solution B would provide: 1920 mL + 250 mL = 2170 mL/day of volume (close to maintenance) AA 2.5% x 1920 mL/day = 48 g of protein (0.96 g/kg) $D_{10}W$ x 1920 mL/day = 192 g of dextrose fat emulsion 20% 250 mL = 50 g of fat Total calories = (48 g x 4 kcal/g) + (192 g x 3.4 kcal/g) + (50 g x 2 kcal/mL) = 1345 kcal/day The above calculations show that Answer B would give the closest and safest requirements for macronutrients, calories, and fluids. The other solutions will either provide too many calories and/or not enough fluids. Patients need to be individually assessed to increase nutrients and fluids to meet their actual goals.

5. The answer is D (1.3.3)

When reviewing the safety and tolerability of peripheral PN solutions, the osmolarity, dextrose concentration, and electrolyte concentrations must be reviewed. Excessive concentrations may be irritating to the vein into which the PN solution is being infused. Hyperosmolar solutions may cause vein collapse and/or infiltration/extravasation. Unlike dextrose solutions, all intravenous fat emulsions, regardless of concentration, are isotonic. Calcium concentrations must be considered for compatibility reasons, but they are dependent on solution pH, phosphate concentration, temperature, and other factors. They are not dependent on the route.

Answers

6. The answer is C (1.3.1)

A normal maintenance requirement for an adolescent male is around 0.8-1.5 g/kg. Answers A and B would provide too little protein for BT, and Answers D and E may provide too much. A 24-hour urine urea nitrogen collection may be helpful in determining BT's nitrogen balance and his true protein requirements.

7. The answer is E (1.3.2)

Patients with enterocutaneous fistulas often have difficulty absorbing nutrients. It is known that some patients may not be reabsorbing zinc (E) and could become deficient. Zinc deficiency is demonstrated as growth failure, diminished food intake, skin lesions, poor wound healing, hair loss, decreased protein synthesis, and deceased immune function. Supplementing above what is in the standard pediatric and/or adult trace element solution may be warranted. In patients with GI fistulae, zinc supplementation has been demonstrated to result in faster resolution of the fistula in addition to the above more general benefits. Aluminum (A) is a contaminant in parenteral nutrition solutions and has no physiologic role. In 2004, the FDA limited the amount of aluminum exposure of patients receiving parenteral nutrition of < 5 µg/kg/d.

8. The answer is B (2.2.1)

It will depend on where BT's fistula is located as to what would be the best replacement fluid. The concentration of fluid draining from the ileum is as follows: Sodium: 140 mEq/L (80-150), Potassium: 5 mEq/L (2-8), Chloride: 104 mEq/L (43-137), Bicarbonate: 30 mEq/L. Therefore, Solution B with 0.45 NS and 30 mEq/L sodium bicarbonate will yield approximately 107 mEq of Na/L, 77 mEq of Cl/L, and 30 mEq bicarbonate/L. These will ensure that the patient does not become depleted. The differences will be made up with appropriate TPN solution, with the minimal amount of potassium being lost. However, it is prudent to change the replacement fluid as laboratory values dictate and not change the TPN frequently, because of cost and workload issues. Dextrose 5% without electrolytes should not be used as a maintenance or replacement fluid because as its dextrose is metabolized, the fluid quickly becomes hypotonic. In fact, dextrose 5% is a good source of free water. As with other hypotonic fluids, water quickly shifts out of the vascular bed and into the cells by way of osmosis.

9. The answer is A (2.3.0)

Since the pediatric specialty formulations were developed for neonatal patients, they are not appropriate for this patient. He should be able to use a standard adult formulation, such as Answer A, a formulation available from B. Braun. Baxter and Hospira also make appropriate adult amino acid solutions. RenAmin (E) is expensive, does not include all amino acids, and is usually reserved for patients in renal dysfunction who require dialysis but cannot tolerate it (i.e., critical illness, severe hypotension). Similarly, Aminosyn-HF (D) is also expensive,

not all-inclusive, and is usually reserved for patients with hepatic dysfunction severe enough that encephalopathy has or could occur. The value of these specialty amino acid solutions is often debated, but standard amino acid solutions suffice for the majority of patients requiring PN.

10. The answer is E (1.3.2)

A common cause of megaloblastic anemia is folate deficiency. Folic acid deficiency is commonly associated with sulfasalazine therapy (E). The medication impairs hydrolysis of dietary intake of folic acid. Taking sulfasalazine between meals and supplementation with folic acid are strategies for preventing deficiency and, thus, megaloblastic anemia. Discontinuation of sulfasalazine is necessary if megaloblastic anemia occurs. The medication may be restarted when anemia is resolved, with close monitoring and efforts to prevent folic acid deficiency. The other answers are not associated with megaloblastic anemia.

Case 62 Pediatric ICU

1. The answer is E (1.2.7)

Vascular access is vital for administration of drugs, fluids, and blood products during a pediatric emergency. However, it is often difficult to achieve adequate access in pediatric patients. In emergent cases, the most accessible site, usually a peripheral venous line (B), must be used. In cases where IV access cannot be readily achieved, an intraosseous line (A) may provide much-needed access. Intraosseous lines are most often inserted in children under the age of 6, although they may be inserted in children and adults alike if the situation warrants. Intraosseus access may be achieved within 1-2 minutes by inserting a rigid, intraosseus or bone marrow needle into the anterior tibia. Alternate sites for insertion include the anterior superior iliac spine, distal femur, and medial malleolus. The intraosseus route is safe for administration of drugs, IV fluids, and blood products. In addition, blood samples may be drawn from this line. An umbilical artery catheter (C) is the preferred route of access in newborns requiring hemodynamic support. Central venous access (D) is usually established after a patient has been stabilized to provide secure access and central venous pressure monitoring. The intrathecal route (E) of administration involves the introduction of a pharmacologic agent directly into the cerebrospinal fluid by injection into the subarachnoid space of the spinal cord. The intrathecal route of administration is most commonly used for select chemotherapy agents, anesthesia, and pain management.

2. The answer is C (3.2.1)

Shock is a clinical state characterized by a significant reduction in tissue perfusion, resulting in oxygen delivery insufficient to meet metabolic demands. The underlying causes of shock are

Answers

often reversible, but if they are not corrected in a timely fashion, may result in irreversible end-organ damage. There are generally four main types of shock, each associated with distinct clinical and cardiovascular signs. Hypovolemic shock (A) is characterized by tachypnea with normal respiratory effort, normal breath sounds, tachycardia, decreased urine output, and a relatively normal level of consciousness. Cardiogenic shock (B) is characterized by tachypnea, increased respiratory effort, abnormal breath sounds (rales, grunting), tachycardia, thready pulses, poor skin perfusion (mottled, prolong capillary refill), lethargy or coma, and markedly decreased urine output. Septic shock (C) is characterized by tachypnea, normal or increased respiratory effort, normal breath sounds (crackles with pneumonia), tachypnea, bounding pulses early in shock followed by thready pulses later on, relatively normal skin perfusion, decreased urine output, and lethargy or coma. Neurogenic shock or distributive shock (D) occurs when a neurologic disturbance causes variation in the distribution of fluids, which may cause acidosis. Hypervolemic shock (E) does not exist. In BA's case, she has tachypnea, increased respiratory effort, crackles in the lungs, tachypnea, normal skin perfusion (pink, capillary refill less than 2 seconds), and coma. Her diagnosis is septic shock.

3. The answer is B (1.1.1)

Acid-base derangements are common in critically ill patients who are experiencing respiratory distress requiring ventilatory support. The first step in analyzing a patient's blood gas is to determine all abnormalities in pH, pCO_2, and bicarbonate. The second step is to calculate the anion gap (anion gap = [Na^+] - ([Cl^-] + [HCO_3^-]). This patient's pH is 7.15, indicating an acidemia is present. BA's pCO_2 is normal, but the bicarbonate level is low, indicating a metabolic acidosis (B) without compensation. The anion gap is 21, indicating an anion gap metabolic acidosis. The causes of an anion gap metabolic acidosis include ketoacidosis (diabetic, alcoholic, starvation), renal failure, drug intoxication (ethylene glycol, methanol, salicylates, paraldehyde), and lactic acidosis (diabetes, hepatic failure, drugs, CHF, and shock).

4. The answer is C (1.2.7)

Intravenous fluids for fluid resuscitation fall into two main categories: crystalloid solutions and colloid solutions. Crystalloids are aqueous solutions containing added electrolytes and minerals to approximate human plasma. Lactated Ringer's solution (A), 0.9% normal saline (B), 5% dextrose (D), 0.45% sodium chloride (E), and any combination of these solutions are considered crystalloids. Colloid solutions, like crystalloids, are also aqueous solutions containing electrolytes and minerals. However, colloids also contain large molecular weight substances that do not easily diffuse across a semipermeable membrane. Because of the added colloidal substances, colloids are able to maintain or improve colloid osmotic pressure. Examples of colloidal solutions include albumin, hetastarch, and Dextran (C). Crystalloid solutions are generally much less expensive than colloids. There continues to be great debate over whether crystalloids or colloids are safer and more efficacious in fluid resuscitation.

5. The answer is D (2.1.3)

The calculated drip rate is 0.38 mL/hour. 10 kg x 0.02 µg/kg/min = 0.2 µg/min = 0.012 mg/hour x bag concentration of 8 mg in 250 mL = 0.375 mL/hour rounded to 0.38 mL/hour.

6. The answer is D (3.2.1)

According to the Clinical Practice Parameters for Hemodynamic Support of Pediatric and Neonatal Septic Shock 2007 Update from the American College of Critical Care Medicine, dopamine (D) remains the preferred vasopressor for the treatment of pediatric fluid-refractory hypotensive shock. Dopamine, a precursor to norepinephrine, produces dose-dependent hemodynamic effects. Published studies provide evidence that patients treated with dopamine may experience worse outcomes than those treated with norepinephrine. However, until further studies indicate a clear advantage of norepinephrine over dopamine, dopamine remains the preferred agent in this setting. Fentanyl (A) is a potent pain medication often used in the ICU setting as a continuous infusion for sedation. Cisatracurium (B) is a neuromuscular blocker used for drug-induced paralysis for ventilated patients. Phenylephrine (C) is a potent vasopressor with weak beta-adrenergic activity. While phenylephrine improves blood pressure, its role in septic shock is limited due to its ability to reduce blood flow by increasing systemic vascular resistance. Ketamine (E) is generally used for sedation for invasive procedures. Ketamine releases endogenous catecholamines to help maintain blood pressure and heart rate. It can be used as a continuous infusion for sedation or analgesia in mechanically ventilated patients to help maintain cardiovascular stability.

7. The answer is C (1.2.2)

Dopamine produces dose-dependent hemodynamic effects. At doses of 0.5-2 µg/kg/min, dopamine stimulates dopaminergic receptors (A), resulting in renal and mesenteric vasodilation. The effect of dopamine at doses of 2-10 µg/kg/min is stimulation of $beta_1$-adrenergic receptors (B), resulting in a positive inotropic effect on myocardial tissue with increased cardiac output. Dopamine has no activity at $beta_2$ receptors (D). At high doses (greater than 10 µg/kg/dose), alpha-adrenergic receptors (C) are stimulated, resulting in increased peripheral resistance and renal vasoconstriction. This vasoconstriction results in increased systolic and diastolic blood pressures due to increased cardiac output and increased peripheral resistance. Omega-adrenergic receptors (E) do not exist.

8. The answer is C (1.3.2)

In order to accurately assess aminoglycoside drug levels, a number of things need to be closely evaluated. First, it is important to examine the timing of the drug samples (B, E) and their relation to dose administration (A, D), the duration of the infusion, and the site of infusion. If the sample is drawn from the same site as the drug infusion, it may lead to inappropriately high peak levels secondary to residual drug left in the line from the dose and picked up on sampling. Second, it is important to look at laboratory markers of infection, including temperature, heart rate, radiology results, and CRP. Finally, it is important to consider the patient's clinical status. You must treat the patient, not just the level. Aminoglycosides, including tobramycin, are renally eliminated, so monitoring of renal function would be more important than hepatic function monitoring (C).

9. The answer is A (1.2.6)

You are told in the question that BA's levels are accurate, which leads you to the conclusion that the levels were drawn from a site other than the site of infusion, the levels were drawn once the drug had reached steady state (usually the third dose with aminoglycosides), and the peak and trough levels were drawn appropriately in relation to the dose. This patient's laboratory markers of infection indicate that BA is still actively fighting pneumonia. In addition, her clinical markers of infection indicate her infection is still quite severe. Her trough level is within the desired range (less than 2), indicating the dosing interval of q8 h is appropriate at this time. In order to appropriately treat pneumonia, a higher peak level may be needed (often 8-10). In this case, it would be appropriate to recommend an increase in the dose (A) to achieve a higher peak level.

10. The answer is B (1.3.0)

Vecuronium is a nondepolarizing neuromuscular blocker that provides skeletal muscle relaxation during mechanical ventilation. The dose of vecuronium is usually titrated to achieve appropriate response, often measured with a peripheral nerve stimulator. All skeletal muscle is affected by this blockade, including the muscles in the eyelids. Because patients receiving neuromuscular blockade are not able to blink, the eyes may become very dry. As a result, artificial tears (B), often in combination with ocular lubricant ointment, are used on an as-needed basis to keep the eyes adequately hydrated. Medical restraints (A) are unnecessary for patients who are chemically paralyzed. Because neuromuscular blockers exhibit no effect on the nasal passages, saline nasal spray (C) is considered nonessential therapy. Patients who are mechanically ventilated and chemically paralyzed are unable to perform incentive spirometry (D). Physical therapy (E) may be considered once the patient has recovered from her acute insult, the paralyzing agent has been discontinued, and she is able to begin activity.

Case 63 Conjunctivitis

1. The answer is C (1.2.3)

Patanol (C) is an antihistamine. Xibrom (A) is an ophthalmic anti-inflammatory, Crolom (B) is a mast-cell stabilizer, Azopt (D) is a carbonic anhydrase inhibitor and Vigamox (E) is an ophthalmic antibiotic.

2. The answer is B (1.1.1)

Trifluridine, ketotifen and olopatadine are not used for bacterial infections. Blephamide contains sodium sulfacetamide and would not be appropriate for a patient with a sulfonamide allergy. Tobramycin is appropriate for some ophthalmic bacterial infections.

3. The answer is A (1.1.3)

Itching is the most common symptom of allergic conjunctivitis while irritation is typically most common in bacterial conjunctivitis. Bacterial and allergic conjunctivitis can be either acute or chronic. Bacterial conjunctivitis typically causes purulent discharge instead of allergic conjunctivitis. Neither type of conjunctivitis is associated with rash or typically causes headaches.

4. The answer is D (3.2.1)

Touching or rubbing the eye would aid transfer of infection if the patient doesn't immediately wash his/her hands. The other options help prevent the spread of pink eye.

5. The answer is C (2.2.2)

For bacterial conjunctivitis, also known as pink eye, antibiotic eye drops are required to treat the infection.

6. The answer is C (3.2.4)

Ketotifen would be most appropriate to treat allergic conjunctivitis.

7. The answer is E (1.1.3)

Conjunctivitis can be allergic, bacterial or viral.

8. The answer is D (1.1.3)

Iris color change is not a symptom of conjunctivitis. Itchy, red, watery eyes with a gritty feeling and crusting are symptoms of conjunctivitis.

9. The answer is B (1.1.2)

Blepharitis is inflammation of the eyelash follicles and acanthamoeba keratitis is a rare infection that inflames the cornea in some contact lens users.

10. The answer is E (2.2.5)

In children it is recommended that the child lie down comfortably and place the drops in the inner corner of the closed eyes. The child can slowly open their eyes allowing the drops to flow in. Excess liquid may be wiped away and light pressure may be applied to the inner corner of the eye to minimize drainage. Pulling down the lower lid and placing drops into the conjunctival sac (C) may be difficult in uncooperative children. The other options are not recommended drop administration techniques.

Answers

Case 64 Otitis Media Externa

1. The answer is E (1.1.2)

Otitis externa is also called swimmer's ear because it can occur in swimmers (or anyone else with prolonged contact with water). Earache usually refers to otitis media.

2. The answer is E (1.1.0)

Otitis externa affects all age groups.

3. The answer is A (1.2.4)

Ofloxacin otic solution is the only otic solution that is approved for use with a perforated tympanic membrane. Antipyrine-benzocaine (B) should be avoided if the tympanic membrane is ruptured. Ciprofloxacin-hydrocortisone (C) is contraindicated because it is non-sterile. Neomycin-hydrocortisone-polymyxin B (D) is contraindicated because it can cause ototoxicity, burning and stinging. Acetic acid solution (E) can cause burning and stinging when used with a perforated tympanic membrane.

4. The answer is B (1.3.3)

Topical antibiotics can sensitize the skin, resulting in a dermatitis, which may exacerbate the symptoms of otitis externa and/or interfere with healing.

5. The answer is D (3.2.3)

These are methods that facilitate prolonged contact of the solution with the affected areas of the ear canal and are particularly useful in small children who cannot/will not stay still. Warming the solution, usually by holding in hands for 1-2 minutes, does not increase the contact of the solution with the affected area but may help minimize dizziness that can occur from instillation of cold drops.

6. The answer is D (1.2.5)

Being a weak acid, acetic acid lowers the pH of the ear canal and creates a local medium that is unfavorable for the growth of organisms.

7. The answer is C (1.1.3)

Excessive cleaning, with cotton swabs for example, can injure the ear canal, making it more susceptible to maceration from water trapped by compacted cerumen, inflammation, and infection. A short ear canal (A) would make it more difficult for water to be trapped therefore decreasing the risk of acute otitis externa (AOE). Diabetes mellitus (B), family history (D) and history of perforated tympanic membrane (E) are not related to AOE.

8. The answer is A (3.2.4)

Chronic use of antibiotics (B or C) will only lead to drug resistance and possible drug hypersensitivity; corticosteroids (D) are only helpful in the presence of inflammation; and ear plugs (E) will work only if the patient adheres to meticulous aural hygiene.

9. The answer is C (1.1.2)

Malignant external otitis can be life threatening. Invasive external otitis (A) does not exist. Suppurative (B) means discharge or pus, which would not affect the surrounding tissues. Regional (D) means around the ear, but doesn't affect the surrounding tissues. Temporal (E) means near the temple on the head, but it isn't a diagnosis.

10. The answer is A (1.2.5)

Antipyrine helps to reduce the ear pain commonly associated with otitis externa.

Case 65 Acne

1. The answer is D (1.2.3)

Carbamazepine (Tegretol) is a strong inducer of several cytochrome P450 enzymes, including 3A4. It is also a major 3A4 substrate. Erythromycin both inhibits and is metabolized by 3A4 enzymes. This eliminates answers B and C. Erythromycin does not affect carbamazepine absorption (E). The most significant aspect of this drug interaction is that when erythromycin is added to a patient stable and therapeutic on carbamazepine, 3A4 will be inhibited, carbamazepine metabolism will slow, and carbamazepine levels will rise to toxic levels (D). Since the patient has been on the current dose of Tegretol for some time, carbamazepine's induction of 3A4 enzymes and effects on its own metabolism will have reached a steady state; erythromycin will throw off this balance. Since erythromycin is a 3A4 substrate and the patient on carbamazepine has more 3A4 enzyme than he otherwise would, one could argue that there is also a risk that a standard dose of erythromycin would be too low in a patient better able to metabolize it. But this would be a reduction in erythromycin efficacy, not a cause of toxicity (A).

2. The answer is B (1.1.3)

A comedo is a pore plugged by keratinocytes and sebum. In an open comedo, this plug is exposed to air at the pore opening, oxidizing and darkening it. Due to the dark plug, such a lesion is called a blackhead (B). In a closed comedo or whitehead, the pore opening is closed off, and the plug remains white (A). Comedones are non-inflammatory lesions. As the plug continues to grow, the pore lining may rupture and allow foreign material into the surrounding dermis, provoking an inflammatory response. Now containing pus, the lesion has become a pustule (E), an inflammatory lesion. A nodule is a large (e.g., greater than 1 cm in diameter) papule (raised lesion) (D).

3. The answer is A (1.3.3)

Most patients will experience at least some skin irritation from benzoyl peroxide (A). Intolerable irritation can be avoided by using a lower concentration product. Sensitive patients can also start out using a product qod and gradually increasing the application frequency to the qd or bid recommended. Benzoyl peroxide does not cause hepatotoxicity (B); allergic reactions, characterized by contact dermatitis (C), occur in approximately 1% of patients; benzoyl peroxide is not thought to significantly contribute to the risk of skin cancer (D); benzoyl peroxide may cause transient skin discoloration when used with a PABA-containing sunscreen, but not by itself (E).

4. The answer is E (1.2.3)

The antibacterial effects of clindamycin are complemented by the keratinolytic effects of benzoyl peroxide (E). Benzoyl peroxide's nonspecific antibacterial mechanism helps reduce the development of specific resistance to clindamycin. The combination, marketed as BenzaClin, has been shown to have greater effects than the individual agents. Adapalene and tretinoin have similar keratinolytic mechanisms of action and therefore are not synergistic (A). Salicylic acid, a weak keratinolytic agent, adds no advantages to azelaic acid or benzoyl peroxide monotherapy, both of which have antibacterial and keratinolytic effects (B, C). Clindamycin and erythromycin are both antibiotics, so they do not achieve the synergy obtained when therapy attacks multiple etiologies of acne (D).

5. The answer is D (1.2.2)

Differin (adapalene) is a topical retinoid most similar to tretinoin (D). Benzoyl peroxide (A) has no vitamin A properties; clindamycin (B), erythromycin (C), and tetracycline (E) are all antibiotics.

6. The answer is D (3.2.2)

Exposure to volatilized grease at his fast-food job may be the reason AD's acne has gotten worse over the last few months (D). Severe acne tends to run in families, but no family history is reported in AD's case (A). Despite the common belief to the contrary, greasy, high-fat foods have not been convincingly linked to acne in well-conducted trials (B). Acne vulgaris is common in all ethnic groups, possibly more common in whites than in African Americans or Asian Americans (C). While acne is more common in obese patients, at 5' 9" and 146 lb, AD's body mass index is only 21.6, well within the normal range (E).

7. The answer is C (2.2.5)

Jars of Benzamycin (benzoyl peroxide plus erythromycin) should be refrigerated after reconstitution. They should also be discarded 3 months after reconstitution. The Benzamycin Pak packets, however, do not require refrigeration. The other products do not require refrigeration: Ziana (clindamycin/tretinoin), Azelex (azelaic acid), Aczone (dapsone), and Epiduo (benzoyl peroxide/adapalene).

8. The answer is D (3.2.2)

For best results, topical treatments should be applied all over acne-prone areas, not only on lesions (D). Acne cannot be controlled until comedones and resulting inflammatory lesions are prevented from forming in the first place. Since it takes a month or so to turn over a new layer of skin, patients should allow at least 6 weeks before concluding a treatment is having no effect. However, AD has been using this regimen for several months, so he has allowed enough time for an adequate trial (A). Benzoyl peroxide is available over the counter in the same strengths it is available by prescription and would be expected at least to improve AD's acne, even if it could not control it alone (B). Acne is not caused by poor hygiene, and increasing use of the cleanser to twice a day, while acceptable, is unlikely to have dramatically more impact than daily cleansing (C). In fact, overly aggressive cleansing can needlessly aggravate the skin. Although it is a good idea to wait until skin has dried completely after cleansing to apply benzoyl peroxide or other treatments, salicylic acid does not specifically deactivate or affect the activity of benzoyl peroxide (E); in fact, combination products containing benzoyl peroxide and salicylic acid exist.

9. The answer is C (1.3.3)

Skin irritation is the most common adverse effect with topical therapies. Antibiotics are the least irritating topical treatments because they do not have keratinolytic effects. Clindamycin is the only treatment listed without keratinolytic effects (C). As for the others, Azelex (azelaic acid) is less irritating than benzoyl peroxide or tretinoin. The Retin-A Micro formulation of tretinoin is less irritating than formulations in plain vehicles. Tazorac (tazarotene) is generally a more irritating retinoid than tretinoin.

10. The answer is A (2.2.5)

A pledget is an absorbent cloth pad used to apply medication, remove exudate, or dress a wound.

Case 66 Rosacea

1. The answer is D (3.2.1)

It is important for patients with rosacea to avoid triggers for skin flushing, such as sun, heat, cold, wind, emotional upset, alcohol, and spicy foods (D). Therefore, heating or treating the face with steam would be counterproductive (C). Astringents or toners will not help and can actually further irritate the skin (A). Weight (B) and intake of high glycemic load foods (E) are not associated with rosacea.

2. The answer is D (3.2.2)

Patients with rosacea have sensitive skin and should avoid any potential irritants. Exfoliating scrubs offer no benefit—the disorder is not one of excessive or abnormal keratinization—and can needlessly traumatize and irritate the skin (D). Op-

Answers

tions A, B, and C, however, should be encouraged. Protecting the skin from burning is important, and NC should routinely use a sunscreen with sun protection factor (SPF) at least 15 and broad-spectrum ultraviolet (UV)-A as well as UV-B protection (A). A mild cleanser such as Cetaphil will keep the skin clean without stripping protective oils or introducing irritants (B). Moisturizing the skin when needed will help it not become further irritated by dryness (C). When selecting sunscreens, cleansers, and moisturizers, NC should choose gentle, noncomedogenic products free of perfumes, alcohol, and dyes to avoid doing more harm than good. Sertraline should not affect NC's rosacea (E).

3. The answer is C (1.1.3)

Thickening and deformity of the nose associated with rosacea is known as the phymatous presentation (C). This is a commonly recognized form, not atypical (B). Other recognized presentations include papulopustular (A), characterized by erythematous papules and pustules; erythematotelangiectatic (D), characterized by erythema and telangiectasia (chronically dilated superficial capillaries); and ocular, a presentation including blepharitis (inflamed eyelids) and conjunctivitis. The category of glandular rosacea (E) has also been proposed (Crawford GH et al. J *Am Acad Dermatol* Sep 2004; 51(3):327-41). This presentation includes papules, pustules, and even nodules resulting from hyperplasia of sebaceous glands of the face; patients lack the increased skin sensitivity most rosacea patients have.

4. The answer is B (1.1.3)

Telangiectasia is chronic dilation of superficial skin capillaries, producing red spider-like clusters or linear patterns of visible small blood vessels.

5. The answer is E (1.2.2)

Tetracycline antibiotics, including doxycycline, exert anti-inflammatory effects, such as reducing neutrophil chemotaxis and inhibiting cytokines, that are as or more important than their antibiotic effects in treating rosacea and acne vulgaris (E). Rosacea is not an infectious disease, and the role of *Demodex* mites is unclear. Although rosacea patients have higher *Demodex* populations than controls, effective treatments do not affect mite populations and reduction of mite populations does not effect treatment (A, B, D). Oracea is approved for use as monotherapy (C).

6. The answer is C (1.2.5)

The least irritating treatment listed is metronidazole cream (C). Topical antibiotics are less irritating than azelaic acid (B), the retinoid adapalene (D), or benzoyl peroxide (E). Creams are less drying and therefore less irritating for NC than gels or solutions, eliminating clindamycin solution (A) and further discounting answers B and D.

7. The answer is B (3.2.1)

Male gender (B) is not a risk factor for rosacea; overall, rosacea may be more prevalent in women, although the phymatous subtype is more common in men. Middle age is a risk factor (A); the condition is usually worst between the ages of 30 and 60. Fair-skinned people with light hair and eye color (C) are at higher risk, although darker-skinned people can get rosacea as well. A tendency to blush easily (D) is associated with development of rosacea. Lastly, although one cannot assume that patients with rosacea drink alcohol, it is true that alcohol consumption causes flushing and thus tends to exacerbate rosacea (E).

8. The answer is E (1.1.3)

Rosacea, unlike acne, does not feature comedones (clogged pores) (E). In general, rosacea, not acne, features persistent erythema (not just erythematous papules or pustules) and telangiectasia (chronically dilated superficial capillaries) (D). Acne has no known positive or negative correlation with rosacea later in life (A, B). Both rosacea and acne usually require maintenance therapy to maintain improvements realized with drug therapy (C).

9. The answer is D (1.2.1)

Finacea, azelaic acid gel, is FDA-approved to treat rosacea (D); Azelex, azelaic acid cream, is not (although it is used for this purpose off-label). The mechanism of action of azelaic acid is unclear, but it seems to normalize skin cell keratinization and reduce inflammation, two actions that could improve rosacea. Tazorac (A) contains tazarotene, a retinoid indicated for acne and psoriasis, which normalizes skin cell differentiation and keratinization and reduces inflammation. Cleocin T (B) contains the antibiotic clindamycin, which is sometimes used off-label for rosacea. Protopic (C) is tacrolimus ointment, a calcineurin inhibitor decreasing T-lymphocyte activation, indicated for moderate-to-severe atopic dermatitis. DUAC (E) contains benzoyl peroxide, indicated for acne, and clindamycin.

10. The answer is C (1.3.1)

Pharmacotherapy for rosacea provides the most benefit in resolving inflammatory lesions such as papules and pustules. Erythema (redness) and telangiectasia (chronically dilated superficial capillaries) are less affected. (This is why erythematotelangiectatic presentations usually improve little with available treatments.) Improvement is gradual and should not be assessed until at least 4-6 weeks into therapy. Rosacea is a chronic condition that waxes and wanes; patients usually need maintenance therapy.

Case 67 Psoriasis

1. The answer is E (1.2.7)

Acute flare-ups of the nature described in this patient are best managed initially with a high-potency topical corticosteroid such as Lidex (fluocinonide). The ointment form is occlusive and offers better drug penetration for the thickened plaques and relatively thick-skinned body areas involved (E). Anthralin cream (A) will not likely be as effective in the short term, nor does the cream offer as much drug penetration. Dovonex (calcipotriene) (B) is best reserved for maintenance therapy for mild-to-moderate psoriasis. Elidel (pimecrolimus) (C) is not indicated for psoriasis; its off-label use is not first-line therapy. Hydrocortisone (D) is too low-potency for this patient, given the areas of skin involvement and severity; furthermore, ointment would be a better choice.

2. The answer is A (1.3.3)

With extended use, high-potency topical corticosteroid therapy may cause skin atrophy that results in striae (A). The effect has been observed after as few as 3 weeks of therapy with a very high-potency agent in a thin-skinned or otherwise highly absorptive area. Paradoxical exacerbation known as "rebound flare" may occur with abrupt withdrawal of potent topical corticosteroid therapy but not during use (B). Skin sensitization (C) would be an idiosyncratic and unusual patient reaction rather than a predictable result of excessively long therapy. Hyperpigmentation (D) and hypoesthesia (reduced sensation (E)) are also not observed, although hypopigmentation can be.

3. The answer is E (1.1.3)

Unlike the other disorders, psoriasis commonly appears at the sites of former trauma (Koebner's phenomenon). Scale, pruritus, and involvement of the scalp are common to psoriasis and seborrheic dermatitis, although the latter often has a more yellowish scale than the silvery scale seen in psoriasis. Erythema and pruritus are common to psoriasis and atopic dermatitis (eczema), as is the importance of maintaining adequate skin hydration with emollients.

4. The answer is A (1.2.1)

PUVA therapy, used in severe psoriasis, calls for patients to apply methoxsalen topically if plaques are confined to a small portion of the body surface area, or to take it by mouth if plaques are widespread (the "P" stands for psoralen). The patient is then exposed to UV-A light, which excites the psoralen molecules to form toxic activated compounds. Although controlled doses of UV-B light have been used with coal tar therapy, patients using coal tars are generally counseled to avoid sunlight exposure due to the increased risk of photosensitivity. Also, coal tars are used only topically, not systemically. Calcipotriene is also solely a topical therapy. Adalimumab and methotrexate are usually reserved for severe, refractory plaques or for patients with manifestations in the joints or nails; they are not used in conjunction with UV light.

5. The answer is C (1.1.4)

Beta blockers may trigger psoriasis, as can lithium. Angiotensin-converting-enzyme (ACE) inhibitors and nonsteroidal anti-inflammatory drugs (NSAIDs) have also been implicated.

6. The answer is C (3.2.2)

Only diet (C) has no known or suspected effect on psoriasis. Exposure to ultraviolet light in sunlight may improve psoria-

sis (A); however, sunbathing is not prescribed and exposure to controlled doses at the dermatologist's office is preferred. Stress (B); dyes, fragrances, and other irritants in skin products (D); and cold weather (E) can all exacerbate psoriasis.

7. The answer is D (2.2.1)

AmLactin (D) contains ammonium lactate, a keratinolytic that breaks up thickened skin and allows drugs and moisture to penetrate more easily. Campho-Phenique (A) contains camphor and phenol, counterirritants that relieve itch by causing mild additional irritation to counter it. However, as they are irritating by nature, they are poor choices to apply to sensitive psoriatic skin. Caladryl (B) contains calamine, a protectant/astringent, and pramoxine, a local anesthetic. Eucerin (C) is a moisturizer. Cortaid (E) contains hydrocortisone.

8. The answer is B (1.2.2)

Dovonex (calcipotriene) is a vitamin D analog that slows skin cell hyperproliferation (B). Tazarotene (e.g., Tazorac and Avage brands) is a synthetic retinoid (A), which also slows hyperproliferation and normalizes keratinization. Coal tars are antimitotic agents (C). Calcineurin inhibitors (D) such as pimecrolimus (Elidel) and tacrolimus (Protopic) reduce the autoimmune response. Keratinolytics (E) such as lactic acid and urea help break up thickened plaques to promote moisturization and drug penetration.

9. The answer is D (1.3.2)

Because it may take 48 hours for full evidence of phototoxicity to appear, treatments should be spaced at least 48 hours apart (D). Due to risks of cataracts, squamous cell skin cancer, and melanoma, patients should not receive more than 200 PUVA treatments over a lifetime (A). Once treatment response is established, treatment frequency can be reduced from 3 treatments per week to 1-2 per week (B). Generating erythema is not a goal of therapy or marker of adequate therapy intensity (C); rather, patients should protect their skin from any ultraviolet light exposure beyond the treatment, avoiding sunbathing or sun exposure through windows. Response to therapy is assessed by reduction of the psoriatic plaques. Patients do not have to discontinue therapy if there is no response after 10 treatments (E); instead, the intensity of UV-A light applied may be increased.

10. The answer is D (3.2.3)

Aloe (D) may soothe psoriatic plaques and improve their appearance if used regularly for several weeks. Zinc (A) can safely be taken orally in reasonable doses but does not improve psoriasis. Colloidal silver (B), while historically used for psoriasis, can cause bluish discoloration or hyperpigmentation when applied topically and should not be used. Pregnenolone (C), a steroid precursor, has been touted for psoriasis, but the risk of taking this pro-hormone outweighs the unproven benefit. Gotu kola (E) has been used topically, not orally, to treat psoriasis, but the evidence supporting this use is scant.

Answers

Case 68 Cardiac Transplantation

1. The answer is C (3.2.1)

Adults exposed to second-hand smoke have an increased risk for heart disease (A) and lung cancer (B). Infants exposed to second-hand smoke in utero or after birth have an increased risk for sudden infant death syndrome (D). Even brief exposure to second-hand smoke can increase the risk for smoking-related diseases (E). Diabetes mellitus has not been linked to exposure to second-hand smoke (C).

CDC website on second-hand smoke. www.cdc.gov/tobacco/data_statistics/fact_sheets/secondhand_smoke/health_effects/index.htm (accessed 2010 Jul 27).

2. The answer is A (3.2.2)

Both behavioral and medication therapies have been shown to help with smoking cessation. Examples of non-drug therapies include individual or group counseling (D) and behavioral cessation therapies (E). Some medications to treat nicotine dependence include Zyban (bupropion) (B) and Chantix (varenicline) (C). Amitriptyline (A) is not commonly used for smoking cessation.

1. CDC website on smoking cessation. www.cdc.gov/tobacco/data_statistics/fact_sheets/cessation/quitting/index.htm#methods (accessed 2010 Jul 27).

2. CDC website on smoking cessation. www.cdc.gov/tobacco/data_statistics/fact_sheets/secondhand_smoke/general_facts/index.htm#adults (accessed 2010 Jul 27).

3. The answer is C (1.1.1)

The pack-year history is calculated by multiplying the number of packs per day by the total years smoked. The patient smoked half-a-pack for 20 years, so (0.5 X 20) is a 10-year pack history (C). Another formula for pack-year history is (# cigarettes smoked in 1 day) X (years smoking)/20.

Smoking pack years. www.smokingpackyears.com (accessed 2010 Jul 27).

4. The answer is A (1.3.3)

Corticosteroids (A) increase the risk for gastrointestinal ulcers by decreasing the protective mucous lining of the stomach. The other transplant medications (B, C, D, E) are not commonly associated with gastrointestinal ulcers.

KS Schonder, HJ Johnson. Solid organ transplantation. In: JT DiPiro, ed. *Pharmacotherapy: A Pathophysiologic Approach*, 7th edition. McGraw-Hill Co., Inc.; 2008: 1459-82.

5. The answer is D (1.2.1)

Micafungin (A), itraconazole (B), posaconazole (C), and voriconazole (E) either have FDA-labeled or unlabeled indications for treating *Aspergillus* infections. Fluconazole does not have clinical activity for treating *Aspergillus*.

ES Dodds Ashley, R Lewis, JS Lewis, C Martin, D Andes. Pharmacology of systemic antifungal agents. CID 2006; 43:S28-S39.

6. The answer is C (1.3.3)

Tacrolimus (C) is associated with certain neurotoxicities including hand tremors. The remaining medications (A, B, D, E) are not commonly associated with this side effect.

1. KS Schonder, HJ Johnson. Solid organ transplantation. In: JT DiPiro, ed. *Pharmacotherapy: A Pathophysiologic Approach*, 7th edition. McGraw-Hill Co., Inc.; 2008: 1459-82.

2. Sporanox (itraconazole solution) package insert. Janssen Pharmaceutica N.V., September 2003.

7. The answer is C (1.2.3)

Nonsteroidal anti-inflammatory drugs (NSAIDs) such as indomethacin inhibit prostaglandin synthesis, resulting in renal arteriolar vasoconstriction, which may increase the risk for nephrotoxicity in patients taking calcineurin inhibitors such as tacrolimus (C). Therefore, it is not recommended to use the two agents concomitantly.

Lexi-Comp Online Interaction Monograph. Lexi-Comp, Inc. Accessed on 7/27/2010.

8. The answer is B (1.3.3)

Both calcineurin inhibitors, such as tacrolimus, and corticosteroids (B) can increase the risk for post-transplant diabetes mellitus. Mycophenolate mofetil (A, C), valganciclovir (D, E), and itraconazole (E) are not commonly associated with increased diabetes risk.

1. KS Schonder, HJ Johnson. Solid organ transplantation. In: JT DiPiro, ed. *Pharmacotherapy: A Pathophysiologic Approach*, 7th edition. McGraw-Hill Co., Inc.; 2008: 1459-82.

2. Sporanox (itraconazole solution) package insert. Janssen Pharmaceutica N.V., September 2003.

9. The answer is B (1.3.2)

The formula for ideal body weight (IBW) in men is IBW = 50 kg + (2.3) X (height in inches greater than 60 inches). The patient's height is 67 inches, so 50 + (7) X (2.3) = 66 kg (B).

TD Dowling. Quantification of renal function. In: JT DiPiro, ed. *Pharmacotherapy: A Pathophysiologic Approach*, 7th edition. McGraw-Hill Co., Inc.; 2008: 714.

10. The answer is A (1.3.2)

The patient's actual body weight is not more than 30% greater than his ideal body weight. Therefore, his actual body weight can be used to calculate his creatinine clearance (CrCl). The patient's CrCl is estimated to be 90 mL/min using the Cockcroft and Gault formula. Valganciclovir requires renal adjustment when the CrCl is estimated to be less than 60 mL/min. Since the patient's CrCl does not require renal adjustment, the regular dose of 900 mg PO daily or the full dose center-specific protocol should be recommended. Therefore, Choice A is the correct answer.

1. TD Dowling. Quantification of renal function. In: JT DiPiro, ed. *Pharmacotherapy: A Pathophysiologic Approach*, 7th edition. McGraw-Hill Co., Inc.; 2008: 714.

2. Valcyte (valganciclovir) package insert. Genetech USA Inc.; November 2009.

Answers

Case 69 Renal Transplantation

1. The answer is C (1.3.3)

Sirolimus (C) increases the risk for elevated total cholesterol and triglycerides. Mycophenolate (A), ranitidine (B), tacrolimus (D), and valganciclovir (E) do not commonly cause elevations in cholesterol or triglycerides.

Rapamune (sirolimus) package insert. Wyeth Pharmaceuticals, Inc.; April 2010.

2. The answer is D (1.2.3)

Tacrolimus is metabolized via cytochrome P450 3A4 (CYP3A4). Cimetidine (A) and grapefruit juice (C) are CYP3A4 inhibitors, and St. John's wort (B) is a CYP3A4 inducer. Therefore, all three of these options could alter the tacrolimus blood concentration. Nonsteroidal anti-inflammatory drugs (NSAIDs) such as ibuprofen (E) inhibit prostaglandin synthesis, thereby increasing the risk for nephrotoxicity in patients taking calcineurin inhibitors. Therefore, it is not recommended to use the agents concomitantly. Apple juice (D) has no interactions with tacrolimus.

1. Prograf (tacrolimus) package insert. Astellas Pharma U.S., Inc.; August 2009

2. Lexi-Comp Online Interaction Monograph. Lexi-Comp, Inc. Accessed on 7/27/2010.

3. The answer is B (1.3.3)

Sirolimus (B) can cause mouth ulcers in transplant recipients. Valganciclovir (A), mycophenolate (C), tacrolimus (D), and prednisone (E) are not commonly associated with this adverse event.

Rapamune (sirolimus) package insert. Wyeth Pharmaceuticals, Inc.; April 2010.

4. The answer is D (1.2.5)

Sirolimus is dosed once daily based on the half-life of the drug (D) (mean half-life = 62 hours). Sirolimus requires therapeutic drug monitoring to target a specific blood concentration (B), can cause impaired wound healing (A) and peripheral edema (C), and may have better compliance as a once daily drug (E); however, these factors do not alter the indicated dosage interval.

1. Rapamune (sirolimus) package insert. Wyeth Pharmaceuticals, Inc.; April 2010.

2. Lexi-Comp Online Database. Lexi-Comp, Inc. Accessed on 7/27/2010.

5. The answer is C (1.1.2)

Serum creatinine (SCr) (A), blood urea nitrogen (BUN) (B), the urine chemical analysis (D), and creatinine clearance (CrCl) (E) all help determine and distinguish the variations of renal insufficiency. The alanine aminotransferase (ALT) (C) is an enzyme measured in the blood that helps assess liver function, so it is not used to assess renal function.

TD Dowling. Quantification of renal function. In: JT DiPiro, ed.

Pharmacotherapy: A Pathophysiologic Approach, 7th edition. McGraw-Hill Co., Inc.; 2008: 705-22.

6. The answer is B (3.1.2)

Absolute risk reduction describes the difference between the incidence rate of an outcome for two treatment arms, the experimental group and control group. CMV disease occurred in 6% of recipients in the valganciclovir group versus 23% in the ganciclovir group. Therefore, 0.23 minus 0.06 is 0.17 or 17% (B), the absolute risk reduction between treatment agents.

1. C Paya, A Humar, E Dominguez et al. Efficacy and safety of valganciclovir vs. oral ganciclovir for prevention of cytomegalovirus disease in solid organ transplant recipients. *AJT*. 2004; 4:611-20.

2. Summarizing data and presenting data in tables and graphs. In: B Dawson, ed. *Basic and Clinical Biostatistics*, 3rd edition. Lange Medical Books/McGraw-Hill Co., Inc.; 2001: 53.

7. The answer is E (3.1.2)

The number-needed-to-treat (NNT) describes the number of patients needing to be on the experimental agent to prevent one patient from having the specified outcome. It is equal to the inverse of the absolute risk reduction (0.17). Therefore, 1 divided by 0.17 is equal to 5.88. Rounding to the nearest whole number without exceeding the calculated NNT shows that 5 patients (E) need to be on valganciclovir prophylaxis to prevent one patient from developing CMV disease.

1. C Paya, A Humar, E Dominguez et al. Efficacy and safety of valganciclovir vs. oral ganciclovir for prevention of cytomegalovirus disease in solid organ transplant recipients. *AJT*. 2004; 4:611-20.

2. Summarizing data and presenting data in tables and graphs. In: B Dawson, ed. *Basic and Clinical Biostatistics*, 3rd edition. Lange Medical Books/McGraw-Hill Co., Inc.; 2001: 53.

8. The answer is E (3.1.2)

The relative risk reduction describes the incidence rate difference for an outcome between an experimental and control group relative to the incidence of the outcome in the control group. It is equal to the absolute risk reduction divided by the incidence in the control group. CMV disease occurred in 6% of recipients in the valganciclovir group versus 23% in the ganciclovir group. Therefore, the relative risk reduction for CMV disease for patients taking valganciclovir was $(0.23 - 0.06)/(0.23) = 0.739$ or roughly 74% (E).

1. C Paya, A Humar, E Dominguez et al. Efficacy and safety of valganciclovir vs. oral ganciclovir for prevention of cytomegalovirus disease in solid organ transplant recipients. *AJT*. 2004; 4:611-20.

2. Summarizing data and presenting data in tables and graphs. In: B Dawson, ed. *Basic and Clinical Biostatistics*, 3rd edition. Lange Medical Books/McGraw-Hill Co., Inc.; 2001: 53.

9. The answer is A (3.2.1)

Renal transplant recipients 1 to 6 months after transplant are at risk for developing opportunistic infections (B) from bacterial, fungal, protozoal, or viral pathogens. One such example is polyomavirus infection (C). During this time period they are also at risk for reactivating donor-derived (D) or recipient-derived (E) latent infections. The risk for wound infections (A)

Answers

from the transplant surgery is more common within the first month after transplant.

JA Fishman. Infection in solid organ transplant recipients. *N Engl J Med.* 2007; 357:2601-14.

10. The answer is D (1.2.2)

Sirolimus and everolimus are immunosuppressants classified as mammalian target of rapamycin (mTOR) inhibitors (D).

KS Schonder, HJ Johnson. Solid organ transplantation. In: JT DiPiro, ed. *Pharmacotherapy: A Pathophysiologic Approach*, 7th edition. McGraw-Hill Co., Inc.; 2008: 1459-82.

Case 70 Geriatric Dementias

1. The answer is A (1.1.3)

Symptoms of Alzheimer's disease include memory loss (A), dysphagia, dyspraxia, disorientation, impaired calculation, and impaired judgment. Behavioral symptoms may include personality changes, anxiety, and mood disorders. Tremor (B), hallucinations (C), shuffling gait (D), and acute onset (E) are not characteristic of Alzheimer's type dementia.

2. The answer is E (1.1.1)

Various disease states can present themselves as dementia in the elderly with symptoms such as confusion and decreased cognition. These should be ruled out before a diagnosis of dementia can be made because they may be treatable.

3. The answer is A (1.2.2)

The mechanism of Aricept's action is theorized to be an enhancement of cholinergic function. This is likely due to a reversible inhibition of acetylcholinesterase, which is an enzyme that breaks down acetylcholine.

4. The answer is B (1.2.4)

Temazepam (Restoril) is a benzodiazepine. These drugs have been associated with causing confusion and disorientation. The elderly may be at increased risk for this. Additional side effects include hallucinations and somnolence. It is most often used for its sedative/hypnotic effects. Confusion and disorientation are not reported with Aricept or vitamin E. Aricept has been reported to be associated with many other CNS side effects such as gastrointestinal distress, hypersalivation, bradycardia, insomnia, dizziness, aphasia, ataxia, restlessness, and abnormal dreams. CNS side effects reported with vitamin E include dizziness and headache.

5. The answer is C (1.2.1)

Antipsychotic medications are useful for extreme symptoms such as physical aggression, extreme agitation, hallucinations, and hostility. Thus, there is a role for antipsychotic drug therapy in some Alzheimer's dementia patients. Because CC does not demonstrate these symptoms, antipsychotic therapy (A) would

not yet be recommended. None of the symptoms that CC exhibits (disorientation, confusion, memory loss, and tremor) are likely to respond to antipsychotic therapy. Thus, answer B is incorrect, and answer (C is correct. The FDA requires a black-box warning on Risperdal regarding a potential increased risk of cardiac events when used in elderly dementia patients. Thus, answer (D is incorrect. Geodon has been associated with QT prolongation and the manufacturer recommends a baseline ECG prior to initiating therapy.

6. The answer is A (1.1.2)

The HamD exam (B) assesses presence or severity of depression not dementia. The ECG (C) measures electrical cardiac conduction, which is not a predictor or indicator of dementia. The CT (D) may identify a potential origin of the cognitive impairment, but doesn't evaluate for the presence of cognitive impairment. The GCS (E) is a neurological scale that measures the level of consciousness, not cognitive impairment.

7. The answer is A (1.1.4)

The exact etiology of dementia and Alzheimer's disease (AD) is unknown. Theories include genetics (alterations on chromosome 1, 14 or 21) and/or environmental factors (stroke, alcohol abuse, head trauma). CC himself does not have a history of stroke (E). Although AD appears to be idiopathic, some families have several members afflicted with the disease as appears to be the case with CC (A). He does not and has not used alcohol, so his social history (D) does not have any significant findings known to increase risk of AD. Hyperlipidemia (B) and hyperkalemia (C) have not been linked to AD.

8. The answer is D (3.2.2)

Caregiver "burn-out" is very common among first-line providers caring for a loved one with Alzheimer's disease. Self-care is important to the caregiver as much as to the patient. Exercise, weekly outings, support groups, private counseling sessions, and remembering past events with the patient can all mitigate the frustration with caring for the patient alone. Discussing past familial events with the patient may provide comfort to the patient and caregiver, depending upon the severity of Alzheimer's disease.

9. The answer is C (1.3.3)

Dry mouth (A) would not be expected because cholinesterase inhibitors inhibit the breakdown of acetylcholine and therefore cause procholinergic effects such as diarrhea (C) rather than anticholinergic effects such as dry mouth and constipation. Other side effects include nausea, insomnia, vomiting, muscle cramps, and anorexia. Cholinesterase inhibitors are not associated with cough (B), thrombocytopenia (D), or hypokalemia (E).

10. The answer is A (3.2.3)

The combination of aspirin and gingko biloba may result in additive adverse drug reactions. Gingko (A) has been associated with such bleeding events as subdural hematoma and subarachnoid hemorrhage. In an additional case report, a patient on only aspirin and gingko experienced bleeding from the iris into the anterior chamber of the eye. These suggest additive adverse effects with the combination of aspirin and gingko. Selenium (C), glucosamine (B), saw palmetto (D), and green tea (E) have not been reported to cause problems when combined with CC's other medications.

Case 71 Benign Prostatic Hyperplasia

1. The answer is D (1.1.2)

RB presents with the symptoms of urinary hesitancy (II) and enlarged rubbery prostate (III). The most commonly associated symptoms of benign prostatic hypertrophy are abdominal tenderness and enlarged, firm, and rubbery prostate. Patients may also present with an enlarged bladder and urinary retention. Urinary hesitancy may also be accompanied by a decrease in urinary force, stream interruption, postvoiding dribbling, and sensations of the bladder not fully emptying. A normal PSA (<4 ng/mL) is usually present. However it can be elevated in BPH even if there is no indication of carcinoma. Hypertension (I) does not play a role in BPH.

2. The answer is B (1.1.3)

Urinary stents are not used in the initial treatment of BPH (A). Watchful waiting, which is close observation of the patient without interventions, is effective in 42% of patients (B). Fluid and salt restriction (C), diet and exercise (D), and physical therapy (E) have no role in BPH treatment.

3. The answer is C (1.2.2)

Transurethral prostatectomy (TURP) (C) is an acceptable and readily performed treatment for BPH. It has been shown to provide clinical improvement of symptoms in nearly 90% of patients. TURP is considered the gold standard of BPH treatment—the one against which other therapeutic measures are compared. More than 90% of simple prostatectomies for BPH are performed transurethrally by TURP. TURP involves removal of tissue from the inner portion of the prostate with a long, thin instrument called a resectoscope, which is passed through the urethra into the bladder. A wire loop attached to the end of the resectoscope cuts away prostate tissue and seals blood vessels with an electric current. The loose bits of tissue are collected in the bladder and flushed out of the body through the resectoscope. A sample of this tissue is sent to the laboratory to be examined for prostate cancer. The procedure is typically performed under general or spinal anesthesia. In carefully selected cases (patients with no medical problems and smaller prostates), TURP may be done as an outpatient procedure. Improvement in symptoms is noticeable almost immediately after surgery, and is greatest in those with the worst symptoms. Marked improvement occurs in about 93% of men with

severe symptoms and in about 80% of those with moderate symptoms—a likelihood of improvement that is significantly better than that achieved with medication or watchful waiting. Also, more than 95% of men who undergo TURP require no further treatment over the next 5 years. Hormone therapy is not utilized at this early stage of the disease (A, B, D). Radiation therapy is only used after a diagnosis of cancer (E).

4. The answer is B (1.2.2)

Alpha-1-adrenergic blockers have efficacy in BPH because of the relaxation of smooth muscle in the bladder neck, prostate capsule, and prostatic urethra.

5. The answer is A (1.1.4)

Coffee, alcohol, and other fluids should be avoided after dinner to prevent nocturnal urination (A). Increasing fluid will require more urination (B). Avoiding smoked meats and cheeses may help prevent issues with MAOIs, but not in BPH (C). Low purine diets may reduce the occurrence of gout, but not BPH (D). Reducing refined sugar intake may help carbohydrate metabolism, but not BPH (E).

6. The answer is D (1.2.4)

Of the drugs listed above, tamsulosin has no effect on blood pressure. Since RB has hypertension and is noncompliant, it would be advantageous to treat both conditions with one medication that can be given only once or twice a day.

7. The answer is A (1.3.1)

TURP and prostatectomy are considered the most effective surgical interventions for BPH. Finasteride is also used to treat benign prostatic hypertrophy (BPH). Finasteride can shrink the prostate and relieve symptoms. The accumulating information on finasteride treatment of BPH is giving more clear indications of which men can benefit (those with prostate volumes >40 mL), and that the benefits seen in 1-year studies continue at least to 2 years. Finasteride seems to have less positive responses with smaller enlargements of the prostate. This patient does not have a grossly enlarged prostate and the efficacy of finasteride would be questionable.

8. The answer is C (3.2.1)

The major adverse effect of alpha-1-adrenergic blockers is hypotension. This is why it is recommended that the first dose be given at bedtime.

9. The answer is E (1.1.2)

TURP, the gold standard of effective treatment for BPH, involves removal of the core of the prostate using an instrument passed through the urethra. High-frequency current flowing through a wire loop allows removal of chips of prostatic tissue and coagulation of blood vessels. The prostate tissue is removed through the cystoscope used to visually guide and monitor this process. Patients require a urethral catheter for 2 days and usually stay in the hospital for 2 days. Most patients

Answers

(80%-90%) experience dramatic improvement in their symptoms and urinary flow rates after TURP. Possible side effects include bleeding requiring transfusion, salt imbalances from fluid absorption, impotence (less than 5%), bladder neck contractures that develop over time (3%), and urinary incontinence (1%-2%).

10. The answer is B (2.2.3)

No dosage adjustment is necessary in the elderly. Although the elimination rate of finasteride is decreased in the elderly, these findings are of no clinical significance. No dosage adjustment is necessary in patients with renal insufficiency. In patients with chronic renal impairment, with creatinine clearances ranging from 9.0 to 55 mL/min, AUC, maximum plasma concentration, half-life, and protein binding after a single dose of 14C-finasteride were similar to values obtained in healthy volunteers. Urinary excretion of metabolites was decreased in patients with renal impairment. This decrease was associated with an increase in fecal excretion of metabolites. Plasma concentrations of metabolites were significantly higher in patients with renal impairment (based on a 60% increase in total radioactivity AUC). However, finasteride has been well tolerated in BPH patients with normal renal function receiving up to 80 mg/day for 12 weeks, where exposure of these patients to metabolites would presumably be much greater. The effect of hepatic insufficiency on finasteride pharmacokinetics has not been studied. Caution should be used in the administration of finasteride in those patients with liver function abnormalities, as finasteride is metabolized extensively in the liver. The study of 15 healthy young subjects, the mean bioavailability of finasteride 5-mg tablets was 63% (range 34%-108%), based on the ratio of area under the curve relative to an intravenous reference dose. Maximum finasteride plasma concentration averaged 37 ng/mL (range, 27-49 ng/mL) and was reached 1-2 hours postdose. Bioavailability of finasteride was not affected by food.

Case 72 Neurogenic Bladder

1. The answer is B (3.2.2)

Urinary tract infections are one of the most common complications of neurogenic bladder. Patients need to void frequently through out the day to avoid retaining urine and change indwelling catheters frequently. Smoking is not proven to make symptoms worse.

2. The answer is C (1.1.4)

All other choices are possible causes of neurogenic bladder. The term neurogenic bladder describes a process of dysfunctional voiding as the result of neurologic injury.

3. The answer is C (3.2.2)

Frequent voiding is important to avoid complications. If medications don't work or if patients cannot tolerate their side effects, intermittent catherization is an effective way to deal with neurogenic bladder. Patients like RJ should avoid situations that increase her bladder volume as she has a problem with urinary retention. It is suggested that these patients should limit their water intake to less than 2 liters a day and if they are diabetic, avoid high blood sugars as it can cause osmotic diuresis. Valsalva maneuver can be used to initiate voiding as well. Kegel exercises are good for those that have urinary incontinence, not retention problems.

4. The answer is B (1.3.3)

Cholinergics like bethanechol can induce bronchospasms, especially in asthma patients. Cholinergics will cause bradycardia and hypotension and increase gastric motility and help with glaucoma as they activate the parasympathetic system.

5. The answer is A (1.2.2)

Muscarinic receptor agonist works on the bladder M_2 and M_3 receptors. M_3 receptors are responsible for normal detrusor contraction.

6. The answer is E (1.2.1)

All the rest are used except sildenafil. Oxybutynin and solifenacin are used for hyperreflexic bladder. Baclofen is used for extremity spasticity with detrusor-sphincter dyssynergia. Doxazosin is used for smooth sphincter dyssynergia where there is a non-relaxing bladder neck.

7. The answer is C (1.2.3)

Amitriptyline has anticholinergic properties that directly oppose the cholinergic properties of bethanechol.

8. The answer is A (1.1.3)

Patients at risk for degenerative neurogenic bladders, particularly those with (or at risk for) sensory neuropathies (e.g., diabetic patients), should have a timed voiding schedule to prevent overdistention and progression to bladder areflexia. RJ has bladder areflexia.

9. The answer is D (1.3.3)

Oxybutynin can cause urinary retention in patients. It is used for patients that have hyperreflexic bladder and not areflexic bladders.

10. The answer is C (1.3.5)

All the options are appropriate therapeutic options to try to control RJ's symptoms. Switching to tolterodine is not appropriate because it can make urinary retention worse by antagonizing the muscarinic receptors in the bladder and cause increased residual urine volume and decreased detrusor muscle pressure.

Reference: *Frontera: Essentials of Physical Medicine and Rehabilitation*, 2nd ed. –"Neurogenic bladder." 2008.

Answers

Case 73 Anesthesia Agents

1. The answer is A (1.2.1)

Since AP is in congestive heart failure, an IV anesthetic agent with a stable cardiovascular profile needs to be used. Of the agents listed, thiopental (B), methohexital (D), and propofol (C) produce hypotension, while ketamine (E) results in hypertension. Etomidate (A) produces minimal hemodynamic changes and is the best agent to use in AP.

2. The answer is E (1.3.3)

Of the commonly used IV anesthetic agents, etomidate has the highest incidence of nausea and vomiting on emergence from anesthesia (>10%) (II), myoclonus (6%-33%) (I), and pain on injection (30%-80%) (III). As a result, etomidate should be reserved for use in patients who will benefit from its stable cardiovascular profile and not be used indiscriminately.

3. The answer is B (1.3.3)

Pretreatment with fentanyl, a synthetic opioid, has been shown to reduce the incidence of myoclonus. In addition, midazolam, a benzodiazepine, has been shown to be effective in reducing this. Esmolol and metoprolol, selective beta-1 blockers, and labetalol, a beta blocker with alpha-blocking activity, are used perioperatively to treat hypertension and/or for cardiac rate control. They have not been shown to prevent myoclonus when administered prior to etomidate. Famotidine, a histamine-2 receptor blocker, also has not been shown to prevent myoclonus.

4. The answer is B (1.2.5)

Pregnant patients have delayed gastric emptying and an increased risk of regurgitation of stomach contents. Aspiration of the stomach contents can result in aspiration pneumonitis, which is a potentially fatal condition. In rapid sequence induction, the goal is to intubate the patient within 60 seconds, thereby minimizing the amount of time the airway is unprotected. To accomplish this, medications with a fast onset of action are required. Of all the medications that can be used to induce general anesthesia, midazolam (B) has the slowest onset of action (30-60 seconds vs. < 30 seconds for the other agents [A, C, D, E]). Based on this fact, midazolam is not a good choice for AP.

5. The answer is A (1.2.1)

Ketamine is the only IV anesthetic agent with good analgesic properties (A). Analgesia is seen at relatively low doses and outlasts the anesthetic component. Ketamine is an excellent agent to use in short, painful procedures requiring sedation (e.g., dressing changes in burn patients). It can be given IM, which may prevent the need for an IV to be started in the patient. Other uses of ketamine include induction of anesthesia in patients in hemodynamic shock, induction of anesthesia in patients with active asthma, and to supplement local or regional anesthesia. Etomidate, thiopental, methohexital, and propofol do not have analgesia properties (B, C, D, E).

6. The answer is B (1.2.2)

Sevoflurane is a volatile inhalation agent. There are currently three volatile inhalation agents commercially available in the United States: desflurane, isoflurane, and sevoflurane. They are halogenated hydrocarbons that are liquid at room temperature. The volatile inhalation agents are readily vaporized in the anesthesia machine.

7. The answer is A (1.2.5)

The IV anesthetic agents all have half-lives ranging from 1 hour (ketamine) to 11 hours (thiopental). As such, one would not expect their clinical duration of action, which is the time from injection of the agent to the return of consciousness, to range between 3 and 15 minutes. This short duration can be attributed to the fact that the concentration of these agents in the brain, which is their site of action, decreases quickly secondary to the rapid redistribution of the agent to other tissues, such as the skeletal muscle. Metabolism has virtually no role in the short clinical duration of action of these agents.

8. The answer is C (1.1.2)

The Bispectral Index (BIS) monitor can be used to assess the degree of hypnosis in a patient receiving general anesthesia. Sensors are placed on the patient's head, which then attach to the monitor. The monitor uses derived values from the electroencephalogram (EEG) and provides a numeric value ranging from 0 to 100. This number indicates the degree of hypnosis in the patient. For example, with the BIS monitor, a BIS value of 0 equals EEG silence, a value near 100 is seen in a fully awake adult, and a value between 40 and 60 indicates a level for general anesthesia recommended by the manufacturer of the monitor.

9. The answer is A (1.2.5)

Approximately 3% of sevoflurane is metabolized hepatically. Sevoflurane's low blood-gas solubility limits the degree of its metabolism as a greater amount of the agent is removed from the blood in one passage through the lungs when compared to a more soluble agent such as isoflurane. Only 0.2% of isoflurane and 0.02% of desflurane are metabolized in the liver. None of these agents would be expected to demonstrate a prolonged duration of action in AP.

10. The answer is C (1.2.6)

The presence of various physiologic and/or pharmacologic factors can influence the amount of volatile inhalation agent that is required to maintain general anesthesia in a patient. Medications such as ketamine, diazepam, pancuronium, lidocaine, verapamil, chlorpromazine, and hydroxyzine have all been reported to reduce the concentration of volatile inhalation agent required to maintain general anesthesia. The barbiturates, opioids, alpha-2 agonists, and opioid agonist-antagonists have also been shown to produce the same effect. In addition, pregnancy, acute ethanol administration, anemia, hypoxia, increasing age, metabolic acidosis, induced hypotension, hypothermia, hyponatremia, acute ethanol administration, and

Answers

decreased central neurotransmitter levels can result in less volatile inhalation agent being required to maintain general anesthesia. Since AP is pregnant, a lower concentration of sevoflurane may be able to be used to maintain her general anesthesia. In addition, as mentioned above, AP's anemia may also result in a need for less sevoflurane for maintenance of her general anesthesia.

Case 74 Neuromuscular Blocking Agents

1. The answer is A (1.1.2)

Drugs that affect skeletal muscle function and decrease the muscle tone are termed skeletal muscle relaxants. There are two major therapeutic categories of skeletal muscle relaxants: neuromuscular blocking agents (NMBAs) and spasmolytics. NMBAs block the effect of acetylcholine at the motor end plate of the neuromuscular junction and therefore interfere with neuromuscular transmission at the motor end plate (A, C). Therapeutic uses of neuromuscular blocking drugs such as rocuronium include facilitating endotracheal intubation. Spasmolytic skeletal muscle relaxants act primarily in the brain, producing sedative and musculoskeletal relaxant properties. These drugs are used to treat musculoskeletal spasm/pain (D, E). Drugs that block the effects of acetylcholine at the muscarinic receptor produce anticholinergic effects such as dry mouth, constipation, confusion, memory impairment, etc. (B).

2. The answer is A (1.3.2)

Train-of-Four (TOF) testing is performed to measure the degree of neuromuscular blockade using a peripheral nerve stimulator. The goal is to ensure that the patient is adequately paralyzed with NMBA using TOF monitoring. MP will exhibit anywhere from zero to four twitches in response to electrical nerve stimulation. If MP were to exhibit one twitch, this would indicate that 90% of his nicotinic receptors at the motor endplate of the neuromuscular junction are blocked by the agent. One or two twitches usually gives conditions suitable for surgery or long-term mechanical ventilation in the intensive care unit. Four twitches would indicate that up to 75% of the receptors are blocked, permitting spontaneous respirations. TOF should be assessed every 30 minutes or until desired twitches are achieved, then every 1 hour once goal TOF is achieved (A). EEG is the recording of electrical activity along the scalp produced by the firing of neurons within the brain (B). ECG or EKG is a transthoracic interpretation of the electrical activity of the heart (C). NCS is a test to evaluate the ability of electrical conduction of the motor and sensory nerves (D). Myelogram detects the pathology of the spinal cord, including the location of a spinal cord injury, cysts, and tumors (E).

3. The answer is D (1.2.1)

Succinylcholine (Quelicin) remains the NMBA of choice for the emergency control of the airway. It has the most rapid on-

set and shortest duration of the currently available NMBAs. It's also the only NMBA that can be given by a nonintravenous route of administration. Succinylcholine can be administered intramuscularly, often combined with atropine to prevent significant bradycardia (D). Versed (midazolam) is benzodiazepine used to provide sedation and amnesia (B). Propofol (Diprivan) is a hypnotic for induction and maintenance of general anesthesia, sedation of mechanically ventilated patients, and sedation for procedures (C). Remifentanil (Ultiva) is potent ultra-short-acting opioid analgesic (E). Cisatracurium (Nimbex) is a neuromuscular blocking agent used to provide muscle paralysis to facilitate intubation, surgery, and mechanical ventilation (A).

4. The answer is D (1.2.2)

Non-depolarizing NMBAs can be reversed with acetylcholinesterase (AChE) inhibitors such as neostigmine, pyridostigmine, and edrophonium. These agents increase the concentration of acetylcholine at the neuromuscular junction, which reduces the effect of the competitive blocking drugs, thus restoring muscle activity (muscle contraction). AChE inhibitors may also cause bradycardia, increased secretions, peristalsis, and bronchoconstriction. To combat these troublesome side effects, AChE inhibitors are combined with anticholinergic drugs such as glycopyrrolate and atropine (D). Naloxone and flumazenil reverse the effects of opioids and benzodiazepines, respectively (A). Diphenhydramine and famotidine block histamine type 1 and type 2 receptors, respectively (C). Midazolam produces anxiolysis, sedation, and amnesia; fentanyl is an analgesic (E). Epinephrine and vasopressin are vasopressors administered during cardiac arrest to promote the return of spontaneous circulation (B).

5. The answer is C (2.2.5)

NBMAs are considered high-alert drugs because misuse can lead to catastrophic injuries or death. These drugs should be given your highest attention, just as you've done with cancer chemotherapeutic agents. To reduce the risk of harm from neuromuscular blocking agents, the following recommendations are given by ISMP.

Limit access. When possible, dispense neuromuscular blocking agents from the pharmacy as prescribed for patients. Allow floor stock of these agents only in the OR, ED, and critical care units where patients can be properly ventilated and monitored.

Segregate storage. When these agents must be available as floor stock, have pharmacy assemble the vials in a sealed box with warnings affixed as noted below. Sequester the boxes in both refrigerated and nonrefrigerated locations.

Warning labels. Affix labels that note: "Warning: Paralyzing Agent-Causes Respiratory Arrest" on each vial, syringe, bag, and storage box of neuromuscular blocking agents.

Safeguard storage in the pharmacy. Sequester and affix warning labels to vials of neuromuscular blocking agents stocked in the pharmacy. Be sure they do not obscure the vial label in any way (C).

The other labels are not appropriate. Cisatracurium and succinylcholine, for example, should be stored in the refrigerator (A). None of the NMBAs are light-sensitive or act in the central nervous system to cause drowsiness (B, D). Although NMBAs may be diluted prior to continuous infusion, they do not have to be diluted prior to IV push administration (which is their main route of administration) (E).

6. The answer is A (2.2.4)

Rocuronium has the fastest onset of action (60-90 seconds). Atracurium, cisatracurium, and vecuronium have intermediate onsets of action (2-3 minutes). Pancuronium has the longest onset of action (>3 minutes).

7. The answer is E (1.3.3)

Succinylcholine is the only depolarizing NMBA available commercially. Succinylcholine may cause many adverse effects including muscle fasciculations; myalgias; increased intraocular, intragastric, or intracranial pressure; anaphylaxis; bradycardia; and hyperkalemia leading to arrhythmias and/or cardiac arrest. Succinylcholine is also a trigger for a malignant hyperthermia (MH) crisis (A, B, C, D). One of the signs of a MH crisis is metabolic acidosis. Metabolic acidosis in not an adverse effect of succinylcholine (E).

8. The answer is B (1.2.1)

The only action of NMBAs is to block neuromuscular transmission at the motor end plate of the neuromuscular junction, causing paralysis of the affected skeletal muscles. This resulting skeletal muscle paralysis facilitates endotracheal intubation, performing the surgery, and long-term mechanical ventilation (A). NMBAs do not provide sedation or pain relief. Patients are still aware of pain even after a full muscle paralysis has occurred. A general anesthetic agent (e.g., sevoflurane, propofol) and/or a benzodiazepine must be given to prevent patient awareness while under anesthesia. An opioid (e.g., fentanyl, morphine) must be given to provide intra- and postoperative analgesia (B, C).

9. The answer is E (1.1.4)

Malignant hyperthermia (MH) is a genetic disorder that affects calcium regulation in the muscle cells. MH is triggered by the administration of a known triggering agent–succinylcholine or any of the inhaled anesthetic agents (sevoflurane, desflurane, isoflurane). Characteristic symptoms of a MH crisis typically include elevated carbon dioxide production, tachycardia, tachypnea, jaw muscle or body rigidity, respiratory and metabolic acidosis, and elevated body temperature. An elevated temperature is typically a late sign that the process is fulminant. Therefore, the physician shouldn't wait for an elevated temperature to initiate the MH protocol. Appropriate management of an MH crisis includes issuing an immediate call for help, discontinuing the inhaled anesthetic agent or succinylcholine (triggering agents), administering dantrolene (Dantrium), and instituting body cooling measures. Respiratory acidosis, metabolic acidosis, reduced urinary output, and any electrolyte or coagulation abnormality are treated in a standard manner. A dose of dantrolene 2.5 mg/kg should be given intravenously as soon as the syndrome of MH is recognized. This dose may be repeated until a total dose of 10 mg/kg is administered.

10. The answer is A (3.1.2)

The Malignant Hyperthermia Association of the United States (MHAUS) (I) is a nonprofit organization for malignant hyperthermia (MH) susceptible patients and their families, health care professionals, corporations, or anyone with an interest in MH. MHAUS is dedicated to providing the best scientific advice to all patients and health care professionals. Information is available on their website (www.mhaus.org) and a 24/7 staffed hot-line for health care professionals (1-800-MH HYPER or 1-800-644-9737; outside the US dial 001-1-315-464-7079). Although there are other resources for the management of an MH crisis, they do not contain information for patients (e.g., medical ID program with wallet cards and warning letters to health care providers, genetic counseling, etc.) (II, III).

Case 75 Allergy

1. The answer is C (1.1.4)

The presence or lack of fever (I) and possible concurrent medications (II) are important factors in assessing patients as described in the case and making appropriate therapeutic recommendations. A response to III will not provide helpful information prior to making a recommendation.

2. The answer is A (1.1.2)

The symptoms as presented, especially the sudden onset and allergy forecast reports, are consistent with seasonal allergic rhinitis. The remaining answers (B, C, D, E) are not consistent with the symptoms or environmental factors as described.

3. The answer is B (1.2.1)

This patient presents with several symptoms, all of which should be addressed with separate agents, although not all are listed in the choices given. According to the evidence-based cough guidelines published by the American College of Chest Physicians in the January 2006 issue of *Chest*, a first-generation antihistamine should be employed as first-line therapy to treat post-nasal drip, which is often an underlying cause of cough in colds and allergies. Nonsedating antihistamines (E) are not effective for treating coughs. Cough suppressants (D) are not proven to relieve coughs. Expectorants (A) are used to loosen congestion, but will not treat the cough. Decongestants (C) are used to relieve nasal congestion.

4. The answer is C (1.2.4)

Cetirizine (B), an H1-receptor antagonist second-generation antihistamine, became available over the counter in November 2007. Although it can produce somnolence at recommended doses, it nevertheless produces less drowsiness than first-gen-

Answers

eration antihistamines. Loratadine (D) is a nonsedating second-generation antihistamine that is also available over the counter. Chlorpheniramine (A) and dexbrompheniramine (E) are of the alkylamine class of antihistamines, which are the least sedating of the first-generation antihistamines. Diphenhydramine (C) is OTC but more sedating (ethanolamine) than any of the others.

5. The answer is C (1.2.2)

Nasalcrom (C), or cromolyn sodium, is the only mast-cell stabilizer in the given list of drugs. Afrin (A) and Neo-Synephrine (B) are both topical decongestants. Flonase (D) and Vanceril (E) are both prescription drugs.

6. The answer is C (1.2.5)

Muscarinic cholinergic blockade (C) contributes to the side effects of dry mouth and eyes and urinary retention. Antihistamines do not act as alpha or beta agonists or antagonists (A, B, D, E).

7. The answer is B (1.2.1)

Vasocon-A is a combination decongestant-antihistamine eye drop and is appropriate for initial treatment of the patient's eye symptoms. Tobrex (A) is a prescription antibiotic eye medication, Visine Original (C) is a decongestant alone, Refresh (D) is an artificial tear preparation, and Collyrium (E) is an eye wash. None of these address the initial allergic symptoms.

8. The answer is C (3.2.1)

Allergy shots are a treatment in which small doses of substances to which a patient is allergic (allergens) are injected under your skin. Over time, the body may become less responsive to the allergens, which will result in fewer symptoms. During initial treatment, allergy shots are given once or twice a week. At first, a small amount of allergens is used. The amount of allergen injected is increased slightly each time, unless there is a serious allergic reaction. Once reaching maintenance, you get the same dose in shots every 2 to 4 weeks for another 4 to 6 months. The shots reduce symptoms in people allergic to pollens, animal dander, dust mites, mold, and cockroaches. Children younger than 2 should not have allergy shots. Older adults may be taking medications or have other medical conditions that may increase the risk of a severe reaction to allergy shots. Allergy shots should not be used when the patient has had a recent heart attack, unstable angina, or other heart conditions or are taking beta-blockers. Allergy shots are also contraindicated in patients with an immune system disease such as AIDS (C); people who have immune system diseases such as systemic lupus or multiple sclerosis should be evaluated individually. None of the other conditions are contraindications for allergy shots (A, B, D, E).

9. The answer is E (3.2.1)

Allergy sufferers may know when it is allergy season, but often have very limited knowledge about allergy awareness in general.

Specifically, patients generally know very little about allergy prevention. When it comes to prevention, there are many therapies that can prevent symptoms from occurring. It is important to check your local allergy forecast (I) to know when pollen counts are elevated. As the pollen count rises, patients may want to take prophylactic medication. Also, when the allergy forecast is high, patients should try to spend more time inside, especially in the morning when the outdoor pollen levels are highest. If patients must go outside or work outdoors, they should wear a facemask to limit the amount of pollen that they inhale. Changing clothes frequently will also help reduce pollen transfer. Using a high-efficiency particulate air (HEPA) filter when cleaning and keeping windows closed can also help (II). Dusting with a damp cloth will also help keep dust mites at bay (III).

10. The answer is C (2.2.1)

Chlor-Trimeton (C) is a first-generation antihistamine appropriate for treatment of a hacking cough associated with colds or allergies according to the 2006 American College of Chest Physician guidelines. The patient should be counseled to take the antihistamine only at night; or, if the cough is irritating during the day, the pharmacist should warn the patient about drowsiness. Delsym (E) is a nonprescription, 12-hour formulation of dextromethorphan, a relatively nonsedating antitussive that is now not recommended as first-line treatment. Robitussin DM Max (A) and Triaminic Cough and Sore Throat (B) contain ingredients that are not needed to treat present symptoms. Robitussin AC (D) contains codeine, which may cause more drowsiness than chlorpheniramine and may also be prescription only (depending on state laws).

Case 76 Dermatitis

1. The answer is B (2.2.1)

Betamethasone valerate 0.1% cream (Valisone) is available by prescription only (B). Aluminum acetate 1:40 solution (C) (Burow's solution) (A) is commercially available on an OTC basis as Domeboro powder packets for reconstitution. Topical hydrocortisone preparations in strengths of 0.5%-1% are available on a nonprescription basis (D), as are diphenhydramine 25-mg capsules (Benadryl) (E).

2. The answer is E (1.1.3)

Nonprescription topical corticosteroids such as hydrocortisone cream 0.5%-1% are safe and effective for treatment of mild-to-moderate contact dermatitis (I). Dilute aluminum acetate solution (1:40) applied topically or as a soak for 30 minutes 3-4 times a day is effective in soothing pain or itching associated with poison ivy or oak of any degree of severity (III). Tepid tub baths using commercially available nonprescription colloidal oatmeal provide soothing relief for patients with mild-to-moderately severe rhus dermatitis (II).

3. The answer is C (3.2.2)

Although oral antihistamine use may be associated with drowsiness and with anticholinergic adverse effects, the topical use of antihistamines does not result in anticholinergic effects, drowsiness, or systemic toxicity (A, B, D, E). Their topical use is associated with a significant incidence of sensitization (C).

4. The answer is C (1.1.3)

Patients sensitized to urushiol, the allergenic constituent of poison ivy, poison oak, and poison sumac plants, should be counseled that avoidance of the allergen or minimization of exposure to the allergen is the best way to prevent future recurrences of rhus dermatitis (A, B, D, E). The points listed are important preventative measures, except that having the skin exposed can increase the likelihood of coming in contact with the allergen. Staying covered up is best (C).

5. The answer is A (1.1.0)

Severe dermatitis, including widespread reaction involving significant swelling of body parts or any eye involvement, is an indication for physician referral for prescription therapy with more potent topical steroids or systemic antiinflammatory corticosteroids (A). Mild rhus dermatitis may be characterized by linear streaks of papules and vesicles along with intense itching or pain (B, C). Moderate dermatitis includes the addition of small or large fluid-filled bullae, which are not necessarily an indication for physician referral (D). Presence of lesions on the hands is not in itself an indication for physician referral (E).

6. The answer is D (1.3.1)

All goals are correct and involve symptomatic relief or prevention of complications except desensitization (D) is not effective for prevention.

7. The answer is C (1.3.3)

Neomycin applied topically produces a relatively high rate (3.5%-6%) of hypersensitivity or allergic contact dermatitis (I). Prolonged use of topical nonprescription antibiotic agents may result in secondary fungal infection, so their use for longer than 5 days should be avoided (II). Topical application of neomycin is not associated with skin hyperpigmentation (III).

8. The answer is E (1.2.1)

All agents listed are OTC products that contain FDA category I ingredients with antifungal activity. With the exception of Betadine, each carries an indication in its labeling for the treatment of athlete's foot (tinea pedis). Betadine is povidone-iodine solution (A). Micatin contains miconazole nitrate (B), Lotrimin AF contains either miconazole nitrate or clotrimazole depending on dosage form (C), and Lamisil AT contains terbinafine (D). Tinactin Spray Liquid contains tolnaftate 1% as its active ingredient (E).

9. The answer is B (3.2.3)

Treatment of tinea cruris (jock itch) with terbinafine 1% cream results in a low rate of recurrent infection if the therapy is continued for 7-10 days (B). Other nonprescription topical antifungals require more lengthy treatment regimens of 2-4 weeks. Terbinafine 1% cream is also effective in the treatment of tinea pedis, for which a 7-day course of therapy is also appropriate; however, complete resolution of symptoms may require up to 4 weeks therapy. Other nonprescription antifungals require treatment regimens of 2-6 weeks for tinea pedis.

10. The answer is A (1.1.3)

Effective treatment of cutaneous fungal infections such as tinea cruris or tinea pedis requires adequate ventilation of the skin, and the use of occlusive clothing, shoes, or bandages should be avoided (A). Selenium sulfide lotion is not used in the treatment of fungal infections; it is effective for treatment of scaly dermatoses such as dandruff or seborrhea (B). Emollients act as a skin barrier, and do not provide adequate ventilation of the skin, and therefore should be avoided (D). The use of occlusive clothing, shoes, or bandages should be avoided (C, E).

Case 77 Vaginal Preparations

1. The answer is C (1.1.3)

Insufficient vaginal lubrication can be caused from a variety of factors, including low estrogen concentrations (menopause, oophorectomy, or postpartum), Sjögren's syndrome, diabetes mellitus, systemic lupus erythematosus, stress, fatigue, strenuous exercise, endometriosis, and medications (I, II). The use of a male condom with or without lubrication will not contribute to the patient's vaginal dryness (III).

2. The answer is D (1.2.1)

A douche is generally used for vaginal hygiene and would be inappropriate for improving vaginal dryness (D). All of the other products listed (A, B, C, E) contain active ingredients in appropriate dosage forms that make them all options for treating vaginal dryness.

3. The answer is A (1.2.6)

Vaginal lubricants can be used as often as needed for the patient. The patient should also use the quantity that is needed to keep them comfortable.

4. The answer is C (1.3.5)

The patient could try a different vaginal lubricant to see if symptoms improve (C). If changing products does not work, then the patient should be referred. If the patient chooses to see a physician, a vaginal estrogen product would be the next step (B). HRT rather than ERT would be recommended orally since the patient's uterus is intact (A). Condoms that are prelubricated with a spermicide are not recommended for use (D).

Answers

A spermicidal sponge would be an appropriate form of birth control; however, the sponge is not useful for treating vaginal dryness (E).

5. The answer is B (1.1.4)

Regular sexual activity will help maintain the vaginal lining so that it is more capable of producing adequate vaginal lubrication during sexual arousal (B). Both baths and sitz baths can flush lubrication from the vaginal area (C, E). Petroleum jelly is not recommended as a lubricant (A), and regular exercise has not been proven to increase lubrication (D).

6. The answer is D (2.2.3)

Glycerin is safe for use with latex condoms (D). All of the other choices are unsafe and will harm the integrity of the latex condom (A, C, E). Miconazole (B) is a vaginal antifungal and would not be used with a condom as a lubricant.

7. The answer is E (3.2.4)

All of the options would be appropriate. The sponge might require additional lubrication, but would be an appropriate alternative.

8. The answer is D (3.2.4)

The onset of action of the sponge is immediate upon insertion; therefore, 15 minutes lead time is not needed prior to use (D). All of the other answers are correct counseling points regarding use of a contraceptive sponge (A, B, C, E).

9. The answer is E (2.2.3)

Astroglide is a lubricant and does not contain any spermicide (E). The other options all contain nonoxynol-9 as a spermicide (A, B, C, D).

10. The answer is C (3.2.4)

Additional lubrication may be necessary and can be used without removing the condom (C). The female condom should only be used once, and should be discarded after use (A). Combination of a male and female condom can increase friction and cause displacement of the female condom (B). It should be removed soon after use (D). It is effective in preventing the spread of sexually transmitted diseases (E).

Federal Law Review

1. The answer is C (1.0.2)

Under the PDMA, federal legend drug samples may be distributed by manufacturer's representatives only when a prescriber requests the samples in writing. Community pharmacies are not allowed to have any samples of federal legend drugs. Hospital pharmacies are allowed to possess samples, but only when they are requested to do so by a prescriber.

2. The answer is C (1.0.4)

All of the listed individuals must obtain a DEA registration number to prescribe controlled substances except a medical resident who is employed by a teaching or research hospital. The resident uses the hospital's DEA registration number when prescribing controlled substances.

3. The answer is B (1.0.1)

The term "pharmacist-in-charge" is used most frequently to indicate which individual pharmacist can be held legally responsible for complying with the applicable laws. A few states do not use this term and instead elect to hold any "pharmacist on duty" responsible for legal compliance. The other terms are usually used in conjunction with employment status.

4. The answer is C (2.0.2)

Drug product interchange (generic selection or generic substitution), monitoring drug therapy, counseling patients, and interpreting prescriptions are all activities associated with core pharmacy practice. Making a physical assessment of a patient for the purpose of diagnosis is considered the practice of medicine and is generally outside the legal scope of pharmacy practice in the vast majority of practice settings.

5. The answer is D (1.0.4)

With the exception of a pharmacist who owns a pharmacy solely in his or her own name (a "sole practitioner"), pharmacists do not register with the DEA as a predicate to handling or dispensing controlled substances. Most, but not all, states issue a separate controlled substances license to pharmacists and other practitioners who handle these drugs. Physicians, hospitals, pharmacies, and nursing homes that dispense or otherwise handle controlled substances do need to obtain a DEA registration.

6. The answer is B (1.0.4)

The issue of who is allowed to prescribe which drugs is determined by state law. Most state laws make these determinations by defining the scope of practice of the practitioner. In the vast majority of cases, podiatry is limited to the treatment of feet and nails (including fingernails). Prescribing contraceptive drugs is outside the scope of the practice of podiatry.

7. The answer is C (1.0.5)

Originally, OBRA-90 mandated that state law require pharmacists or their agents to offer to counsel in certain situations. That counseling requirement has been expanded to include new prescriptions for all patients. The laws are specific that while others may make the offer to counsel, only a pharmacist (or perhaps a pharmacist intern under the supervision of a pharmacist) may actually provide the counseling. Under the concept of professional discretion or judgment, a pharmacist may advise any patient at any time about the use of OTC and prescription-only medication.

8. The answer is D (2.0.2)

CMS administers Medicare and Medicaid programs. JCAHO only certifies institutions as complying with its standards of practice. DHHS is the federal administrative agency that oversees the FDA. The FDA does not license or register pharmacies even though, to a limited extent, it does have regulatory authority over some pharmacy activities. The states, through the board of pharmacy or an equivalent body, actually grant a pharmacy authority to operate and the DEA registers pharmacies to handle and dispense controlled substances.

9. The answer is A (3.0.2)

Controlled substances are placed into one of five schedules by the DEA. Federal legend drugs are those designated by the FDA as available only with the prescription of a licensed prescriber. INDs are drugs authorized for research uses by the FDA. A sample drug is one designated by a manufacturer or wholesaler as available for distribution without charge. A generic drug is one that is made by more than one manufacturer.

10. The answer is A (3.0.1)

Federal law requires pharmacies to keep controlled substances prescriptions at least 2 years after the date most recently dispensed. Having dispensed a refill on July 1, 2011, First Community must keep it on file until at least June 30, 2013.

11. The answer is C (3.0.1)

Using the same rule explained in the previous question, because ABC last dispensed the controlled substance on November 1, 2011, it must keep the prescription on file until at least October 31, 2013.

12. The answer is B (3.0.2)

Federal law limits refills on Schedule III and IV drugs to five times within a 6-month period from the date the prescription is issued. This five refill limit applies even though a physician indicates, as in this case, that more than five refills are authorized. Here, because the patient has already obtained five refills, the pharmacy must refuse to dispense any additional medication. Likewise, no other pharmacy could dispense any other refills on the authority of this prescription. In any event, the prescription could not be transferred back to the original pharmacy or any other pharmacy because DEA regulations limit the transfer of controlled substance prescriptions to one time only between unrelated pharmacies. Although not listed as a possible answer, the pharmacist could call the physician to obtain a new prescription authorization.

13. The answer is A (2.0.3)

DEA regulations allow a hospital pharmacy to supply a limited number of doses of controlled substances drugs to the emergency room if the drugs are stored in a locked cabinet. Procedures must be established under an approved protocol for stocking, restocking, and logging out all drugs stored in the cabinet. The pharmacy director must approve the protocol.

14. The answer is E (3.0.2)

Most states issue controlled substances licenses, in addition to other kinds of licenses, to pharmacists, pharmacies, physicians, and other authorized prescribers. The board of pharmacy or an equivalent agency usually issues the licenses.

15. The answer is A (3.0.1)

The FDA makes the determination that drugs are safe and effective for intended purposes when it approves an NDA for an individual drug. The DEA determines if FDA-approved drugs should be controlled and how they should be scheduled. DHHS is the parent agency of the FDA but does not make determinations about drugs directly. CMS administers Medicare and Medicaid and, at least in part, pays suppliers for those drugs used by beneficiaries of those programs. The BNDD is the predecessor to the DEA and no longer exists.

16. The answer is B (3.0.1)

As explained in the answer to question 15, the DEA determines which drugs should be designated as controlled substances.

17. The answer is D (3.0.1)

Both the federal and individual state governments have authority to regulate controlled substances. The World Trade Federation is not a government agency. Local municipalities usually do not have direct authority to regulate controlled substances.

18. The answer is C (3.0.2)

Authority to designate which schedule a controlled substance will be placed in is vested in the U.S. Attorney General under federal statute. This cabinet-level presidential appointee is in charge of the Department of Justice, which is the parent agency of the DEA.

19. The answer is A (2.0.2)

Pharmacists and pharmacy interns are not required to register with the DEA before handling controlled substances. Neither police officers nor employees of manufacturers of controlled substances are required to obtain DEA registration. Pharmacies, however, must register with the DEA if controlled substances are handled.

20. The answer is C (1.0.4)

The federal transfer warning ("Federal law prohibits the transfer of this drug to any person other than the patient for whom it was prescribed") must appear on the pharmacy label of dispensed controlled substances listed in Schedules II, III, and IV. The warning is not required for Schedule V controlled substances.

21. The answer is E (2.0.3)

DEA regulations allow pharmacies to either stock controlled substances in a locked cabinet in the pharmacy or disperse these medications throughout the other drug inventory. A combi-

Answers

nation of both methods is also permissible. For example, many pharmacies lock up Schedule II controlled substances while dispensing Schedule III-V drugs with the rest of the pharmacy inventory.

22. The answer is A (1.0.4)

The term "purported prescription" is used in DEA regulation 21 CFR 1306.04 to describe an order for a controlled substance that may originate from a physician and appear to be a prescription in all other regards but is not deemed to be a prescription because it was issued for a nonlegitimate reason. For example, a prescription that is sold to a patient by a physician outside of a normal patient-physician relationship for purposes of diversion is a purported prescription. Note that even though a pharmacist might verify that an authorized prescriber issued a prescription, it is no less an unlawful purported prescription if issued for a reason that is not a legitimate medical purpose.

23. The answer is D (1.0.4)

Unlike the limits on refills of Schedule III and IV controlled substances (five times in 6 months), Schedule V prescriptions may be refilled as many times as authorized by the prescriber or allowed by state law (usually 1 year from the date of issuance).

24. The answer is D (1.0.6)

Federal law limits the transfer of controlled substance prescriptions to one time between unrelated pharmacies. For purposes of this rule, "unrelated" means not under common ownership. For example, an independently owned pharmacy and a chain store pharmacy corporation are unrelated.

25. The answer is D (1.0.4)

Two chain store pharmacies owned by the same corporation are related and may transfer controlled substances prescriptions as often as refills are authorized, but only if the two pharmacies are linked by a real-time online network. Chain pharmacies, even though owned by one corporation, are limited to the one-time transfer rule if they are not linked by a real-time online computer network.

26. The answer is B (1.0.6)

Schedule II controlled substances may be distributed (i.e., transferred) between DEA registrants only by use of DEA Form 222 or the electronic equivalent. Schedule II drugs cannot be dispensed by a pharmacy to a prescriber by use of a prescription that indicates the drugs will be used for the prescriber's office. Form 106 is used to report stolen or missing controlled substances.

27. The answer is D (1.0.2)

In contrast to the procedure for transferring Schedule II controlled substances between DEA registrants, Schedule III and IV drugs are to be distributed using an invoice that is to be filed with other Schedule III and IV records.

28. The answer is C (1.0.7)

Federal law requires pharmacies to complete a controlled substance inventory every 2 years. Note that many states require inventories to be taken more frequently. A 1-year period is common.

29. The answer is B (1.0.7)

Federal law requires pharmacies to maintain records of controlled substances prescriptions, invoices, and transfer records as well as inventories for at least 2 years. Note that many states have requirements that at least some of these records be kept for a longer period. For example, some states require that all prescriptions be kept a minimum of 5 years.

30. The answer is E (3.0.2)

Penalties for willful or knowing violations of the controlled substances laws may include criminal and civil sanctions as well as administrative actions against the pharmacy's DEA registration. Therefore, all of the answers are correct.

Compounding

Powders

1. The answer is A (3.2.3)

As listed in the directions for the patient, "bid" is the Latin abbreviation for two times daily or twice daily.

2. The answer is C (2.1.1)

By subtracting the ingredients, excluding corn starch, from the total amount to be dispensed, you obtain the required quantity of corn starch. Therefore, for 20 g:

Tolnaftate   1% w/w = 0.2 g
Zinc oxide   5% w/w = 1.0 g
Talc 20% w/w = 4 g
Total ingredients   5.2 g
20 g - 5.2 g = 14.8 g corn starch

3. The answer is A (2.1.1)

By subtracting the ingredients, excluding corn starch, from the total amount to be dispensed, this gives the required quantity of corn starch. Therefore, for 30 g:

Tolnaftate   1% w/w = 0.3 g
Zinc Oxide   5% w/w = 1.5 g
Talc 20% w/w = 6 g
7.8 g total ingredients
30 g - 7.8 g = 22.2 g corn starch

4. The answer is B (2.1.1)

1% tolnaftate = (1 g tolnaftate/100 g total) × 30 g total= 0.3 tolnaftate

5. The answer is B (2.1.1)

(0.2 g tolnaftate/20 g total)=1:100::tolnaftate:total

6. The answer is B (3.2.3)

Since this preparation is in powder form and will be administered to the feet, the only auxiliary label required is "not to be taken by mouth."

7. The answer is E (2.1.4)

0.0014 g/10 g × 300 g = 0.042 g

8. The answer is B (2.1.4)

1.4 mg/10 g × 10 g = 1.4 mg = 0.0014 g

9. The answer is D (2.1.4)

0.0014 g/10 g × 100 g = 0.014%

10. The answer is C (3.2.3)

The Latin abbreviation "au" in the patient instructions is translated as administration in both ears.

11. The answer is A (3.2.3)

The Latin abbreviation "tid" in the patient instructions is translated to mean administration of the drug product three times daily.

12. The answer is E (2.1.1)

2% = (2 g/100 g) × 100 g = 2 g Miconazole

13. The answer is D (2.1.1)

Since 2 grams of the total 100-gram preparation are made up of miconazole, the remaining 98 grams (100 g - 2 g) will be boric acid powder.

14. The answer is E (3.2.3)

Based on the patient instructions and on the formulation type, the auxiliary labels include "for external use only" and "for the ear."

15. The answer is E (2.1.1)

(400 µg/15 g) × (1 mg/1000 µg) × 30 g = 0.8 mg

16. The answer is A (2.1.1)

Since 0.8 mg is required for a 30-gram preparation, twice that, or 1.6 mg would be required for the 60-gram preparation. 1.6 mg or 0.0016 g.

17. The answer is C (2.1.1)

30 g × (15.432 gr/1 gr) = 462.96 gr

18. The answer is D (2.1.1)

30 g × (1 mL/1.3 g)=23.1 mL

19. The answer is A (3.2.3)

The Latin abbreviation for powder is "pulv."

20. The answer is B (2.1.1)

Since misoprostol and polyethylene oxide are in a ratio of 0.4 mg:200 mg, dividing 200 mg by 0.4 reduces the ratio.

21. The answer is D (2.1.1)

(0.0004 g misoprostol/15 g total) × 100=0.0027% w/w

Capsules

1. The answer is E (2.1.1)

Assuming that there is no overage, the total six capsules will contain 60 mg pseudoephedrine and 12 mg chlorpheniramine, both of which are below SAW of the balance.

2. The answer is B (2.1.1)

8 capsules × (160 acetaminophen/1 capsule) × (1 g/1000 mg) × (15.432 gr/1 g) = 19.8 gr

3. The answer is A (2.1.1)

10 capsules × (10 mg pseudoephedrine/1 capsule) × (1 g/ 1000 mg) × (15.432 gr/1 g) = 1.54 gr

4. The answer is A (2.1.1)

(350 mg/1 capsule) × 6 capsules = 2100 mg or 2.1 g

5. The answer is C (2.1.1)

350 mg - 10 mg - 2 mg - 160 mg = 178 mg lactose

6. The answer is A (2.1.1)

(160 mg acetaminophen/350 mg total) × 100 = 45.7%

7. The answer is C (3.2.3)

The Latin abbreviations "tid" and "prn" are translated as three times daily as needed.

8. The answer is E (3.2.3)

None of the auxiliary labels listed there are required for this type of formulation.

9. The answer is C (3.2.3)

The Latin abbreviation "qid" is translated as four times daily.

10. The answer is B (2.1.1)

(50 mg dehydropiandosterone/350 mg total) × 100 = 14.3%

Answers

11. The answer is A (2.1.1)

350 mg - 50 mg = 300 mg/capsule of lactose

10 capsules × (300 mg/1 capsule) = 3000 mg or 3 g

12. The answer is C (2.1.1)

50 mg × 12 = 600 mg or 0.6 g dehydroepiandrosterone

13. The answer is C (2.1.1)

Since 300 mg lactose are required for each capsule, 10 capsules would require three grams of lactose

3 g × (15.432 gr/1 g) = 46.296 gr

14. The answer is B (2.1.1)

300 mg lactose/50 mg dehydroepiandrosterone = 6; therefore, there is 1 part dehydroepiandrosterone per 6 parts lactose.

15. The answer is C (2.1.1)

(280 - 1 - 8 - 1 - 150) × 100 = 12,000 mg or 12 g

16. The answer is C (2.1.1)

8 mg/280 mg × 100 mg = 2.857% w/w

17. The answer is C (2.1.1)

60 capsules × 150 mg/capsule = 9000 mg or 9 g

Tablets

1. The answer is B (2.1.1)

150 mg × 200 tablets = 30 g

30 g + 0.01 (30 g) = 30.3 g

2. The answer is C (3.2.3)

The Latin abbreviation "tid prn" in the patient instructions is translated as three times daily as needed.

3. The answer is B (2.1.1)

(15 mg pseudoephedrine/150 mg total) × 100 = 10% w/w

4. The answer is A (2.1.1)

15 mg pseudoephedrine × 200 tablets = 3000 mg or 3 g

3 g + 0.01(3 g) = 3.03 g

3.03 g × (15.432 gr/1 g) = 46.75 gr

5. The answer is A (2.1.1)

10 mg loratadine × 200 tablets = 2000 mg or 2 g

2 g + 0.01 (2 g) = 2.02 g

6. The answer is B (2.1.1)

150 mg total/10 mg loratadine = 1.5; so, 1 part loratadine per 1.5 parts total or 1:1.5

Troches and Lozenges

1. The answer is B (3.2.3)

The Latin abbreviation "bid" in the patient instructions is translated as twice daily.

2. The answer is B (2.1.1)

50 mg sodium fluoride × 10 lozenges = 500 mg or 0.5 g

0.5 g + 0.2 (0.5 g) = 0.60 g

3. The answer is A (2.1.1)

(2 g/mold) × (1 mL/0.98 g) = 2.04 mL/mold

4. The answer is B (2.1.1)

10 lozenges × (2 g/lozenge) = 20 g

20 g - (10 × 0.05 g sodium fluoride) = 19.5 g sorbitol

5. The answer is A (2.1.1)

(50 mg sodium fluoride/2000 mg total) × 100 = 2.5% w/w

Solutions

1. The answer is C (2.1.1)

Since one fluid ounce is 30 mL, the amount dispensed will be 60 mL (2 × 30 mL).

(Q.27 in CBT)

2. The answer is B (2.1.1)

(20 mg phenobarbital/5 mL) × 60 mL = 240 mg phenobarbital

240 mg × (1 mL/25 mg) = 9.6 mL stock solution

3. The answer is C (2.1.1)

60 mL total × (10 mL simple syrup/100 mL total) × (1.3 g simple syrup/1 mL simple syrup) = 7.8 g simple syrup

4. The answer is C (2.1.1)

Since each teaspoon is 5 mL and the instructions call for two teaspoons per dose, the total dose in milliliters is 10 mL.

5. The answer is C (3.2.3)

The Latin abbreviation "tid" in the patient instructions is translated as three times daily.

6. The answer is B (2.1.1)

(20 mg phenobarbital/5 mL) × 60 mL = 240 mg phenobarbital

7. The answer is A (2.1.1)

60 mL total × (10 mL simple syrup/100 mL total) = 6 mL

8. The answer is A (2.1.1)

(0.1 g methylparaben/100 mL) × 5 mL = 0.005 g or 5 mg methylparaben

20 mg phenobarbital/5 mg methylparaben = 4

9. The answer is B (2.1.1)

2.5 g/100 mL = 2.5% w/v

10. The answer is A (2.1.1)

(2.5 g/100 mL) × 15 mL = 0.375 g or 375 mg meperidine

11. The answer is D (2.1.1)

(200 mg/100 mL) × 15 mL = 30 mg

12. The answer is B (3.2.3)

The Latin abbreviation "qid prn" in the patient instructions translates to four times daily as needed.

13. The answer is D (3.2.3)

The preparation should not be taken by mouth and is intended for use in the nose.

Suspensions

1. The answer is A (2.1.1)

(0.9 g/100 mL) × 100 mL = 0.9 g

2. The answer is A (2.1.1)

(0.24 g/250 mL) × 100 = 0.096% w/v

3. The answer is A (2.1.1)

(0.24 g/250 mL) × 150 mL = 0.144 g

0.144 g × (15.432 gr/1 g) = 2.2 gr

4. The answer is B (3.2.3)

The Latin abbreviation "bid" in the patient instructions translates to twice daily.

5. The answer is C (2.1.1)

(0.24 g/250 mL) × 100 mL = 0.096 g or 96 mg

6. The answer is B (2.1.1)

10.5 lb × (1 kg/2.2 lb) × (0.5 mg/1 kg) × 250 mL/240 mg) = 2.48 mL

7. The answer is A (3.2.3)

Since the preparation is a suspension, the required auxiliary label is "Shake Well."

8. The answer is C (2.1.1)

Each fluid ounce is 30 mL, so two fluid ounces is 60 mL.

9. The answer is A (2.1.1)

(5 mL/100 mL) × 60 mL = 3 mL 2N sodium hydroxide

3 mL × (1.2 g/1 mL) = 3.6 g

10. The answer is A

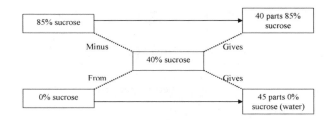

The parts given in the above allegation can be reduced to 4:4.5 (2.1.1)

11. The answer is B (2.1.1)

3/4 tsp × (5 mL/1 tsp) = 3.75 mL

12. The answer is A (3.2.3)

The Latin abbreviation "qd" given in the patient instructions is translated to once daily

13. The answer is B (2.1.1)

(5 mL/100 mL) × 60 mL=3 mL 2N sodium hydroxide

14. The answer is A (2.1.1)

(0.02 g/100 mL) × 60 mL=0.012 g or 12 mg sodium lauryl sulfate

12 mg × (100 mL/1000 mg)=1.2 mL stock solution

Sterile Solutions

1. The answer is B (2.1.1)

(1 mg/1 mL) × 2 mL = 2 mg albuterol per dose

2. The answer is C (3.2.3)

According to the patient instructions, the Latin abbreviation tqid prn is translated as "three to four times daily as needed."

3. The answer is A (2.1.1)

(0.01 g/100 mL) × 20 mL = 2 mg benzalkonium chloride

4. The answer is B (2.1.1)

(0.01 g/100 mL) × 20 mL = 2 mg benzalkonium chloride

2 mg × (100 mL/100 mg) = 2 mL stock solution

Answers

Ointments

1. The answer is A (2.1.1)

(0.5 g/100 g) × 10 g = 0.05 g hydrocortisone

2. The answer is A (2.1.1)

10 g × (1 mL/1.1 g) = 9.09 mL

3. The answer is A (2.1.1)

Hydrocortisone 0.5% w/w = 0.05 g
Methylparaben 0.1% w/w = 0.01 g
Propylparaben 0.01% w/w = 0.001 g
0.05 g + 0.01 g + 0.001 g = 0.06 g
So, the total amount of white petrolatum needed is 10 g - 0.06 g = 9.94 g

4. The answer is B (2.1.1)

(0.1 g/100 g) × 10 g = 0.01 g methylparaben

5. The answer is D (3.2.3)

According to the patient instructions, the Latin abbreviation "qod" is translated as "every other day."

6. The answer is D (3.2.3)

The Latin abbreviation "ung" is translated as ointment.

7. The answer is E (3.2.3)

Ointments are for external use only and should not be taken by mouth. There is no need to shake semisolid dosage forms.

8. The answer is C (3.2.3)

The Latin abbreviation "q2–3h prn" in the patient instructions are translated as "every 2–3 hours as needed."

9. The answer is C (2.1.1)

(10g/100g) × 15g = 1.5g anhydrous lanolin

10. The answer is B (2.1.1)

(18 g/100 g) × 15g = 2.7 g cetyl esters wax

11. The answer is E (2.1.1)

(30 g/100 g) × 15g = 4.5 g yellow wax

12. The answer is C (2.1.1)

(42 g/100 g) × 15g = 6.3 g liquid petrolatum

13. The answer is B (2.1.1)

(42 g/100 g) × 15g = 6.3 g liquid petrolatum
6.3 g × (1 mL/0.89 g) = 7.08 mL

14. The answer is C (2.1.1)

42% liquid petrolatum/18% cetyl esters wax = 2.33

Therefore, there is 1 part cetyl esters wax per 2.33 parts liquid petrolatum

15. The answer is E (3.2.3)

Ointments are for external use only and should not be taken by mouth. There is no need to shake semisolid dosage forms.

Pastes

1. The answer is B (2.1.1)

(53 g/100 g) × 30 g = 15.9 zinc oxide ointment

2. The answer is A (2.1.1)

(17 g/100 g) × 30 g = 5.1 g white petrolatum
Plus
((100 g - (20 g zinc oxide + 15 g mineral oil))/100 g) × (53 g/100 g) × 30 g = 10.34 g white petrolatum (zinc oxide ointment) So, 10.34 + 5.1 = 15.44 g total white petrolatum

3. The answer is D (2.1.1)

(17 g/100 g) × 30 g = 5.1 g white petrolatum

4. The answer is C (2.1.1)

(25 g/100 g) × 30 g = 7.5 g mineral oil
7.5 g (1 mL/0.89 g) = 8.4 mL

5. The answer is C (2.1.1)

(5 g/100 g) × 30 g = 1.5 g white wax

6. The answer is B (2.1.1)

53 g zinc oxide ointment/5 g white wax = 10.6
Therefore, there is 1 part white wax per 10.6 parts zinc oxide ointment.

Creams

1. The answer is C (2.1.1)

15 g × (1 mL/1.1 g) = 13.6 mL

2. The answer is B (2.1.1)

(5 g/1000 g) × 15 g = 0.075 g or 75 mg boric acid
75 mg × (100 mL/5000 mg) = 1.5 mL stock solution

3. The answer is E (3.2.3)

The Latin abbreviation "q2–3 h prn" in the patient instructions is translated "every 2–3 hours as needed."

Answers

4. The answer is A (2.1.1)

(125 g/1000 g) × 15 g = 1.875 g cetyl esters wax

5. The answer is C (2.1.1)

(125 g/1000 g) × 100 = 12.5% cetyl esters wax

6. The answer is C (2.1.1)

(560 g/1000 g) × 15 g = 8.4 g mineral oil
8.4 g × (1 mL/0.89 g) = 9.4 mL

7. The answer is B (2.1.1)

100% cream/12.5% cetyl esters wax = 8
Therefore, there is 1 part cetyl esters wax per 8 parts cream

Lotions

1. The answer is A (2.1.1)

15 g × (1 mL/1.2 g) = 12.5 mL

2. The answer is A (2.1.1)

(0.5 g/100 g) × 15 g = 0.075 g or 75 mg lactic acid
75 mg × (1 mL/25 mg) = 3 mL stock solution

3. The answer is B (2.1.1)

Since 0.5 g are contained in 100 g of the total preparation, the concentration of lactic acid is 0.5% w/w.

4. The answer is D (2.1.1)

0.5 g lactic acid/0.1 g methylparaben = 5
Therefore, there is 1 part methylparaben per 5 parts lactic acid.

5. The answer is C (2.1.1)

(6 g/100 g) × 15 g = 0.9 g mineral oil
0.9 g × (1 mL/0.89 g) = 1.01 mL

Gels

1. The answer is B (2.1.1)

(0.02 g/15 g) × 100 = 0.133% capsaicin

2. The answer is C (2.1.1)

50 mg × (100 mL/1250 mg) = 4 mL stock solution

3. The answer is D (2.1.1)

Dissolving 100 mg capsaicin in 10 mL ethanol will form a 10-mg/mL solution; 2 mL will contain the correct amount of capsaicin for the preparation.

4. The answer is B (2.1.1)

5 drops × (1 mL/20 drops) = 0.25 mL TEA

5. The answer is B (3.2.3)

According to the patient instructions, the Latin abbreviation qod prn is translated "every other day as needed."

6. The answer is C (2.1.1)

(0.3 g/100 mL) × 0.3 mL = 0.9 mg scopolamine HBr

7. The answer is A (2.1.1)

0.1 mL × (1.2 g/1 mL) = 0.12 g

8. The answer is A (2.1.1)

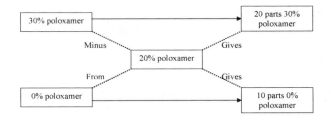

The ratio of 10 parts water to 20 parts 30% poloxamer can be reduced to 1:2.

9. The answer is D (2.1.1)

(0.1 g/100 mL) × 0.3 mL = 0.3 mg methylparaben

10. The answer is C (3.2.3)

The Latin abbreviation ud is translated "as directed."

Aqueous Nasal Sprays

1. The answer is A (2.1.1)

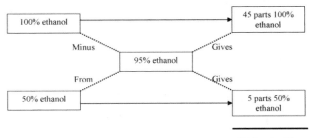

Total parts = 50

(5 parts 50% ethanol/50 parts total) × 1000 mL = 100 mL 50% ethanol

Answers

2. The answer is A (2.1.1)

(0.2 g/100 mL) × 30 mL = 0.06 g or 60 mg methylparaben 60 mg × (100 mL/3000 mg) = 2 mL stock solution

3. The answer is C (2.1.1)

(0.25 g/100 mL) × 100 = 0.25% dihydroergotamine mesylate

4. The answer is A (2.1.1)

(5 mL/100 mL) × 30 mL = 1.5 mL glycerin
1.5 mL × (0.92 g/1 mL) = 1.38 g

5. The answer is E (2.1.1)

(250 mg/10 sprays) × (1 mL/1000 mg) = 0.025 mL

6. The answer is E (2.1.1)

(0.25 g/100 mL) × (0.025 mL/spray) = 0.0625 mg

7. The answer is B (2.1.1)

(30 g - 28.4 g)/10 sprays × (1 mL/1 g) = 0.16 mL/spray
2 mg Morphine Sulfate/mL × 0.16 mL/spray = 0.32 mg/ actuation or 320 mcg/actuation

8. The answer is A (2.1.1)

(30 g - 29.1 g)/10 sprays × 1 mL/0.8 g = 0.1125 mL/ spray
0.02 mg naltrexone/mL × 0.1125 mL/spray = 0.00225 mg/ actuation or 2.25 mcg/actuation

9. The answer is B (2.1.1)

0.115 mL × 2 mg/mL × 12 actuations/day = 2.76 mg

Rectal Suppositories

1. The answer is B (3.2.3)

According to the patient instructions listed on the prescription order, the Latin abbreviation q 8 h prn can be translated "every 8 hours as needed."

2. The answer is A (2.1.1)

(10 mg/1 suppository) × 6 suppositories = 60 mg
If balance SAW is 100 mg, needs an aliquot
100 mg/60 mg = 200 mg/120 mg
So, weigh out 100 mg resorcin, dilute to 200 mg with zinc oxide and remove 120 mg of that mixture.

3. The answer is A (2.1.1)

3 mL × (1.1 g/1 mL) = 3.3 g for each suppository
3.3 g × 6 suppositories = 19.8 g total

19800 mg - 6 (50 mg + 20 mg + 10 mg + 300 mg) = 17520 mg or 17.52 g

4. The answer is B (2.1.1)

(50 mg/1 suppository) × 4 suppositories = 200 mg

5. The answer is A (2.1.1)

2 g × 4 suppositories = 8 g total
8000 mg - 4 (50 mg + 20 mg + 10 mg + 300 mg) = 6480 mg or 6.48 g

Vaginal Suppositories

1. The answer is C (2.1.1)

2 g × 4 suppositories = 8 g total

2. The answer is D (3.2.3)

According to the patient instructions listed on the prescription drug order, the Latin abbreviation qhs is translated "before bedtime."

3. The answer is A (2.1.1)

2 g × 4 suppositories = 8 g total
8000 mg - 4[40 mg + ((5 g/100 g) × 2000 mg)] = 7440 mg or 7.44 g

4. The answer is C (2.1.1)

(5 g/100 g) × 2 g = 0.1 g or 0.1 mL water

Solutions

1. The answer is B (2.1.1)

0.2 g/100 mL = 0.2% w/v

2. The answer is C (2.1.1)

100 mL - (200 mg × 1 mL/50 mg) - (25 mg × 1 mL/25 mg) = 95 mL of saline required, such that 5 mL of saline must be removed from the 100 mL bag.

3. The answer is C (2.1.1)

0.025 mg/100 mL = 0.025%

4. The answer is A (2.1.1)

0.9 g/100 mL × 90 mL = 0.81 g NaCl
0.81 g/100 mL = 0.81% w/v

Calculations

Basic Principles of Pharmaceutical Calculations

1. The answer is E (2.1.4)

$1.45 \text{ mg} \times (1 \times 10^9 \text{ pg}/1 \text{ mg}) = 1.45 \times 10^9 \text{ picograms}$

2. The answer is C (2.1.4)

$5 \text{ quarts} \times (32 \text{ fluid ounces}/1 \text{ quart}) = 160 \text{ fluid ounces}$

3. The answer is A (2.1.4)

$3 \text{ lb} \times (1 \text{ kg}/2.2 \text{ lb}) \times (1000 \text{ g}/1 \text{ kg}) \times (15.432 \text{ gr}/1 \text{ g}) = 2.1 \times 10^4 \text{ g r}$

4. The answer is C (2.1.4)

$110 \text{ lb} \times (1 \text{ kg}/2.2 \text{ lb}) \times (2.5 \text{ mg}/1 \text{ kg}) = 125 \text{ mg}$

5. The answer is D (2.1.4)

$94 \text{ g}/100 \text{ mL} = 0.94 \text{ g/mL}$

6. The answer is E (2.1.4)

$2 \text{ g} \times (1 \text{ mL}/0.976 \text{ g}) = 2.05 \text{ mL}$

7. The answer is C (2.1.4)

$2 \text{ g} \times (1 \text{ mL}/1.02 \text{ g}) = 1.96 \text{ mL}$

8. The answer is A (2.1.4)

Specific volume $= (1/\text{specific gravity}) = (1/0.956) = 1.05$

9. The answer is A (2.1.1)

$1.5 \text{ kg} \times (1000 \text{ g}/1 \text{ kg}) \times (15.432 \text{ gr}/1 \text{ g}) = 23148 \text{ gr}$

10. The answer is A (2.1.1)

Specific Gravity $= 6.5 \text{ g}/30 \text{ mL} = 0.22$

11. The answer is B (2.1.4)

$1 \text{ mL}/6.5 \text{ g} \times 9 \text{ g} = 1.38 \text{ mL}$

Basic Pharmaceutical Calculations

1. The answer is C (2.1.4)

$20 \text{ g}/1000 \text{ mL} = 5 \text{ g}/X$
$X = 250 \text{ mL}$

2. The answer is C (2.1.4)

Only C is correct because the answer for B requires measurement below the SAW for the balance.

3. The answer is B (2.1.4)

Dissolving 90 mg methylparaben in 12 mL forms a 7.5 mg/mL solution, which 2 mL will contain 15 mg.

4. The answer is A (2.1.4)

$(50 \text{ mg}/1 \text{ mL}) \times (1000 \text{ μg}/1 \text{ mg}) \times (1000 \text{ mL}/1 \text{ L}) = 5 \times 10^7 \text{ μg/ mL}$

5. The answer is C (2.1.1)

$(750 \text{ mL}/5 \text{ hr}) = (150 \text{ mL/hr})$
$(150 \text{ mL/hr}) \times (1 \text{ hr}/60 \text{ min}) = (2.5 \text{ mL/min})$

6. The answer is D (2.1.1)

$(700 \text{ drops/hr}) \times 8 \text{ hr} = 5600 \text{ drops}$
$(5600 \text{ drops}/1000 \text{ mL}) = 5.6 \text{ drops/mL}$

Dosage Calculations

1. The answer is A (2.1.4)

Using Fried's Rule for infants,
$(3 \text{ months}/150 \text{ months}) \times 500 \text{ mg} = 10 \text{ mg}$

2. The answer is E (2.1.4)

Using Clark's Rule,
$15 \text{ kg} \times (2.2 \text{ lb}/1 \text{ kg}) = 33 \text{ lb}$
$(33 \text{ lb}/150) \times 65 \text{ mg} = 14.3 \text{ mg}$

3. The answer is A (2.1.4)

$200 \text{ lb} \times (1 \text{ kg}/2.2 \text{ lb}) \times (2 \text{ mg}/1 \text{ kg}) = 182 \text{ mg}$

4. The answer is C (2.1.4)

Drawing a line from the 300-lb mark to the 71-inch mark on the nomogram for body surface area, the surface area of this patient is 2.5 m^2

$(2.5 \text{ m}^2/1.73 \text{ m}^2) \times 300 \text{ mg} = 434 \text{ mg}$

5. The answer is A (2.1.4)

Since each teaspoon is 5 mL, 30 mL is 6 teaspoons.

6. The answer is B (2.1.4)

$(2 \text{ tablespoons}/1 \text{ day}) \times (15 \text{ mL}/1 \text{ tablespoon}) \times 30 \text{ days} = 900 \text{ mL}$

7. The answer is B (2.1.4)

$(30 \text{ drops}/5 \text{ mL}) = 6 \text{ drops/mL}$

Answers

8. The answer is A (2.1.4)
$1.2 \text{ mL} \times (5 \text{ drops}/1 \text{ mL}) = 6 \text{ drops}$

9. The answer is B (2.1.4)
$30 \text{ mL} \times (5 \text{ drops}/1 \text{ mL}) \times (1 \text{ dose}/15 \text{ drops}) = 10 \text{ doses}$

10. The answer is A (2.1.4)
$1.5 \text{ mg} \times (1 \text{ g}/1000 \text{ mg}) \times (1000 \text{ mL}/1 \text{ g}) = 1.5 \text{ mL}$

11. The answer is B (2.1.4)
$0.8 \text{ mg} \times (1000 \text{ mcg}/1 \text{ mg}) \times (2 \text{ mL}/500 \text{ mcg}) = 3.2 \text{ mL}$

Concentration

1. The answer is C (2.1.4)
$(0.05 \text{ g}/500 \text{ mL}) \times 100 \text{ mL} = 0.01\% \text{ w/v}$

2. The answer is B (2.1.4)
$20 \text{ g ZnO}/100 \text{ g mixture} = 20\% \text{ w/w}$

3. The answer is A (2.1.4)
50% w/v is a ratio of 50 g of substance to 100 mL solution, so the ratio can be reduced to 1:2.

4. The answer is C (2.1.4)
Since the lidocaine HCl solution is diluted in half, the resulting concentration is 0.5%, or:
$1(250) = x(500)$, where $x = 0.5$

5. The answer is C (2.1.4)
$90(500 \text{ mL}) = 50(X \text{ mL})$ where $X = 900 \text{ mL}$ total solution
However, since 500 mL of the final solution is taken from the ethanol, only 400 mL of water are needed.

6. The answer is B (2.1.4)
$5 \times 300 \quad 1500$
$2 \times 400 \quad 800$
$8 \times 250 \quad 2000$
$7.5 \times 400 \quad 3000$
$1350 \quad 7300 \div (1350 \text{ mL}) = 5.4\%$

7. The answer is E (2.1.4)
$5\% = 5 \text{ g}/100 \text{ mL} = 50 \text{ mg/mL}$
$200 \text{ mL} \times (50 \text{ mg}/1 \text{ mL}) = 10{,}000 \text{ mg}$
$(10{,}000 \text{ mg} \times 1)/74.5 = 134.23 \text{ mEq}$

8. The answer is A (2.1.4)
$5\% = (5 \text{ g}/100 \text{ mL}) \times 1000 \text{ mL} = 50 \text{ g/L}$
$((50 \text{ g/L})/74.5 \text{ g}) \times 2 \text{ species} \times 1000 = 1342 \text{ mOsm/L}$

9. The answer is A (2.1.4)
0.9% sodium chloride solution is considered to be isotonic.

10. The answer is A (2.1.4)
$0.9 \text{ g}/100 \text{ mL} \times 100 \text{ mL} = 0.9 \text{ g}$
$0.9 \text{ g} - 0.01 \times 0.16 = 0.8984 \text{ g} = 898.4 \text{ mg}$

11. The answer is D (2.1.4)
$2.5 \text{ mL} \times 20 \text{ mEq}/5 \text{ mL} = 10 \text{ mEq}$
$10 \text{ mEq}/1000 \text{ mL} = 0.01 \text{ mEq/mL}$

12. The answer is B (2.1.4)
$25 \text{ drops/min} \times 1 \text{ mL}/15 \text{ drops} = 1.67 \text{ mL/min}$
$1.67 \text{ mL/min} \times 22.5 \text{ mEq}/1000 \text{ mL} \times 60 \text{ min}/1 \text{ hr} = 2.25 \text{ mEq/hr}$

13. The answer is B (2.1.4)
$0.8 \text{ g}/100 \text{ mL} \times 50 \text{ mL/hr} = 0.4 \text{ g/hr} = 400 \text{ mg/hr}$

Calculations For Sterile Products

1. The answer is C (2.1.4)
$0.8 \text{ mg} \times 1 \text{ mL}/0.4 \text{ mg} = 2 \text{ mL}$

2. The answer is A (2.1.4)
$50 \text{ units} \times 1 \text{ mL}/100 \text{ units} = 0.5 \text{ mL}$

3. The answer is A (2.1.4)
$1000 \text{ mL}/4 \text{ hr} \times 1 \text{ hr}/60 \text{ min} \times 8 \text{ drops/mL} = 33.3 \text{ drops/min}$

4. The answer is E (2.1.4)
$500 \text{ mL} \times 1 \text{ hr}/55 \text{ mL} = 9 \text{ hr}$

5. The answer is D (2.1.4)
$450 \text{ mL}/100 \text{ min} \times 10 \text{ drops/mL} = 45 \text{ drops/min}$

6. The answer is B (2.1.4)
$25 \text{ mL/hr} \times 0.5 \text{ hr} = 12.5 \text{ mL}$

7. The answer is A (2.1.4)
The powder has 2 mL of volume
$10 \text{ mL}/12 \text{ mL} \times 400{,}000 \text{ Units/mL} = 333{,}333 \text{ Units/mL}$

8. The answer is A (2.1.4)
$1000 \text{ Units/hr} \times 4 \text{ hr} = 4000 \text{ units}$

9. The answer is C (2.1.4)

500 mg/4 mL = 125 mg/mL

10. The answer is A (2.1.4)

450 mL × 5 g/100 mL = 22.5 g

11. The answer is C (2.1.4)

Flow Rate = 240 mg/hr × 1000 mL/4000 mg = 60 mL/hr

12. The answer is A (2.1.4)

2500 Units/2 hr × 0.5 hr = 625 Units

13. The answer is C (2.1.4)

0.015 g × 1000 mL/10 g = 1.5 mL

14. The answer is D (2.1.4)

0.45 g × 10 mL/0.5 g = 9 mL

15. The answer is B (2.1.4)

(900 mg × 1)/58 = 15.5 mEq

16. The answer is E (2.1.4)

500 mL/1000 mg × 60 mg/hr = 30 mL/hr

17. The answer is E (2.1.4)

30 mL × 10 g/100 mL = 3 g

18. The answer is A (2.1.4)

500 mL/3 hr × 1 hr/60 min × 8 drops/mL = 22 drops/min

19. The answer is D (2.1.4)

6 %w/v = 6 g/100 mL or 60 g/L

20. The answer is C (2.1.4)

4 mL/500 mL × 350 mg/1 mL = 2.8 mg/mL

21. The answer is B (2.1.4)

30 mL × 1 g/10,000 mL = 0.003 = 3 mg